Coronary Vasculature

Robert J. Tomanek

Coronary Vasculature

Development, Structure-Function, and Adaptations

Springer

Robert J. Tomanek
Carver College of Medicine
Cardiovascular Center
University of Iowa
Iowa City, Iowa, USA

ISBN 978-1-4614-4886-0 ISBN 978-1-4614-4887-7 (eBook)
DOI 10.1007/978-1-4614-4887-7
Springer New York Heidelberg Dordrecht London

Library of Congress Control Number: 2012947995

Printed on acid-free paper

Springer is part of Springer Science+Business Media (www.springer.com)

Preface

The fact that ischemic heart disease is the leading cause of morbidity and mortality in the industrial world highlights the importance of the coronary vasculature. Although a wealth of literature regarding coronary vessels and myocardial perfusion exists, by virtue of necessity, most laboratories are highly specialized performing work that is highly focused. As a consequence, cross talk between various areas of this broad field is limited. This publication is intended for an audience of cardiovascular scientists and physicians, and the goal is to provide a single comprehensive publication that reviews, discusses, and integrates findings in the various areas of research pertaining to the coronary vasculature. The chapters were written with some redundancy and include references to other chapters, to present the topics in an integrated manner and in recognition that chapters are often read in isolation. The focus of each of the 12 chapters included in this book is described below.

Chapter 1 is aimed at providing the reader with a basic understanding of the principles of vessel formation and the molecules that regulate this process. This chapter considers the cascade of events that comprise vascular formation and the major signaling pathways that regulate these events. Chapter 2 provides an account of the cells that migrate to the heart to form its outer layer (epicardium) and the mechanisms that promote the related cell transformations and the development of the coronary vasculature. The third chapter is an extension of Chap. 2 and reviews development of the coronary vasculature during postnatal growth. The early postnatal period involves a rapid period of growth that challenges the coronary vasculature to adapt to meet greater metabolic demands.

Chapter 4 dissects the structure of the coronary vasculature in relation to its regulation of coronary flow and myocardial perfusion. This chapter considers the regulation of flow by various components of the coronary hierarchy and examines the structure–function relationships for the various types of vessels. Chapter 5 considers a topic rarely addressed: a historical perspective of the coronary system. One can appreciate some of the most important discoveries in the context of many centuries and come to appreciate that new findings require considerable time to become accepted. Errors of coronary vessel development, i.e., anomalies, and their effects on the coronary circulation are the topics of Chap. 6. Most importantly, this chapter addresses possible mechanisms underlying coronary anomalies and the effect of these anomalies on myocardial ischemia and sudden death. Chapter 7 covers aging of the coronary vasculature and provides contrasts between biological aging and age-related changes; the latter are alterations that are linked to life style and disease (senility) rather than to normal biological aging (senescence).

Chapters 8–11 address adaptations of the coronary vasculature. Exercise training (Chap. 8) represents one of the most important avenues to reducing the risks of cardiovascular disease. Differences in protocols and animal models are discussed with regard to discordant findings. Chapter 9 reviews hypoxic signaling mechanisms, and the role of hypoxia in coronary vessel formation and growth, adaptations to high altitude and cardiac hypertrophy, and the protective effects of hypoxic preconditioning. This chapter is closely related to Chap. 10 on myocardial ischemia and infarction, because hypoxia is a component of ischemia. Chapter 10 addresses both the acute and chronic effects of ischemia on the coronary circulation, vascular growth and remodeling, and pre- and postconditioning. Chapter 11 considers the coronary vasculature with regard to the type of stimulus that evokes the hypertrophy, e.g., pressure overload, volume overload, increased thyroid hormone levels, and cardiomyopathy. The importance of vascular growth during cardiac hypertrophy is that it normalizes myocardial perfusion and oxygen delivery in the context of increased workloads. Chapter 12 (Therapy for the Coronary Circulation) explores the various strategies employed to induce coronary vascular growth and function. Major topics include therapies utilizing (1) genes and proteins, (2) endothelial stem and progenitor cells, and (3) pharmacological agents. Responses of various components of the coronary hierarchy, especially the collateral circulation, are reviewed. The development of the various chapters was aided by consultants with expertise on the topics included in this publication.

Iowa City, Iowa, USA Robert J. Tomanek

Acknowledgements

The author is grateful to the NIH-National Library of Medicine for funding this project via grant award 5 G13 LM010002. The illustrations in this book were prepared by Paul C. Reimann, Department of Anatomy and Cell Biology, University of Iowa. The image on the cover is a water color painting by Rita Svoboda Tomanek. The author also appreciates the numerous conversations with many scientists regarding topics that are included in this publication. Finally, the assistance of Mrs. Laurie Jewell in preparing the manuscript is gratefully acknowledged.

Consultants

Content expertise was provided by the following consultants:

Paolo Angelini, M.D. Cardiologist Leachman Cardiology Associates Houston, TX	James M. Downey, Ph.D. Professor Emeritus of Physiology University of South Alabama Mobile, AL
Robert J. Bache, M.D. Professor of Medicine Division of Cardiology University of Minnesota Minneapolis, MN	David D. Gutterman, M.D. Senior Associate Dean for Research Northwestern Mutual Professor of Cardiology Medical College of Wisconsin Milwaukee, WI
Cristina Basso, M.D., Ph.D. Associate Professor, Pathological Anatomy Consultant, Cardiology Department of Cardiac, Thoracic and Vascular Sciences Pathological Anatomy-Cardiovascular Pathology University of Padua Medical School Padova, Italy	David G. Harrison, M.D. Betty and Jack Bailey Professor of Medicine and Pharmacology Director of Clinical Pharmacology Nashville, TN
Christine M. Blaumueller, Ph.D. Scientific Editor and Writing Consultant The University of Iowa, Roy J. and Lucille A. Carver College of Medicine Department of Anatomy and Cell Biology Department of Molecular Physiology and Biophysics Iowa City, IA	Edward G. Lakatta, M.D., Senior Investigator Chief, Laboratory of Cardiovascular Science and Cardiovascular Function Section National Institute on Aging Baltimore, MD
John M. Canty, Jr., M.D. Albert and Elizabeth Rekate Professor of Medicine and Chief, Division of Cardiovascular Medicine University at Buffalo Buffalo, NY	M. Harold Laughlin, Ph.D. Curators' Professor and Chair Department of Biomedical Sciences College of Veterinary Medicine, and Department of Medical Pharmacology and Physiology, and DCRC University of Missouri Columbia, MO
William M. Chilian, Ph.D. Professor of Physiology Chair, Integrative Medical Sciences College of Medicine Northeast Ohio Medical University Rootstown, OH	Mark W. Majesky, Ph.D. Professor of Pediatrics and Pathology Seattle Children's Research Institute University of Washington Seattle, WA

Karel Rakusan, M.D., Ph.D.
Professor Emeritus
Cellular and Molecular Medicine
University of Ottawa
Ottawa, Ontario, Canada

Takashi Mikawa, Ph.D.
Professor of Anatomy and Cardiovascular Research Institute
University of California San Francisco
San Francisco, CA

Boja Ostadal, DrSc.
Professor, Institute of Physiology
Academy of Sciences of the Czech Republic
Prague, Czech Republic

Gina C. Schatteman, Ph.D.
Associate Professor Emeritus of Health and Human Physiology
The University of Iowa
Iowa City, IA

Gregg L. Semenza, M.D., Ph.D.
C. Michael Armstrong Professor of Pediatrics, Medicine, Oncology, Radiation Oncology, Biological Chemistry and Genetic Medicine
Johns Hopkins University School of Medicine
Baltimore, MD

Michael Simons, M.D.
R.W. Berliner Professor of Medicine and Cell Biology
Chief, Section of Cardiovascular Medicine
Director, Yale Cardiovascular Research Center
Yale University School of Medicine
New Haven, CT

Mervin C. Yoder, M.D.
Professor of Pediatrics
Professor of Biochemistry and Molecular Biology
Indiana University School of Medicine
Indianapolis, IN

Contents

General Concepts of Blood Vessel Formation and Remodeling

1

Introduction

The goal of this chapter is to provide the reader with a basic understanding of the cascade of events that comprise blood vessel formation and remodeling, as well as the extrinsic factors that underlie vascular adaptations. Although vascular patterns and characteristics are organ specific, they nevertheless share many common features and developmental regulators.

Blood vessels are formed by mesoderm-derived progenitor cells that differentiate into endothelial cells (ECs), pericytes, smooth muscle cells, and fibroblasts. During development, de novo vessel formation occurs by a process termed "vasculogenesis." ECs differentiate from precursor cells, migrate, and form vascular channels. Further vessel growth during development and in the adult requires a phenomenon known as "angiogenesis," whereby branches or extensions of these EC-derived channels are formed by sprouting or partitioning (intussusception). The term "arteriogenesis" is used to define the formation of both arterioles and arteries, as well as the remodeling of collateral vessels. Although angiogenesis is frequently used to describe vessel formation and growth, it is a distinct process. Therefore, Simons [1] suggested the use of "neovascularization" to encompass vasculogenesis, angiogenesis, and arteriogenesis, as they apply to new vessel formation in the adult, whether artery, vein, or capillary.

A basic understanding of these processes was nicely summarized by Risau [2] more than a decade ago. His review illustrated the progression of vascular development from the induction of mesoderm and establishment of cell fate through vessel formation and remodeling. As we have learned in recent years, many transcription and growth factor molecules are involved in signaling pathways that regulate the processes noted above. Remodeling is a phenomenon that occurs not only during the prenatal and postnatal developmental periods but also in the adult in response to alterations in the environment, e.g., ischemia, and increases or decreases in perfusion or pressure.

Key molecules and their abbreviations used in this chapter are provided in Table 1.1.

Progenitor Cells

Embryonic Life

Hemangioblast, Angioblast, and Hemogenic Endothelium

As described above and illustrated in Fig. 1.1, ECs, which are derived from mesoderm, form the first vascular channels in both the yolk sac and embryonic tissues. During gastrulation, fibroblast growth factors (FGFs) induce angioblasts and hematopoietic cells that form yolk sac blood islands [9]. The suggestion that ECs and blood cells derive from a common precursor cell was first made a century ago [10]; this progenitor cell was termed "hemangioblast" by Murray in 1932 [9]. The finding that a single vascular endothelial growth factor receptor-2 (VEGFR-2$^+$) cell from a chick gastrula could be induced to give rise to both EC and hematopoietic colonies in vitro provided proof of hemangioblasts [11]. Since that time, additional support for the hemangioblast as progenitor for both ECs and blood cells has been provided (reviewed in [12, 13]).

EC Differentiation

ECs differentiate from endothelial precursor cells, which like hemangioblasts, lack the CD45 surface marker [3]. A study by Drake and Flemming [14] showed that coexpression of TAL1 (a transcription factor) and vascular endothelial growth factor receptor-2 (VEGFR-2) in embryonic mesodermal cells is the major criterion for distinguishing these cells from hematopoietic cells which express TAL1, but not VEGFR-2. In the embryo, a mature EC develops via the following cell lineage: mesodermal cell–hemangioblast–angioblast–proliferating ECs [15]. Embryonic angioblasts form clusters establishing cell to cell contacts that detach

R.J. Tomanek, *Coronary Vasculature: Development, Structure-Function, and Adaptations*,
DOI 10.1007/978-1-4614-4887-7_1, © Springer Science+Business Media New York 2013

Table 1.1 Key molecules involved in vascular morphogenesis

Akt is a serine/threonine kinase that is activated by PI3 kinase downstream of growth factors. It is involved in Ras stimulation and the control of cell survival
ALK5 (activin receptor-like kinase) is the TGF-β type 1 receptor. ALK5 signaling, which results in Smad 2 and 3 phosphorylation, inhibits angiogenesis
Angiopoietin-1 promotes angiogenesis (induces branching), vessel stabilization by tightening of cell junctions and decreasing permeability (maturation)
Angiopoietin-2 promotes vascular remodeling by blocking the stabilizing action of angiopoietin-1
BMPs (bone morphogenic proteins) are members of the TGF-β super family, bind to type II and type I serine–threonine kinase receptors and signal via smad and non-smad proteins. BMP-4 induces EC proliferation and migration and is required for normal heart and vessel development. BMP-4 also enhances VEGFR-2 and Tie-2 expression and phosphorylation. Thus, this BMP acts directly on the endothelium to facilitate angiogenesis
CArG boxes are DNA sequences within SMC genes that are required for SMC-specific transcription. They coordinate regulation of multiple transcriptional programs that control differentiation and plasticity of SMC phenotype
Chordin inhibits BMP-2, -4, and -7 activities by interacting with their cell-surface heparan proteoglycans. Chordin can also inhibit BMPs by binding to biglycan
COUP-TFII-promoter/transcription factor is present in veins that mediate lymphogenesis. Ablation of COUP-TFII in mice results in the failure of pre-lymphatic ECs and lymphatic vessel formation. COUP-TFII also maintains lymphatic identity and VEGF-C induction of lymphogenesis by stimulating neuropilin-2, a co-receptor for VEGF-C
Ephrins/Ephs are ligand/receptor pairs that mediate critical steps in angiogenesis including cell migration cell–cell contacts and cell binding to the ECM. Eph B4/ephrin B2 is a key receptor/ligand pair that defines ECs in arteries and veins. Ephrin B2 is required for VSMC recruitment
ERK (externally regulated kinase)=MAP (mitogen-activated protein kinase). This kinase is activated by mitogens and transmits entry into the cell
Ets transcription factors are central to EC transcriptional programs. At least 19 Ets factors are expressed in human ECs, activating the expression of numerous EC genes by binding to their enhancers and repressing the expression of other genes. Erq, a key Ets transcription factor expressed in all ECs, drives the expression of ICAM-2 and VE-cadherin, which are required for vessel stability and in the transcription of VEGFR-1 and VEGFR-2
FGF-1 and FGF-2 promote vasculogenesis, angiogenesis, and serve as a chemotactic for ECs and smooth muscle cells
FGF-4 promotes the differentiation of embryonic vascular stem cells
FGF-8 promotes angiogenesis in the embryo
FGF-9 promotes angiogenesis in the coronary and pulmonary systems
F-18 is a chemotactic for ECs
Fox (Forkhead) transcription factors. Several members of this family are expressed in ECs and play roles in vascular biology and EC transcription. For example, Fox C family is essential for vascular development and for EC specification
GATA-2 is a zinc finger transcription factor that regulates both EC and hematopoietic cells. GATA-2 is important for the development of Flk-1$^+$/Tal1$^+$ hemangioblast-like cells, as well as EC development
Gridlock transcription repressor is an artery-restricted gene, expressed in the lateral posterior mesoderm, that acts to maintain arterial fate. Reductions in gridlock expression cause an increase in the venous marker EphB4 receptor and a decrease in the arterial marker ephrin-B2
Hedgehog proteins are family of morphogenic proteins that mediate development of various organs. Among the roles of sonic hedgehog during development is upregulation of VEGFs, angiopoietins, and angiogenesis in heart and lungs. Hedgehog signaling is important in ischemic tissues where it upregulates VEGF
HIF-1 (hypoxia inducible factor-1) is a transcriptional complex consisting of HIF-1α and HIF-1β (aryl hydrocarbon receptor nuclear translocator [ARNT]) subunits. HIF-α is the major hypoxia sensor, which binds with HIF-1β to form an activated transcriptional core complex. HIF-1 regulates many genes, including VEGF in which case it evokes enhanced VEGF protein secretion. In continuation, VEGF and hypoxia induce a variety of angiogenesis growth factors and cytokines
HGF (hepatocyte growth factor) promotes EC migration, proliferation, and vascular sprouting
IGF (insulin-like growth factor) comes in two forms (IGFs I and II polypeptides) both of which elicit mitogenesis and increase VEGF mRNA in carcinoma cells
Integrins are members of a superfamily of cell surface proteins, some of which bind to extracellular components. Key integrins for vascular morphogenesis include the $\alpha_v\beta_3$ dimer, which binds vitronectin, fibronectin, collagen, and other ligands, and the $\alpha_5\beta_1$ which binds fibronectin

Krüppel-like factor transcription (KLF) family These transcription factors function in ECs after, rather than prior to, initial EC specification and differentiation. Shear stress leads to Klf2-induced expression of several genes that are required for vascular stabilization and tone. KLF4 inhibits VSMC proliferation by upregulating negative cell-cycle regulatory genes
MCP-1 (monocyte chemotactic protein) is coinduced with interleukin-8 and is a chemotactic for monocytes. MCP-1 plays a key role in arteriogenesis during the development of collateral vessels
Matrix metalloproteinases (MMPs) are proteolytic enzymes that degrade the extracellular matrix and accordingly are required for sprouting angiogenesis. They also activate and modify growth factors and cytokines and generate matrix protein fragments that inhibit angiogenesis
Noggin is a glycosylated protein that binds BMPs 2, 4, 6, and 7 and thereby inhibits BMP activity. During development, NOGGIN, like Chordin, suppresses vessel formation by suppressing the generation of ECs. Noggin is notochord derived
NOTCH-1 receptor and its DELTA-4 ligand. Signaling by these proteins is induced by VEGF and stabilizes EC network formation. Notch receptors are expressed specifically in arterial ECs of the early embryo; it is therefore key to arterial specification of arterial ECs
PlGF (placental growth factor) functions in angiogenesis and bone marrow-derived cell recruitment, and is a ligand for VEGFR-1
Platelet derived growth factor BB (PDGF-BB) promotes capillary stabilization and mural cell recruitment
Platelet endothelial cell adhesion molecule (PECAM-1 or CD31) is expressed on hematopoietic and immune cells including ECs and has been implicated in diverse responses involved in vascular biology and inflammation. These include angiogenesis leukocyte transmigration, vascular permeability, thrombosis, and EC mechanosensing of fluid shear stress
Semaphorin-3E, a ligand for the Plexin-D1 receptor that initiates a signaling pathway involved in growing blood vessels
SRF (serum response factor) is a transcription factor required for early mesoderm formation and specification that is important for differentiation of muscle lineages. SRF is necessary for the activation of SMC-specific transcription during development and for its maintenance in adult vessels. SRF regulates cytoskeleton and cell adhesion molecules, acting as a linker between extracellular stimuli and cellular phenotype
Stromal-derived factor-1 (SDF-1) is a chemokine, and binds exclusively to CXCR4 whereby it promotes progenitor cell recruitment and vascular assembly. SDF-1 is constitutively produced by bone marrow cells and platelets and facilitates retention, growth, and differentiation of hematopoietic stem cells. SDF-1α regulates vascular repair (1) via $CD34^+$ cell recruitment in the circulation and their differentiation into endothelial progenitor cells and (2) by the recruitment of CXCR4-dependent smooth muscle progenitor cell recruitment
Tal1 is a transcription factor that is essential for endothelial and blood cell development and activation of several EC-specific gene enhancers
TGF-β promotes the recruitment and differentiation of vascular mural cells, e.g., during arteriogenesis
TIMP (tissue inhibitors of metalloproteinases) inhibit metalloproteinases by binding to them (e.g., collagenase). Mutations in TIMP-3 are associated with some vascular diseases
VEGF-A promotes vasculogenesis, angiogenesis, EC survival, vascular permeability, and the recruitment of bone marrow cells
VEGF-B promotes angiogenesis and the recruitment of bone marrow cells
VEGF-C promotes lymphogenesis (along with VEGF-D) and angiogenesis involving capillary stabilization
Wnts are secreted proteins that signal via Frizzled family receptors. Wnts thereby regulate cell proliferation differentiation, cell fate specification, and differentiation; Wnt signaling has also been implicated in cross talk with other families of secreted factors, e.g., FGFs, TGF-βs, Hedgehog, and Dll4

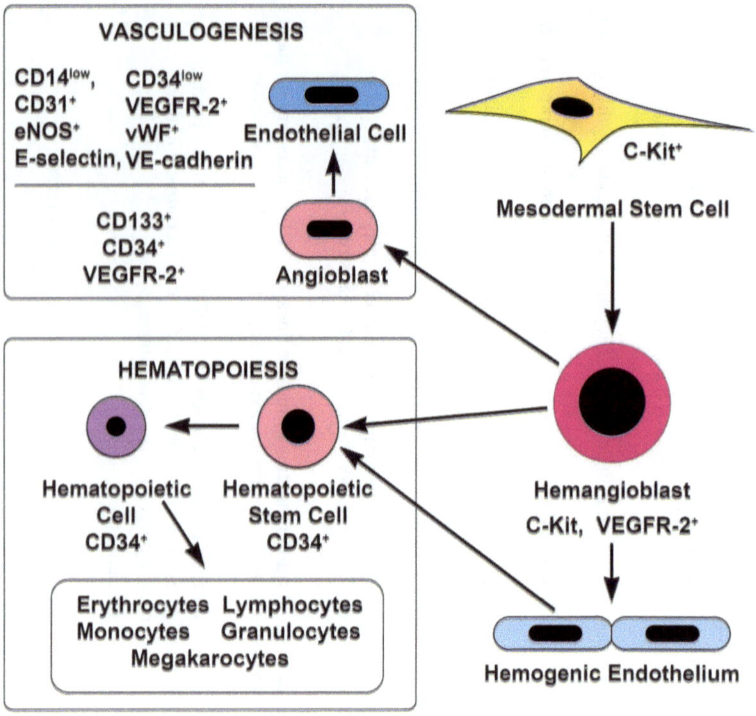

Fig. 1.1 Stem and endothelial progenitor cells. Endothelial cell differentiation occurs in adults as well as during prenatal development. The hemangioblast is a cell that is considered a precursor of angioblasts and hemogenic endothelial stem cells, based on the observation that several surface markers are common to both ECs and hematopoietic cells. VEGFR-2 (Flk-1 or KDR) is common to all cells with hemangioblast properties, including a mesodermal stem cell. Markers expressed by cell types in angiogenic or hematopoietic lineages are still somewhat controversial. Those noted here represent markers frequently reported primarily in humans and/or mice [3–8]

before these cells take on the migratory phenotype. Many molecular mechanisms regulate this and other aspects of the specification of the EC lineage (reviewed by [16]). These involve essential signaling pathways, including those regulated by VEGF, angiopoietin/Tie, wnt/Frizz-led, Delta/Notch, bone morphogenic protein (BMP), Ephrin/Eph, transforming growth factor β (TGF-β), platelet-derived growth factor (PDGF), and FGF. The essential nature of the Notch signaling is not limited to its role in EC proliferation and migration; it is also crucial for the differentiation and maintenance of stem and progenitor populations (reviewed in [17]).

Pathway for Differentiation

The differentiation pathway by which blood cells and ECs are formed appears to be more complex than first appreciated. Hematopoietic cells can arise not only through differentiation of hemangioblasts into hematopoietic stem cells but also from differentiation of hemogenic ECs (reviewed in [18–20]). Hemogenic endothelium is a transitional EC cluster that arises from the hemangioblast and generates blood cells. When hemangioblasts were plated and cultured for 2 days, a population of ECs (Tie-2$^+$ and C-kit$^+$) that lacked the CD45 hematopoietic marker was generated [21]. The emergence of hematopoietic cells from ECs that were progeny of VEGFR-2, E-cadherin mesoderm was observed using time-lapse microscopy and morphological and molecular markers [22]. The hemogenic ECs expressed V-cadherin, formed tight junctions, and internalized acetylated low density lipoprotein. These findings indicated that hemogenic endothelium develops subsequent to hemangioblasts and provides a link between the hemangioblast and hematopoietic cells.

Postnatal Life

Angioblasts

The idea that ECs can differentiate from angioblasts during postnatal life was promoted by studies carried out more than a decade ago that reported that human CD34$^+$ cells obtained from peripheral blood, bone marrow, and umbilical cord blood were EC precursors (EPCs) and could contribute to vascular tube formation both in vitro and in vivo [23, 24]. It was suggested that these precursor cells and hemangioblasts share some antigenemic determinants, i.e., VEGFR-2, Tie 2, c-kit, Sca^{-1}, CD133, and CD34 [23–25], and that both cell types are induced via sonic hedgehog signaling [26]. Since these papers were published, subsequent studies have suggested that bone marrow-derived cells are incorporated into blood vessels during tissue repair and tumor growth (reviewed in [3]). There is a consensus that the EC progenitor cells can arise from the bone marrow; however, the source of these ECs may be from several populations, not necessarily from a single type of bone marrow-derived cell (e.g., myeloid cells, mesenchymal cells), as well as from non-bone marrow cells [27]. Hematopoietic stem cell-associated neovascularization has been shown to occur after ischemia; however, unresolved questions remain. One critical question is the definition of a progenitor cell, since there remain several cell types that are considered to be EPCs [28].

EC and Hematopoietic Lineages

That the hemangioblast is not the exclusive precursor for all endothelial lineages is suggested by studies in mice and zebrafish [4]. In addition to bone marrow, several other stem-cell niches contain vascular progenitor cells that remain quiescent until they are mobilized during injury or disease [29]. A summary of hematopoietic and EC lineages and their surface markers is provided in Fig. 1.1, which focuses on lineages of mesodermal stem cells that give rise to both ECs and blood cells. Many laboratories are pursuing the role of EC precursors in vascular repair [30], a topic that is addressed in Chap. 12.

In conclusion, there are several cell types in adults that may be classified as vascular progenitor cells and that are able to differentiate into ECs and VSMCs (reviewed in [31]). These include bone marrow mononuclear cells, adipose tissue-derived stem cells, and hemangioblasts. At this time, no definitive circulating population of a single EC progenitor in the adult has been documented [32]. Our current state of understanding is limited by (1) the reliance on cell surface markers in the absence of functional tests and (2) possible artifacts arising from in vitro approaches.

Formation of the Primary Capillary Plexus (Vasculogenesis)

Cell Recruitment and Assembly

The formation of a tubular network (vasculogenesis) requires angioblasts in the embryo and EPCs in the adult. The migration of angioblasts, endothelial progenitor cells (EPCs), and ECs is dependent on chemoattractants, growth factors, cytokines, and morphogen interactions between the cell and the extracellular matrix, and interactions among cells [15]. Numerous transcription factors play roles in endothelial gene expression (see recent review by DeVal and Black [33]). TAL1, GATA2, and the Ets protein, Fli, are expressed early and control transcription in both endothelial and hematopoietic cells, whereas Krüppel-like factors activate genes involved in stress or injury responses. Vascular tube formation (tubulogenesis) requires the assembly of ECs and the formation of cell–cell junctions and the basement membrane. Embryonic vasculogenesis, as described by Flamme and Risau [34], is initiated when mesodermal cells migrate and form blood islands (which consist of hematopoietic cells and angioblasts), and provide cells for the primary plexus. Drake [35] elaborated on this process by noting that angioblasts elongate, following their aggregation, to form cords that merge into capillary-like networks. This process, he noted, may be linked to hematopoiesis, especially during extraembryonic vessel formation.

Lumen Formation

Analysis carried out in embryoid bodies from differentiating embryonic stem cells—an in vitro model for studying vasculogenesis and angiogenesis [36, 37]—has suggested that ECs form vascular tubes by (1) their assembly from blood islands; (2) forming intracellular vacuoles which then fuse to form a vascular channel; or (3) joining with free neighboring ECs to form junctions [9, 38, 39]. In the case of lumen formation by the fusion of vesicles within an EC to form a single channel, adjacent ECs must attach by forming junctions so that the central vacuoles are in register. Lumen formation by joining adjacent ECs that lack a central vacuole also requires formation and remodeling of junctions to form a channel or lumen between chords of ECs. Underlying mechanisms are discussed in Zeeb et al. [40] and Strilic et al. [41]. These primitive tubes are stabilized by the deposition of a basement membrane and the incorporation of pericytes under the basement membrane; thus, the tubes are in close contact with ECs. They then undergo branching and fusion (angiogenesis) and, in the case of venous and arterial vessels, recruit additional mural cells to form the two outer layers—the media and adventitia.

Vasculogenesis in Adults

In the adult, EPCs derived from bone marrow and other sites may circulate through the vasculature and can home to sites of neovascularization where they differentiate into ECs (reviewed in Ribatti [13]). EPCs proliferate and migrate in response to growth factors and chemokines and may contribute to neovascularization. The formation of vascular tubes (vasculogenesis) is followed by branching and the fusion of branches to form larger channels (angiogenesis) and then by the recruitment of mural cells (pericytes and smooth muscle cells) to form the tunica media and tunica adventitia of the arterial and venous vessels. These processes are tightly controlled by growth factors that are spatially and temporally expressed.

VEGF–VEGFR and the Vasculogenic Cascade

The vascular endothelial growth factor and receptor (VEGF-VEGFR) axis is central to the migration of angioblasts and EPCs, as evidenced by the finding that heterozygous deletion of VEGF-A, VEGFR-1, or VEGFR-2 nearly completely

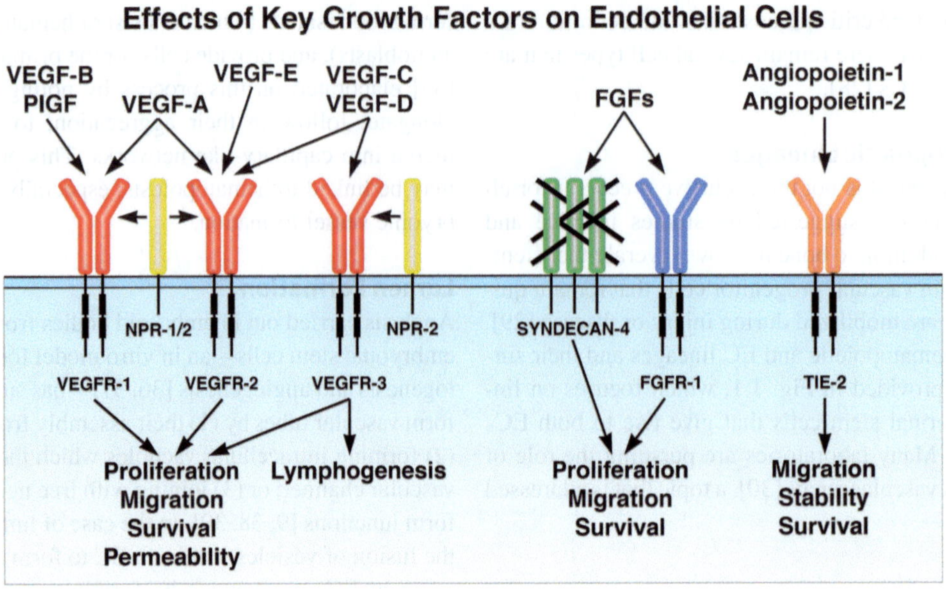

Fig. 1.2 Signaling by key growth factors in vasculogenesis and angiogenesis. Neuropilins function as co-receptors with VEGF receptors. The effects on endothelial cells are noted for 5 tyrosine receptors. Angiopoietin-2 affects endothelial cell migration, whereas Angiopoietin-1 promotes stability and maturation

prevents vessel formation in mouse embryos. Figure 1.2 summarizes the effects of VEGFs, placental growth factor (PIGF), FGFs, and angiopoietins on ECs. Hypoxia, which develops in embryonic tissues as a consequence of tissue expansion prior to a functional circulation, is a powerful stimulus for vasculogenesis. Hypoxia leads to enhanced hypoxia-inducible factor-1 (HIF-1) and the subsequent induction of VEGF and serum-derived factor-1 (SDF-1). This signaling cascade stimulates EC progenitors during vasculogenesis. Erythropoietin and its receptor are important for both vasculogenesis and angiogenesis, as revealed by studies documenting that this ligand receptor pair facilitates EC proliferation and migration, and inhibition of apoptosis in humans and mice [42]. Migration of EPCs is also dependent upon endothelial nitric oxide synthase (eNOS) [43], which facilitates their detachment from each other and from the extracellular matrix, and allows their migration along a path set by attractive and repulsive gradients of soluble factors [15].

VEGF and two of its receptors, VEGFR-1 (flt-1) and VEGFR-2 (flk-1), are well-documented as key regulators of vasculogenesis (see review by Rossant and Howard [44]). The critical importance of VEGFR-2 is indicated by evidence that its absence prevents angioblast development and the failure of primary capillary plexus formation [45]. Moreover, the VEGFR-2 co-receptors, neuropilins 1 and 2, are also required for vasculogenesis as evidenced by embryonic death in neuropilin double mutants [46]. VEGFR-1 mutations are also lethal; the phenotype in the affected embryos is EC overgrowth, suggesting that signaling via this receptor regulates the assembly of these cells. VEGF signaling also plays a role in both physiological and pathological growth in the adult. VEGFR-2 activation requires the NOS-III/NO system as evidenced by the attenuated angiogenic response (in vivo) to VEGF and to Ang-1 in mice deficient in eNOS [47]. NOS-III is the enzyme that regulates the biological availability and activity of NO. eNOS knockout mice are also defective in pericyte recruitment and arteriogenesis, and experience a diminished flow reserve [48].

Fibroblast Growth Factors

The FGF signaling pathways influence a variety of biological processes and involve co-receptors, as well as cell-surface and cytoplasmic proteins [49, 50]. FGFs have long been recognized as inducers of vasculogenesis, angiogenesis, and arteriogenesis. EPCs express FGFR-1 and differentiate into ECs when this receptor is stimulated [51]; FGFR-1 signaling is essential for normal embryonic vascular development [52]. This is evidenced by the fact that FGF signaling influences the migration, proliferation, and maturation of ECs [53]. FGF-2 is likewise important for induction of angioblasts and their assembly into a vascular pattern during embryogenesis [54]. The proangiogenic activities of FGFs include cross talk with VEGFs and inflammatory cytokines/chemokines [55] in which context FGFs are key to arteriogenesis. Specifically, they play a key role in arteriogenesis by stimulating platelet-derived growth factor receptor (PDGFR) and monocyte chemoattractant protein (MCP). Moreover, in combination, FGF-2 and PDGF-BB synergistically stabilize vessels [56].

The cross talk between FGF and VEGF is also important in neovascularization, as evidenced by the finding that the angiogenic response to FGF is lost in the absence of VEGF [57]. FGF-2 has a priming effect on vascular smooth muscle cells (VSMC), most likely the result of its upregulation of PDGFR [58]. These and other observations have led to the conclusion by Murakami and Simons [50] that FGF promotes angiogenesis and arteriogenesis indirectly by regulating the expression of VEGF, PDGFR, monocyte chemotactic protein-1 (MCP-1), and hepatocyte growth factor (HGF). HGF directly enhances EC migration, proliferation, and vascular sprouting [59].

Other Key Growth Factors

The tyrosine kinase receptor, Tie-1, and its ligands, angiopoietins 1 and 2, have preferential expression in ECs and regulate vascular morphogenesis during development and in the adult. In addition, activation of Tie-2 mediates EC survival and recruitment of mural cells, thus promoting vessel assembly and maturation (reviewed in Thomas [60]). During the initial stage of vessel formation, angiopoietin-1 and its tie-2 receptor facilitate cell–cell and cell–matrix interactions [61], and consequently vessel stabilization and EC quiescence. In this way, this growth factor-receptor promotes cell and vessel maturation. In contrast, angiopoietin-2 facilitates the formation of vessels by destabilizing them, allowing EC migration and subsequent branch formation. Thus, angiopoietins 1 and 2 act as agonist and antagonists, respectively, of vessel maturation (reviewed in Pfaff [62]). A high ratio of angiopoietin 1:2 maintains vessels in the quiescence state, whereas a low ratio causes EC destabilization. Along with the angiopoietin-Tie system, Eph receptors and their ephrin ligands modulate cell trafficking in the vascular system and recruitment of mural cells [62]. This receptor/ligand pair signals bidirectionally as Eph receptors signal forward and ephrins signal reverse. Since these receptors and ligands are membrane molecules, their interaction depends on juxtapositional contact among neighboring cells.

Integrins and Other Adhesion Molecules

Cell–cell and cell–ECM (extracellular matrix) interactions are essential for the assembly of ECs into a tubular network (suggested reviews for this topic [63–66]). In this regard, integrins play key roles in a sequence of events that contribute to vessel formation. They are a large family of heterodimeric, transmembrane glycoproteins required for cell–ECM and cell–cell adhesion and signaling. Cell migration, proliferation, and differentiation require interactions with the ECM. Some integrins interact directly with growth factor receptors, thus providing receptor cross talk and optimizing cell stimulation. For example, the key receptor for vasculogenesis, VEGFR-2, interacts with integrin $\alpha_v \beta_3$. EC stimulation with VEGF facilitates formation of a VEGFR-2 complex with this integrin and adhesion to vitronectin and fibrinogen.

Vascular endothelial (VE)-cadherin is the main cell adhesion molecule involved in tight junction formation and is expressed early and exclusively in ECs. This initial expression of VE-cadherin correlates with hemangioblast commitment to the EC lineage and continues to be expressed in the adult. VE-cadherin promotes VEGF-A triggered activation of cell survival signaling. Neural (N)-cadherin is also found in ECs, but is diffusely distributed over the cell surface. PECAM-1 (CD31) is most strongly expressed at cell–cell junctions. However, its role in outside–inside cell signaling has also been indicated.

Suppressors of Vasculogenesis

Although many stimuli of vasculogenic events have been identified, much less is known about suppressors of these events. Such agents are necessary to prevent vascularization of tissues that do not require a blood supply. For example, chondromodulin-1 prevents the vascularization of avascular tissues such as heart valves and cartilage (reviewed in [67]). The region between the paired aortae (midline avascular zone) in the embryonic disk is avascular due to notochord-derived BMP antagonists, such as Noggin and Chordin [68]. BMPs influence EC differentiation from embryonic stem cells [69] and induce VEGFR-2 expression in EC and hematopoietic lineages [70]. The avascular notochord is the result of BMP inhibition, which precludes EC differentiation, migration, and vessel network formation [67]. This inhibitory effect is important for preventing vascularization of the midline region prior to the fusion of the two aortae.

Over-vascularization in adults is also prevented by inhibitors such as angiostatins and endostatins. Because these ligands effectively inhibit migration and tube formation [71, 72], they have therapeutic potential. For example, angiostatin induces and sustains dormancy in human primary tumors in mice [73].

Branching and Fusion (Angiogenesis)

An increase in the number of capillaries or venules requires vascular destabilization, i.e., breaking cell-to-cell contacts, as a requisite for EC migration. Angiopoietin-2 (a Tie-2 receptor ligand), plasminogen activator proteinases, heparanase family members, and matrix metalloproteinases degrade the extracellular matrix, thereby releasing growth factors, e.g., VEGF, FGF-2. These molecules, in turn, induce EC migration

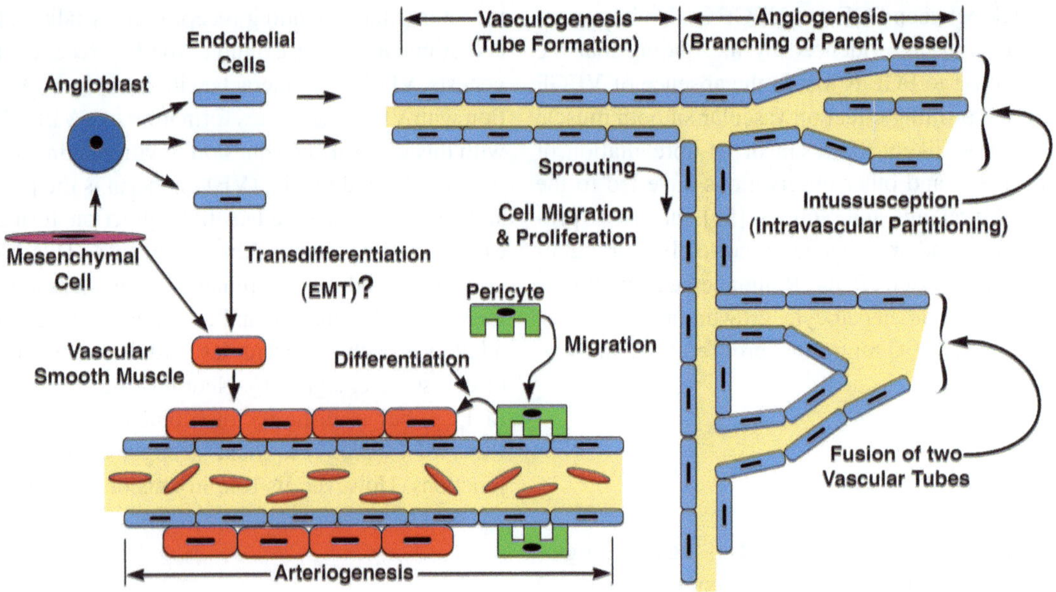

Fig. 1.3 Vascular morphogenesis. The origin and differentiation of vascular cells and the formation of vascular structures are illustrated. Endothelial cells form tubes (vasculogenesis), then branching occurs (angiogenesis) via sprouting or intravascular partitioning. Fusion of vascular tubes increases vessel diameter and is followed by the recruitment of mural cells (pericytes and smooth muscle) and their differentiation. The formation of arterioles and arteries (arteriogenesis) is a response to flow in the vascular plexus

and proliferation. The angiogenic properties of VEGF include the ability to stimulate an increase in vessel permeability, which occurs when vessels dilate in response to nitric oxide. The enhanced permeability facilitates extravasation of plasma proteins that provide migrating ECs with a scaffold. Angiopoietin-1 then stabilizes the vessel by tightening cell–cell junctions, thereby decreasing permeability [74].

Branches Are Formed by Two Distinct Processes: Sprouting and Intussusception (Fig. 1.3)

Sprouting

The long-recognized "sprouting" of vascular channels involves metalloproteinase (MMP) secretion followed by activation of ECs, EMC degradation, and EC migration (reviewed in van Hinsberg and Koolwijk [75, 76]). Such sprouting is normally inhibited by antiangiogenic factors, but these inhibitory proteins are neutralized by proangiogenic growth factors. Specific cell-bound proteases, including MT1-MMP, MMP-2, MMP-9, and u-PA, degrade ECM components, thereby providing a channel for migrating ECs. Sprouting occurs not only during early development but also during remodeling of mature capillaries and small venules. Folkman [77] reviewed EC migration and sprout formation in various models nearly 3 decades ago. Subsequent studies have illuminated a series of events that generate a vascular branch by sprouting (1) fragmentation of the basal lamina via proteolysis; (2) migration of EC into the perivascular space; (3) bipolar alignment of EC; and (4) mitosis of distal ECs to elongate the sprout (Fig. 1.3). The subsequent recruitment of pericytes inhibits further sprouting.

Tip Cells: The Sprout's Leading Edge

Once the basement membrane is degraded, ECs migrate and proliferate to form capillary sprouts (Fig. 1.4). The sprout is composed of stalk cells, which proliferate and form a capillary lumen. The leading edge consists of ECs called "tip cells," which are regulated by pro- and antiangiogenic factors. As noted in several reviews [78–81], VEGF is essential for the initiation of angiogenic sprouting, as well as for migration and proliferation of the cells comprising the sprout. The sprout consists of stalk cells which proliferate and form the capillary lumen. Thus, the spatial expression of VEGF initiates sprouting and its cross talk with Dll4/Notch signaling ensures that only a limited number of tip cells are formed. Notch and VEGF signaling pathways are the major regulators of tip and stalk cell behaviors, and consequently of the sprouting process. It is the site of the highest VEGF levels that directs tip cell motility. VEGF is upregulated by hypoxia as are a number of other growth factor genes (e.g., angiopoietin-2, (TGF-β), platelet-derived growth factor-B (PDGF-B), and insulin-like growth factors (IGFs) present in the extracellular matrix). Thus, hypoxic regions with high VEGF concentration are sites at which vascular sprouts develop. VEGF-A activation of ECs results in the expression of the Notch ligand Dll4 (Fig. 1.4). The high Notch signaling represses transcription of VEGFR-2, neuropilin, and Flt-4 in

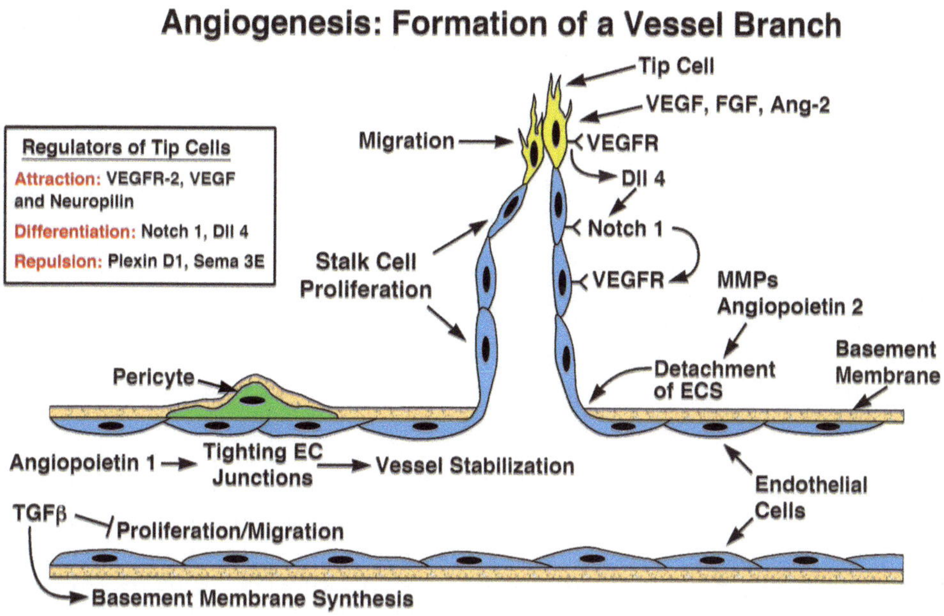

Fig. 1.4 Angiogenesis: formation of a vascular branch (via sprouting). A branch forms by a series of events which include dissolution of the basement membrane, detachment of ECs, proliferation of ECs forming the attached stalk, and migration of Tip cells at the leading edge of the forming branch. The parent vessel is stabilized by angiopoietin-1-induced tightening of EC junctions and the effects of pericyte presence. EC proliferation/migration in the parent vessel is suppressed by TGF-β. Note that various molecules regulate Tip cell migration by attractive or repulsive influences and thereby facilitate Tip cell differentiation. See text for details

some ECs, which acquire the stalk cell phenotype (reviewed in [81]). Thus, the high Notch signaling in stalk cells acts as a brake for excessive tip cell formation as evidenced in mice in which Notch signaling has been suppressed [82]. The tip cells—which are enriched for CXCR4, the stromal cell derived factor-1 (SDF-1) receptor—extend their filopodia and move distally [83]. SDF-1 stimulates capillary formation. Suchting et al. [84], as well as several other laboratories, reported that heterozygous deletion of Dll4 or pharmacological inhibition of Notch signaling inhibited vessel sprouting and branching during development. The data also revealed that blocking Notch signaling results in a loss of sprouting suppression.

Vascular sprouting involving EC migration, actin polymerization, and junction assembly requires serum response factor (SRF), a transcription factor that links extracellular stimuli to the cellular phenotype [85]. Hypoxia not only serves as a stimulus for VEGF and other growth factors that regulate sprouting but also plays a role in ECM composition, deposition, and rearrangement by modulating enzymes that modify the ECM [86]. Tip cells have been found to contain three clusters of enriched genes that encode (1) extracellular matrix degrading enzymes, (2) basement membrane components, and (3) secreted molecules [83, 87]. The secreted molecules include endothelial-specific molecule 1, angiopoietin-2, and apelin, each of which binds to cognate receptors on endothelial stalk cells. Tip cells persist only for a few hours and, by expressing a distinct gene profile, orchestrate capillary outgrowth [88]. Sema-3E (a class III semaphorin)—acting through a single-pass transmembrane receptor, plexin D1—provides a repulsive cue for ECs that express this receptor [89]. Sema-3E causes a rapid disassembly of integrin-mediated adhesive structures and thereby inhibits angiogenesis in tumors. EC polarity is important in blood vessel formations, although its determinants are not well understood (reviewed in [90]). Perturbations of polarity are associated with several pathologies.

EC Migration During Angiogenesis

Three integrated mechanisms: chemotaxis, hypotaxis, and mechanotaxis facilitate EC migration [91]. Chemotactic agents include cytokines and growth factors, of which the most important promoters are VEGF, FGF and angiopoietins, soluble adhesion molecules, ephrins, and angiogens. The second mechanism, haptotaxis (involving contact), occurs as extracellular matrix components influence EC migration independently of chemotactic factors. Haptotaxis requires collagen and integrins, especially the cross talk between integrins and growth factors. Mechanotaxis, discussed in more detail in a subsequent section of this chapter and in Chap. 11, relates to physical forces (such as hemodynamic forces) that act on ECs.

Intussusception

A second type of vascular channel formation is intussusception (invagination or infolding of a part), which occurs by intravascular partitioning via inward movement of ECs within the capillary. This type of branching, reviewed by Djonov and Makanya [92], requires folds from opposite sides of the vessel wall to protrude into the lumen and make contact to form EC bilayers, which are then perforated (Fig. 1.3). Fibroblasts, which produce collagen fibrils, invade the interendothelial junctions along with pericytes. These events allow the vessel to split into two sister vessels. This type of vessel formation, described in many organs, is a type of branching in capillaries, arterioles, and venules [93]. The events comprising vasculogenesis and angiogenesis leading to the recruitment of mural cells are illustrated in Fig. 1.3.

Increases in Lumen Diameter

Increases in vascular lumen diameter can occur not only by cell division of ECs, but also by vascular fusion, as described by Drake and Little [94], who suggested that this growth phenomenon, which is a form of remodeling, occurs in animals both prenatally and postnatally. Moreover, they documented VEGF as the primary stimulus of vascular fusion. Large increases in vessel diameter, in particular, require an increase in EC number [95]. Thus, vessel diameter can be increased by either EC proliferation within the existing vessel or by the fusion of vessels to form a larger vessel. Vessel stability is dependent on the EC tyrosine receptor Tie-2 [96]; as noted earlier, its ligand, angiopoietin 1, stabilizes the vessel, whereas another ligand, angiopoietin 2, causes vessel destabilization (reviewed in Rossant and Howard [44]). As neovascularization proceeds via branching and fusion, excessive vascular channels, i.e., those with low blood flow, are simultaneously pruned.

Assembly of the Vascular Hierarchy

The initial vascular plexus that is formed during development consists of ECs. The formation of the two outer vascular tunics (media and adventitia) requires the recruitment, differentiation, and assembly of additional cell types (Fig. 1.3). Neovascularization, both in the developing organism and adult, also begins with the formation of a vascular tube.

Recruitment and Assembly of Pericytes and Smooth Muscle Cells

Pericyte Signaling

Pericytes are mesenchyme-derived cells that interface with ECs through their peg-like processes and thereby allow communication between the two cell types (Fig. 1.3). As previously reviewed [97], PDGF-B secreted from ECs attracts pericytes by binding to their PDGFR-β receptor. Pericyte mobilization also requires the metalloproteinase MMP-9 which is activated on ECs [75]. Once pericytes reach the vascular wall, they secrete tissue inhibitors of metalloproteinases (e.g., TIMP-3), which inhibit MMP-2 activation on ECs and stabilize vascularization. Ablation of either PDGF-B or PDGFR-β attenuates migration of pericytes to sprouting capillaries and results in capillary microaneurysms [98]. PDGF-B also induces proliferation of VSMC and differentiation of mesenchymal cells. Thus, the PDGF-B/PDGFR-β axis defines paracrine signaling from ECs to pericytes and smooth muscle cells (defined as mural cells).

Pericytes stabilize vessels and, in some cases, differentiate into VSMC; they are stimulated by TGF-β, which also inhibits VEGFR-2 on ECs [99, 100]. EC proliferation then ceases, while the tunica media develops. Signaling from potential mural cells to ECs also occurs when angiopoietin-1 (Ang-1) signals to the Tie-2 receptors on ECs and serves as a stabilization factor, thus facilitating cell adhesion and consequently vessel maturation [61]. During vessel remodeling, Ang-2 levels increase and facilitate EC migration, vessel sprouting, and increases in capillary diameters [91]. Pericytes are also required for vascular integrity in adults. For example, pericyte dropout is the likely cause of retinal capillary microaneurysms and hemorrhage in diabetic patients [101].

Endothelial and Mural Cell Integrins

ECs and pericytes express numerous integrins that constitute a family of heterodimeric glycoprotein adhesion molecules [102]. Integrin subunits bind fibronectin, collagen, laminin, and vitronectin and are expressed on both ECs and pericytes. Fibroblasts and VSMCs also express integrins. Alpha V integrins are increased during angiogenesis and increases in $\alpha V\beta 3$ and $\alpha V\beta 5$ dimers have been noted during vascular sprouting. Key growth factors involved in vascular morphogenesis interact with integrins [66]. Examples include FGFR-3, VEGFR-2, PDGFR (interactions with $\alpha V\beta 3$), and Tie-2 (interactions with $\alpha_5\beta_1$). Cross talk between receptor kinases and integrin receptors plays a key role in vascular morphogenesis. An important example is the reciprocal association between VEGFR-2 and integrin $\alpha_V\beta 3$ [103]. This interaction regulates EC migration, survival, and tubulogenesis, and underscores the importance of integrins in neovascularization.

Vascular Smooth Muscle Cell Assembly

The development of the tunica media requires the recruitment, differentiation, and migration of VSMCs not only during development but also during remodeling and vascular repair. These events require signaling between ECs and mesenchymal cells (see reviews by [104–108]). VSMCs not only proliferate and migrate but also synthesize ECM components such as collagen and elastin, as well as proteoglycans and adhesion molecules including cadherens and integrins. Molecules, e.g., biogenic amines, growth factors, and cytokines, are stored in the ECM and therefore can be activated to facilitate cell migration (reviewed in Gerthoffer [109]), a process that is dependent on local ECM proteolysis, cytoskeletal remodeling, and changes in adhesive molecules. VSMC migration, like that of other migratory cells, requires cell polarity and the generation of propulsive and traction forces. Major signaling pathways include those involving Rho kinase, actin-binding proteins, myosin II motors, and G proteins.

A variety of intrinsic and extrinsic factors facilitate progression of VSMCs to a mature state. These include humoral, neural, and mechanical influences. Since VSMCs are not terminally differentiated, they maintain their high degree of plasticity and are able to change their phenotype. Their differentiation and the expression of numerous markers are dependent on CArG boxes (DNA sequences within SMC genes) and the binding molecule, SRF [110]. SMC differentiation requires an interplay between SRF-CArG, SRF accessory cofactors, and histone modifications [111]. Myocardin, a coactivator of SRF-dependent transcription, activates smooth and cardiac muscle-specific promoters and induces the expression of CArG-dependent markers including calponin, smooth muscle (SM) α-actin, smooth muscle heavy chain, SM22α, and telokin [112, 113]. However, this dependence on myocardin may be limited to specific VSMCs [107].

TGF-β1 signaling induces mesenchymal cells to differentiate into smooth muscle via its Alk-5 receptor and its association with receptor-regulated Smads 2/3 (reviewed in Gaengel [97]). TGF-β regulates proliferation, migration, survival, differentiation, and ECM synthesis in ECs and VSMCs [114]. As noted previously in this chapter, the TGF-β1-ALK5 pathway [115] induces the plasminogen activator inhibitor in ECs, thereby preventing ECM degradation, and thus negating EC proliferation and migration (reviewed in Jain [116]). This endothelial stabilization is requisite for vessel maturation. TGF-β induction of muscle differentiation from mesenchymal cells is characterized by the expression of α-smooth muscle actin, smooth muscle myosin, and calponin. In the embryo, development of VSMCs from stem cells is a function of TGF-β signaling via smad 2/3 [117]. A TGF-β co-receptor, endoglin, is required for VSMC recruitment, as evidenced by the finding that insufficiency of the co-receptor is associated with aberrant VSMC incorporation and vessel fragility [118].

PDGF-BB-induced VSMC proliferation depends on FGF-2 and its activation of FGFR-1 [50, 52]. Inhibition of PDGF-B-mediated FGFR-1 phosphorylation suppresses DNA synthesis and consequently cell proliferation. PDGF-B also promotes pericyte adhesion to the vascular wall. This growth factor is primarily a short-range paracrine factor since it is expressed only at the active sites of vascular sprouts, such as in EC tip cells [119, 120]. It is critical for expansion of the pericyte population in most organs, based on the evidence that PDGF-B and PDGFR-β knockout mice lack a complete investment of mural cells and as a result, the endothelial sprouts hyperproliferate, dilate, and become hyperpermeable [121].

Notch-3 signaling is essential for proper angiogenesis and mural cell investment [122] and differentiation [123]. Because mural cells play a regulatory role during vascular development, their absence results in EC hyperplasia and abnormal cell shape; capillaries become enlarged, more permeable, abnormally remodeled, and exhibit microaneurysms [124, 125]. Small vessels with Notch-3 gene mutations are related to ischemic and hemorrhagic strokes and diffuse white matter disease (reviewed in [126]). An example of this disorder is cerebral autosomal dominant arteriopathy with subcortical infarcts and leukoencephalopathy (CADASIL). The Notch-3 mutation causes degeneration of VSMCs in small arteries and arterioles leading to recurrent infarcts [126, 127].

Specification of Arterial and Venous Vessels

Endothelial Phenotypes Are Specified

Arterial and venous ECs express distinct gene expression profiles [128, 129]. There is now compelling evidence that arteriovenous EC specification is determined in the embryo (reviewed in dela Paz and D'Amore [130]). Arterial and venous ECs are specified by genes that encode transcription factors, ligands, and receptors (Fig. 1.5). A key distinction between ECs in these vessel types is that the transmembrane ligand ephrin B2 is expressed in arteries, whereas the EphB4 receptor is expressed in veins [136]. Thus, the highest ephrin-B2 expression in developing systems is in the arterial endothelium. Microvessel assembly is dependent on ephrin-B2, because this ligand modulates cell spreading and focal adhesion. Thus, ephrin B2-EphB4 signaling functions in both assembly and specification of the vascular wall. Both ephrin B2 and EphB4 are detectable in the primary vascular plexus of the embryo, an indication that arterial and venous ECs are genetically determined [129]. The determination of arterial and venous fates involves interactions between ligand/receptor pairs (ephrin B_2/EphB_4). The signaling from the ephrin B_2 on the future arterial EC maintains its arterial fate, whereas the Eph B_4 signaling in the future venous EC results in its venous fate [137].

Arterial Specificity

As recently reviewed [128, 130], arterial identity requires Notch, VEGF, and sonic hedgehog (Shh) signaling pathways. Arterial, but not venous, ECs express Notch 1 and 4 [138], and a lack of the Notch ligand, Dll4, results in major vascular defects [139]. Jagged 1 and Notch 1/Notch 4 function in the regulation of branching morphogenesis during development, since mice mutant for these proteins have

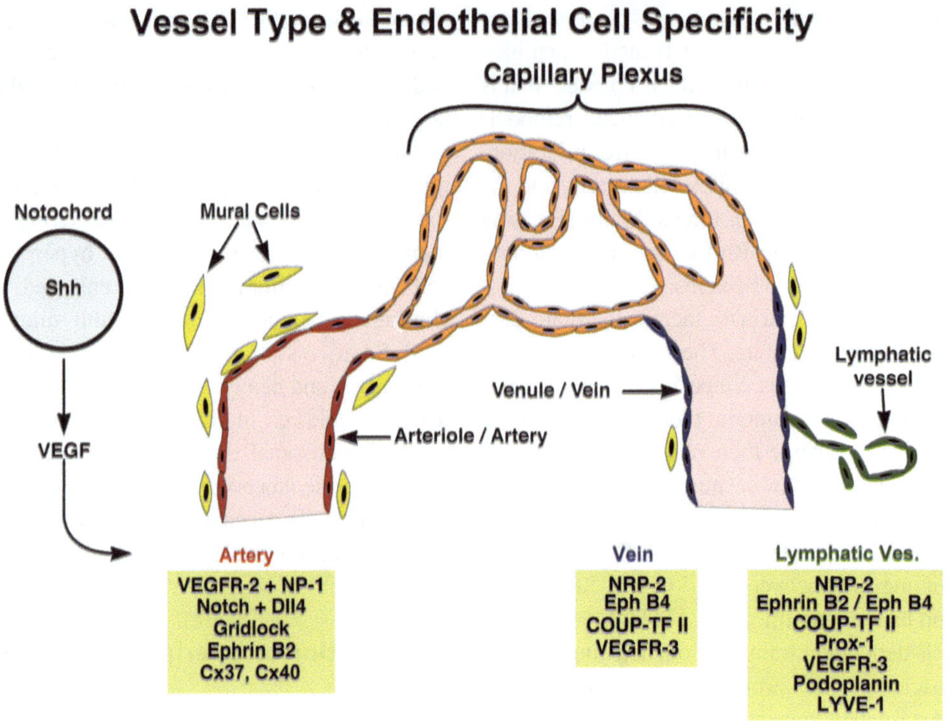

Fig. 1.5 Artery/vein specification occurs early in development and requires specific receptors. Sonic hedgehog (Shh) from the notochord stimulates VEGF-A, which is a ligand for VEGFR-2 and neuropilin-1 (NP-1) in presumptive arterial endothelial cells. Activation of these receptors results in delta-like 4 (Dll4) ligand upregulation and activation of its Notch signaling. Gridlock, an artery-restricted gene, is activated by Notch signaling and serves to inhibit EphB4, the receptor specifying venous endothelial cells. In contrast to arteries, veins express VEGFR-3 and NP-1. Lymphatic vessels develop via venular ECs. Lymphatic endothelial cells require the homeobox gene Prox-1 for lymphatic development and express LYVE-1 (lymphatic endothelial hyaluronan receptor) and podoplanin (a mucoprotein, coexpressed with VEGF-3 in small lymphatic vessels) [128, 131–135]

disorganized vessels with a reduced number of branches [140]. Specification of arterial ECs (Fig. 1.5) is directed by notochord-derived sonic hedgehog (Shh) signaling, which enhances VEGF-A and activates VEGFR-2 and NP-1 (neuropilin-1) EC receptors (reviewed in Dela Paz and Swift [130]). Notch and its Dll4 ligand continue the signaling cascade by activating gridlock (a transcriptional repressor that negatively regulates venous identity) and ephrin B2 (which facilitates arterial EC phenotype) [131, 132].

Venous Specificity

Venous and lymphatic ECs express COUP-TFII, a promoter-transcription factor that is absent in arterial ECs; it suppresses Notch signaling and consequently arterial EC phenotype [141]. A role for two FOX transcription factors in the induction of arterial markers was documented in mouse embryos mutant for Foxc1 and Foxc2. These mice fail to express arterial, but not venous, markers and are characterized by arteriovenous malformations [142]. That selective signaling pathways are required for specification of arteries and veins has also been documented [133]. When ERK (MAP kinase), a stimulator of arterial progenitors, is inhibited, arterial specification is blocked. However, another VEGF stimulated pathway, which involves ART activation by PI3 kinase, continues to promote venous specification. Thus, PI3 kinase and ERK have opposing roles in the specification of arteries and veins.

Lymphatic Specificity

Lymphogenesis is initiated via delamination of a subset of ECs from veins, which form lymph sacs and an early vascular plexus [143, 144]. A key transcriptional hub comprises transcriptional factors Prox-1, CoupTF11, and Sox18 has been identified in mice and is essential for lymphatic EC fate specification (reviewed in [145]). These cells contain the lymphatic vessel hyaluronan-1 receptor. They are induced into the lymphatic cell lineage by the transcription factor Sox18, which induces Prox-1, the main regulator of lymphatic endothelial identity (reviewed in [146]). As illustrated in Fig. 1.5, the lymphatic ECs derived from venous ECs during development, express specific genes that are not found on ECs lining arteries and veins. The developing embryo progressively acquires lymphatic specification after the arterial-venous fate decisions are completed [129]. Prox-1 induces the expression of other lymphatic EC genes, e.g., podoplanin [132]. Prox-1 interacts with COUP-TFII, a promoter/transcription factor, which is expressed in lymphatic, as well as venous vessels [129]. Lymphatic and blood circulation require separation for their specialized functions. This separation is made possible by an adaptor protein SLP-76 and Syk, a thyrosine kinase, both of which are expressed in hematopoietic cells [5, 147]. Since ECs do not express SLP-76 and Syk, hematopoietic cells are able, in some way, to dictate separation of the lymphatic and blood vessels. In the absence of these two molecules, these vessel types are not separated.

Arterial-Venous Segregation By Selective Cell Sprouting

High resolution imaging of zebrafish vascular development has revealed a mode of blood vessel formation for the first embryonic artery and vein via selective migration of progenitor cells from a precursor vessel [148]. This occurred by dorsal and ventral angioblast migration regulated by VEGF, Notch, and EphB4a/Ephrin-B2a signaling. Ephrin-B4α limited the ventral migration of angioblasts. In contrast, EphB4a promoted the ventral migration of venous angioblasts. These data suggest a repulsion between venous and arterial cells that facilitates directional control of angioblast sprouting and thus provides a cellular framework for arterial and venous vascular tubes.

Hemodynamic Forces and EC Plasticity

Although specific markers of arterial and venous ECs are expressed prior to the establishment of blood flow, EC plasticity is maintained until late embryonic development [149]. However, flow is considered the master regulator of arterial-venous differentiation, at least in the yolk sac [134, 150, 151]. This conclusion is based on experiments in which the yolk sac grows in the absence of blood flow, but does not develop arteries and veins [150]. Expression of both ephrin B2 and neuropilin-1 mRNAs is regulated by flow, as demonstrated by experiments that documented disconnection of small caliber vessels that were connected to the stem of the forming vitelline artery and a subsequent connection, by sprouting, to the venular plexus [150, 151]. Although early ECs are prespecified as arteries or veins, they remain plastic and are able to change their gene expression when introduced into a new environment. For example, arterial ECs transplanted into a vein begin to express a venous marker [149]. Further evidence that flow can alter EC markers comes from a study that showed that changing blood flow patterns from arterial to venous causes ECs to cease expressing arterial genes (Ephrin B2) and begin expressing venous genes, such as EphB4 [150]. A review of this topic has been provided by Jones [152].

Coordinated Arterial and Venous Growth

A fully functional circulatory system requires that arteries and veins develop in terms of both number and size via a complimentary program. Proof of this concept arose from a study on mice mutant for Notch, ephrin B2, and Ephb4 [153]. Comparisons of the growth of the developing aorta and cardinal vein revealed that Notch overexpression caused an enlargement of the aorta and underdevelopment of the cardinal vein, due to an increase in the number of arterial ECs. A loss of either ephrin B2 or its EphB4 receptor likewise caused aortic enlargement and underdeveloped cardinal veins. In this situation, ECs with a venous phenotype are "mislocalized" to the aorta. These data indicate that the B2/EphB4 signal serves to sort arterial and venous ECs into their appropriate vessels, a function distinct from that of Notch.

Conclusions: Arterial, Venous and Lymphatic Vessel Specification

The formation of arteries, veins, and lymphatic vessels is specified in the embryo by the selective expression of signaling molecules (Fig. 1.5). This process involves specific EC markers which facilitate the development of the specific vessel type. The key distinction between arteries and veins is determined by the ligand ephrin-B2 and the EphB4 receptor, respectively. Arterial ECs also express Notch1 and 4 and Dll4, the Notch ligand. Venous and lymphatic distinction is attributed, in part, to a promoter-transcription factor (COUP-TFII) that is absent in arterial ECs, and has been shown to suppress NOTCH signaling and therefore the arterial phenotype. The formation of arteries and veins also involves vessel segregation by selective EC sprouting and is influenced by hemodynamic forces that can influence EC phenotype. Lymphatic EC identity occurs with the expression of specific genes as these cells delaminate from veins.

Remodeling

Vascular wall plasticity underlies the adaptability of the vascular wall; see review by Martinez-Lemus [154]. Vascular remodeling is an active process that includes vasculogenesis, angiogenesis, and arteriogenesis, processes that require structural alterations in the ECM, as well as cell growth, migration, and death [155]. Arterial remodeling entails restructuring and reorganizing the mural components including VSMCs, elastin, collagen, and other ECM components [156]. It can occur in response to changing metabolic demands during embryonic, fetal, and postnatal growth, and in vascular pathologies, including hypertension, restenosis, and atherosclerosis. Vessel diameter can change acutely via vasoconstriction and vasodilation, in response to various stimuli. However, when the stimulus (e.g., increased blood flow or arterial pressure) is chronic, adaptation to the new mechanical or metabolic environment requires structural changes.

Remodeling During Development

The developing vasculature must undergo several morphological changes in order to meet the metabolic requirements for rapid tissue expansion. In the embryo, vascular pruning, fusion, and diameter increases facilitate the development of a hierarchy of vessels and provides adequate organ perfusion and O_2 delivery. As noted earlier in this chapter, remodeling plays an important role during development. More than a century ago, Thoma [157] theorized that, in the chick, vessel (1) lumen diameter depends on flow, (2) length depends on longitudinal force, and (3) wall thickness depends on blood pressure. Clark [158] provided support for the first theory by observing that increases in flow (blood volume) in frog larva tail capillaries caused them to remodel into arterioles, whereas decreases in flow caused capillaries to regress. With regard to the second theory (dependence of length on longitudinal force), he subsequently observed that capillary length increased in the direction of tissue growth, a finding that supports current evidence that stretch is a mechanical stimulus for longitudinal vascular growth. Finally, Thomas' third theory that blood pressure during development determines wall thickness is also now well established [159]. A good example of vascular remodeling when flow is no longer needed is that which occurs in the ductus arteriosus, during the late stage of fetal development. This remodeling involves increases in glycosaminoglycan production, which causes fragmentation of elastic fibers and promotes inward movement of VSMCs, resulting in a progressive stenosis (reviewed in Gibbons and Dzau [155]).

Remodeling in the Adult

Even in the adult, the vessel wall is not a static structure, but rather continually adapts to local mechanical, neural, and humoral factors [154]. These adaptations are also influenced and complicated by diseases, e.g., diabetes and atherosclerosis. Although most reviews of vascular remodeling have focused on the roles of shear stress and pressure, stretch is an equally important factor that occurs during tissue or organ growth or when vascular volume increases. Remodeling of an arteriole or artery is characterized by changes in all three layers of the vascular wall (reviewed by McGrath and colleagues [160]). An increase in the number of adventitial cells is an early remodeling change and may initiate other changes in the vascular wall. Adventitial inflammation may also occur in some pathological types, e.g., atherosclerosis. Smooth muscle cell hypertrophy occurs during hypertensive states and may involve repositioning of these cells, via their migration.

Flow and Shear Stress

Luminal diameters of arteries correlate with the magnitude of blood flow and thus shear stress, as evidenced by a decrease in diameter when flow is chronically decreased [161]. This remodeling is associated with heparin-binding dependent activation of epidermal growth factor (EGF) [162]. Similarly, high flows enhance lumen diameter by promoting EC proliferation [163, 164], resulting in an "outward" remodeling adaptation and therefore is EC dependent [165]. EC proliferation and migration have been associated with upregulation of VEGF, $\alpha V\beta 3$ integrin, PECAM-1, and VE-cadherin [25].

Remodeling in Response to Pressure and Decreased Flow

Chronically increased arterial pressure, as occurs in hypertensive states, is a well-known stimulus for remodeling. Because the type of remodeling varies according to the specific segment of the arterial hierarchial tree, the generalization that arteries undergo inward remodeling in hypertensive states [166] is not applicable to all arteries. As reviewed by Prewitt et al. [167], hypertension evokes different adaptations in distinct components of the arterial tree (Fig. 1.6). Large arteries adapt by outward hypertrophy, which results in thickening of the tunica media without a reduction in lumen diameter. In contrast, small arteries adapt to elevated pressure by inward hypertrophy, which reduces lumen diameter and increases resistance. Inward remodeling can also occur during chronically decreased flow, but includes a reduction in vascular smooth muscle. In this low flow model, there is both a reduction in the number of the smallest arterioles and a decrease in arteriolar diameter [168]. Several phenomena may characterize this type of remodeling, e.g., fibrosis, extracellular matrix remodeling, inflammation, and apoptosis (reviewed in Intengan and Schiffrin [169]). Consistent with the role of mechanical factors as determinants of vessel morphology, VSMC apoptosis is a response to marked reductions in blood flow [170, 171]. VSMC apoptosis also occurs during vascular diseases, e.g., restenosis, aneurysms, and atherosclerosis [172].

Remodeling and the Extracellular Matrix

Vascular remodeling is highly dependent on the ECM integrin-cytoskeletal axis, and the events that occur at the cell membrane that link extracellular and cellular events are central to vascular remodeling. These events have been detailed by Martinez-Lemus et al. [154]. Arteriolar remodeling requires several key cellular enzymes: focal adhesion kinase, tissue-type transglutaminase, and other non-receptor tyrosine

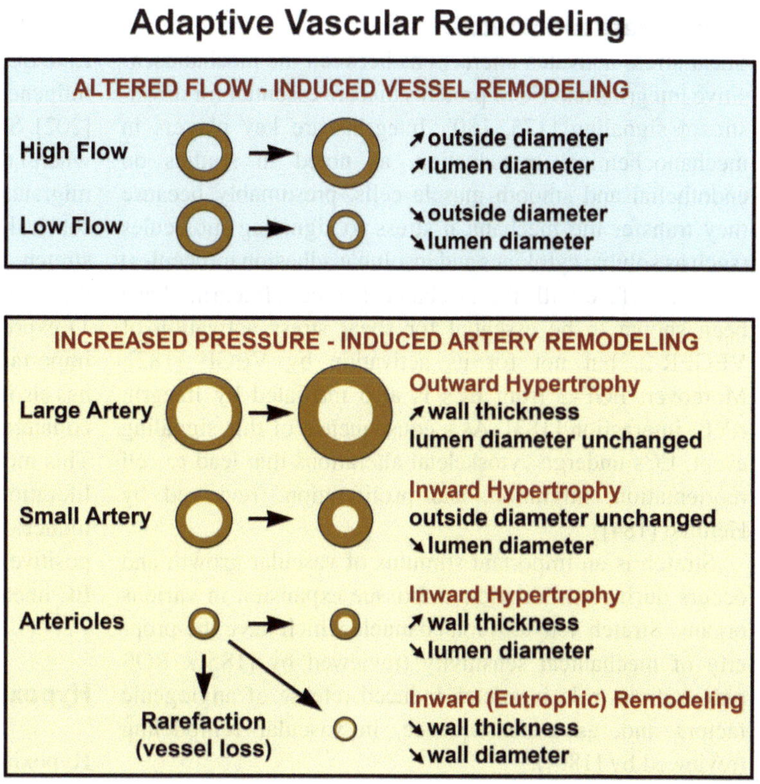

Fig. 1.6 Adaptive vascular remodeling occurs in response to altered flow or pressure. The adaptation to high flow results in increases of overall vessel diameter, as well as inside diameter. Low flow causes the opposite adaptations. Remodeling in response to increased pressure can be either inward or outward, resulting in a decreased or unchanged luminal diameter, respectively. The response depends on the position of the vessel in the arterial hierarchy

kinases that act on the cytoskeleton. Remodeling stimuli (e.g., pressure) activate the cell membrane receptors that link the ECM to the cytoskeleton. MMPs then trigger ECM degradation, which is necessary for cell migration and rearrangement of VSMCs. Finally, integrins act as receptors and thereby control both smooth muscle migration and ECM remodeling.

Primary Stimuli for Vascular Growth and Remodeling

Both metabolic and mechanical factors are able to trigger cellular changes that lead to vascular growth and remodeling. The major metabolic contributor is hypoxia. Mechanical influences include shear stress, stretch, and pressure, all of which influence the cell's shape.

Mechanical Forces

Vascular remodeling occurs when mechanical forces are chronically altered, typically in the arterial vasculature. As noted earlier, even vessel phenotype can be altered, as occurs in the specification of arterial and venous identity [173]. Several review papers have addressed the role of mechanical forces in vascular remodeling [174–176]. Increases in blood flow (fluid velocity) or hematocrit enhance shear stress, whereas increases in vessel diameter cause cells in the vascular wall to stretch. Shear stress has been documented as the initial signal for arteriogenesis by Eitenmuller et al. [177], who employed an arterio-venous shunt model to demonstrate that enhanced blood flow increased maximal vascular conductance (a measure of vascular volume) in the absence of ischemia or hypoxia.

Hydrostatic Forces

Hydrostatic forces, from both the luminal and abluminal surfaces, affect vascular cells and play critical roles in both growth and remodeling of blood vessels. When vascular cells are exposed to prolonged changes in flow, reactive oxygen species (ROS) are produced and serve as second messengers to influence remodeling (reviewed by Lehoux [178]). A number of studies have shown that increased blood flow via chronic administration of vasodilator drugs, e.g., dipyridamole, adenosine, ethanol, and nifedipine, stimulates capillary growth [174]. Transduction mechanisms in ECs involve both the cytoskeleton and biochemical signals at sites of mechanotransduction, including the cell membrane [179], and are the primary transducers of hemodynamic forces that initiate events leading to angiogenesis, arteriogenesis, or remodeling. Reviews that focused on shear stress signaling in ECs have highlighted many molecules that function as mechanosensors; these include PECAM-1, G-proteins and G-coupled receptors, and ion channels [176, 180, 181].

Shear Stress and Stretch

Shear stress activates interactions between the mechanosensitive integrins and ECM proteins that are essential for downstream signaling [175, 180]. Integrins are key players in mechanochemical transduction, as noted in studies on endothelial and smooth muscle cells, presumably because they transfer the mechanical stress to signaling molecules (such as soluble cytokines and insoluble adhesion molecules) at the interface with the mechanical forces. Integrins have been shown to be essential for shear stress activation of VEGFR-2, but not for its activation by VEGF [182]. Moreover, FGF-2 from ECs is also mediated by integrin $\alpha V\beta_3$ interaction [183]. As a consequence of this signaling event, ECs undergo cytoskeletal alterations that lead to cell reorientation, migration, and proliferation (reviewed by Helmke [184]).

Stretch is an important stimulus of vascular growth and occurs during vasodilation and tissue expansion in various organs. Stretch activates ion channels which have the property of mechanical sensitivity (reviewed by [185]). ROS play a direct role in stretch-induced release of angiogenic factors and, as a consequence, in vascular remodeling (reviewed by [186]).

Specific Endothelial Cell Responses

Many studies have documented EC proliferation in response to shear stress [175, 187], and cyclic stretch and pressure [188]. EC responses to fluid shear stress involve a complex interplay between structural and biochemical signaling [189]. Distortion of cell shape and the accompanying alterations in the cytoskeleton modulate the cell cycle in a Rho-dependent manner. Cyclic stretch-induced proliferation is associated with upregulation of Angiopoietins 1 and 2, Tie-2, and VEGFR-2 [190, 191], and is dependent on VEGF for proliferation, migration, and tube formation [192]. Similar to the response to cyclic stretch, ECs exposed to shear stress undergo Tie-2 phosphorylation [193] and proliferation [194]. EC proliferation is also stimulated by chronic tangential load shear stress [187, 195] and flattening of ECs (compression) increases their sensitivity to growth factors [196]. ECs exposed to pulsatile flow migrate and form tubes [197], whereas fluid shear stress differentially modulates endothelial cell genes, encoding two key growth factors, namely FGF-2 and PDGF-B, which regulate arterial growth and remodeling via their paracrine signaling to smooth muscle [198]. In contrast, human umbilical vein ECs exposed to laminar shear stress or pressure are characterized by a decline in VEGF expression [199], suggesting the role of EC specialization according to its location in a specific vessel. It has also been shown that physiological levels of shear stress reduce EC loss by interfacing CPP32-like proteases and thereby inhibit apoptosis of these cells [200].

Specific Vascular Smooth Muscle Cell Responses

Like ECs, VSMCs also proliferate in response to mechanical influences, e.g., enhanced pressure in vivo [201] and in vitro [202]. Smooth muscle cells situated in vascular bifurcations, where they are exposed to non-laminar flow, frequently migrate [203]. In addition, exposure to stretch enhances their survival [204]. More recent evidence indicates that cyclic stretch, but not shear stress, induces activator protein-1-mediated increases in monocyte chemoattractant protein (MCP-1) expression in vascular smooth muscle [205]. MCP-1 is important in collateral vessel development. Fluid shear stress has also been documented as a trigger for the development of collateral vessels [206, 207], a topic addressed in Chap. 12. This mechanical factor correlates with increases in the proliferation of both ECs and VSMCs. Fluid shear stress also induces the proliferation and differentiation of VEGFR-2 positive embryonic stem cells and shepherds them into the EC lineage [208].

Hypoxia

Hypoxia is a major trigger of vascular morphogenesis, not only during development but also in the adult. This is the topic of Chap. 9. The following sections provide a brief review of the topic.

Hypoxia Inducible Factor

The key molecule in the cascade of events activated by hypoxia is the transcription factor, hypoxia inducible factor-1 (HIF-1), which activates other transcription and growth factors and consequently angiogenesis (reviewed by Semenza [209]). Under normoxic conditions, HIF-1 is degraded by hydroxylation of HIF-1α subunits by a family of oxygen-sensing prolyl hydroxylase domain proteins (PHDs). During hypoxia, the hydroxylase activity is inhibited and degradation does not occur. HIF-1 binds to specific cis-acting sequences (hypoxia response elements) and can activate over 40 genes, including VEGF. In the context of hypoxia, HIF-1-activated VEGF triggers the expression of other growth factors and cytokines, e.g., Placenta Growth Factor (PlGF), SDF-1, angiopoietins 1 and 2, PDGF-B, and TGF-β3. The key role of HIF-1 in O_2 homeostasis is supported by data documenting its ability to stimulate the expression of many of the genes that are upregulated in a hypoxic environment [210]. These genes encode cytokines, growth factors and growth factor receptors, and a variety of signaling molecules.

The mechanisms underlying hypoxia-induced neovascularization are discussed in a review by Fong [211]. These include upregulation of a number of angiogenic proteins that can be upregulated both directly and indirectly via molecules activated by HIF-1. ECs proliferate and migrate in response to hypoxia-upregulated VEGF-A and eNOS [212–214], findings that underscore the importance of hypoxia in vascular morphogenesis. However, hypoxia, if sufficiently severe, can also attenuate these angiogenic responses by facilitating an accumulation of HIF-1α, which can stabilize p53 and promote apoptosis [215] and may trigger the generation of ROS that damage cell membranes and DNA [216].

Response of VSMCs and Monocytes

VSMC proliferate when PDGF-β receptor expression is elevated by hypoxia [217]. The ensuing VSMC migration is likely facilitated by attenuating focal adhesion of VSMC via a hypoxia-induced decrease in focal adhesion kinase phosphorylation [218]. In the context of hypoxia, monocytes migrate into tissues where they differentiate into macrophages, cells that secrete several molecules important for activation of angiogenesis, such as granulocyte-colony stimulating factor, PDGF, TGF-α, FGF-2, and IGF-1 [219].

Vascular Morphogenesis in the Embryo/Fetus

The presence of hypoxia in various tissue regions in embryos and fetuses has been demonstrated with markers for low O_2 [220, 221]. Failure to activate genes that respond to O_2 tension was noted in mice homozygous mutant for aryl hydrocarbon-receptor nuclear translocator (ARNT) gene, which forms 50% of HIF-1 complex [222]. These embryos displayed yolk sac vessel abnormalities resembling those of VEGF-deficient mice and were not viable past embryonic day 10.5. Similarly, HIF-1α null mutants displayed insufficient vascularization by embryonic day 8 [223]. Hypoxic regions in quail embryos were characterized by increases in both HIF-1 and VEGF, and vessel density was increased in these regions [224].

Hypoxia is also a major stimulus for angiogenesis in the adult, as detailed in Fong's review [211], which documents hypoxia-induced neovascularization in several pathological conditions, e.g., ischemia in heart and skeletal muscle, atherosclerosis, wound healing, tumors, rheumatoid arthritis, and ocular diseases. The role of increased HIF-1α in these various conditions indicates that it is a prime candidate for clinical interventions. Although in vitro studies have documented a direct role of hypoxia in angiogenesis, in vivo analysis reveals that hypoxia also increases blood flow, which constitutes a mechanical stimulus.

Vascular Integrity

Vascular hemostasis depends on vascular integrity, which requires continuous blood flow and the interactions of vascular cells and the extracellular matrix; see reviews by Murakami [225] and Dejana [226]. Endothelial cell junction organization is critical for normal permeability. Alterations in these structures are the basis of edema, inflammation, and hemorrhage.

Cell–Cell Junctions

ECs have three specialized junctions: adherens, tight, and gap. Permeability is primarily regulated by adherens junctions, whereas tight junctions serve as gatekeepers for solutes and ions across the endothelium [227, 228]. Gap junctions function primarily in cell–cell signaling. At the adherens junctions, VE-cadherins mediate cell–cell contacts extracellularly and also link actin-binding proteins intracellularly. A prime function of cadherins is to stabilize the adherens junctions and thus maintain the "gatekeeper" function. Vascular permeability is increased by VEGF, but decreased by FGF [225].

Extracellular Matrix

The interstitial matrix that lies between cells contains collagens; of these, collagen I plays a major role in support of the endothelium, and along with type III, supports blood vessels. Studies in mouse knockouts have revealed that the absence of either of these collagens is lethal as it leads to vascular rupture [229, 230]. Disorders of these collagens, i.e., Ehlers-Danlos and osteogenesis imperfecta, often result in aortic aneurysms [231]. The basal lamina—which contains type IV collagen, laminins, nidogens, and the heparin sulfate proteoglycan, perlecan—is not only a physical barrier to macromolecules and migrating cells but also a scaffold for pericytes and ECs. The basal lamina is tethered to fibrils via collagen type VII, and together, these fibrils and the basal lamina constitute the "basement membrane." Laminins and type IV collagens are important for microvascular integrity as evidenced by the finding that genetic disruption of these components causes microvascular hemorrhage (reviewed in [225]).

Pericytes and the Endothelium

As noted earlier, pericytes and ECs are in close contact. The pericyte lies under the basement membrane of ECs, and accordingly, the membrane mediates communication between the two cell types. In addition to their role in vascular morphogenesis, pericytes provide vascular stability in adult vessels via their close association with the endothelium. Perhaps the best example of this role for pericytes is found in retinal vessels where these cells form an extensive mural component. Diabetic retinopathy is characterized by early loss of pericytes and is associated with microvessel aneurysms and hemorrhage [101, 232].

References

1. Simons M. Angiogenesis: where do we stand now? Circulation. 2005;111:1556–66.
2. Risau W. Mechanisms of angiogenesis. Nature. 1997;386:671–4.
3. Timmermans F, Plum J, Yoder MC, Ingram DA. Endothelial progenitor cells: identity defined? J Cell Mol Med. 2009;13:87–102.
4. Xiong JW. Molecular and developmental biology of the hemangioblast. Dev Dyn. 2008;237:1218–31.
5. Rafii S, Lyden D. Therapeutic stem and progenitor cell transplantation for organ vascularization and regeneration. Nat Med. 2003;9:702–12.
6. Ema M, Rossant J. Cell fate decisions in early blood vessel formation. Trends Cardiovasc Med. 2003;13:254–9.
7. Ribatti D. Hemangioblast does exist. Leuk Res. 2008;32:850–4.
8. Eguchi M, Masuda H, Asahara T. Endothelial progenitor cells for postnatal vasculogenesis. Clin Exp Nephrol. 2007;11:18–25.
9. Risau W, Flamme I. Vasculogenesis. Annu Rev Cell Dev Biol. 1995;11:73–91.
10. Sabin FR. Preliminary note on the differentiation of angioblasts and the method by which they produce blood vessels, blood plasma and red blood cells as seen in the living chick. Anat Rec. 1917;13:199–204.
11. Eichmann A, Corbel C, Nataf V, Vaigot P, Breant C, Le Douarin NM. Ligand-dependent development of the endothelial and hemopoietic lineages from embryonic mesodermal cells expressing vascular endothelial growth factor receptor 2. Proc Natl Acad Sci USA. 1997;94:5141–6.
12. Schatteman GC. Adult bone marrow-derived hemangioblasts, endothelial cell progenitors, and EPCs. Curr Top Dev Biol. 2004;64:141–80.
13. Ribatti D. The discovery of endothelial progenitor cells. An historical review. Leuk Res. 2007;31:439–44.
14. Drake CJ, Fleming PA. Vasculogenesis in the day 6.5 to 9.5 mouse embryo. Blood. 2000;95:1671–9.
15. Schmidt A, Brixius K, Bloch W. Endothelial precursor cell migration during vasculogenesis. Circ Res. 2007;101:125–36.
16. Jin SW, Patterson C. The opening act: vasculogenesis and the origins of circulation. Arterioscler Thromb Vasc Biol. 2009;29:623–9.
17. Kwon SM, Alev C, Asahara T. The role of notch signaling in endothelial progenitor cell biology. Trends Cardiovasc Med. 2009;19:170–3.
18. Lancrin C, Sroczynska P, Serrano AG, Gandillet A, Ferreras C, Kouskoff V, et al. Blood cell generation from the hemangioblast. J Mol Med (Berl). 2010;88:167–72.
19. Huber TL. Dissecting hematopoietic differentiation using the embryonic stem cell differentiation model. Int J Dev Biol. 2010;54:991–1002.
20. Sugiyama D, Tsuji K. Definitive hematopoiesis from endothelial cells in the mouse embryo; a simple guide. Trends Cardiovasc Med. 2006;16:45–9.
21. Lancrin C, Sroczynska P, Stephenson C, Allen T, Kouskoff V, Lacaud G. The haemangioblast generates haematopoietic cells through a haemogenic endothelium stage. Nature. 2009;457:892–5.
22. Eilken HM, Nishikawa S, Schroeder T. Continuous single-cell imaging of blood generation from haemogenic endothelium. Nature. 2009;457:896–900.
23. Asahara T, Murohara T, Sullivan A, Silver M, van der Zee R, Li T, et al. Isolation of putative progenitor endothelial cells for angiogenesis. Science. 1997;275:964–7.
24. Shi Q, Rafii S, Wu MH, Wijelath ES, Yu C, Ishida A, et al. Evidence for circulating bone marrow-derived endothelial cells. Blood. 1998;92:362–7.
25. Asahara T, Kawamoto A. Endothelial progenitor cells for postnatal vasculogenesis. Am J Physiol Cell Physiol. 2004;287:C572–9.
26. Baron M. Induction of embryonic hematopoietic and endothelial stem/progenitor cells by hedgehog-mediated signals. Differentiation. 2001;68:175–85.
27. Urbich C, Dimmeler S. Endothelial progenitor cells: characterization and role in vascular biology. Circ Res. 2004;95:343–53.
28. Brixius K, Funcke F, Graf C, Bloch W. Endothelial progenitor cells: a new target for the prevention of cardiovascular diseases. Eur J Cardiovasc Prev Rehabil. 2006;13:705–10.
29. Jevon M, Dorling A, Hornick PI. Progenitor cells and vascular disease. Cell Prolif. 2008;41 Suppl 1:146–64.
30. Zampetaki A, Kirton JP, Xu Q. Vascular repair by endothelial progenitor cells. Cardiovasc Res. 2008;78:413–21.
31. Kumar AH, Caplice NM. Clinical potential of adult vascular progenitor cells. Arterioscler Thromb Vasc Biol. 2010;30:1080–7.
32. Becher MU, Nickenig G, Werner N. Regeneration of the vascular compartment. Herz. 2010;35:342–51.
33. De Val S, Black BL. Transcriptional control of endothelial cell development. Dev Cell. 2009;16:180–95.
34. Flamme I, von Reutern M, Drexler HC, Syed-Ali S, Risau W. Overexpression of vascular endothelial growth factor in the avian embryo induces hypervascularization and increased vascular permeability without alterations of embryonic pattern formation. Dev Biol. 1995;171:399–414.
35. Drake CJ. Embryonic and adult vasculogenesis. Birth Defects Res C Embryo Today. 2003;69:73–82.
36. Risau W, Sariola H, Zerwes HG, Sasse J, Ekblom P, Kemler R, et al. Vasculogenesis and angiogenesis in embryonic-stem-cell-derived embryoid bodies. Development. 1988;102:471–8.
37. Wang R, Clark R, Bautch VL. Embryonic stem cell-derived cystic embryoid bodies form vascular channels: an in vitro model of blood vessel development. Development. 1992;114:303–16.
38. Rongish BJ, Torry RJ, Tucker DC, Tomanek RJ. Neovascularization of embryonic rat hearts cultured in oculo closely mimics in utero coronary vessel development. J Vasc Res. 1994;31:206–15.
39. Tomanek RJ, Yue X, Zheng W. Vascular development of the heart. In: Tomanek RJ, editor. Assembly of the vasculature and its regulation. Boston: Birkhauser; 2002. p. 133–55.
40. Zeeb M, Strilic B, Lammert E. Resolving cell-cell junctions: lumen formation in blood vessels. Curr Opin Cell Biol. 2010;22:626–32.
41. Strilic B, Kucera T, Lammert E. Formation of cardiovascular tubes in invertebrates and vertebrates. Cell Mol Life Sci. 2010;67:3209–18.
42. Muller-Ehmsen J, Schmidt A, Krausgrill B, Schwinger RH, Bloch W. Role of erythropoietin for angiogenesis and vasculogenesis: from embryonic development through adulthood. Am J Physiol Heart Circ Physiol. 2006;290:H331–40.
43. Tsutsui M, Shimokawa H, Morishita T, Nakashima Y, Yanagihara N. Development of genetically engineered mice lacking all three nitric oxide synthases. J Pharmacol Sci. 2006;102:147–54.
44. Rossant J, Howard L. Signaling pathways in vascular development. Annu Rev Cell Dev Biol. 2002;18:541–73.
45. Shalaby F, Rossant J, Yamaguchi TP, Gertsenstein M, Wu XF, Breitman ML, et al. Failure of blood-island formation and vasculogenesis in Flk-1-deficient mice. Nature. 1995;376:62–6.
46. Takashima S, Kitakaze M, Asakura M, Asanuma H, Sanada S, Tashiro F, et al. Targeting of both mouse neuropilin-1 and neuropilin-2 genes severely impairs developmental yolk sac and embryonic angiogenesis. Proc Natl Acad Sci USA. 2002;99:3657–62.
47. Babaei S, Teichert-Kuliszewska K, Zhang Q, Jones N, Dumont DJ, Stewart DJ. Angiogenic actions of angiopoietin-1 require endothelium-derived nitric oxide. Am J Pathol. 2003;162:1927–36.
48. Yu J, deMuinck ED, Zhuang Z, Drinane M, Kauser K, Rubanyi GM, et al. Endothelial nitric oxide synthase is critical for ischemic

remodeling, mural cell recruitment, and blood flow reserve. Proc Natl Acad Sci USA. 2005;102:10999–1004.
49. Itoh N. The Fgf families in humans, mice, and zebrafish: their evolutional processes and roles in development, metabolism, and disease. Biol Pharm Bull. 2007;30:1819–25.
50. Murakami M, Nguyen LT, Zhuang ZW, Moodie KL, Carmeliet P, Stan RV, et al. The FGF system has a key role in regulating vascular integrity. J Clin Invest. 2008;118:3355–66.
51. Burger PE, Coetzee S, McKeehan WL, Kan M, Cook P, Fan Y, et al. Fibroblast growth factor receptor-1 is expressed by endothelial progenitor cells. Blood. 2002;100:3527–35.
52. Lee SH, Schloss DJ, Swain JL. Maintenance of vascular integrity in the embryo requires signaling through the fibroblast growth factor receptor. J Biol Chem. 2000;275:33679–87.
53. Presta M, Dell'Era P, Mitola S, Moroni E, Ronca R, Rusnati M. Fibroblast growth factor/fibroblast growth factor receptor system in angiogenesis. Cytokine Growth Factor Rev. 2005;16:159–78.
54. Cox CM, Poole TJ. Angioblast differentiation is influenced by the local environment: FGF-2 induces angioblasts and patterns vessel formation in the quail embryo. Dev Dyn. 2000;218:371–82.
55. Murakami M, Simons M. Fibroblast growth factor regulation of neovascularization. Curr Opin Hematol. 2008;15:215–20.
56. Cao R, Brakenhielm E, Pawliuk R, Wariaro D, Post MJ, Wahlberg E, et al. Angiogenic synergism, vascular stability and improvement of hind-limb ischemia by a combination of PDGF-BB and FGF-2. Nat Med. 2003;9:604–13.
57. Seghezzi G, Patel S, Ren CJ, Gualandris A, Pintucci G, Robbins ES, et al. Fibroblast growth factor-2 (FGF-2) induces vascular endothelial growth factor (VEGF) expression in the endothelial cells of forming capillaries: an autocrine mechanism contributing to angiogenesis. J Cell Biol. 1998;141:1659–73.
58. Kano MR, Morishita Y, Iwata C, Iwasaka S, Watabe T, Ouchi Y, et al. VEGF-A and FGF-2 synergistically promote neoangiogenesis through enhancement of endogenous PDGF-B-PDGFRbeta signaling. J Cell Sci. 2005;118:3759–68.
59. Morishita R, Ogihara T. Hepatocyte growth factor. In: Simons M, Rubanyi GM, editors. Modern concepts in angiogenesis. London: Imperial College Press; 2007. p. 367–84.
60. Thomas M, Augustin HG. The role of the angiopoietins in vascular morphogenesis. Angiogenesis. 2009;12:125–37.
61. Saharinen P, Eklund L, Miettinen J, Wirkkala R, Anisimov A, Winderlich M, et al. Angiopoietins assemble distinct Tie2 signalling complexes in endothelial cell-cell and cell-matrix contacts. Nat Cell Biol. 2008;10:527–37.
62. Pfaff D, Fiedler U, Augustin HG. Emerging roles of the Angiopoietin-Tie and the ephrin-Eph systems as regulators of cell trafficking. J Leukoc Biol. 2006;80:719–26.
63. Robson P, Pichla S, Zhou B, Baldwin HS. The role of cell adhesion receptors in vascular development. An overview. In: Tomanek RJ, editor. Assembly of the vasculature and its regulation. Boston: Birkhauser; 2002. p. 97–110.
64. Hodivala-Dilke KM, Reynolds AR, Reynolds LE. Integrins in angiogenesis: multitalented molecules in a balancing act. Cell Tissue Res. 2003;314:131–44.
65. Stupack DG, Cheresh DA. Integrins and angiogenesis. Curr Top Dev Biol. 2004;64:207–38.
66. Somanath PR, Ciocea A, Byzova TV. Integrin and growth factor receptor alliance in angiogenesis. Cell Biochem Biophys. 2009;53: 53–64.
67. Bressan M, Davis P, Timmer J, Herzlinger D, Mikawa T. Notochord-derived BMP antagonists inhibit endothelial cell generation and network formation. Dev Biol. 2009;326:101–11.
68. Reese DE, Hall CE, Mikawa T. Negative regulation of midline vascular development by the notochord. Dev Cell. 2004;6:699–708.
69. Park C, Afrikanova I, Chung YS, Zhang WJ, Arentson E, Fong Gh G, et al. A hierarchical order of factors in the generation of FLK1- and SCL-expressing hematopoietic and endothelial progenitors from embryonic stem cells. Development. 2004;131:2749–62.
70. Nimmagadda S, Geetha Loganathan P, Huang R, Scaal M, Schmidt C, Christ B. BMP4 and noggin control embryonic blood vessel formation by antagonistic regulation of VEGFR-2 (Quek1) expression. Dev Biol. 2005;280:100–10.
71. Eriksson K, Magnusson P, Dixelius J, Claesson-Welsh L, Cross MJ. Angiostatin and endostatin inhibit endothelial cell migration in response to FGF and VEGF without interfering with specific intracellular signal transduction pathways. FEBS Lett. 2003;536:19–24.
72. Troyanovsky B, Levchenko T, Mansson G, Matvijenko O, Holmgren L. Angiomotin: an angiostatin binding protein that regulates endothelial cell migration and tube formation. J Cell Biol. 2001;152:1247–54.
73. O'Reilly MS, Holmgren L, Chen C, Folkman J. Angiostatin induces and sustains dormancy of human primary tumors in mice. Nat Med. 1996;2:689–92.
74. Suri C, Yancopoulos GD. The ties that bind: emerging concepts about the structure and function of angiopoietins and their receptors in angiogenesis. In: Tomanek RJ, editor. Assembly of the vasculature and its regulation. Boston: Birkhauser; 2002. p. 55–66.
75. van Hinsbergh VW, Koolwijk P. Endothelial sprouting and angiogenesis: matrix metalloproteinases in the lead. Cardiovasc Res. 2008;78:203–12.
76. van Hinsbergh VW, Engelse MA, Quax PH. Pericellular proteases in angiogenesis and vasculogenesis. Arterioscler Thromb Vasc Biol. 2006;26:716–28.
77. Folkman J. Angiogenesis: initiation and control. Ann N Y Acad Sci. 1982;401:212–27.
78. Holderfield MT, Hughes CC. Crosstalk between vascular endothelial growth factor, notch, and transforming growth factor-beta in vascular morphogenesis. Circ Res. 2008;102:637–52.
79. Gerhardt H. VEGF and endothelial guidance in angiogenic sprouting. Organogenesis. 2008;4:241–6.
80. le Noble F, Klein C, Tintu A, Pries A, Buschmann I. Neural guidance molecules, tip cells, and mechanical factors in vascular development. Cardiovasc Res. 2008;78:232–41.
81. Phng LK, Gerhardt H. Angiogenesis: a team effort coordinated by notch. Dev Cell. 2009;16:196–208.
82. Hellstrom M, Phng LK, Hofmann JJ, Wallgard E, Coultas L, Lindblom P, et al. Dll4 signalling through Notch1 regulates formation of tip cells during angiogenesis. Nature. 2007;445:776–80.
83. Strasser GA, Kaminker JS, Tessier-Lavigne M. Microarray analysis of retinal endothelial tip cells identifies CXCR4 as a mediator of tip cell morphology and branching. Blood. 2010;115:5102–10.
84. Suchting S, Freitas C, le Noble F, Benedito R, Breant C, Duarte A, et al. The Notch ligand Delta-like 4 negatively regulates endothelial tip cell formation and vessel branching. Proc Natl Acad Sci USA. 2007;104:3225–30.
85. Franco CA, Li Z. SRF in angiogenesis: branching the vascular system. Cell Adh Migr. 2009;3:264–7.
86. Germain S, Monnot C, Muller L, Eichmann A. Hypoxia-driven angiogenesis: role of tip cells and extracellular matrix scaffolding. Curr Opin Hematol. 2010;17:245–51.
87. del Toro R, Prahst C, Mathivet T, Siegfried G, Kaminker JS, Larrivee B, et al. Identification and functional analysis of endothelial tip cell-enriched genes. Blood. 2010;116:4025–33.
88. Jakobsson L, Franco CA, Bentley K, Collins RT, Ponsioen B, Aspalter IM, et al. Endothelial cells dynamically compete for the tip cell position during angiogenic sprouting. Nat Cell Biol. 2010;12:943–53.
89. Sakurai A, Gavard J, Annas-Linhares Y, Basile JR, Amornphimoltham P, Palmby TR, et al. Semaphorin 3E initiates antiangiogenic signaling through plexin D1 by regulating Arf6 and R-Ras. Mol Cell Biol. 2010;30:3086–98.

90. Lee CY, Bautch VL. Ups and downs of guided vessel sprouting: the role of polarity. Physiology (Bethesda). 2011;26:326–33.
91. Lamalice L, Le Boeuf F, Huot J. Endothelial cell migration during angiogenesis. Circ Res. 2007;100:782–94.
92. Djonov V, Makanya AN. New insights into intussusceptive angiogenesis. In: Class M, Breier G, editors. Mechanisms of angiogenesis. Switzerland: Birkhauser Verlag; 2005. p. 17–33.
93. Burri PH, Hlushchuk R, Djonov V. Intussusceptive angiogenesis: its emergence, its characteristics, and its significance. Dev Dyn. 2004;231:474–88.
94. Drake CJ, Little CD. VEGF and vascular fusion: implications for normal and pathological vessels. J Histochem Cytochem. 1999; 47:1351–6.
95. LaRue AC, Mironov VA, Argraves WS, Czirok A, Fleming PA, Drake CJ. Patterning of embryonic blood vessels. Dev Dyn. 2003;228:21–9.
96. Dumont DJ, Gradwohl G, Fong GH, Puri MC, Gertsenstein M, Auerbach A, et al. Dominant-negative and targeted null mutations in the endothelial receptor tyrosine kinase, tek, reveal a critical role in vasculogenesis of the embryo. Genes Dev. 1994;8:1897–909.
97. Gaengel K, Genove G, Armulik A, Betsholtz C. Endothelial-mural cell signaling in vascular development and angiogenesis. Arterioscler Thromb Vasc Biol. 2009;29:630–8.
98. Lindahl P, Johansson BR, Leveen P, Betsholtz C. Pericyte loss and microaneurysm formation in PDGF-B-deficient mice. Science. 1997;277:242–5.
99. Sato Y, Rifkin DB. Inhibition of endothelial cell movement by pericytes and smooth muscle cells: activation of a latent transforming growth factor-beta 1-like molecule by plasmin during co-culture. J Cell Biol. 1989;109:309–15.
100. Mandriota SJ, Menoud PA, Pepper MS. Transforming growth factor beta 1 down-regulates vascular endothelial growth factor receptor 2/flk-1 expression in vascular endothelial cells. J Biol Chem. 1996;271:11500–5.
101. Motiejunaite R, Kazlauskas A. Pericytes and ocular diseases. Exp Eye Res. 2008;86:171–7.
102. Silva R, D'Amico G, Hodivala-Dilke KM, Reynolds LE. Integrins: the keys to unlocking angiogenesis. Arterioscler Thromb Vasc Biol. 2008;28:1703–13.
103. Somanath PR, Malinin NL, Byzova TV. Cooperation between integrin alphavbeta3 and VEGFR2 in angiogenesis. Angiogenesis. 2009;12:177–85.
104. Majesky MW, Dong XR, Lu J. Development and differentiation of vascular smooth muscle. In: Tomanek RJ, editor. Assembly of the vasculature and its regulation. Boston: Birkhauser; 2002. p. 111–31.
105. Majesky MW. Development of coronary vessels. Curr Top Dev Biol. 2004;62:225–59.
106. Owens GK, Kumar MS, Wamhoff BR. Molecular regulation of vascular smooth muscle cell differentiation in development and disease. Physiol Rev. 2004;84:767–801.
107. Kawai-Kowase K, Owens GK. Multiple repressor pathways contribute to phenotypic switching of vascular smooth muscle cells. Am J Physiol Cell Physiol. 2007;292:C59–69.
108. Mack CP. Signaling mechanisms that regulate smooth muscle cell differentiation. Arterioscler Thromb Vasc Biol. 2011;31:1495–505.
109. Gerthoffer WT. Mechanisms of vascular smooth muscle cell migration. Circ Res. 2007;100:607–21.
110. Chen J, Kitchen CM, Streb JW, Miano JM. Myocardin: a component of a molecular switch for smooth muscle differentiation. J Mol Cell Cardiol. 2002;34:1345–56.
111. McDonald OG, Owens GK. Programming smooth muscle plasticity with chromatin dynamics. Circ Res. 2007;100:1428–41.
112. Wang D, Chang PS, Wang Z, Sutherland L, Richardson JA, Small E, et al. Activation of cardiac gene expression by myocardin, a transcriptional cofactor for serum response factor. Cell. 2001;105: 851–62.
113. Wang DZ, Olson EN. Control of smooth muscle development by the myocardin family of transcriptional coactivators. Curr Opin Genet Dev. 2004;14:558–66.
114. Bertolino P, Deckers M, Lebrin F, ten Dijke P. Transforming growth factor-beta signal transduction in angiogenesis and vascular disorders. Chest. 2005;128:585S–90.
115. Bobik A. Transforming growth factor-betas and vascular disorders. Arterioscler Thromb Vasc Biol. 2006;26:1712–20.
116. Jain RK. Molecular regulation of vessel maturation. Nat Med. 2003;9:685–93.
117. Sinha S, Hoofnagle MH, Kingston PA, McCanna ME, Owens GK. Transforming growth factor-beta1 signaling contributes to development of smooth muscle cells from embryonic stem cells. Am J Physiol Cell Physiol. 2004;287:C1560–8.
118. Mancini ML, Terzic A, Conley BA, Oxburgh LH, Nicola T, Vary CP. Endoglin plays distinct roles in vascular smooth muscle cell recruitment and regulation of arteriovenous identity during angiogenesis. Dev Dyn. 2009;238:2479–93.
119. Betsholtz C. Insight into the physiological functions of PDGF through genetic studies in mice. Cytokine Growth Factor Rev. 2004;15:215–28.
120. Armulik A, Abramsson A, Betsholtz C. Endothelial/pericyte interactions. Circ Res. 2005;97:512–23.
121. Hoch RV, Soriano P. Roles of PDGF in animal development. Development. 2003;130:4769–84.
122. Liu H, Zhang W, Kennard S, Caldwell RB, Lilly B. Notch3 is critical for proper angiogenesis and mural cell investment. Circul Res. 2010;107:860–70.
123. Liu H, Kennard S, Lilly B. NOTCH3 expression is induced in mural cells through an autoregulatory loop that requires endothelial-expressed JAGGED1. Circul Res. 2009;104:466–75.
124. Hellstrom M, Gerhardt H, Kalen M, Li X, Eriksson U, Wolburg H, et al. Lack of pericytes leads to endothelial hyperplasia and abnormal vascular morphogenesis. J Cell Biol. 2001;153:543–53.
125. Uemura A, Ogawa M, Hirashima M, Fujiwara T, Koyama S, Takagi H, et al. Recombinant angiopoietin-1 restores higher-order architecture of growing blood vessels in mice in the absence of mural cells. J Clin Invest. 2002;110:1619–28.
126. Yamamoto Y, Craggs L, Baumann M, Kalimo H, Kalaria RN. Review: molecular genetics and pathology of hereditary small vessel diseases of the brain. Neuropathol Appl Neurobiol. 2011;37:94–113.
127. Joutel A. Pathogenesis of CADASIL: transgenic and knock-out mice to probe function and dysfunction of the mutated gene, Notch3, in the cerebrovasculature. Bioessays. 2011;33:73–80.
128. Swift MR, Weinstein BM. Arterial-venous specification during development. Circ Res. 2009;104:576–88.
129. Kume T. Specification of arterial, venous, and lymphatic endothelial cells during embryonic development. Histol Histopathol. 2010;25:637–46.
130. dela Paz NG, D'Amore PA. Arterial versus venous endothelial cells. Cell Tissue Res. 2009;335:5–16.
131. Lin FJ, Tsai MJ, Tsai SY. Artery and vein formation: a tug of war between different forces. EMBO Rep. 2007;8:920–4.
132. Rocha SF, Adams RH. Molecular differentiation and specialization of vascular beds. Angiogenesis. 2009;12:139–47.
133. Hong CC, Peterson QP, Hong JY, Peterson RT. Artery/vein specification is governed by opposing phosphatidylinositol-3 kinase and MAP kinase/ERK signaling. Curr Biol. 2006;16:1366–72.
134. Eichmann A, Yuan L, Moyon D, Lenoble F, Pardanaud L, Breant C. Vascular development: from precursor cells to branched arterial and venous networks. Int J Dev Biol. 2005;49:259–67.
135. Zhong TP, Childs S, Leu JP, Fishman MC. Gridlock signalling pathway fashions the first embryonic artery. Nature. 2001;414: 216–20.
136. Pasquale EB. Eph receptor signalling casts a wide net on cell behaviour. Nat Rev Mol Cell Biol. 2005;6:462–75.

137. Aitsebaomo J, Portbury AL, Schisler JC, Patterson C. Brothers and sisters: molecular insights into arterial-venous heterogeneity. Circ Res. 2008;103:929–39.
138. Villa N, Walker L, Lindsell CE, Gasson J, Iruela-Arispe ML, Weinmaster G. Vascular expression of Notch pathway receptors and ligands is restricted to arterial vessels. Mech Dev. 2001;108:161–4.
139. Gale NW, Dominguez MG, Noguera I, Pan L, Hughes V, Valenzuela DM, et al. Haploinsufficiency of delta-like 4 ligand results in embryonic lethality due to major defects in arterial and vascular development. Proc Natl Acad Sci USA. 2004;101:15949–54.
140. Xue Y, Gao X, Lindsell CE, Norton CR, Chang B, Hicks C, et al. Embryonic lethality and vascular defects in mice lacking the Notch ligand Jagged1. Hum Mol Genet. 1999;8:723–30.
141. You LR, Lin FJ, Lee CT, DeMayo FJ, Tsai MJ, Tsai SY. Suppression of Notch signalling by the COUP-TFII transcription factor regulates vein identity. Nature. 2005;435:98–104.
142. Seo S, Fujita H, Nakano A, Kang M, Duarte A, Kume T. The forkhead transcription factors, Foxc1 and Foxc2, are required for arterial specification and lymphatic sprouting during vascular development. Dev Biol. 2006;294:458–70.
143. Wigle JT, Oliver G. Prox1 function is required for the development of the murine lymphatic system. Cell. 1999;98:769–78.
144. Wilting J, Neeff H, Christ B. Embryonic lymphangiogenesis. Cell Tissue Res. 1999;297:1–11.
145. Francois M, Harvey NL, Hogan BM. The transcriptional control of lymphatic vascular development. Physiology (Bethesda). 2011;26:146–55.
146. Atkins GB, Jain MK, Hamik A. Endothelial differentiation: molecular mechanisms of specification and heterogeneity. Arterioscler Thromb Vasc Biol. 2011;31:1476–84.
147. Abtahian F, Guerriero A, Sebzda E, Lu MM, Zhou R, Mocsai A, et al. Regulation of blood and lymphatic vascular separation by signaling proteins SLP-76 and Syk. Science. 2003;299:247–51.
148. Herbert SP, Huisken J, Kim TN, Feldman ME, Houseman BT, Wang RA, et al. Arterial-venous segregation by selective cell sprouting: an alternative mode of blood vessel formation. Science. 2009;326:294–8.
149. Moyon D, Pardanaud L, Yuan L, Breant C, Eichmann A. Plasticity of endothelial cells during arterial-venous differentiation in the avian embryo. Development. 2001;128:3359–70.
150. le Noble F, Moyon D, Pardanaud L, Yuan L, Djonov V, Matthijsen R, et al. Flow regulates arterial-venous differentiation in the chick embryo yolk sac. Development. 2004;131:361–75.
151. Nguyen TH, Eichmann A, Le Noble F, Fleury V. Dynamics of vascular branching morphogenesis: the effect of blood and tissue flow. Phys Rev E Stat Nonlin Soft Matter Phys. 2006;73:061907.
152. Jones EA. Mechanical factors in the development of the vascular bed. Respir Physiol Neurobiol. 2011;178(1):59–65.
153. Kim YH, Hu H, Guevara-Gallardo S, Lam MT, Fong SY, Wang RA. Artery and vein size is balanced by Notch and ephrin B2/EphB4 during angiogenesis. Development. 2008;135:3755–64.
154. Martinez-Lemus LA, Hill MA, Meininger GA. The plastic nature of the vascular wall: a continuum of remodeling events contributing to control of arteriolar diameter and structure. Physiology (Bethesda). 2009;24:45–57.
155. Gibbons GH, Dzau VJ. Mechanisms of disease: the emerging concept of vascular remodeling. N Engl J Med. 1994;330:1431–8.
156. Langille BL. Arterial remodeling: relation to hemodynamics. Can J Physiol Pharmacol. 1996;74:834–41.
157. Thoma R. Untersuchungren Über die Histogenese und histomechanik des Gefässytems. Enkverlag, Stuttgart. 1893
158. Clark ER. Studies on the growth of blood-vessels in the tail of the frog larva: observation and experiment on the living animal. Am J Anat. 1918;23:37–88.
159. Gerrity RG, Cliff WJ. The aortic tunica media of the developing rat. I. Quantitative stereologic and biochemical analysis. Lab Invest. 1975;32:585–600.
160. McGrath JC, Deighan C, Briones AM, Shafaroudi MM, McBride M, Adler J, et al. New aspects of vascular remodelling: the involvement of all vascular cell types. Exp Physiol. 2005;90:469–75.
161. Guyton JR, Hartley CJ. Flow restriction of one carotid artery in juvenile rats inhibits growth of arterial diameter. Am J Physiol. 1985;248:H540–6.
162. Zhang H, Sunnarborg SW, McNaughton KK, Johns TG, Lee DC, Faber JE. Heparin-binding epidermal growth factor-like growth factor signaling in flow-induced arterial remodeling. Circ Res. 2008;102:1275–85.
163. Sho E, Komatsu M, Sho M, Nanjo H, Singh TM, Xu C, et al. High flow drives vascular endothelial cell proliferation during flow-induced arterial remodeling associated with the expression of vascular endothelial growth factor. Exp Mol Pathol. 2003;75:1–11.
164. Korshunov VA, Berk BC. Flow-induced vascular remodeling in the mouse: a model for carotid intima-media thickening. Arterioscler Thromb Vasc Biol. 2003;23:2185–91.
165. Langille BL, O'Donnell F. Reductions in arterial diameter produced by chronic decreases in blood flow are endothelium-dependent. Science. 1986;231:405–7.
166. Folkow B, Hallback M, Lundgren Y, Sivertsson R, Weiss L. Importance of adaptive changes in vascular design for establishment of primary hypertension, studied in man and in spontaneously hypertensive rats. Circ Res. 1973;32 Suppl 1:2–16.
167. Prewitt RL, Rice DC, Dobrian AD. Adaptation of resistance arteries to increases in pressure. Microcirculation. 2002;9:295–304.
168. Wang DH, Prewitt RL. Alterations of mature arterioles associated with chronically reduced blood flow. Am J Physiol. 1993;264: H40–4.
169. Intengan HD, Schiffrin EL. Vascular remodeling in hypertension: roles of apoptosis, inflammation, and fibrosis. Hypertension. 2001;38:581–7.
170. Cho A, Mitchell L, Koopmans D, Langille BL. Effects of changes in blood flow rate on cell death and cell proliferation in carotid arteries of immature rabbits. Circ Res. 1997;81:328–37.
171. Kumar A, Lindner V. Remodeling with neointima formation in the mouse carotid artery after cessation of blood flow. Arterioscler Thromb Vasc Biol. 1997;17:2238–44.
172. Korshunov VA, Berk BC. Smooth muscle apoptosis and vascular remodeling. Curr Opin Hematol. 2008;15:250–4.
173. Jones EA, le Noble F, Eichmann A. What determines blood vessel structure? Genetic prespecification vs. hemodynamics. Physiology (Bethesda). 2006;21:388–95.
174. Hudlicka O, Brown M. Physical forces and angiogenesis. In: Rubanyi GM, editor. Mechanoreception by the vascular wall. Mount Kisko: Futura Publishing Co; 1993. p. 197–241.
175. Shyy JY, Chien S. Role of integrins in endothelial mechanosensing of shear stress. Circ Res. 2002;91:769–75.
176. Li YS, Haga JH, Chien S. Molecular basis of the effects of shear stress on vascular endothelial cells. J Biomech. 2005;38:1949–71.
177. Eitenmuller I, Volger O, Kluge A, Troidl K, Barancik M, Cai WJ, et al. The range of adaptation by collateral vessels after femoral artery occlusion. Circ Res. 2006;99:656–62.
178. Lehoux S. Redox signalling in vascular responses to shear and stretch. Cardiovasc Res. 2006;71:269–79.
179. Davies PF, Tripathi SC. Mechanical stress mechanisms and the cell. An endothelial paradigm. Circ Res. 1993;72:239–45.
180. Ingber DE, Tensegrity I. Cell structure and hierarchical systems biology. J Cell Sci. 2003;116:1157–73.
181. Davies PF. Hemodynamic shear stress and the endothelium in cardiovascular pathophysiology. Nat Clin Pract Cardiovasc Med. 2009;6:16–26.
182. Wang Y, Miao H, Li S, Chen KD, Li YS, Yuan S, et al. Interplay between integrins and FLK-1 in shear stress-induced signaling. Am J Physiol Cell Physiol. 2002;283:C1540–7.
183. Gloe T, Sohn HY, Meininger GA, Pohl U. Shear stress-induced release of basic fibroblast growth factor from endothelial cells is

mediated by matrix interaction via integrin alpha(v)beta3. J Biol Chem. 2002;277:23453–8.
184. Helmke BP. Molecular control of cytoskeletal mechanics by hemodynamic forces. Physiology (Bethesda). 2005;20:43–53.
185. Sachs F. Stretch-activated ion channels: what are they? Physiology (Bethesda). 2010;25:50–6.
186. Birukov KG. Cyclic stretch, reactive oxygen species, and vascular remodeling. Antioxid Redox Signal. 2009;11:1651–67.
187. Davies PF, Remuzzi A, Gordon EJ, Dewey Jr CF, Gimbrone Jr MA. Turbulent fluid shear stress induces vascular endothelial cell turnover in vitro. Proc Natl Acad Sci USA. 1986;83:2114–7.
188. Huttner I, Gabbiani G. Vascular endothelium: recent advances and unanswered questions. Lab Invest. 1982;47:409–11.
189. Mammoto A, Mammoto T, Ingber DE. Rho signaling and mechanical control of vascular development. Curr Opin Hematol. 2008; 15:228–34.
190. Chang H, Wang BW, Kuan P, Shyu KG. Cyclical mechanical stretch enhances angiopoietin-2 and Tie2 receptor expression in cultured human umbilical vein endothelial cells. Clin Sci (Lond). 2003;104:421–8.
191. Zheng W, Christensen LP, Tomanek RJ. Differential effects of cyclic and static stretch on coronary microvascular endothelial cell receptors and vasculogenic/angiogenic responses. Am J Physiol Heart Circ Physiol. 2008;295:H794–800.
192. Zheng W, Christensen LP, Tomanek RJ. Stretch induces upregulation of key tyrosine kinase receptors in microvascular endothelial cells. Am J Physiol Heart Circ Physiol. 2004;287:H2739–45.
193. Lee HJ, Koh GY. Shear stress activates Tie2 receptor tyrosine kinase in human endothelial cells. Biochem Biophys Res Commun. 2003;304:399–404.
194. Sumpio BE, Banes AJ, Levin LG, Johnson Jr G. Mechanical stress stimulates aortic endothelial cells to proliferate. J Vasc Surg. 1987;6:252–6.
195. Hume WR. Proline and thymidine uptake in rabbit ear artery segments in vitro increased by chronic tangential load. Hypertension. 1980;2:738–43.
196. Folkman J, Greenspan HP. Influence of geometry on control of cell growth. Biochim Biophys Acta. 1975;417:211–36.
197. Cullen JP, Sayeed S, Sawai RS, Theodorakis NG, Cahill PA, Sitzmann JV, et al. Pulsatile flow-induced angiogenesis: role of G(i) subunits. Arterioscler Thromb Vasc Biol. 2002;22:1610–6.
198. Malek AM, Gibbons GH, Dzau VJ, Izumo S. Fluid shear stress differentially modulates expression of genes encoding basic fibroblast growth factor and platelet-derived growth factor B chain in vascular endothelium. J Clin Invest. 1993;92:2013–21.
199. Gan L, Miocic M, Doroudi R, Selin-Sjogren L, Jern S. Distinct regulation of vascular endothelial growth factor in intact human conduit vessels exposed to laminar fluid shear stress and pressure. Biochem Biophys Res Commun. 2000;272:490–6.
200. Dimmeler S, Haendeler J, Rippmann V, Nehls M, Zeiher AM. Shear stress inhibits apoptosis of human endothelial cells. FEBS Lett. 1996;399:71–4.
201. Bevan RD, van Marthens E, Bevan JA. Hyperplasia of vascular smooth muscle in experimental hypertension in the rabbit. Circ Res. 1976;38:58–62.
202. Haudenschild CC, Grunwald J, Chobanian AV. Effects of hypertension on migration and proliferation of smooth muscle in culture. Hypertension. 1985;7:I101–4.
203. Liu SQ. Focal expression of angiotensin II type 1 receptor and smooth muscle cell proliferation in the neointima of experimental vein grafts: relation to eddy blood flow. Arterioscler Thromb Vasc Biol. 1999;19:2630–9.
204. Cheng G, Wessels A, Gourdie RG, Thompson RP. Spatiotemporal and tissue specific distribution of apoptosis in the developing chick heart. Dev Dyn. 2002;223:119–33.
205. Demicheva E, Hecker M, Korff T. Stretch-induced activation of the transcription factor activator protein-1 controls monocyte chemoattractant protein-1 expression during arteriogenesis. Circ Res. 2008;103:477–84.
206. Ito WD, Arras M, Scholz D, Winkler B, Htun P, Schaper W. Angiogenesis but not collateral growth is associated with ischemia after femoral artery occlusion. Am J Physiol. 1997;273: H1255–65.
207. Gimbrone Jr MA, Anderson KR, Topper JN, Langille BL, Clowes AW, Bercel S, et al. Special communicationthe critical role of mechanical forces in blood vessel development, physiology and pathology. J Vasc Surg. 1999;29:1104–51.
208. Yamamoto K, Sokabe T, Watabe T, Miyazono K, Yamashita JK, Obi S, et al. Fluid shear stress induces differentiation of Flk-1-positive embryonic stem cells into vascular endothelial cells in vitro. Am J Physiol Heart Circ Physiol. 2005;288: H1915–24.
209. Semenza GL. Regulation of oxygen homeostasis by hypoxia-inducible factor 1. Physiology (Bethesda). 2009;24:97–106.
210. Manalo DJ, Rowan A, Lavoie T, Natarajan L, Kelly BD, Ye SQ, et al. Transcriptional regulation of vascular endothelial cell responses to hypoxia by HIF-1. Blood. 2005;105:659–69.
211. Fong GH. Mechanisms of adaptive angiogenesis to tissue hypoxia. Angiogenesis. 2008;11:121–40.
212. Namiki A, Brogi E, Kearney M, Kim EA, Wu T, Couffinhal T, et al. Hypoxia induces vascular endothelial growth factor in cultured human endothelial cells. J Biol Chem. 1995;270: 31189–95.
213. Murohara T, Witzenbichler B, Spyridopoulos I, Asahara T, Ding B, Sullivan A, et al. Role of endothelial nitric oxide synthase in endothelial cell migration. Arterioscler Thromb Vasc Biol. 1999; 19:1156–61.
214. Phillips PG, Birnby LM, Narendran A. Hypoxia induces capillary network formation in cultured bovine pulmonary microvessel endothelial cells. Am J Physiol. 1995;268:L789–800.
215. Stempien-Otero A, Karsan A, Cornejo CJ, Xiang H, Eunson T, Morrison RS, et al. Mechanisms of hypoxia-induced endothelial cell death. Role of p53 in apoptosis. J Biol Chem. 1999;274: 8039–45.
216. Covello KL, Simon MC. HIFs, hypoxia, and vascular development. Curr Top Dev Biol. 2004;62:37–54.
217. Sheares KK, Jeffery TK, Long L, Yang X, Morrell NW. Differential effects of TGF-beta1 and BMP-4 on the hypoxic induction of cyclooxygenase-2 in human pulmonary artery smooth muscle cells. Am J Physiol Lung Cell Mol Physiol. 2004;287:L919–27.
218. Corley KM, Taylor CJ, Lilly B. Hypoxia-inducible factor 1alpha modulates adhesion, migration, and FAK phosphorylation in vascular smooth muscle cells. J Cell Biochem. 2005;96:971–85.
219. Sunderkotter C, Goebeler M, Schulze-Osthoff K, Bhardwaj R, Sorg C. Macrophage-derived angiogenesis factors. Pharmacol Ther. 1991;51:195–216.
220. Lee YM, Jeong CH, Koo SY, Son MJ, Song HS, Bae SK, et al. Determination of hypoxic region by hypoxia marker in developing mouse embryos in vivo: a possible signal for vessel development. Dev Dyn. 2001;220:175–86.
221. Nanka O, Valasek P, Dvorakova M, Grim M. Experimental hypoxia and embryonic angiogenesis. Dev Dyn. 2006;235:723–33.
222. Maltepe E, Schmidt JV, Baunoch D, Bradfield CA, Simon MC. Abnormal angiogenesis and responses to glucose and oxygen deprivation in mice lacking the protein ARNT. Nature. 1997; 386:403–7.
223. Ryan HE, Lo J, Johnson RS. HIF-1 alpha is required for solid tumor formation and embryonic vascularization. Embo J. 1998;17:3005–15.
224. Nanka O, Krizova P, Fikrle M, Tuma M, Blaha M, Grim M, et al. Abnormal myocardial and coronary vasculature development in experimental hypoxia. Anat Rec (Hoboken). 2008;291:1187–99.
225. Murakami M, Simons M. Regulation of vascular integrity. J Mol Med. 2009;87:571–82.

226. Dejana E, Tournier-Lasserve E, Weinstein BM. The control of vascular integrity by endothelial cell junctions: molecular basis and pathological implications. Dev Cell. 2009;16:209–21.
227. Dejana E. Endothelial cell-cell junctions: happy together. Nat Rev Mol Cell Biol. 2004;5:261–70.
228. Taddei A, Giampietro C, Conti A, Orsenigo F, Breviario F, Pirazzoli V, et al. Endothelial adherens junctions control tight junctions by VE-cadherin-mediated upregulation of claudin-5. Nat Cell Biol. 2008;10:923–34.
229. Lohler J, Timpl R, Jaenisch R. Embryonic lethal mutation in mouse collagen I gene causes rupture of blood vessels and is associated with erythropoietic and mesenchymal cell death. Cell. 1984;38:597–607.
230. Liu X, Wu H, Byrne M, Krane S, Jaenisch R. Type III collagen is crucial for collagen I fibrillogenesis and for normal cardiovascular development. Proc Natl Acad Sci USA. 1997;94:1852–6.
231. Kivirikko KI. Collagens and their abnormalities in a wide spectrum of diseases. Ann Med. 1993;25:113–26.
232. Bjarnegard M, Enge M, Norlin J, Gustafsdottir S, Fredriksson S, Abramsson A, et al. Endothelium-specific ablation of PDGFB leads to pericyte loss and glomerular, cardiac and placental abnormalities. Development. 2004;131:1847–57.

Prenatal Coronary Morphogenesis

2

Abbreviations

BMP	Bone morphogenic protein
EC	Endothelial cells
ECM	Extracellular matrix
EMT	Epithelial–mesenchymal-transition
EPDCs	Epithelial progenitor derived cells
FGF	Fibroblast growth factor
HH	Hamburger–Hamilton stages (chick development)
PDGF	Platelet-derived growth factor
PE	Proepicardium
TGF-β	Transforming growth factor-β
VEGF	Vascular endothelial growth factor
VSMC	Vascular smooth muscle cell
Wt-1	Wilm's tumor gene

Introduction

The coronary vasculature is formed by precursor cells that (1) originate outside the heart; (2) migrate to form the epicardium and subepicardium; (3) differentiate into endothelial cells, smooth muscle, and fibroblasts; and (4) migrate and assemble into vascular structures. This is an elaborate process involving vasculogenesis, angiogenesis, and arteriogenesis. Since the heart chambers are initially thin-walled, consisting primarily of a trabecular network of cardiomyocytes, O_2 diffusion from the chamber lumens is sufficient. However, the thickening of the compact regions makes this diffusion inadequate and sets into motion a cascade of events that facilitate the formation of a coronary vasculature. The initial set of vascular channels consists of endothelial-lined tubes that are not yet perfused because they lack connections to the aorta. Part of this network penetrates the root of the aorta just above the left and right cusps, establishing a functional coronary circulation. This event is followed by the development of larger coronary vessels. This chapter addresses these events and the factors that precipitate and regulate coronary vessel development.

Proepicardium

The generally accepted assumption that the progenitor cells of the coronary vasculature were derived from cardiac mesoderm was shown to be false nearly a half century ago by Manasek [1]. This assumption had already been challenged by His in 1885 [2], and later by Kurkiewicz [3], who noted that the pericardial mesothelium, known as pericardial villi, was the source of epicardial cells. A transient, grape-like cluster of cells called proepicardium (PE) develops from splanchnic mesoderm that is the source of the proepicardium, which in turn generates cells that form the epicardium and subepicardium, and subsequently, the coronary vasculature (Fig. 2.1). As described in mouse and rat [4–10], cells from the pericardial surface of the septum transversum form multicellular villi which reach the dorsal surface of the heart where they detach and adhere to the myocardium. Most of these studies, as well as one on the tree shrew [11], noted free floating vesicles that detach from the villi. The motion of the heart pulling on the vesicles when they attach has been proposed as the mechanism for their detachment [8]. In avian embryos, which have been extensively studied, the proepicardium forms at the ventral wall of the sinus venosum [1, 12, 13]. A simple cuboidal mesothelium with microvilli covers an extracellular matrix (ECM) core and forms villi that project as outgrowths [6, 14, 15]. The ECM core contains mesenchymal cells [16]. The villi project a bridge to the right atrioventricular myocardium, which contains an ECM of heparin sulfate and fibronectin between the proepicardial cells and the myocardium [16]. The tips of the villi adhere to the dorsal wall of the atrioventricular canal and proepicardial cells spread over the surface of the heart, forming a monolayer cover.

Origin of Proepicardium

The proepicardium is thought to arise from the lateral margins of the heart fields because it develops next to the sinus

R.J. Tomanek, *Coronary Vasculature: Development, Structure-Function, and Adaptations*,
DOI 10.1007/978-1-4614-4887-7_2, © Springer Science+Business Media New York 2013

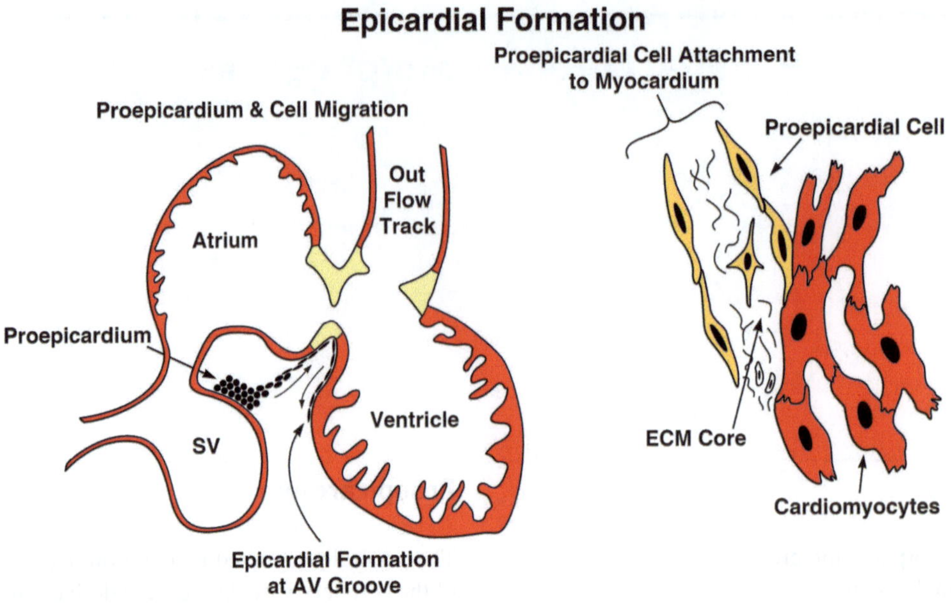

Fig. 2.1 Epicardial formation. In avians, proepicardial cells migrate from the ventral surface of the sinus venosus (SV) into the AV groove and then along the surface of the heart (*left illustration*). The proepicardial cells form multiple villi with an extracellular matrix (ECM) core containing mesenchymal cells (*right illustration*). In mice, the proepicardium is inferior to the sinus venosus and adjacent to the liver bud.

venosus in the peripheral mesoderm [17]. Mesoderm overlying the liver bud endoderm has been documented as a source of proepicardial cells, suggesting a role for the liver as an inducer of the proepicardium [18]. The influence appears to be reciprocal in that the mesoderm acts as an inducer for hepatic cell differentiation and liver bud formation. In avians, the proepicardium develops on the wall of the sinus venosus, as seen in Fig. 2.1 [19]. In mouse embryos, the proepicardium is located on the pericardial surface of the septum transversum adjacent to the liver bud [20]. The role of proepicardium as a cell source for the epicardium and the coronary vasculature has been documented in a variety of vertebrates, a finding that suggests that this entity has been conserved through evolution. In addition to the studies on birds [13, 15, 21–23] and mammals [6–8, 24, 25], the proepicardium and epicardium have been studied in fish [10, 26, 27] and amphibians [28, 29]. The proepicardium consists of bilateral primordia. In avians, the right side persists while the left side regresses; whereas in mice, both primordia develop [30]. A key study documenting the proepicardium as the cell source of coronary vessels used replication-defective retrovirus expressing β-galactosidase injected into embryonic chick hearts [31]. Retroviral injections revealed that endothelial and smooth muscle cells first entered the heart at Stage 17, substantially after the myocardium has developed contractions. Subsequently, it was shown that the proepicardium includes a lineage of smooth muscle progenitor cells that migrate to the epicardium [32].

Specification of Proepicardial Cells

More recently, questions regarding the induction and specification of the proepicardium in the mesoderm have been addressed [33]. Induction of the proepicardial marker genes Wt-1 (Wilm's Tumor gene), capsulin, and Tbx18 in chick mesothelial cells was shown, both in vitro and in vivo, to be a function of the liver and did not occur until (Hamburger–Hamilton) HH stage 12 (about 15 somites). Thus, this induction involves paracrine signaling at a specific developmental stage. The Wt-1 positive epicardial progenitor cells appear to originate from precursors that express transcription factors Isl1 and NKX2-5, which are required for the normal development of the proepicardium [34]. Capsulin, a transcription factor also called epicardin, is expressed in the septum transversum mesenchyme, then in the proepicardium, and subsequently, in the epicardium [35]. GATA-4 [36], α4-integrin [37, 38], and BMP4 [39] are also expressed in proepicardial cells and are required for epicardial formation.

In the chick, bone morphogenic protein 4 (BMP4) appears in the right sinus horn and then in the proepicardium, whereas BMP2 occurs in the sinus venosus [39]. Ishii et al. [40] showed that proepicardial explants migrate toward the cocultured myocardium and that this preferential direction can be mimicked by BMP2/4 and inhibited by Noggin. Differentiation into epicardial and myocardial lineages is mediated by BMP-2 and fibroblast growth factor-2 (FGF-2) signaling [41]. FGF-2 stimulates differentiation into the epicardial lineage, whereas coexpression of BMP-2 and FGF-2 inhibits differentiation into both myocardium and epicardium. FGF ligands maintain proliferation and prevent apoptosis of proepicardial cells [42].

Epicardium

Proepicardial Migration and Epicardial Formation

As illustrated in Fig. 2.1, proepicardial (PE) cells in both avians and mammals reach the dorsal surface of the heart, proliferate, and spread over the rest of the myocardial surface [4, 22, 43–45]. Their attachment to the myocardium, via an extracellular bridge in the multicellular villous projections of the proepicardium that reach the posterior myocardial surface at the atrioventricular junction, has been shown to be similar in both mammal and avian models [16, 25]. This conclusion was based on serial section reconstructions, electron microscopy, and immunofluorescence. Upon proepicardial attachment, the proteoglycan-rich extracellular bridge lies between the epicardium and myocardium. Based on experiments with chimeric chick embryos and quail PE transplants, the inner curvature of the heart has been shown to be selectively permissive for the penetration of endothelial progenitor cells [46]. These mesothelial cells express cytokeratins, a distinguishing marker for epithelial cells [43]. The epicardial cells undergo a spatiotemporal migration over the surface of the heart in avian, amphibian, and mammalian species. They spread radially to the right and left from the AV sulcus, then cranially, caudally to the atria [5]. Epicardial formation is complete at embryonic (E) day 10.5 in mice [47], E13.5 in rats [25], and HH23 in chick [15]. Subsequently, the proepicardium disappears and the epicardium undergoes epithelial–mesenchymal transition (EMT). Thus, the fate of these epicardial (mesothelial) cells is to differentiate into coronary smooth muscle cells, fibroblasts, endothelial cells, and atrioventricular cushion mesenchyme, or remain in an undifferentiated state in the subepicardium [48].

Regulation of Epicardial Formation (Fig. 2.2)

As already discussed, proepicardial cells require a number of genes to migrate and form an epicardium. Coupling of proepicardial cells on the surface of the myocardium requires the gap junction protein connexin 43 (Cx43), since its

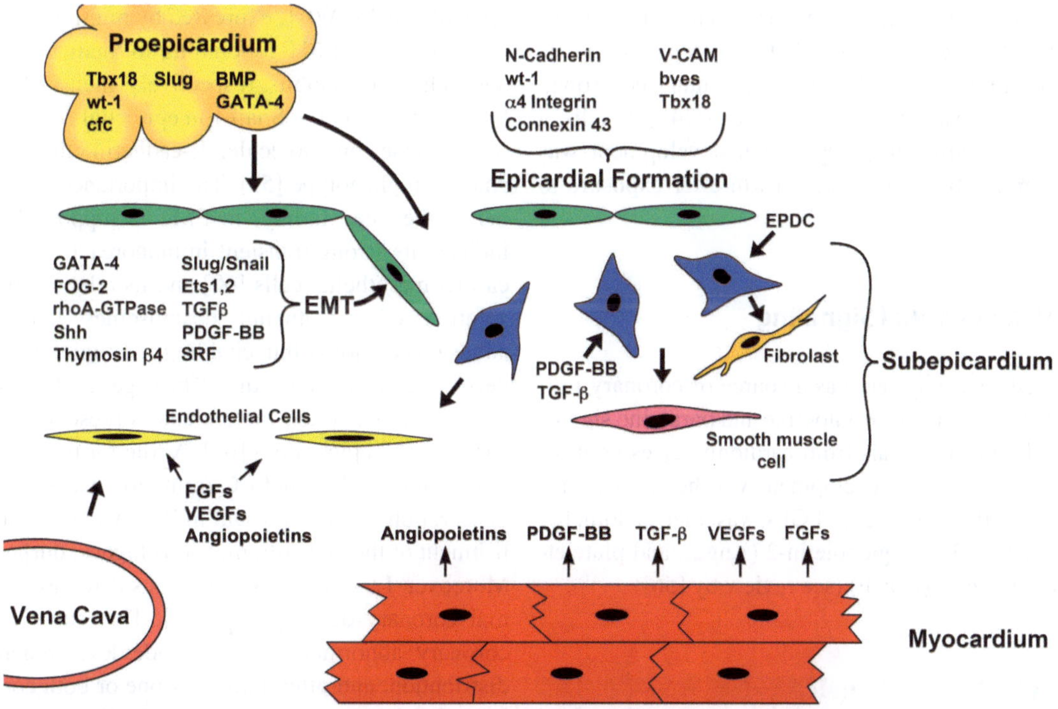

Fig. 2.2 A summary of epicardial formation, epicardial mesenchymal transition (EMT) and vascular cell differentiation. Proepicardial cell migration results in the formation of an epicardium and is influenced by a variety of transcription factors and adhesion molecules. EMT is also influenced by a wide range of molecules. The main source of vascular cells is the epicardium/subepicardium; however, some endothelial cells may also originate in the vena cava. Subepicardial cells derived from the epicardium (EPDC) undergo differentiation to vascular phenotypes (endothelial, smooth muscle, fibroblasts) in response to growth factors. These events are influenced by signaling from the myocardium

absence results in coronary patterning defects, such as anomalous origins of coronary arteries [49]. These findings are not surprising since gap junctions are membrane channels enabling cell–cell communication. The major adhesion molecule, N-cadherin, is required for the formation of both gap and adherens junctions, as well as the Cx43α1 protein subunit expression [50]. Decreases in N-cadherin are associated with a loss of cell–cell contact in the epicardium, which occurs when angiopoietin-1 is overexpressed [51]. Epicardial attachment and proliferation are dependent upon transforming growth factor β (TGF-β) signaling, as documented in epithelial-specific Alk5 (a TGF-β receptor) mutant mice [52]. Erythropoietin is essential for proliferation, differentiation, and survival of erythroid progenitor cells and is also required for adhesion of the epicardium to the heart and for capillary formation in the myocardium [53]. Mice homozygous for either erythropoietin or its receptor experience epicardial detachment and vascular abnormalities, as well as ventricular hypoplasia.

When the α4-integrin ligand, vascular cell adhesion molecule (VECAM-1) gene is disrupted, epicardial formation is prevented [54]. Similarly, GATA-4 null embryos lack a proepicardium and therefore fail to develop an epicardium [36]. WT-1 is also expressed by proepicardial cells and is critical for epicardial development [47]. A role for retinoic acid is suggested by its presence in both intact epicardial cells and in those that migrate to the heart to form the epicardium [55]. The development of the proepicardium is influenced by FGF-2 as evidenced by its enhanced growth during ex vivo exposure to this growth factor [41]. Finally, a role for FGF signaling in proepicardial development was also demonstrated by its reduced growth after exposure to FGFR-1 inhibitors.

Epicardial–Myocardial Signaling

Epicardial cells not only serve as a source of coronary progenitor cells but also provide autocrine and paracrine signals (Fig. 2.2). Moreover, signals from cardiomyocytes contribute to coronary vascular development via the release of a number of growth factors, e.g., FGFs, vascular endothelial growth factor (VEGF), angiopoietin-2 (Ang2), and platelet-derived growth factor (PDGF) (see review by [56]).

> Signals from the epicardium are important for the induction of cardiomyocyte proliferation. Thus, the symbiotic relationship between the epicardium and myocardium facilitates the development of both vascular cells and cardiomyocytes.

Epithelial–Mesenchymal Transition and Cell Fate

Epicardial cells undergo epithelial–mesenchymal transition (EMT), specification, and differentiation into various cell lineages (Fig. 2.2). This process includes their delamination, that is, detachment of cell–cell junctions, a change in phenotype, and migration. EMT occurs during several developmental processes, as well as during tumor progression and metastases, and nonmalignant degenerative disorders. Three events characterize EMT [57]. First, epithelial cell release occurs when cell–cell contacts disintegrate, epithelial markers are repressed, and cell polarity is lost. Second, the change in phenotype, with loss of polarity, involves cytoskeletal remodeling—a phenomenon that includes a transformation of cortical actin into actin stress fibers. This transformation to actin stress fibers (which are composed of polymerized F-actin and myosin II filaments) provides the molecular basis for contraction, and thus motility. Finally, the invasive characteristic of these transformed cells requires their ability to degrade adjacent basal laminae and extracellular matrices, and subsequently to synthesize a new ECM.

Activation of EMT (Fig. 2.2)

Signaling pathways implicated for EMT include Wnt, Hedgehog, TGF-β, and Notch. Snail 1 transcription factors repress adhesion molecules, which allows delamination of epicardial cells; Wt-1, expressed by migrating mesenchymal cells, promotes EMT by binding to Snail 1 and E-cadherin and induces or inhibits, respectively, their cell activity [58]. Stabile expression of Snail 1 in epithelial cells induces a loss of the adhesion molecule, E-cadherin, thus facilitating a change in phenotype [59]. The importance of Slug (a member of the Snail family) in EMT is supported by data that indicate its strong transient immunoreactivity in avian epicardial mesothelial cells [60] and its relationship to the dissolution of mesothelial desmosomes (strong cell–cell adhesion junctions), thus enabling cell migration. Epicardium-derived cells express the T-box gene, Tbx18 [61], that encodes transcription factors and is present in both proepicardium and epicardium [62]. A role for the Ets-1 transcription factor in EMT and EC formation was suggested by the observation that it is present in PE, increases with the establishment of the epicardium, and is highest during EMT [63]. Moreover, Ets-1 and Ets-2 are considered essential for normal coronary development [64]. That study revealed that coronary abnormalities (i.e., underdevelopment, irregular distribution, and often failure of one or both coronary arteries to form) were due to defective EMT. In embryonic avian hearts, EMT activation has been found to occur in response to hypoxia and HIF-1α; the latter was elevated by the active form of Notch 1 [65]. These authors suggested that this effect is most notable in the hypoxic sulcus regions of the heart which experience the first signs of vasculogenesis; they proposed that the hypoxia-HIF1-VEGF-Notch pathway may play a role in EMT and coronary progenitor cell differentiation.

Proepicardium–Epicardium–Coronary Vessels: A Continuum

The transformation of cells from the proepicardium to epicardium to the coronary vasculature can be considered a continuum. For example, GATA-4 is essential for the formation of the proepicardium, epicardium and EMT, as well as for coronary vessel formation [66]. Communication between cells and the ECM constitutes another signaling process that activates EMT. For example, β-catenin, an intracellular anchor protein that links cadherens with actin is essential for epicardial function [67]. Mice homozygous for β-cadherin do not undergo expansion of the subepicardium and experience impaired of EPC differentiation into coronary smooth muscle cells. The gap junction protein Cx43 is required not only for epicardial formation but also for coronary vasculogenesis. Cell motility, and consequently migration of epithelial-derived cells in Cx43 knockout mice, is blunted due to cytoarchitectural perturbations; these mice exhibit defects in the vascular plexus [68].

Cell Fate

From the foregoing, one can conclude that the fate of proepicardial cells is to (1) remain as epicardial cells or (2) invade the subepicardium and undergo assembly into blood vessels. Thus, there must be both intrinsic and extrinsic factors that determine which of the three fates a cell will experience. One important intrinsic factor is the ATP-dependent SWI/SNF chromatin remodeling complex, BAF180 [69]. Ablation of this regulator results in impaired EMT, arrested epicardial remodeling, limited migration of epicardial cells, and failure to develop a coronary plexus. Signaling by FGFs and TGFβs has been shown to stimulate EMT and cell migration and invasion [70–74]. In this regard, TGFβs weaken epithelial intercellular adhesion molecules [70, 75, 76]. Thus, the ability of cells to undergo EMT, and consequently invasion and migration, requires attenuation of V-CAM-1, β catenin, and E-cadherin [70]. It has been proposed that a transmembrane glycoprotein, podoplanin, stimulates EMT by downregulating E-cadherin and thereby facilitating the detachment of epicardial progenitor-derived cells (EPDCs) from the epicardium [77]. That study documented a reduced EMT and enhanced E-cadherin in podoplanin knockout mice. The repression of adhesion molecules is facilitated by Slug and Snail transcription factors which, as previously noted, are essential for EMT [59, 78]. A decrease in the adhesion molecule α4-integrin, which normally restrains EMT, enhances the invasiveness of EPDCs [76]. That study concluded that α4-integrin levels may determine the molecule's effect, i.e., high levels inhibit, while low levels stimulate invasiveness of EPDCs.

Progenitor Cell Migration and the Subepicardium

Thymosin β4 (Tβ4), a G-actin binding protein, has been found to induce mobilization of EPDCs and their inward migration and differentiation into endothelial cells (ECs) and vascular smooth muscle cells (VSMCs) [79, 80]. These studies revealed that progenitor cells in Tβ4 knockout mice persisted in or near the epicardium, indicating a loss of paracrine signaling from the myocardium where Tβ4 is normally expressed. Embryonic and postnatal day 1 epicardial explants produced outgrowths comprising smooth muscle α-actin and Tie-2 (angiopoietin receptor) positive cells, characteristic of smooth muscle and endothelial cells, respectively. Addition of Tβ4 to the cultured explants increased the numbers of these cells, with additional increases occurring when VEGF and FGF-7 were added. Establishment of cell polarity is requisite for the development of many tissue types. Cardiomyocytes in the developing heart express the cell polarity gene, Vang12, which is disrupted in loop tail (Lp) mutants. In these hearts, limited EPDC migration is due to actin cytoskeletal disruptions and a reduction in subepicardial fibronectin causes a decrease in VSMCs in coronary vessels, a consequence of RhoA/Rho kinase signaling defects [81].

> These findings taken together illustrate that several molecules facilitate EPDC activation, migration, and differentiation, and they underscore the importance of myocardial signaling for coronary vessel formation.

The Subepicardium

This region, illustrated in Fig. 2.3, contains EPDCs, has a rich ECM containing collagens I, IV, V, and VI [7, 82], proteoglycans and laminin [7], vitronectin, fibrillin-2, elastin [83], and the extracellular glycoprotein, tenascin-X [84]. The migration of EPDCs is also associated with vitronectin and fibronectin deposition since migratory sites in both the subepicardium and myocardium are positive for these ECM components [83]. With the formation of a rich ECM and the infiltration of many cells, the subepicardium expands and accumulates types I and III collagens [82]. Following its early expression in the subepicardium, tenascin-X is then expressed in the myocardium in association with developing blood vessels [84]. Its pattern of expression suggests a role in the migration of connective tissue cells. Blood islands (endothelial and blood cells that form a vesicular-like structure) are seen during the early stages of coronary vessel development, primarily in the subepicardium, but also in the myocardium [15, 44, 85, 86].

Myocardial Influences

The myocardium, an important source of growth factors such as FGFs, VEGFs, and angiopoietins, provides para-

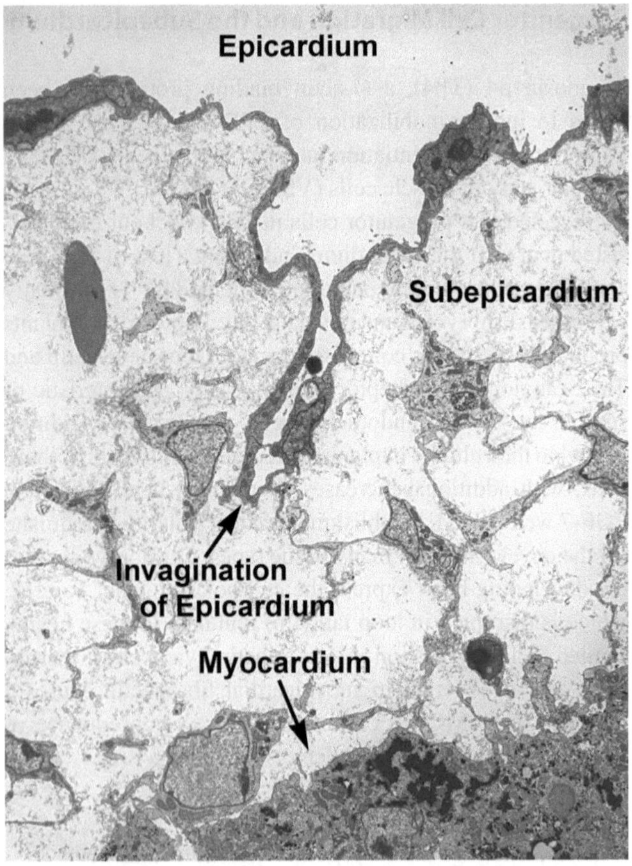

Fig. 2.3 Electron micrograph of cells of the epicardium and subepicardium of a quail heart. The epicardial invagination is a step in delamination of epicardial cells during their transformation into mesenchymal cells. Subepicardial cells often appear linked by long cytoplasmic processes (as seen here). Red blood cells are common in this region. The rich extracellular matrix contains many collagens, proteoglycans, laminin, vitronectin, fibrillin-2, tenascin, and elastin

crine signaling to the epicardium and EPDCs (Fig. 2.2). Not surprisingly, EMT is stimulated by FGFs [73, 79], VEGF, and epidermal growth factor [73]. Consistent with FGF's role in this process is an upregulation of FGFR-1, the major receptor for FGF signaling; its overexpression increases EMT [72]. FGFR-1 plays a key role in EPDCs invasiveness of the subepicardium, as well as their migration to the myocardium. This study also revealed that FGFR-1 is already expressed in a subset of proepicardial cells as well as epicardial cells and that FGFR-1 signaling activation increases delamination of epicardial cells and their invasiveness. Moreover, FGFR-1 overexpression increased the proportion of ECs in the FGFR-1 overexpressing progeny. Angiopoietin-1 is a stabilization factor for developing vessels by facilitating "tight" vessels that are resistant to leakage [87]. However, its overexpression in embryonic mice caused decreases in N-cadherin, a loss of cell–cell contact and defective development of the epicardium [51].

Coronary Cell Lineages and Differentiation

Knowing that subepicardial cell differentiation provides coronary ECs and VSMCs, as well as fibroblasts (summarized in Fig. 2.2), a number of investigators have addressed factors that predetermine or subsequently regulate cell fate. That smooth muscle cells and fibroblasts are derived from EPDCs has been consistently documented [31, 32, 88–95] and is based on data from several types of experimental approaches, including interspecies chimeras [88, 91, 96] and retroviral tagging of the proepicardium [31, 32]. Several reviews of this topic have been published [5, 10, 33]. Although the derivation of coronary endothelial cells has been more controversial, their derivation from the proepicardium is now documented [20, 97]. In the following sections, the origins of smooth muscle and endothelial cells are discussed in more detail.

Coronary Endothelial Cells

Data from Avians

In avians, the coronary EC precursor, the angioblast, is VEGFR-2 positive and is first recognized as such when the proepicardium attaches to the heart [98]. Epicardial markers cytokeratin, Wt1, RALDH2, and the retinoid X receptor are expressed in angioblasts found in either the epicardium or subepicardium. RALDH2 is the major retinoic acid dehydrogenase that catalyzes retinaldehyde conversion into retinoic acid during avian embryonic cardiac development and is expressed in epicardial derived cells [55]. Cells derived from the PE migrate from a rich retinoic acid environment into the myocardium to form endothelial tubes [90]. Epicardial retinoid receptor α mutant ventricles in E15 mice have tortuous vessels and altered branching patterns indicative of defective arteriogenesis [99]. The vasculogenic potential of proepicardial cells prior to epicardial attachment is indicated by experiments that transplanted the proepicardium onto collagen gels and found angioblastic differentiation, as revealed by the QH1 marker specific for quail ECs [98]. The differentiation process was markedly enhanced when the proepicardia were exposed to VEGF and FGF-2.

Data from Mice

In mouse embryos, angiogenic sprouts from the sinus venosus have been shown to be a source of ECs for capillaries, arteries, and veins [100]. The study used endothelial markers to establish the origin of the expanding vascular plexus at E11.5 on the dorsal cardiac surface near the sinus venosus. The plexus spread around the atrioventricular canal and outflow tract to the ventricular groove. Additional in vitro experiments revealed that if the sinus venosus and atrium

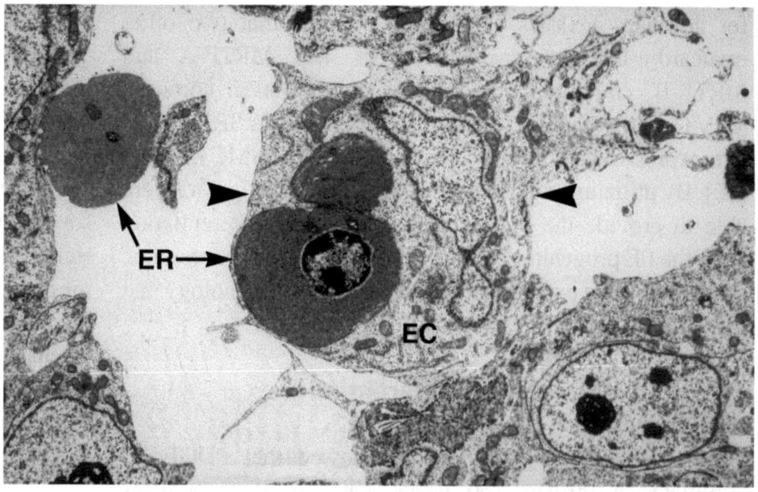

Fig. 2.4 Electron micrograph of blood island (between *arrowheads*) from an embryonic rat heart. *EC* endothelial cell; *ER* erythrocyte. The endothelial cells in blood islands are not fully differentiated

were removed, vascular sprouts did not develop. Recent work on the proepicardium indicates that it contains distinct cell compartments which give rise to coronary ECs, both in vitro and in vivo [97]. Cells that express scleraxis and semaphoring 3D also contribute to the early sinus venosus and cardiac endocardium, respectively. These findings reconcile earlier avian and mouse data that disputed the contribution of the PE to the coronary endothelium. The presence of ECs in the mouse PE prior to vasculogenesis in the heart had been previously documented [20].

Endothelial Cell Lineage Signaling

As noted in Chap. 1, the specification of endothelial cell lineage involves many signaling pathways such as Wnt/Frizzled, Delta/Notch, Ephrin/Eph, FGF, VEGF, and angiopoietin/Tie. Retroviral tagging experiments in quail proepicardium demonstrated for the first time that coronary ECs, as well as VSMCs and fibroblasts, originated from the structure that forms the epicardium [31, 32]. Support for this conclusion comes from subsequent studies using chick-quail chimeras [89–91, 101] or adenoviral tagging [88]. Since angioblasts are precursors of endothelial cells, the first sign of angioblasts in the formation of coronary vessels has been explored. A review of the subject suggests that all avian coronary cell lineages are segregated in the proepicardium prior to its contact with the heart [18].

Blood Islands and EDPCs

Blood islands (erythrocytes/erythroblasts, together with ECs that form a vesicular-like structure) are seen before and during the early stages of coronary vessel development (Fig. 2.4). Such structures have been described in embryonic hearts of humans [85, 102, 103], rats [104, 105], mice [106], and quail [107–109]. A review of these structures [110], also termed "vascular vesicles," indicates that they are present both prior and during coronary vasculogenesis and angiogenesis and suggests their role in vessel formation. A study on quail hearts documented the presence of hematopoietic, $CD45^+$ precursors prior to blood island formation and concluded that hematopoiesis and vasculogenesis have a close temporal relationship [109]. Subsequently, my colleagues and I [108] used retroviral tagging to document that some erythrocytes in blood islands were progeny of the proepicardium. This finding is consistent with the presence of the $CD45^+$ cells as early as HH23 (embryonic day 3.5–4.0) in the quail [109] and in the finding that red blood cells within blood islands of embryonic mouse hearts express the Terr/119 antigen which specifies the later stages of erythroblast differentiation [110].

Coronary Smooth Muscle Cells

Marker Gene Expression

Differentiation of coronary VSMCs, which are primarily derived from EPDCs [88, 92, 96], requires activation of marker gene expression. Mikawa and Gourdie [32] were the first to document the migration of VSMCs from the proepicardium to the heart. They employed a PE culture system that is still used today. When proepicardial cells are cultured, they initially express smooth muscle α-actin, smooth muscle 22 α, and serum response factor (SRF), and then calponin, smooth muscle α-actin, and smooth muscle myosin heavy chain [92]. SRF is required for most VSMC markers; its role as a DNA-binding protein depends on coactivators and coexpressors [111]. Myocardin is one example of an SRF co-activator of smooth muscle differentiation and like other coactivators and corepressors, modifies CArG box-dependent transcription of SMC marker genes [111–113]. However, more recent data indicate that myocardin is essential for the development of cardiomyocytes and visceral smooth muscle cells, but not for coronary VSMCs [114]. It is possible that two other myocardin-like transcription factors, i.e., MRTF-A and MRTF-B, could play the role of myocardin in coronary VSMCs. Smooth muscle differentiation requires SRF and its overexpression is sufficient for the induction of SMC markers [92]. By utilizing explanted PE cells, these investigators were able to provide the first evidence that SMC differentiation from the PE progenitor cells involves a multistep process, i.e., changes in gene expression patterns and cell morphology and cytoskeletal organization that is SRF dependent.

Signaling Molecules for Differentiation and Migration

Work from Majesky's laboratory showed that PDGF-BB stimulates a rhoA/ρ 160 RhoK pathway that mediates cytoskeletal actin reorganization in PE cells and their differentiation into VSMCs [93]. Thus, these differentiated cells are able to migrate and subsequently are recruited into the coronary vascular wall. Interaction between the notch ligand, jagged 1 (expressed by coronary ECs) and its receptor notch (expressed by coronary smooth muscle myoblasts), further stimulates smooth muscle differentiation and promotes expression of a mature VSMC phenotype [115, 116]. Epicardial cell migration and differentiation require PDGFR-β, as well as the PDGFR-β-driven phosphoinositide 3′-kinase signaling [117]. Epicardial cells in PDGFR-$\beta^{-/-}$ hearts have aberrant migration patterns into the myocardium that are associated with an irregular cytoskeleton. SRF expression in derivatives of the proepicardium is dependent on regulatory sequences that have been identified as an E-box/Ets containing cis-acting module in the SRF promoter that mediates expression in these cells [118]. That study revealed that this module is not expressed in the epicardium, a finding that suggests that these PE-derived cells either bypasses the epicardium or that the cis-acting module is operative only during migration from the epicardium. TGF-β, which is abundant in the developing heart [119], has been shown to induce EMT and VSMC differentiation in chick [75] and mice [120]. Immortalized epicardial cells were found to be dependent upon the TGFβ type I receptor ALK5 kinase activity.

Fibroblasts and Pericytes

The major source of cardiac fibroblasts are EPDCs [121]. During embryonic heart development coronary fibroblasts express many genes important for the development of the ECM and its various components including integrins, fibronectin, transcription factors, cadherins, and growth factors. They, along with differentiating ECs, secrete molecules that comprise the ECM.

Pericytes also contribute to the formation of the myocardial capillary ECM and facilitate EC-pericyte adhesion [122]. It is likely that pericytes and ECs share a common progenitor cell, since stem cell-derived Flk1$^+$ (VEGFR-1$^+$) cells can differentiate into either ECs or mural cells and assemble into to the vasculature [123]. Differentiation into ECs was stimulated by $VEGF_{165}$ exposure. "Mural cells" can be VSMCs or pericytes and the distinction between the two can be problematic during differentiation. Indeed, pericytes may be precursors of VSMCs or they may develop from tissue resident stem cells, fibroblasts/myofibroblasts, or circulating progenitor cells [122]. The specific roles of pericytes in assembly of the vascular wall and role in coronary vascular function are discussed in subsequent sections of this chapter.

Establishing the Primary Coronary Plexus

The Growth Pattern

Vascular tubes form in the subepicardium and in the myocardium. Their formation occurs as ECs differentiate from progenitor cells and assemble to form a tubular network (vasculogenesis). In addition to the ECs in blood islands, some ECs form a large cytoplasmic vacuole (Fig. 2.5), i.e. an intercellular lumen [124, 125]. Vascular tubes fuse and branch (angiogenesis) to form a network that eventually extends throughout the myocardium. ECs in the capillary network mature during the last days of gestation. As observed in the rat, plasmalemmal vesicles increase in numbers and the basal lamina becomes continuous as the endothelial cells become more narrow and pericytes are recruited [126, 127].

The formation of vascular tubes (tubulogenesis) follows a VEGF gradient from the epicardium to the endocardium [128]. This study on rat embryos revealed that the highest VEGF concentration is initially in the epicardial region and then increases toward the epicardium between E13 and birth. Tubulogenesis follows the VEGF gradient. Moreover, the rate of myocardial growth, as evidenced in an avian embryo, influences the rate of myocardial vascularization [129]. Increased growth of the ventricular compact region was accomplished by banding the outflow tract of HH Stage 21 (3.5 days) chicken hearts, i.e., prior to the onset of coronary vasculogenesis and resulted in a 64% greater ventricular mass by HH stage 29 (6 days). However, vascular volume and numerical density were similar to the nonbanded hearts, indicating that vascular growth in the banded embryos increased in proportion to the increase in heart mass. Thus, vascularization in the embryonic heart is accelerated when myocardial growth is enhanced.

Relationship of Coronary Tubulogenesis and Extracellular Matrix

Extracellular matrix (ECM) molecules serve as an anchoring scaffold and provide signals for growth and differentiation.

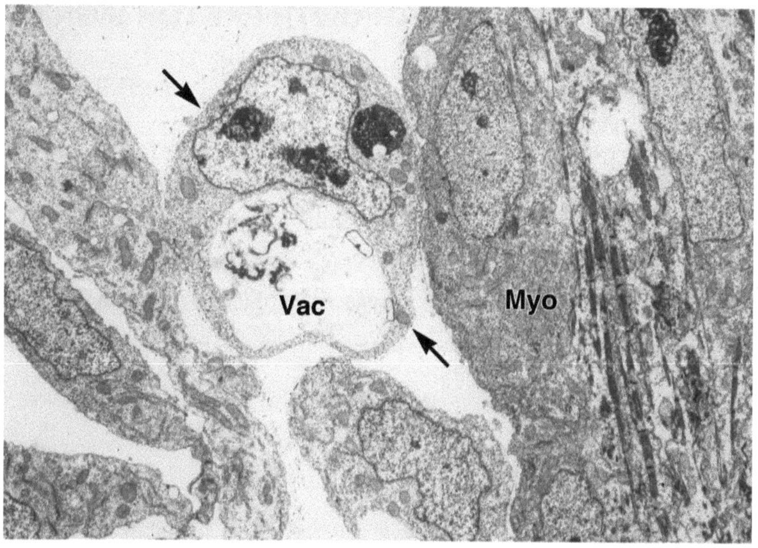

Fig. 2.5 This electron micrograph of an endothelial cell (between *arrows*) illustrates a large vacuole (Vac) containing debris. This vacuole appears to constitute a lumen as endothelial cells assemble to form a vascular plexus. The micrograph is from a rat embryonic heart. *Myo* myoblast

My colleagues and I used immunohistochemistry to elucidate the relationship of specific ECM components to vessel formation in embryonic rat hearts [125]. We found that fibronectin precedes vasculogenesis and appears to provide the extracellular milieu for EC precursor migration. Laminin deposition coincided with tube formation and was closely followed by type IV collagen. Collagens I and III first appeared in the adventitia of forming arterioles and venules.

Hypoxia Is an Initiator of Tubulogenesis

My colleagues and I have used a heart explant model in numerous studies on coronary vasculogenesis and angiogenesis first described by Bolander et al. [130]. When a portion of the heart, e.g., ventricular apex, is explanted onto a collagen gel, the epicardium delaminates to form tubes in the gel consisting entirely of endothelial cells. When embryonic quail hearts were cultured in a hypoxic environment, VEGF mRNA was upregulated and tubulogenesis was increased [131]. In contrast, when O_2 was increased to hyperoxic levels, VEGF mRNA was downregulated and coincided with a limited tubulogenesis. Several splice variants of VEGF-A are upregulated by hypoxia and $VEGF_{165}$ induced tubulogenesis [132]. The role of hypoxia in a quail in vivo model was also documented [133]. That study demonstrated that hypoxic regions of the embryonic heart were characterized by hypoxia inducible factor-1α and 1β (HIF-1α, HIF-1β) and VEGF expression. Capillary growth was notable in the areas of high VEGF expression. Subsequently, this group showed that experimental hypoxia in this model resulted in a higher capillary density, but also failure of the compact region of the myocardium to develop, coronary abnormalities, and embryonic death [134].

Further evidence that hypoxia plays a significant role in the developing heart comes from work on chick eggs subjected to a hypoxic environment [135]. Using EF5 (a fluorinated derivative of etanidazole, a marker for hypoxia), the pattern of greatest levels of hypoxia was found in or near regions which later contained major coronary vessels. This included the region where the peritruncal network surrounded the aortic root. In human embryos, EPAS1, a transcription factor that responds to hypoxia, overlaps to some extent with VEGFR-1 and Tie-2 in the myocardium and other tissues, and is often colocalized with HIF-1α [136]. The link between hypoxia and VEGF in coronary vessels was documented in adult mice by exposing them to 6% ambient O_2 for 6 h [137]. This exposure caused an upregulation of VEGF and VEGFR-1 mRNA. Hypoxia has also been shown to increase the number of hemangioblasts [138] and ECs [139] in stem cell cultures.

Multiple Growth Factors Regulate Tubulogenesis (Fig. 2.6)

The importance of three major vasculogenic/angiogenic growth factors in coronary morphogenesis was established by in vitro experiments in my lab over a decade ago [140–142]. We documented a role for both VEGF and FGF-2 in enhancing tube formation in vitro [140] and in vivo [124, 141] models. Explanted embryonic ventricles were cultured on collagen gels and the vascular tubes outgrowing from the epicardium were quantified. Tubulogenic inhibition occurred when antibodies to VEGF-A, FGF-2, or soluble Tie-2 receptors (a receptor for angiopoietins) were added to the culture media. The greatest inhibition occurred with FGF-2 antibodies, which was, in part, attributed to a reduction of ECs.

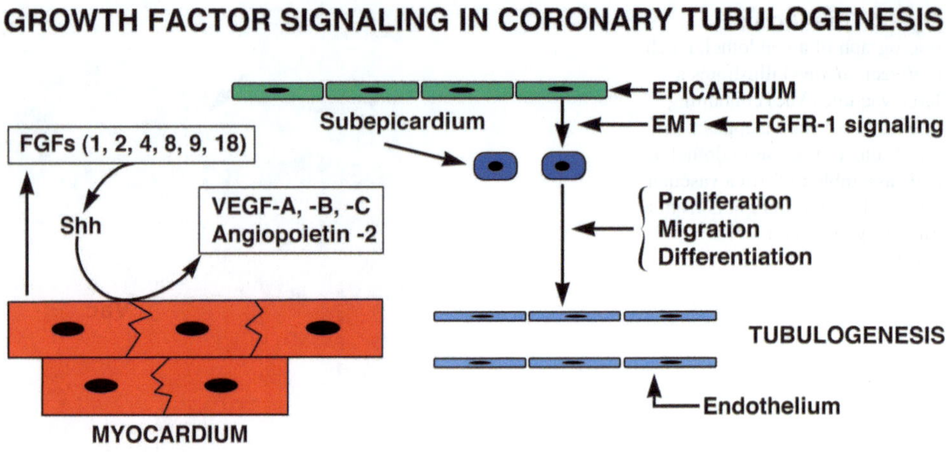

Fig. 2.6 A summary of growth factor regulation of tubulogenesis in the embryonic heart. Sonic hedgehog, FGFs, VEGFs, and angiopoietin-2 provide important signals that are required for tubulogenesis. FGFR-1 signaling plays a key role in epithelial mesenchymal transition (EMT). As also shown in Fig. 2.2, the myocardium is a source of growth factors involved in tubulogenesis

That multiple growth factors are indeed effective in stimulating tubulogenesis was further supported by our data that indicated a greater (80–90%) inhibition of tube formation when two of the three growth factors were inhibited. The interdependency of angiopoietins, FGF-2, and VEGF-A was shown by experiments that included a protein for one growth factor in combination with inhibition of another growth factor. Under this condition, there was a threefold to fivefold reduction in tube formation.

VEGF Family Members Play Key Roles

VEGF ligands comprise a large family and include splice variants and three receptors. Although deletion of the VEGF-A gene is embryonic lethal in mice [143], its overexpression results in aberrant coronary development [144], a finding that supports the concept of a narrow window of its expression. However, in addition to VEGF-A, the developing heart also expresses an abundance of VEGF-B [145, 146], as well as detectable levels of VEGF-C [145] and VEGF-D [147]. Moreover, 3 VEGF receptors, 1, 2, and 3, are expressed in the developing heart along with neuropilin-1, a receptor that overlaps with VEGFR-1 (flt-1) [148]. VEGF-C synergizes with VEGF-A and enhances plasminogen activator activity in endothelial cell lines [149].

To specify the effects of VEGF family members on tubulogenesis in the embryonic heart, we inhibited various VEGFs by adding neutralizing antibodies to quail heart explants [124]. Surprisingly, inhibition of VEGF-B attenuated tubulogenesis the most, followed by anti-VEGF-C and then anti-VEGF-A. Consistent with a major role for VEGF-B in tubulogenesis was the finding that addition of soluble VEGFR-1, which binds VEGFs A and B and placental growth factor (PIGF), inhibited tube formation by 87%. Addition of soluble receptor VEGFR-2, which does not bind VEGF-B and PIGF, but binds VEGFs A, C, D, and E, gave only half the effect of soluble VEGFR-1.

These data indicate that VEGF-B is an effective inducer of tubulogenesis in the embryonic heart. Indeed, work by Lavine and Ornitz [150] suggests that both VEGF-B and VEGF-A, along with angiopoietin 2, affect coronary tube formation and are activated by hedgehog signaling. The interactions involving multiple growth factors are discussed in the next section.

FGFs and Hedgehog Signaling (Fig. 2.6)

FGFs play many roles during development, including myocardial proliferation and coronary morphogenesis. In this regard, the epicardium regulates myocardial growth in response to erythropoietin signals [151]. By using both genetically engineered mice and organ cultures, Lavine et al. [152] were able to show how FGFs and hedgehog signaling drive coronary morphogenesis. This finding is consistent with the evidence that loss of hedgehog signaling decreases or eliminates vascular assembly in mice and avians, respectively [153]. The wave of hedgehog signaling required for VEGFs A, B, and C, and angiopoietin-2 expression occurs in response to FGF signaling. Thus, FGF signaling to the cardiomyocyte regulates hedgehog signaling, which then dictates the level of VEGF expression [154]. This work also documented FGF-9 as an essential growth factor for coronary development by noting that FGF-9$^{-/-}$ embryonic hearts failed to develop a complete vascular plexus. Among the impairments in these mice were a poorly developed subepicardial mesenchyme and a delay in subepicardial and myocardial blood vessels. These impairments were not associated with any notable abnormalities of the epicardium.

FGFs and VEGFs Cooperate in Tubulogenesis

Most FGF proteins activate FGFR-1, which is required for blood vessel development [155]. The role of this receptor in epicardial cell transition and differentiation of coronary lineages has been documented [72]. During EMT, FGFR-1 is upregulated and its overexpression increases EMT and epicardial cell delamination [72]. These data fit with the finding that FGF-2 is abundant in developing avian and rodent hearts [156–158] and with the data indicating a peak in FGF-2 transcripts during the early stage of myocardial vascularization [141]. Since FGFR-1 is a receptor for most FGFs, it is not surprising that other FGFs, in addition to 1, 2, and 9, are angiogenic. For example, FGF-1 or FGF-4 retroviral infection of the ventricular wall of quail embryos affected upregulation of FGFR-1 and VEGFR-2 in epicardial and subepicardial cells [159]. Experiments on embryonic quail and mouse heart explants in my lab revealed that FGFs 1, 2, 4, 8, 9, and 18 contribute to tubulogenesis primarily via FGFR-1 signaling and that the optimal tubulogenic response occurs when multiple FGF proteins are available [103]. FGF proteins enhanced three key elements of capillary plexus formation, i.e., EC proliferation, migration, and assembly into tubes. This work also documented the interdependence of the various FGFs on VEGF-A for their vasculogenic/angiogenic efficacy. Further documentation of the FGF–VEGF relationship comes from the finding that VEGF inhibition in mice results in decreased expression of FGF-9 and decreased myocardial vascularization [160]. Another finding demonstrating the importance of FGFR-1 signaling is that addition of mouse embryonic stem cells to embryonic heart explants, which enhances tubulogenesis, is negated when FGFR-1-dominant negative inhibitor is added to the culture medium [103].

> In conclusion, multiple FGFs may play a role in coronary tubulogenesis. FGFR-1 plays an early role in the vascularization process by enhancing EMT and epicardial delamination. Finally, FGFs depend on VEGF-A for their angiogenic effects in the myocardium.

Other Key Molecules for Tubulogenesis

FOG-2, a cofactor for GATA transcription factors, is required for heart morphogenesis and formation of the coronary vasculature as documented in FOG-$2^{-/-}$ embryos [161]. Coronary vessels are absent in these embryos despite the formation of an epicardial layer and markers of cardiac vessel development (ICAM-2 and VEGFR-2). Transgenic reexpression of FOG-2 rescues the vascular phenotype. Thus, failure of coronary vessel formation is linked to the inability to activate EMT. FOG-2 and its interaction with GATA-4 were found to be essential in mouse hearts prior to E12.5 and for maintenance of the coronary vasculature in the adult heart [162]. The importance of both spatial and temporal expression in coronary morphogenesis is also recognized in calcineurin-NFAT signaling [163]. Calcineurin is activated by Ca^{2+} signals that are outcomes of tyrosine kinase activity. Coronary morphogenesis (tube formation) was induced by calcineurin-NFAT signaling in ECs between E10.5 and E11.5, while deletion of this signaling at later time points had no effect [163]. Moreover, deletion of calcineurin in either epicardial or myocardial cells had no effect. These data indicate specific temporal and spatial requirements of NFAT signaling for coronary angiogenesis, and the importance of the transcription factor NFAT in this process.

Formation of the Coronary Ostia and Onset of Coronary Circulation

Vascular Tube Ingrowth into the Aorta

As the primary capillary plexus expands throughout the heart, a capillary ring encircles the root of the aorta (Fig. 2.7). The ECs that form this ring penetrate the aorta just above the left and right coronary cusps and form channels through the aortic wall. Formation of coronary ostia via ingrowth, rather than outgrowth, was not established until 1989 [164]. This work in chick hearts was verified in both avian and rodent models [23, 156, 165], as well as in human hearts (unpublished data from my lab). This process is characterized by aortic penetration of multiple capillary strands which fuse to form the left and right coronary ostia [166]. Redundant channels are eliminated by apoptosis at the time of ostial formation [167]. The fusion of the capillary strands occurs at E7 in quail and this event is associated with VSMC recruitment at the sites of penetration followed by the formation of coronary trunks at E8–E9 [166]. Similar observations on rat heart serial sections document the formation of a plexus of epithelial cords or capillary-like channels formed at the aorta root, followed by recruitment of mesenchymal cells that became smooth muscle α-actin positive after ostial formation [168]. Remodeling of the coronary stems involves a fourfold diameter increase between E18 and E21 [169]. The formation of coronary ostia is dependent on epicardial cell-derived Fas ligand, which induces apoptosis at the sites in the aorta where the two ostia are formed [170]. Thus, apoptosis forms a channel that becomes lined by ECs.

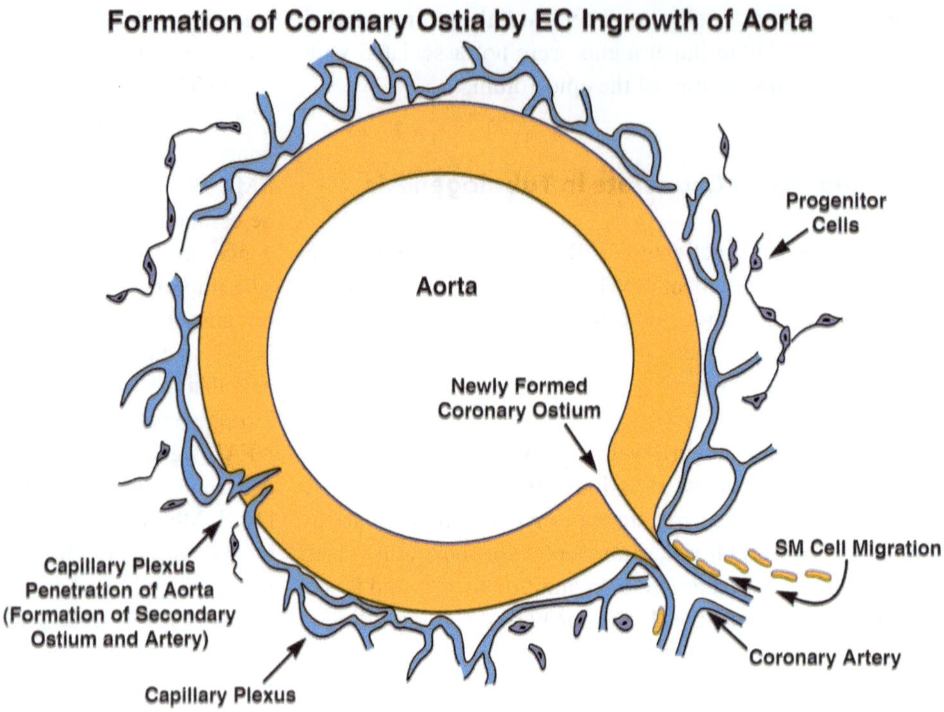

Fig. 2.7 The coronary ostia are formed by the ingrowth of a capillary plexus. The endothelial-lined ostium is connected to the tubular network. The coronary artery stems recruit smooth muscle cells (SM). In this cartoon, one coronary artery (seen on *the right of the illustration*) has already formed (usually the *left*) and the second is in the early stages of formation, as indicated by penetration of endothelial strands into the aortic wall. The penetration of the endothelial strands requires apoptosis in the aortic wall to form the coronary ostium

Signals for Coronary Ostial and Stem Formation

The mechanisms that limit aortic ingrowth of the capillary plexus to only two sites, i.e., above the left and right coronary cusps, are not well understood. This event requires not only spatial but also temporal regulation, as noted by formation of the left ostium prior to the right in humans [102], chickens [171], and rats [168].

Onset of Coronary Blood Flow Triggers Arteriogenesis

Arteriogenesis (formation of arterioles) has long been recognized as a response to mechanical stimuli and was discussed in Chap. 1. Experiments in fetal lambs documented a relationship between coronary development and blood flow [172]. After 4 days of intermittent adenosine into the circumflex artery, maximal coronary flow nearly doubled in the absence of any change in oxygen content, tension, or arterial pressure. The authors noted that blood flow regulates vessel growth via endothelial signaling in response to shear stress, stretch, and pulsatile strain. These factors can induce vascular growth by several mechanisms, for example NO stimulation of FGF-2 [173] or VEGF expression [174]. Fluid shear stress induces the differentiation of Flk-1 positive (VEGF-R2^{+}) embryonic stem cells in ECs [175]. Flow affects cells via a mechanical (shear) force and by enhancing rate-dependent mass transport. In these experiments, the former was found to be the mechanism inducing stem cell differentiation.

The addition of ECs into the developing artery or arteriole is but one component of the process. Differentiation and recruitment of mural cells (VSMCs and pericytes) are the second component, which requires their interaction with ECs. Smooth muscle cells are recruited in response to PDGF-BB secreted by ECs, a topic discussed later in this chapter. This recruitment is regulated by the extracellular glycoprotein, tenascin C [176]. In avian embryonic hearts, tenascin immunohistochemistry revealed that tenascin was deposited around the developing coronary stem and that it colocalized with VSMC α-actin. Tenascin C has been shown to enhance PDGFR-β and promote PDGF-induced proliferation and migration of VSMCs [177]. This was a result of enhanced crosstalk signaling of the integrin αVβ3-PDGFR-β complex. The muscularization process of endothelial channels destined to become coronary arteries and arterioles begins at the aortic root (Figs. 2.7 and 2.8) and spreads distally. Thus, the tunica media is developed last in the smallest branches. This pattern was quantified in our studies on quail coronary arteries/arterioles [178].

> These data fit with the observation that arteries and arterioles develop only after the establishment of coronary flow and that the developmental pattern proceeds in a proximal to distal sequence.

Parasympathetic Nerves

The sites of coronary ostia are associated with parasympathetic ganglia, as described in chicks [165], quail [107], and humans (Tomanek, unpublished data). The idea that parasympathetic nerves promote growth of the coronary vessels at their origins was suggested by Bogers et al. [179] and is supported by the finding that neural crest ablation limits the number of coronary artery stems or alters their position [180].

VEGF Signaling

One clue that the sites of coronary ostial and arterial stem formation are influenced by VEGF signaling came from a study in my lab that discovered intense VEGFR-2 and VEGFR-3 transcripts at the sites of the arterial stems [124]. This region is also characterized by intense VEGF staining of precursor cells. A subsequent study documented the dependency of coronary ostia and arterial stem formation on VEGF signaling [108]. When a soluble VEGFR-1/VEGFR-2 chimera was administered to embryonic chicks, the treatment either prevented coronary artery stem formation or limited formation to one stem. Moreover, antibodies to VEGF-B, but not VEGF-A, limited coronary artery stem formation. These data demonstrate that 1) VEGF signaling is not only important for tubulogenesis but also for coronary ostial and artery stem formation, and 2) VEGF-B is important for both tubulogenesis and coronary artery stem formation.

> Based on these in vivo and on the in vitro studies detailed earlier in this chapter and above, VEGF-B appears to be the most significant VEGF ligand in the avian heart since its inhibition attenuates the formation of vascular tubes and prevents the formation of coronary ostia and arterial stems.

FGF-2 and PDGF Signaling

Coronary artery stem formation and arterial growth are also influenced by FGF-2 and PDGF signaling [178]. Neutralizing antibodies to FGF-2 and/or PDGF-BB were injected into the vitelline vein of quail embryos at various stages of development. If administered prior to ostial formation, the embryos usually developed only one or lacked both coronary artery stems. When coronary arteries were formed, as occurred more frequently when the neutralizing antibodies were administered at the onset of coronary ostial formation, arterial segments were characterized by a thinner tunica media and VSMC investment did not extend as far distally as in the controls. Moreover, administration of VEGF-trap (the VEGFR-1/VEGFR-2 chimera that binds ligands for either of these receptors) administered after ostial formation also limited medial development of coronary arteries.

> In conclusion, these data indicate that VEGFs, FGF-2, and PDGF-BB facilitate the development of coronary arteries.

VSMC Recruitment and Assembly

Coronary VSMCs in avians have been shown to be derived entirely from the epicardium as demonstrated by labeling proepicardial cells [32, 88, 90, 91, 101]. In mice, however, VSMCs in a short segment of the proximal coronary stem are derived from the neural crest while the remaining coronary VSMCs are derived from the epicardium [181]. VSMCs are recruited either de novo from mesenchymal progenitors adjacent to the vessel or from a pool of preexisting VSMCs. The initial phase involves induction of VSMC and pericyte progenitors followed by their migration and proliferation [182]. An absence of PDGF-B signaling attenuates the number of coronary VSMCs and pericytes. These data fit with the finding that PDGF-B inhibition limits coronary artery stems and the development of the tunica media of coronary arteries as well as the assembly of VSMCs distal to the origins of the coronary arteries [178].

As stated earlier, the earliest appearance of coronary VSMC markers in the artery stems occurs only after the establishment of a coronary circulation. In the rat, smooth muscle α-actin (SM α-actin) was observed on E16 and smooth muscle-myosin heavy chain on E17 [183]. In quail embryonic hearts, SM α-actin becomes detectable around E8 [180], corresponding to the first signs of coronary ostial and stem formation. The visualization of smooth muscle cell markers also occurs in a proximal to distal sequence as noted in chick hearts [180] and fits with the sequence of tunica media formation. This study also documented the importance of the presence of the neural crest for an orderly development of coronary VSMCs.

VSMC recruitment is also influenced by signaling via the TGF-β type I receptor, Alk5 [52]. Alk5/Gata5-Cre mutant mouse hearts experience defective development of the VSMC layer surrounding coronary arteries, but contain a higher number of small vessels lacking VSMCs. Since the main coronary arteries were similar in the mutants and controls, the authors concluded that the role of Ak5-mediated signaling is to recruit VSMCs during remodeling of vascular tubes downstream of the major coronary artery stems.

The processes of VSMC recruitment into coronary arteries via PDGF and Angiopoietin/Tie-2 signaling pathways require the transcription factor CHF1/Heg 2 [184]. Knockout of this transcription factor in mice resulted in sparse VSMCs in coronary arteries and abnormally remodeled venous networks. Fibronectin and laminin may also affect VSMCs migration and coronary artery formation. Data from quail embryos indicate VSMC association with fibronectin strands and the presence of fibronectin in the developing tunica media. These glycoproteins are generously expressed in embryonic human coronary arteries [185].

Inhibition of VSMC Differentiation

A delay in epicardial VSMC differentiation and migration is necessary because the EC vascular tube network must be in place prior to VSMC recruitment. It has been established that early vasculogenesis in the mammalian heart occurs in a rich retinoic acid environment [186]. More recent work has shown that VSMC differentiation is prevented by the high levels of both retinoic acid and VEGF, which are characteristic of the early stage of vascular tube formation [187]. The study revealed that in quail proepicardial cultures, VEGF decreases the number of SMα-actin expressing cells and concomitantly increases the EC cell phenotype. Similarly, retinoic acid abrogated smooth muscle α-actin expression. My colleagues and I have shown that VEGFR-2 and VEGFR-3 receptor density in quail hearts is highest at E6 corresponding to the onset of tubulogenesis and falls by E8–E9, when coronary ostia and stems are formed [124]. However, some VEGF level is required for the formation of the coronary ostia [108] and also the subsequent optimal formation of the tunica media of coronary arteries [178].

Assembly of the Coronary Arterial Tree

Recruitment of VSMCs in the arterial tree, as already noted, occurs in a base-apex direction. Work from my lab [178] showed that VSMC incorporation in embryonic day 9 quail hearts is limited to a distance of 500–900 μm from the origin of the main coronary artery. By day 10 all hearts had VSMCs 800 μm to more than 1 mm from the origin of the major coronary artery. The study also documented the importance of FGF-2, PDGF-BB, and VEGF in facilitating the muscularization of arteries. For example, administration of anti-FGF-2 or anti-PDGF reduced the distance of muscularization by more than 60% when administered at the time the main coronary artery stems were being formed. The extent of muscularization was also impaired. VEGF-Trap (the VEGFR-1/VEGFR-2 chimera) also reduced the extent of arterial development during this time period. The assembly of the coronary arterial tree follows a similar course in mice (unpublished data). Arterioles are formed during late gestation and in the early postnatal period.

Development of the Arterial Wall

Because of the rapid growth of the heart, remodeling of the larger vessels is an early event. This allows the growth of the vasculature to parallel the growth of the ventricular wall, as documented in chick embryos [129]. Innervation of the arterial wall is also progressive, i.e., larger vessels are innervated first, as documented in the quail [178]. Nerve fibers appear initially on the tunica adventitia (E10) and later (E12–E15) in contact with the tunica media; the number of nerve fibers associated with blood vessels increased significantly between E10 and E15. We also found a close association between VSMCs and both fibronectin and laminin; the former is generously distributed at sites of vessel formation and aligned with VSMCs. Fibronectin forms a fine network in the tunica adventitia and extends into the media. Laminin forms a ring around the artery or arteriole in addition to its fine network within the media.

Formation of Coronary Veins and Lymphatics

Coronary Veins

Compared to coronary arteriogenesis, the formation and development of the coronary venous system have received much less attention. A study utilizing chicken quail chimeras reported that precursor cells formed small vessels that grew into the sinus venosus and contradicted the assumption that veins developed as outgrowths of the sinus venosus [23]. Thus, this observation suggests that like capillary ingrowth into the aorta to form the coronary arteries, venous formation also constitutes a process of ingrowth. As demonstrated in the dog fish, progenitor cells from the subepicardial mesenchyme migrate, form capillary-like structures, and coalesce to form veins [9]. A system of venules at the atrioventricular sulcus is evident at E16 in rat heart and the larger veins are already positioned posteriorly during this development period [188].

As discussed previously, hedgehog signaling plays a key role in coronary vascularization. Moreover, hedgehog signaling regulates the formation of specific cell types as revealed by a study that used conditioned gene targeting to document that (1) cardiomyoblasts and perivascular cells are targets of hedgehog signaling and (2) these two cell types control development of distinct vascular subtypes [154].

> Most significantly, these experiments showed that hedgehog signaling to the cardiomyoblast is essential for the development of coronary veins, while its signaling to perivascular cells is essential for arterial development. As discussed in Chap. 1, venous and arterial fates are established at the time of, or prior to, vascular plexus formation.

Lymphogenesis in the Heart

Lymphatic vessels in the human heart have been found to often accompany subendocardial branches of the coronary arteries along their adventitia [189]. These vessels are present in the subepicardium, myocardium, and subendocardium [190]. Although the development of the chick cardiac lymphatic vessels was described more than 4 decades ago [191, 192], only more recently has the topic received much attention. The availability of antibodies for lymphatic ECs, e.g., Prox1 (a homeobox transcription factor) and LYVE-1 (the hyaluronan receptor), has provided the opportunity to explore the derivation and assembly of lymphatic cells in the heart. Wilting and colleagues [193] demonstrated the presence of lymphatic vessels in the subepicardial mesenchyme in E9 chicks and noted their attachment to lymphatic trunks. Using quail-chick chimeras, these authors showed that the lymphatic ECs are not derived from the proepicardium. Additionally, they noted a lymphatic collecting vessel that appeared to have venous anastomoses. Lymphatic vessel formation in mice involves a phenotype change in ECs; their precursors stem from leukocytes and monocytes (A. Ratajska, personal communication). Cardiac lymphatic vessel formation begins simultaneously at the arterial and venous poles.

Juszynski et al. [194] followed the progression of Lyve-1 positive lymphatic ECs throughout embryonic/fetal and early postnatal development in mice. This detailed study showed that isolated Lyve-1 positive cells occur at E11 in the venous pole and in systemic veins, a finding that suggests their venous origin in the heart as in other organs (reviewed in Chap. 1). These cells are most numerous at the base of the heart and form tubules and collecting vessels by E14.5. The development of a lymphatic capillary plexus at E16.5 is followed by coalescence of vascular structures to form larger structures and the development of 2 collecting ducts from the right and left ventricles. A subsequent study that examined lymphatic markers during development in chick, quail, and mouse hearts documented Prox-1 positive cells on the developing aorta and pulmonary artery, which contribute to a branching lymphatic network that spreads over the heart [195]. The cells that form lymphatic vessels then express LYVE-1, VEGFR-3, and podoplanin. The data indicate that three cell types express lymphatic markers in the heart (1) Prox-1-positive cells, derived from an extracardiac source; (2) epicardial LYVE-1-positive cells that may incorporate into the lymphatic vasculature; and (3) LYVE-1-positive cells in the myocardium that do not become Prox-1-positive. VEGF-C and VEGF-D play key roles in lymphogenesis by activation of VEGFR-3 and its co-receptor neuropilin (reviewed by [196]).

Coronary Development in Humans

As noted in the previous sections, most of our knowledge regarding coronary vessel development is based on experimental animals. This raises the question: how similar is the process in humans to that of other mammalian and avian models? The following section summarizes what is known regarding the formation of coronary vessels in humans.

Early Development

Stages (S) 14–18 (32–44 days) are a period during which the premature vascular plexus forms and precedes the establishment of the coronary arteries (S18–19). Septation of the 4 heart chambers is completed by S18 [197]. The loose epicardial cells, blood islands, and subepicardial capillaries, characteristic of mammalian and avian coronary development, appear in humans during these developmental stages [85, 102, 198]; and Tomanek (unpublished data). Figure 2.8a, b is a micrograph of subepicardial blood islands and an expanded subepicardium with a network of loose cells at the A–V junction. The loose network of cells surrounding the aorta and pulmonary artery and parasympathetic ganglia is observed at the roots of these vessels [103]. That the subepicardial tubular plexus contributes to the formation of the coronary arteries was noted by Conte and Pelligrini [198]. They also described subepicardial vessels connected to the sinus venosus at S15 and noted that like in mammalian and avian models, these are developing veins. Hirakow [102] described the development of the cardiac vein at the sinus venosus from serially sectioned hearts. He found that the vascular structures were present in the wall of the sinus venous at S16 (E37) and formed at least one channel by S17 (E41).

The formation of the coronary ostia and main coronaries occurs between S18 (E44) and S20 (E57) [85, 102, 103, 198]. Again, as in the case of venous formation at the sinus venosus, an invagination is seen at the aorta. The capillary-like network that penetrates the aorta in all other species studied is similar in humans (Tomanek, unpublished data). The left coronary artery develops first and was found to be present in 67% of S18 embryos, whereas both left and right were present by S19 [199] or S20 [102] and Tomanek (unpublished data). The coronary arterial tree develops rapidly. By the ninth week, the right coronary artery has sprouted branches to the sinoatrial node and the left coronary has divided into the left anterior descending and circumflex arteries [200]. VEGF receptors are present in coronary vessels as early as 5–6 weeks [201]. Their localization in the

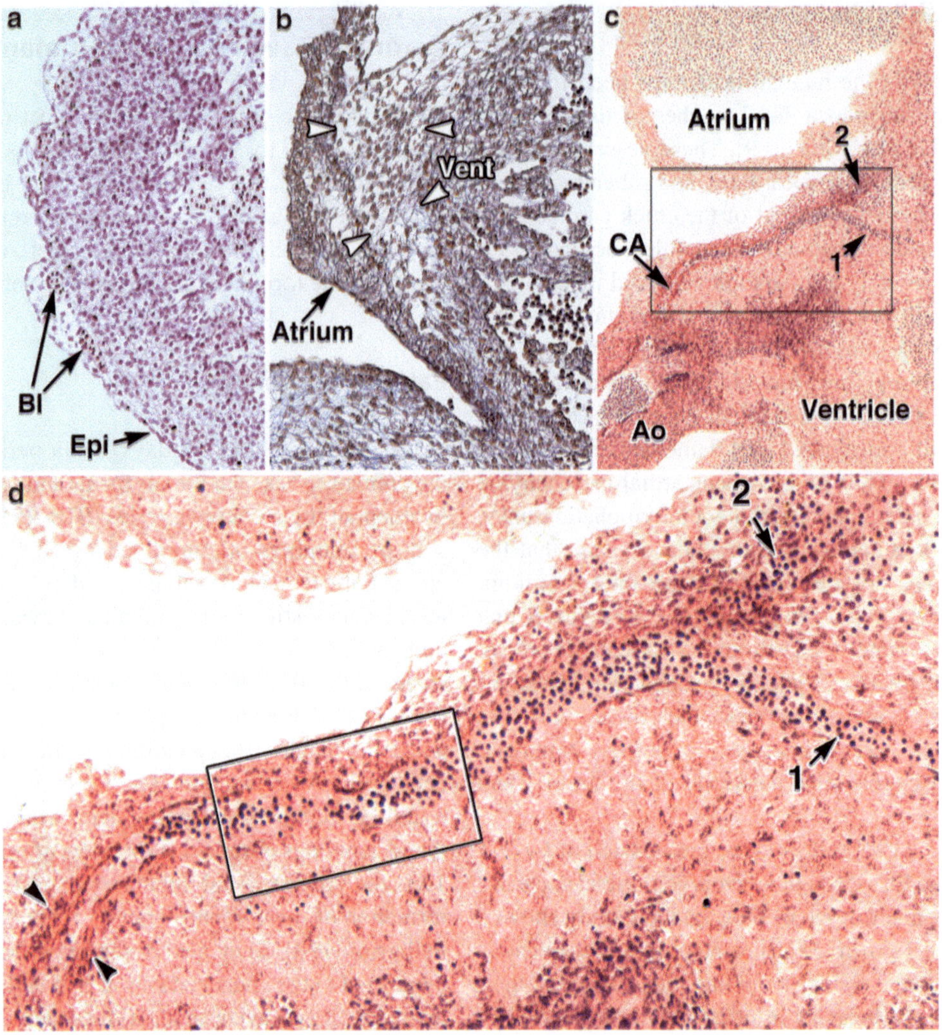

Fig. 2.8 Human embryonic hearts. (**a**) Blood islands (*arrows*) precede and accompany formation of the primary vascular plexus as seen here in a 41-day embryonic heart. (**b**) An expanded subepicardium between the atrium and ventricle is seen between the *arrowheads*. It contains a network of cells, many of which are progenitors of the coronary vasculature. This image is from a 44-day embryo. (**c**) Formation of a main coronary artery in a 48-day embryo. Near its origin (CA) at the aorta (Ao), smooth muscle has enveloped the endothelial tube. More distally, smooth muscle has not yet completely covered the endothelial tube. Two branches (1 & 2) of the main coronary artery are seen. (**d**) This is an enlargement of the area in the *rectangle* in (**c**). The smooth muscle layer is complete at the root of the coronary artery (between *arrowheads*). Just distal to this region (indicated by the *rectangle*), the media of the artery is incomplete. In the branches (1 & 2), some smooth muscle is present in 2, but not in 1

hearts of different gestational ages is similar. VEGFR-1 and VEGFR-2 were documented in capillaries, myocardial arteries and veins, and epicardial veins. Epicardial arteries lacked VEGFR-2. Neuropilin, Tie-1, and Tie-2 were noted in all vessel types. Vascularization of the human heart occurs earlier in the left than in the right ventricle [202].

Later Development

The formation of the two main coronary arteries, late in the second month, establishes a coronary circulation and the onset of an arterial hierarchy (Tomanek, unpublished data). Figure 2.8c is an image that illustrates the base to apex progression of medial development in a main coronary artery. During the subsequent 2 months, numerous endothelial-lined tubes become muscularized as branches of the arterial tree. Transmural arteries are evident by the fourth month. The remainder of in utero development is characterized by remodeling of the main coronary vessels into larger vessels to accommodate the increasing ventricular mass.

A collateral coronary circulation in human embryonic hearts has been described based on angiographic findings [203]. Collaterals were noted in 19–39 week embryos and

Synopsis of Prenatal Coronary Morphogenesis

The coronary vasculature is formed by proepicardial cells that originate outside the heart and migrate to form the epicardium and subepicardium. Epicardial cells undergo epithelial–mesenchymal transition, a process that involves many signaling molecules that determine cell fate. Formation of a coronary endothelial plexus precedes the development of coronary arteries and veins and is evoked by a relative hypoxia as the myocardium expands. The capillary plexus penetrates the aorta, a process that is VEGF dependent, and forms two coronary ostia. The onset of coronary blood flow evokes recruitment of VSMCs to the coronary stems; the media of the arteries then forms in a base to apex progression. This process is regulated by FGFs and PDGF. Veins develop as ingrowths of the sinus venosus. Venous and arterial fates are influenced by hedgehog signaling. The prenatal development of the coronary vasculature is strikingly similar in avians, mammals, and humans.

they were found to be more abundant and larger in diameter in the septum and subepicardium. The anastomoses were 3–50 μm in diameter and were observed in all regions of the heart.

References

1. Manasek FJ. Embryonic development of the heart. I. A light and electron microscopic study of myocardial development in the early chick embryo. J Morphol. 1968;125:329–65.
2. His W. Anatomic Menschlicher Embryonen. Leipzig: Vogel; 1885.
3. Kurkiewicz T. ZurKenntnis der histogenese des Hermuskels der wireltiere. Bull Internat Acad D sc De Cravocie. 1909;ii: 148–191.
4. Van den Eijnde SM, Wenink AC, Vermeij-Keers C. Origin of subepicardial cells in rat embryos. Anat Rec. 1995;242:96–102.
5. Ratajska A, Czarnowska E, Ciszek B. Embryonic development of the proepicardium and coronary vessels. Int J Dev Biol. 2008;52: 229–36.
6. Komiyama M, Ito K, Shimada Y. Origin and development of the epicardium in the mouse embryo. Anat Embryol (Berl). 1987;176:183–9.
7. Kalman F, Viragh S, Modis L. Cell surface glycoconjugates and the extracellular matrix of the developing mouse embryo epicardium. Anat Embryol (Berl). 1995;191:451–64.
8. Rodgers LS, Lalani S, Runyan RB, Camenisch TD. Differential growth and multicellular villi direct proepicardial translocation to the developing mouse heart. Dev Dyn. 2008;237:145–52.
9. Munoz-Chapuli R, Macias D, Ramos C, Gallego A, DA V. Development of the subepicardial mesenchyme and the early cardiac vessels in the dogfish (*Scyliorhinus canicula*). J Exp Zool. 1996;275:95–111.
10. Munoz-Chapuli R, Macias D, Ramos C, Fernandez B, Sans-Coma V. Development of the epicardium in the dogfish (*Scyliorhinus Canicula*). Acta Zool (Stockholm). 1997;78:39–46.
11. Kuhn W, Roebroek R, Blom H, van Oppenraaij D, Przuntek H, Kretschmer A, et al. Elevated plasma levels of homocysteine in Parkinson's disease. Eur Neurol. 1998;40:225–7.
12. Viragh S, Gittenberger-de Groot AC, Poelmann RE, Kalman F. Early development of quail heart epicardium and associated vascular and glandular structures. Anat Embryol (Berl). 1993; 188:381–93.
13. Manner J. Experimental study on the formation of the epicardium in chick embryos. Anat Embryol (Berl). 1993;187:281–9.
14. Viragh S, Challice CE. The origin of the epicardium and the embryonic myocardial circulation in the mouse. Anat Rec. 1981;201:157–68.
15. Hiruma T, Hirakow R. Epicardial formation in embryonic chick heart: computer-aided reconstruction, scanning, and transmission electron microscopic studies. Am J Anat. 1989;184:129–38.
16. Nahirney PC, Mikawa T, Fischman DA. Evidence for an extracellular matrix bridge guiding proepicardial cell migration to the myocardium of chick embryos. Dev Dyn. 2003;227:511–23.
17. Moorman AF, Christoffels VM, Anderson RH, van den Hoff MJ. The heart-forming fields: one or multiple? Philos Trans R Soc Lond B Biol Sci. 2007;362:1257–65.
18. Ishii Y, Langberg J, Rosborough K, Mikawa T. Endothelial cell lineages of the heart. Cell Tissue Res. 2009;335:67–73.
19. Schulte I, Schlueter J, Abu-Issa R, Brand T, Manner J. Morphological and molecular left-right asymmetries in the development of the proepicardium: a comparative analysis on mouse and chick embryos. Dev Dyn. 2007;236:684–95.
20. Cossette S, Misra R. The identification of different endothelial cell populations within the mouse proepicardium. Dev Dyn. 2011;240: 2344–53.
21. Shimada Y, Ho E, Toyota N. Epicardial covering over myocardial wall in the chicken embryo as seen with the scanning electron microscope. Scan Electron Microsc. 1981;(Pt 2):275–80.
22. Manner J. The development of pericardial villi in the chick embryo. Anat Embryol (Berl). 1992;186:379–85.
23. Poelmann RE, Gittenberger-de Groot AC, Mentink MM, Bokenkamp R, Hogers B. Development of the cardiac coronary vascular endothelium, studied with antiendothelial antibodies, in chicken-quail chimeras. Circ Res. 1993;73:559–68.
24. Munoz-Chapuli R, Macias D, Ramos C, de Andres V, Gallego A, Navarro P. Cardiac development in the dogfish (*Scyliorhinus canicula*): a model for the study of vertebrate cardiogenesis. Cardioscience. 1994;5:245–53.
25. Nesbitt T, Lemley A, Davis J, Yost MJ, Goodwin RL, Potts JD. Epicardial development in the rat: a new perspective. Microsc Microanal. 2006;12:390–8.
26. Icardo JM, Guerrero A, Duran AC, Colvee E, Domezain A, Sans-Coma V. The development of the epicardium in the sturgeon *Acipenser naccarii*. Anat Rec (Hoboken). 2009;292:1593–601.
27. Serluca FC. Development of the proepicardial organ in the zebrafish. Dev Biol. 2008;315:18–27.
28. Fransen ME, Lemanski LF. Epicardial development in the axolotl, Ambystoma mexicanum. Anat Rec. 1990;226:228–36.
29. Jahr M, Schlueter J, Brand T, Manner J. Development of the proepicardium in Xenopus laevis. Dev Dyn. 2008;237:3088–96.
30. Majesky MW. Development of coronary vessels. Curr Top Dev Biol. 2004;62:225–59.
31. Mikawa T, Fischman DA. Retroviral analysis of cardiac morphogenesis: discontinuous formation of coronary vessels. Proc Natl Acad Sci USA. 1992;89:9504–8.
32. Mikawa T, Gourdie RG. Pericardial mesoderm generates a population of coronary smooth muscle cells migrating into the heart along with ingrowth of the epicardial organ. Dev Biol. 1996;174: 221–32.
33. Ishii Y, Langberg JD, Hurtado R, Lee S, Mikawa T. Induction of proepicardial marker gene expression by the liver bud. Development. 2007;134:3627–37.

34. Zhou B, von Gise A, Ma Q, Rivera-Feliciano J, Pu WT. Nkx2-5- and Isl1-expressing cardiac progenitors contribute to proepicardium. Biochem Biophys Res Commun. 2008;375:450–3.
35. Robb L, Mifsud L, Hartley L, Biben C, Copeland NG, Gilbert DJ, et al. Epicardin: a novel basic helix-loop-helix transcription factor gene expressed in epicardium, branchial arch myoblasts, and mesenchyme of developing lung, gut, kidney, and gonads. Dev Dyn. 1998;213:105–13.
36. Watt AJ, Battle MA, Li J, Duncan SA. GATA4 is essential for formation of the proepicardium and regulates cardiogenesis. Proc Natl Acad Sci USA. 2004;101:12573–8.
37. Yang JT, Rayburn H, Hynes RO. Cell adhesion events mediated by α_4 integrins are essential in placental and cardiac development. Development. 1995;121:549–60.
38. Pinco KA, Liu S, Yang JT. alpha4 integrin is expressed in a subset of cranial neural crest cells and in epicardial progenitor cells during early mouse development. Mech Dev. 2001;100:99–103.
39. Schlueter J, Manner J, Brand T. BMP is an important regulator of proepicardial identity in the chick embryo. Dev Biol. 2006;295: 546–58.
40. Ishii Y, Garriock RJ, Navetta AM, Coughlin LE, Mikawa T. BMP signals promote proepicardial protrusion necessary for recruitment of coronary vessel and epicardial progenitors to the heart. Dev Cell. 2010;19:307–16.
41. Kruithof BP, van Wijk B, Somi S, Kruithof-de Julio M, Perez Pomares JM, Weesie F, et al. BMP and FGF regulate the differentiation of multipotential pericardial mesoderm into the myocardial or epicardial lineage. Dev Biol. 2006;295:507–22.
42. Torlopp A, Schlueter J, Brand T. Role of fibroblast growth factor signaling during proepicardium formation in the chick embryo. Dev Dyn. 2010;239:2393–403.
43. Vrancken Peeters M, Mentink MMT, Poelmann RE, G-dG AC. Cytokeratins as a marker for epicardial formation in the quail embryo. Anat Embryol (Berl). 1995;191:503–8.
44. Perez-Pomares JM, Macias D, Garcia-Garrido L, Munoz-Chapuli R. Contribution of the primitive epicardium to the subepicardial mesenchyme in hamster and chick embryos. Dev Dyn. 1997;210: 96–105.
45. Manner J, Perez-Pomares JM, Macias D, Munoz-Chapuli R. The origin, formation and developmental significance of the epicardium: a review. Cells Tissues Organs. 2001;169:89–103.
46. Lie-Venema H, Eralp I, Maas S, Gittenberger-De Groot AC, Poelmann RE, DeRuiter MC. Myocardial heterogeneity in permissiveness for epicardium-derived cells and endothelial precursor cells along the developing heart tube at the onset of coronary vascularization. Anat Rec A Discov Mol Cell Evol Biol. 2005; 282:120–9.
47. Moore AW, McInnes L, Kreidberg J, Hastie ND, Schedl A. YAC complementation shows a requirement for Wt1 in the development of epicardium, adrenal gland and throughout nephrogenesis. Development. 1999;126:1845–57.
48. Wessels A, Perez-Pomares JM. The epicardium and epicardially derived cells (EPDCs) as cardiac stem cells. Anat Rec. 2004;276A: 43–57.
49. Li WE, Waldo K, Linask KL, Chen T, Wessels A, Parmacek MS, et al. An essential role for connexin43 gap junctions in mouse coronary artery development. Development. 2002;129: 2031–42.
50. Wei CJ, Francis R, Xu X, Lo CW. Connexin43 associated with an N-cadherin-containing multiprotein complex is required for gap junction formation in NIH3T3 cells. J Biol Chem. 2005;280: 19925–36.
51. Ward NL, Van Slyke P, Sturk C, Cruz M, Dumont DJ. Angiopoietin 1 expression levels in the myocardium direct coronary vessel development. Dev Dyn. 2004;229:500–9.
52. Sridurongrit S, Larsson J, Schwartz R, Ruiz-Lozano P, Kaartinen V. Signaling via the Tgf-beta type I receptor Alk5 in heart development. Dev Biol. 2008;322:208–18.
53. Wu H, Lee SH, Gao J, Liu X, Iruela-Arispe ML. Inactivation of erythropoietin leads to defects in cardiac morphogenesis. Development. 1999;126:3597–605.
54. Kwee L, Baldwin HS, Shen HM, Stewart CL, Buck C, Buck CA, et al. Defective development of the embryonic and extraembryonic circulatory systems in vascular cell adhesion molecule (VCAM-1) deficient mice. Development. 1995;121:489–503.
55. Xavier-Neto J, Shapiro MD, Houghton L, Rosenthal N. Sequential programs of retinoic acid synthesis in the myocardial and epicardial layers of the developing avian heart. Dev Biol. 2000;219:129–41.
56. Olivey HE, Svensson EC. Epicardial-myocardial signaling directing coronary vasculogenesis. Circ Res. 2010;106:818–32.
57. Zavadil J, Bottinger EP. TGF-beta and epithelial-to-mesenchymal transitions. Oncogene. 2005;24:5764–74.
58. Chau YY, Brownstein D, Mjoseng H, Lee WC, Buza-Vidas N, Nerlov C, Jacobsen SE, Perry P, Berry R, Thornburn A, Secton D, Morton N, Hohenstein P, Freyer E, Samuel K, Van't Hof R, Hastie N. Acute multiple organ failure in adult mice deleted for the developmental regulator Wt1, PLoS. 2011;7:e1002404.
59. Cano A, Perez-Moreno MA, Rodrigo I, Locascio A, Blanco MJ, del Barrio MG, et al. The transcription factor snail controls epithelial-mesenchymal transitions by repressing E-cadherin expression. Nat Cell Biol. 2000;2:76–83.
60. Carmona R, Gonzalez-Iriarte M, Macias D, Perez-Pomares JM, Garcia-Garrido L, Munoz-Chapuli R. Immunolocalization of the transcription factor Slug in the developing avian heart. Anat Embryol (Berl). 2000;201:103–9.
61. Cai H, Reed RR. Cloning and characterization of neuropilin-1-interacting protein: a PSD-95/Dlg/ZO-1 domain-containing protein that interacts with the cytoplasmic domain of neuropilin-1. J Neurosci. 1999;19:6519–27.
62. Kraus F, Haenig B, Kispert A. Cloning and expression analysis of the mouse T-box gene Tbx18. Mech Dev. 2001;100:83–6.
63. Macias D, Perez-Pomares JM, Garcia-Garrido L, Carmona R, Munoz-Chapuli R. Immunoreactivity of the ets-1 transcription factor correlates with areas of epithelial-mesenchymal transition in the developing avian heart. Anat Embryol (Berl). 1998;198:307–15.
64. Lie-Venema H, Gittenberger-de Groot AC, van Empel LJ, Boot MJ, Kerkdijk H, de Kant E, et al. Ets-1 and Ets-2 transcription factors are essential for normal coronary and myocardial development in chicken embryos. Circ Res. 2003;92:749–56.
65. Yang K, Doughman YQ, Karunamuni G, Gu S, Yang YC, Bader DM, et al. Expression of active Notch1 in avian coronary development. Dev Dyn. 2009;238:162–70.
66. Crispino JD, Lodish MB, Thurberg BL, Litovsky SH, Collins T, Molkentin JD, et al. Proper coronary vascular development and heart morphogenesis depend on interaction of GATA-4 with FOG cofactors. Genes Dev. 2001;15:839–44.
67. Zamora M, Manner J, Ruiz-Lozano P. Epicardium-derived progenitor cells require beta-catenin for coronary artery formation. Proc Natl Acad Sci USA. 2007;104:18109–14.
68. Rhee DY, Zhao XQ, Francis RJ, Huang GY, Mably JD, Lo CW. Connexin 43 regulates epicardial cell polarity and migration in coronary vascular development. Development. 2009;136:3185–93.
69. Huang X, Gao X, Diaz-Trelles R, Ruiz-Lozano P, Wang Z. Coronary development is regulated by ATP-dependent SWI/SNF chromatin remodeling component BAF180. Dev Biol. 2008;319:258–66.
70. Dokic D, Dettman RW. VCAM-1 inhibits TGFbeta stimulated epithelial-mesenchymal transformation by modulating Rho activity and stabilizing intercellular adhesion in epicardial mesothelial cells. Dev Biol. 2006;299:489–504.

71. Lavine KJ, White AC, Park C, Smith CS, Choi K, Long F, et al. Fibroblast growth factor signals regulate a wave of Hedgehog activation that is essential for coronary vascular development. Genes Dev. 2006;20:1651–66.
72. Pennisi DJ, Mikawa T. FGFR-1 is required by epicardium-derived cells for myocardial invasion and correct coronary vascular lineage differentiation. Dev Biol. 2009;328:148–59.
73. Morabito CJ, Dettman RW, Kattan J, Collier JM, Bristow J. Positive and negative regulation of epicardial-mesenchymal transformation during avian heart development. Dev Biol. 2001;234:204–15.
74. Olivey HE, Mundell NA, Austin AF, Barnett JV. Transforming growth factor-beta stimulates epithelial-mesenchymal transformation in the proepicardium. Dev Dyn. 2006;235:50–9.
75. Compton LA, Potash DA, Mundell NA, Barnett JV. Transforming growth factor-beta induces loss of epithelial character and smooth muscle cell differentiation in epicardial cells. Dev Dyn. 2006; 235:82–93.
76. Dettman RW, Pae SH, Morabito C, Bristow J. Inhibition of alpha4-integrin stimulates epicardial-mesenchymal transformation and alters migration and cell fate of epicardially derived mesenchyme. Dev Biol. 2003;257:315–28.
77. Mahtab EA, Wijffels MC, Van Den Akker NM, Hahurij ND, Lie-Venema H, Wisse LJ, et al. Cardiac malformations and myocardial abnormalities in podoplanin knockout mouse embryos: correlation with abnormal epicardial development. Dev Dyn. 2008;237: 847–57.
78. Savagner P, Yamada KM, Thiery JP. The zinc-finger protein slug causes desmosome dissociation, an initial and necessary step for growth factor-induced epithelial-mesenchymal transition. J Cell Biol. 1997;137:1403–19.
79. Smart N, Risebro CA, Melville AA, Moses K, Schwartz RJ, Chien KR, et al. Thymosin beta4 induces adult epicardial progenitor mobilization and neovascularization. Nature. 2007;445:177–82.
80. Smart N, Risebro CA, Melville AA, Moses K, Schwartz RJ, Chien KR, et al. Thymosin beta-4 is essential for coronary vessel development and promotes neovascularization via adult epicardium. Ann NY Acad Sci. 2007;1112:171–88.
81. Phillips HM, Hildreth V, Peat JD, Murdoch JN, Kobayashi K, Chaudhry B, et al. Non-cell-autonomous roles for the planar cell polarity gene Vangl2 in development of the coronary circulation. Circ Res. 2008;102:615–23.
82. Tidball JG. Distribution of collagens and fibronectin in the subepicardium during avian cardiac development. Anat Embryol (Berl). 1992;185:155–62.
83. Bouchey D, Drake CJ, Wunsch AM, Little CD. Distribution of connective tissue proteins during development and neovascularization of the epicardium. Cardiovasc Res. 1996;31:Spec No: E104–15.
84. Burch GH, Bedolli MA, McDonough S, Rosenthal SM, Bristow J. Embryonic expression of tenascin-X suggests a role in limb, muscle, and heart development. Dev Dyn. 1995;203:491–504.
85. Hutchins GM, Kessler-Hanna A, Moore GW. Development of the coronary arteries in the embryonic human heart. Circulation. 1988;77:1250–7.
86. Viragh SZ, Kalman F, Gittenberger-de Groot AC, Poelmann RE, AFM M. Angiogenesis and hematopoiesis in the epicardium of the vertebrate embryo heart. Ann NY Acad Sci. 1990;588: 455–8.
87. Suri C, Yancopoulos GD. The ties that bind: emerging concepts about the structure and function of angiopoietins and their receptors in angiogenesis. In: Tomanek RJ, editor. Assembly of the vasculature and its regulation. Boston: Birkhauser; 2002. p. 55–66.
88. Dettman RW, Denetclaw Jr W, Ordahl CP, Bristow J. Common epicardial origin of coronary vascular smooth muscle, perivascular fibroblasts, and intermyocardial fibroblasts in the avian heart. Dev Biol. 1998;193:169–81.
89. Manner J. Does the subepicardial mesenchyme contribute myocardioblasts to the myocardium of the chick embryo heart? A quail-chick chimera study tracing the fate of the epicardial primordium. Anat Rec. 1999;255:212–26.
90. Gittenberger-de Groot A, Vrancken Peeters M-P, Mentink M, Gourdie R, Poelmann R. Epicardium-derived cells contribute a novel population to the myocardial wall and the atrioventricular cushions. Circ Res. 1998;82:1043–52.
91. Vrancken Peeters M-P, Gittenberger-de Groot AC, Mentink MM, Poelmann RE. Smooth muscle cells and fibroblasts of the coronary arteries derive from epithelial-mesenchymal transformation of the epicardium. Anat Embryol (Berl). 1999;199:367–78.
92. Landerholm TE, Dong XR, Lu J, Belaguli NS, Schwartz RJ, Majesky MW. A role for serum response factor in coronary smooth muscle differentiation from proepicardial cells. Development. 1999;126:2053–62.
93. Lu J, Landerholm TE, Wei JS, Dong XR, Wu SP, Liu X, et al. Coronary smooth muscle differentiation from proepicardial cells requires rhoA-mediated actin reorganization and p160 rho-kinase activity. Dev Biol. 2001;240:404–18.
94. Sun Y, Liang X, Najafi N, Cass M, Lin L, Cai CL, et al. Islet 1 is expressed in distinct cardiovascular lineages, including pacemaker and coronary vascular cells. Dev Biol. 2007;304:286–96.
95. Moretti A, Caron L, Nakano A, Lam JT, Bernshausen A, Chen Y, et al. Multipotent embryonic isl1+ progenitor cells lead to cardiac, smooth muscle, and endothelial cell diversification. Cell. 2006;127:1151–65.
96. Perez-Pomares JM, Macias D, Garcia-Garrido L, Munoz-Chapuli R. Immunolocalization of the vascular endothelial growth factor receptor-2 in the subepicardial mesenchyme of hamster embryos: identification of the coronary vessel precursors. Histochem J. 1998;30:627–34.
97. Katz TC, Singh MK, Degenhardt K, Rivera-Feliciano J, Johnson RL, Epstein JA, et al. Distinct compartments of the proepicardial organ give rise to coronary vascular endothelial cells. Dev Cell. 2012;22:639–50.
98. Guadix JA, Carmona R, Munoz-Chapuli R, Perez-Pomares JM. In vivo and in vitro analysis of the vasculogenic potential of avian proepicardial and epicardial cells. Dev Dyn. 2006;235: 1014–26.
99. Merki E, Zamora M, Raya A, Kawakami Y, Wang J, Zhang X, et al. Epicardial retinoid X receptor alpha is required for myocardial growth and coronary artery formation. Proc Natl Acad Sci USA. 2005;102:18455–60.
100. Red-Horse K, Ueno H, Weissman IL, Krasnow MA. Coronary arteries form by developmental reprogramming of venous cells. Nature. 2010;464:549–53.
101. Perez-Pomares JM, Carmona R, Gonzalez-Iriarte M, Atencia G, Wessels A, Munoz-Chapuli R. Origin of coronary endothelial cells from epicardial mesothelium in avian embryos. Int J Dev Biol. 2002;46:1005–13.
102. Hirakow R. Development of the cardiac blood vessels in staged human embryos. Acta Anat (Basel). 1983;115:220–30.
103. Tomanek RJ, Christensen LP, Simons M, Murakami M, Zheng W, Schatteman GC. Embryonic coronary vasculogenesis and angiogenesis are regulated by interactions between multiple FGFs and VEGF and are influenced by mesenchymal stem cells. Dev. Dyn. 2010;239:3182–3191.
104. Heintzberger CF. Development of myocardial vascularisation in the rat. Acta Morphol Neerl Scand. 1983;21:267–84.
105. Rongish BJ, Torry RJ, Tucker DC, Tomanek RJ. Neovascularization of embryonic rat hearts cultured in oculo closely mimics in utero coronary vessel development. J Vasc Res. 1994;31:206–15.
106. Ratajska A, Czarnowska E, Kolodzinska A, Kluzek W, Lesniak W. Vasculogenesis of the embryonic heart: origin of blood island-like

structures. Anat Rec A Discov Mol Cell Evol Biol. 2006;288: 223–32.
107. Tomanek RJ, Hansen HK, Dedkov EI. Vascular patterning of the quail coronary system during development. Anat Rec A Discov Mol Cell Evol Biol. 2006;288:989–99.
108. Tomanek RJ, Ishii Y, Holifield JS, Sjogren CL, Hansen HK, Mikawa T. VEGF family members regulate myocardial tubulogenesis and coronary artery formation in the embryo. Circ Res. 2006;98:947–53.
109. Kattan J, Dettman RW, Bristow J. Formation and remodeling of the coronary vascular bed in the embryonic avian heart. Dev Dyn. 2004;230:34–43.
110. Ratajska A, Czarnowska E, Kolodzinska A, Jablonska A, Stachurska E. New morphological aspects of blood islands formation in the embryonic mouse hearts. Histochem Cell Biol. 2009;131:297–311.
111. Majesky MW. Developmental basis of vascular smooth muscle diversity. Arterioscler Thromb Vasc Biol. 2007;27:1248–58.
112. Wang D, Chang PS, Wang Z, Sutherland L, Richardson JA, Small E, et al. Activation of cardiac gene expression by myocardin, a transcriptional cofactor for serum response factor. Cell. 2001; 105:851–62.
113. Creemers EE, Sutherland LB, McAnally J, Richardson JA, Olson EN. Myocardin is a direct transcriptional target of Mef2, Tead and Foxo proteins during cardiovascular development. Development. 2006;133:4245–56.
114. Hoofnagle MH, Neppl RL, Berzin EL, Teg Pipes GC, Olson EN, Wamhoff BW, et al. Myocardin is differentially required for the development of smooth muscle cells and cardiomyocytes. Am J Physiol Heart Circ Physiol. 2011;300:H1707–21.
115. Gries Kamp T, Rudat C, LÜdkte TH, Norden J, Kispert A. Notch signaling regulates smooth muscle differentiation of epicardium-derived cells. Circ Res. 2011;108:813–23.
116. del Monte G, Casanova JC, Guadix JA, MacGrogan D, Burch JB, Pérez-Pomares JM, de la Pompa JL. Differential notch signaling in the epicardium is required for cardiac inflow development and coronary vessel morphogenesis. Circ Res. 2011;108:824–36.
117. Mellgren AM, Smith CL, Olsen GS, Eskiocak B, Zhou B, Kazi MN, et al. Platelet-derived growth factor receptor beta signaling is required for efficient epicardial cell migration and development of two distinct coronary vascular smooth muscle cell populations. Circ Res. 2008;103:1393–401.
118. Nelson TJ, Duncan SA, Misra RP. Conserved enhancer in the serum response factor promoter controls expression during early coronary vasculogenesis. Circ Res. 2004;94:1059–66.
119. Akhurst RJ, Lehnert SA, Faissner A, Duffie E. TGF beta in murine morphogenetic processes: the early embryo and cardiogenesis. Development. 1990;108:645–56.
120. Austin AF, Compton LA, Love JD, Brown CB, Barnett JV. Primary and immortalized mouse epicardial cells undergo differentiation in response to TGFbeta. Dev Dyn. 2008;237:366–76.
121. Snider P, Standley KN, Wang J, Azhar M, Doetschman T, Conway SJ. Origin of cardiac fibroblasts and the role of periostin. Circ Res. 2009;105:934–47.
122. Diaz-Flores L, Gutierrez R, Madrid JF, Varela H, Valladares F, Acosta E, et al. Pericytes. Morphofunction, interactions and pathology in a quiescent and activated mesenchymal cell niche. Histol Histopathol. 2009;24:909–69.
123. Yamashita J, Itoh H, Hirashima M, Ogawa M, Nishikawa S, Yurugi T, et al. Flk1-positive cells derived from embryonic stem cells serve as vascular progenitors. Nature. 2000;408:92–6.
124. Tomanek RJ, Holifield JS, Reiter RS, Sandra A, Lin JJ. Role of VEGF family members and receptors in coronary vessel formation. Dev Dyn. 2002;225:233–40.
125. Rongish BJ, Hinchman G, Doty MK, Baldwin HS, Tomanek RJ. Relationship of the extracellular matrix to coronary neovascularization during development. J Mol Cell Cardiol. 1996;28:2203–15.
126. Oštádal B, Schiebler T, Rychter Z. Relations between the development of the capillary wall and myoarchitecture of the rat heart. Adv Exp Med Biol. 1975;53:375–88.
127. Porter GA, Bankston PW. Functional maturation of the capillary wall in the fetal and neonatal rat heart: permeability characteristics of developing myocardial capillaries. Am J Anat. 1987;180: 323–31.
128. Tomanek RJ, Ratajska A, Kitten GT, Yue X, Sandra A. Vascular endothelial growth factor expression coincides with coronary vasculogenesis and angiogenesis. Dev Dyn. 1999;215:54–61.
129. Tomanek RJ, Hu N, Phan B, Clark EB. Rate of coronary vascularization during embryonic chicken development is influenced by the rate of myocardial growth. Cardiovasc Res. 1999;41:663–71.
130. Bolender D, Olson M, Markwald R. Coronary vessel vasculogenesis. Ann NY Acad Sci. 1990;588:340–4.
131. Yue X, Tomanek RJ. Stimulation of coronary vasculogenesis/angiogenesis by hypoxia in cultured embryonic hearts. Dev Dyn. 1999;216:28–36.
132. Yue X, Tomanek RJ. Effects of VEGF(165) and VEGF(121) on vasculogenesis and angiogenesis in cultured embryonic quail hearts. Am J Physiol Heart Circ Physiol. 2001;280:H2240–7.
133. Nanka O, Valasek P, Dvorakova M, Grim M. Experimental hypoxia and embryonic angiogenesis. Dev Dyn. 2006;235:723–33.
134. Nanka O, Krizova P, Fikrle M, Tuma M, Blaha M, Grim M, et al. Abnormal myocardial and coronary vasculature development in experimental hypoxia. Anat Rec (Hoboken). 2008;291:1187–99.
135. Wikenheiser J, Doughman YQ, Fisher SA, Watanabe M. Differential levels of tissue hypoxia in the developing chicken heart. Dev Dyn. 2006;235:115–23.
136. Favier J, Kempf H, Corvol P, Gasc JM. Coexpression of endothelial PAS protein 1 with essential angiogenic factors suggests its involvement in human vascular development. Dev Dyn. 2001;222: 377–88.
137. Marti HH, Risau W. Systemic hypoxia changes the organ-specific distribution of vascular endothelial growth factor and its receptors. Proc Natl Acad Sci USA. 1998;95:15809–14.
138. Ramirez-Bergeron DL, Runge A, Dahl KD, Fehling HJ, Keller G, Simon MC. Hypoxia affects mesoderm and enhances hemangioblast specification during early development. Development. 2004; 131:4623–34.
139. Han Y, Kuang SZ, Gomer A, Ramirez-Bergeron DL. Hypoxia influences the vascular expansion and differentiation of embryonic stem cell cultures through the temporal expression of vascular endothelial growth factor receptors in an ARNT-dependent manner. Stem Cells. 2010;28:799–809.
140. Ratajska A, Torry RJ, Kitten GT, Kolker SJ, Tomanek RJ. Modulation of cell migration and vessel formation by vascular endothelial growth factor and basic fibroblast growth factor in cultured embryonic heart. Dev Dyn. 1995;203:399–407.
141. Tomanek RJ, Lotun K, Clark EB, Suvarna PR, Hu N. VEGF and bFGF stimulate myocardial vascularization in embryonic chick. Am J Physiol. 1998;274:H1620–6.
142. Tomanek RJ, Sandra A, Zheng W, Brock T, Bjercke RJ, Holifield JS. Vascular endothelial growth factor and basic fibroblast growth factor differentially modulate early postnatal coronary angiogenesis. Circ Res. 2001;88:1135–41.
143. Carmeliet P, Ferreira V, Breier G, Pollefeyt S, Kieckens L, Gertsenstein M, et al. Abnormal blood vessel development and lethality in embryos lacking a single VEGF allele. Nature. 1996; 380:435–9.
144. Miquerol L, Langille BL, Nagy A. Embryonic development is disrupted by modest increases in vascular endothelial growth factor gene expression. Development. 2000;127:3941–6.
145. Lagercrantz J, Farnebo F, Larsson C, Tvrdik T, Weber G, Piehl F. A comparative study of the expression patterns for vegf, vegf-b/vrf and vegf-c in the developing and adult mouse. Biochim Biophys Acta. 1998;1398:157–63.

146. Ikuta T, Ariga H, Matsumoto KI. Effect of tenascin-X together with vascular endothelial growth factor A on cell proliferation in cultured embryonic hearts. Biol Pharm Bull. 2001;24:1320–3.
147. Achen MG, Jeltsch M, Kukk E, Makinen T, Vitali A, Wilks AF, et al. Vascular endothelial growth factor D (VEGF-D) is a ligand for the tyrosine kinases VEGF receptor 2 (Flk1) and VEGF receptor 3 (Flt4). Proc Natl Acad Sci USA. 1998;95:548–53.
148. Makinen T, Olofsson B, Karpanen T, Hellman U, Soker S, Klagsbrun M, et al. Differential binding of vascular endothelial growth factor B splice and proteolytic isoforms to neuropilin-1. J Biol Chem. 1999;274:21217–22.
149. Pepper M, Mandriota S, Jeltsch M, Kumar V, Alitalo K. Vascular endothelial growth factor (VEGF)-C synergizes with basic fibroblast growth factor and VEGF in the induction of angiogenesis in vitro and alters endothelial cell extracellular proteolytic activity. J Cell Physiol. 1998;177:439–52.
150. Lavine KJ, Ornitz DM. Shared circuitry: developmental signaling cascades regulate both embryonic and adult coronary vasculature. Circ Res. 2009;104:159–69.
151. Lavine KJ, Yu K, White AC, Zhang X, Smith C, Partanen J, et al. Endocardial and epicardial derived FGF signals regulate myocardial proliferation and differentiation in vivo. Dev Cell. 2005; 8:85–95.
152. White AC, Lavine KJ, Ornitz DM. FGF9 and SHH regulate mesenchymal Vegfa expression and development of the pulmonary capillary network. Development. 2007;134:3743–52.
153. Vokes SA, Yatskievych TA, Heimark RL, McMahon J, McMahon AP, Antin PB, et al. Hedgehog signaling is essential for endothelial tube formation during vasculogenesis. Development. 2004;131:4371–80.
154. Lavine KJ, Schmid GJ, Smith CS, Ornitz DM. Novel tool to suppress cell proliferation in vivo demonstrates that myocardial and coronary vascular growth represent distinct developmental programs. Dev Dyn. 2008;237:713–24.
155. Lee SH, Schloss DJ, Swain JL. Maintenance of vascular integrity in the embryo requires signaling through the fibroblast growth factor receptor. J Biol Chem. 2000;275:33679–87.
156. Tomanek RJ, Haung L, Suvarna PR, O'Brien LC, Ratajska A, Sandra A. Coronary vascularization during development in the rat and its relationship to basic fibroblast growth factor. Cardiovasc Res. 1996;31:Spec No: E116–26.
157. Spirito P, Fu YM, Yu ZX, Epstein SE, Casscells W. Immunohistochemical localization of basic and acidic fibroblast growth factors in the developing rat heart. Circulation. 1991;84: 322–32.
158. Joseph-Silverstein J, Consigli SA, Lyser KM, Ver Pault C. Basic fibroblast growth factor in the chick embryo: immunolocalization to striated muscle cells and their precursors. J Cell Biol. 1989; 108:2459–66.
159. Pennisi DJ, Mikawa T. Normal patterning of the coronary capillary plexus is dependent on the correct transmural gradient of FGF expression in the myocardium. Dev Biol. 2005;279:378–90.
160. Montano MM, Doughman YQ, Deng H, Chaplin L, Yang J, Wang N, et al. Mutation of the HEXIM1 gene results in defects during heart and vascular development partly through downregulation of vascular endothelial growth factor. Circ Res. 2008;102: 415–22.
161. Tevosian SG, Deconinck AE, Tanaka M, Schinke M, Litovsky SH, Izumo S, et al. FOG-2, a cofactor for GATA transcription factors, is essential for heart morphogenesis and development of coronary vessels from epicardium. Cell. 2000;101:729–39.
162. Zhou B, Ma Q, Kong SW, Hu Y, Campbell PH, McGowan FX, et al. Fog2 is critical for cardiac function and maintenance of coronary vasculature in the adult mouse heart. J Clin Invest. 2009;119: 1462–76.
163. Zeini M, Hang CT, Lehrer-Graiwer J, Dao T, Zhou B, Chang CP. Spatial and temporal regulation of coronary vessel formation by calcineurin-NFAT signaling. Development. 2009;136:3335–45.
164. Bogers AJ, Gittenberger-de Groot AC, Poelmann RE, Peault BM, Huysmans HA. Development of the origin of the coronary arteries, a matter of ingrowth or outgrowth? Anat Embryol (Berl). 1989;180:437–41.
165. Waldo KL, Kumiski DH, Kirby ML. Association of the cardiac neural crest with development of the coronary arteries in the chick embryo. Anat Rec. 1994;239:315–31.
166. Ando K, Nakajima Y, Yamagishi T, Yamamoto S, Nakamura H. Development of proximal coronary arteries in quail embryonic heart: multiple capillaries penetrating the aortic sinus fuse to form main coronary trunk. Circ Res. 2004;94:346–52.
167. Velkey JM, Bernanke DH. Apoptosis during coronary artery orifice development in the chick embryo. Anat Rec. 2001;262:310–7.
168. Ratajska A, Fiejka E. Prenatal development of coronary arteries in the rat: morphologic patterns. Anat Embryol (Berl). 1999;200: 533–40.
169. Ratajska A, Fiejka E, Sieminska J. Prenatal development of coronary arteries in the rat: morphometric patterns. Folia Morphol (Warsz). 2000;59:297–306.
170. Eralp I, Lie-Venema H, DeRuiter MC, van den Akker NM, Bogers AJ, Mentink MM, et al. Coronary artery and orifice development is associated with proper timing of epicardial outgrowth and correlated fas ligand associated apoptosis patterns. Circ Res. 2005;96: 526–34.
171. Rychter Z, Ostadal B. Fate of "sinusoidal" intertrabecular spaces of the cardiac wall after development of the coronary vascular bed in chick embryo. Folia Morphol (Praha). 1971;19:31–44.
172. Wothe D, Hohimer A, Morton M, Thornburg K, Giraud G, Davis L. Increased coronary blood flow signals growth of coronary resistance vessels in near-term ovine fetuses. Am J Physiol Regul Integr Comp Physiol. 2002;282:R295–302.
173. Ziche M, Parenti A, Ledda F, Dell'Era P, Granger HJ, Maggi CA, et al. Nitric oxide promotes proliferation and plasminogen activator production by coronary venular endothelium through endogenous bFGF. Circ Res. 1997;80:845–52.
174. Gu JW, Brady AL, Anand V, Moore MC, Kelly WC, Adair TH. Adenosine upregulates VEGF expression in cultured myocardial vascular smooth muscle cells. Am J Physiol. 1999;277: H595–602.
175. Yamamoto K, Sokabe T, Watabe T, Miyazono K, Yamashita JK, Obi S, et al. Fluid shear stress induces differentiation of Flk-1-positive embryonic stem cells into vascular endothelial cells in vitro. Am J Physiol Heart Circ Physiol. 2005;288:H1915–24.
176. Ando K, Takahashi M, Yamagishi T, Miyagawa-Tomita S, Imanaka-Yoshida K, Yoshida T, et al. Tenascin C may regulate the recruitment of smooth muscle cells during coronary artery development. Differentiation. 2011;81:299–306.
177. Ishigaki T, Imanaka-Yoshida K, Shimojo N, Matsushima S, Taki W, Yoshida T. Tenascin-C enhances crosstalk signaling of integrin alphavbeta3/PDGFR-beta complex by SRC recruitment promoting PDGF-induced proliferation and migration in smooth muscle cells. J Cell Physiol. 2011;226:2617–24.
178. Tomanek RJ, Hansen HK, Christensen LP. Temporally expressed PDGF and FGF-2 regulate embryonic coronary artery formation and growth. Arterioscler Thromb Vasc Biol. 2008;28:1237–43.
179. Bogers AJ, Bartelings MM, Bokenkamp R, Stijnen T, van Suylen RJ, Poelmann RE, et al. Common arterial trunk, uncommon coronary arterial anatomy. J Thorac Cardiovasc Surg. 1993;106: 1133–7.
180. Hood LC, Rosenquist TH. Coronary artery development in the chick: origin and deployment of smooth muscle cells, and the effects of neural crest ablation. Anat Rec. 1992;234:291–300.

181. Jiang X, Rowitch DH, Soriano P, McMahon AP, Sucov HM. Fate of the mammalian cardiac neural crest. Development. 2000;127: 1607–16.
182. Hellstrom M, Kalen M, Lindahl P, Abramsson A, Betsholtz C. Role of PDGF-B and PDGFR-beta in recruitment of vascular smooth muscle cells and pericytes during embryonic blood vessel formation in the mouse. Development. 1999;126:3047–55.
183. Ratajska A, Zarska M, Quensel C, Kramer J. Differentiation of the smooth muscle cell phenotypes during embryonic development of coronary vessels in the rat. Histochem Cell Biol. 2001;116:79–87.
184. Watanabe T, Koibuchi N, Chin MT. Transcription factor CHF1/ Hey2 regulates coronary vascular maturation. Mech Dev. 2010;127:418–27.
185. Kim H, Yoon CS, Rah B. Expression of extracellular matrix components fibronectin and laminin in the human fetal heart. Cell Struct Funct. 1999;24:19–26.
186. Moss JB, Xavier-Neto J, Shapiro MD, Nayeem SM, McCaffery P, Drager UC, et al. Dynamic patterns of retinoic acid synthesis and response in the developing mammalian heart. Dev Biol. 1998;199:55–71.
187. Azambuja AP, Portillo-Sanchez V, Rodrigues MV, Omae SV, Schechtman D, Strauss BE, et al. Retinoic acid and VEGF delay smooth muscle relative to endothelial differentiation to coordinate inner and outer coronary vessel wall morphogenesis. Circ Res. 2010;107:204–16.
188. Ratajska A, Ciszek B, Sowinska A. Embryonic development of coronary vasculature in rats: corrosion casting studies. Anat Rec. 2003;270A:109–16.
189. Eliska O, Eliskova M, Miller AJ. The absence of lymphatics in normal and atherosclerotic coronary arteries in man: a morphologic study. Lymphology. 2006;39:76–83.
190. Sacchi G, Weber E, Agliano M, Cavina N, Comparini L. Lymphatic vessels of the human heart: precollectors and collecting vessels. A morpho-structural study. J Submicrosc Cytol Pathol. 1999;31: 515–25.
191. Rychter Z, Jelinek R, Klika E, Antalikova L. Development of the lymph bed in the wall of the chick embryo heart. Physiol Bohemoslov. 1971;20:533–9.
192. Klika E, Antalikova L, Rychter Z, Jelinek R. Inception and manner of development of the lymph vessels in the chick embryo heart. Lymphology. 1972;5:137–48.
193. Wilting J, Buttler K, Schulte I, Papoutsi M, Schweigerer L, Manner J. The proepicardium delivers hemangioblasts but not lymphangioblasts to the developing heart. Dev Biol. 2007;305:451–9.
194. Juszynski M, Ciszek B, Stachurska E, Jablonska A, Ratajska A. Development of lymphatic vessels in mouse embryonic and early postnatal hearts. Dev Dyn. 2008;237:2973–86.
195. Karunamuni G, Yang K, Doughman YQ, Wikenheiser J, Bader D, Barnett J, et al. Expression of lymphatic markers during avian and mouse cardiogenesis. Anat Rec (Hoboken). 2010;293:259–70.
196. Jussila L, Alitalo K. Vascular growth factors and lymphangiogenesis. Physiol Rev. 2002;82:673–700.
197. Yamada S, Samtani RR, Lee ES, Lockett E, Uwabe C, Shiota K, et al. Developmental atlas of the early first trimester human embryo. Dev Dyn. 2010;239:1585–95.
198. Conte G, Pellegrini A. On the development of the coronary arteries in human embryos, stages 14-19. Anat Embryol (Berl). 1984;169:209–18.
199. Mandarim-de-Lacerda CA. Development of the coronary arteries in staged human embryos (the Paris Embryological Collection revisited). An Acad Bras Cienc. 1990;62:79–84.
200. Licata R. The human embryonic heart in the ninth week. Am J Anat. 1954;94:73–125.
201. Partanen TA, Makinen T, Arola J, Suda T, Weich HA, Alitalo K. Endothelial growth factor receptors in human fetal heart. Circulation. 1999;100:583–6.
202. Rychter Z, Jirasek JE, Rychterova V, Uher J. Vascularization of heart in human embryo: location and shape of non-vascularized part of cardiac wall. Folia Morphol (Praha). 1975;23:88–96.
203. Cortis BS, Serratto M. The collateral coronary circulation in the human fetus: angiographic findings. Cardiologia. 1998;43:77–81.

3 Postnatal Coronary Morphogenesis and Growth

Abbreviations

EC	Endothelial cell
FGF	Fibroblast growth factor
LV	Left ventricle
L_V	Length density (length/mm^3)
N_A	Numerical density (number/mm^2)
RV	Right ventricle
S_V	Surface density (surface area/mm^3)
TGF-β	Transforming growth factor β
VEGF	Vascular endothelial factor
V_V	Volume density (volume/mm^3)

Introduction

The early postnatal stage of development is characterized by a rapid growth of the myocardium, which occurs by increases in both cardiomyocyte volume and number. This marked and rapid myocardial growth requires a rapid and substantial expansion of the coronary vasculature. In this regard, it has been documented that in the rat heart, approximately 50% of the capillary bed present in the adult is formed during the first 3 or 4 weeks of life [1]. Many studies have addressed capillary growth using quantitative methods to assess various capillary parameters. These approaches are explained in the following section.

Methods for Quantitative Assessment of Vessel Growth

Vascular growth may involve several types of changes. The absolute volume or volume density of the vasculature can occur as a consequence of changes in absolute vessel number or numerical density. Moreover, surface area may be altered. Because myocardial volume increases during postnatal growth and during hypertrophy in the adult, vascular parameters are expressed as densities, i.e., number, length, volume, or surface area per tissue volume. The use of morphometry has enabled investigators to specify changes in specific vessel types, as well as the magnitude of the changes. The parameters assessed as indices of vascular growth are described below.

Numerical, Length, Volume, and Surface Densities

Numerical density is perhaps the most widely used parameter to estimate vessel growth, but is also one that can be prone to error since vessels in the heart are not sufficiently anisotropic, i.e., not all vessels are present in the same plane. If sufficient sampling is done with care regarding the polarity of cardiomyocytes, numerical density of capillaries may be a reasonable estimate of capillary growth. Numerical density is expressed as number per mm^2 (N_A). However, length density, expressed as the total vessel length in a mm^3 of tissue (L_V), is a more accurate measure of vascularity in that it is adjusted for vessel orientation. L_V estimated in my lab is based on the major (a) and minor (b) axes of the vessel profile according to the formula: $L_V = a/b$ x number of vessel profiles/mm^2. Volume density (V_V), i.e., total vessel volume/mm^3, provides an index of flow potential of the vascular system, while surface density (S_V), i.e., surface area/mm^3, relates to the area of the vessel's lumen available for O_2 exchange between blood and tissue.

Cell Proliferation, Diffusion Distance and Capillary/Myocardial Cell Ratio

Proliferation of vascular cells is estimated by DNA labeling and expressed as percent of cells labeled. A limitation of this approach is that the estimate may be obtained during a period when proliferation has ceased or has not yet begun. This problem may be overcome by obtaining measurements at multiple time points. Capillary/cardiomyocyte ratios are an approximation of capillary proliferation only if cardiomyocyte proliferation is no longer occurring.

Diffusion Distance and Capillary Domain

Diffusion distance, defined as 0.5 X mean intercapillary distance, provides an index of the maximal distance for O_2 diffusion. Because capillary spacing in the myocardium is

R.J. Tomanek, *Coronary Vasculature: Development, Structure-Function, and Adaptations*,
DOI 10.1007/978-1-4614-4887-7_3, © Springer Science+Business Media New York 2013

heterogeneous, diffusion distance varies. For this reason, an index of heterogeneity is used to quantify the degree of heterogeneity of spacing. Computerized images are employed to demonstrate capillary domains, and the Log SD of the domains provides an index of heterogeneity. Capillary domain is defined as the tissue area supplied by an individual capillary.

Capillary Growth

Early Postnatal Growth

One of the earliest studies to address postnatal capillary growth utilized hearts from neonatal-adult rabbits [2]. The data revealed that a sufficient capillary proliferation compensated for the cardiomyocyte growth, thus maintaining a fairly constant capillary density. Studies on rats [3] and humans [4] also provided evidence that capillary proliferation exceeds that of cardiomyocytes during the early postnatal period. The overall vascular capacity of the rat heart, as determined by albumin ^{131}I perfusions, was found to be characterized by large increases during the first 4 weeks of postnatal life, and diffusion distance and heart weight were found to be closely related (r=0.81) [5]. Subsequently, Rakusan and colleagues [6] found that three stages of growth were evident in the rat heart (1) proliferation of both cardiomyocytes and capillaries (1–4 weeks); (2) cessation of cardiomyocyte proliferation, but continuation of capillary proliferation (4–7 weeks);and (3) cessation of capillary proliferation, resulting in a constant capillary/cardiomyocyte ratio (after 7 weeks). The robust extent of capillary growth during the first 3 weeks is indicated by the finding that the capillary/cardiomyocyte ratio nearly doubles during this time period. Thus, during the early postnatal period, the addition of new capillaries exceeds the addition of new cardiomyocytes. The first week of postnatal life includes an organization of the capillary bed so that the major orientation of most capillaries is along the long axis of cardiomyocytes [7].

In lambs, the first few days after birth are characterized by a large increase in ventricular work and O_2 consumption, especially in the left ventricle (LV) [8]. For this reason, it is not surprising that capillary growth is substantial during this time period. Data from rat hearts denote that capillary growth reaches a peak during the first 11 days of postnatal life as evidenced by a morphometric study that based measurements on electron micrographs [9]. During this time period capillary/cardiomyocyte ratio increased fivefold and diffusion distance decreased by 45% in the LV (Fig. 3.1). Total capillary length increased 19-fold from day 1 to day 11 and the capillary growth in each ventricle was proportional to the increase in muscle volume. Capillary growth in the right ventricle (RV) was less than that of the LV. For instance, capillary surface areas in the RV and LV between day 1 and day 11 increased 7.6- and 15.0-fold, respectively. These values are consistent with the data that show a volume increase of the LV free wall between 1 and 11 days that is double that of the RV. Another study [10] reported that between birth and 13 days, the rat myocardial capillary volume density is increased by 60% and surface density is doubled.

The high metabolic rate noted at the time of birth in lambs remains elevated for the next 2 weeks and then declines gradually to adult values [8]. Diffusion distance in the rat myocardium, of importance for the maintenance of tissue PO_2, decreases during the first 11 days of postnatal life as capillary angiogenesis peaks [9]. Intussusceptive angiogenesis during early postnatal growth of the heart has been documented as a mechanism that contributes to the increase in capillary numbers [11]. Coronary capillary endothelial cells (ECs) undergo a maturation process during postnatal growth, as observed during the first 5 weeks in dogs [12]. An increase in capillary vesicles and a decrease in EC thickness were noted; the study concluded that blood flow may act as a molding force for vascular lumens.

The changes in vascularity that occur during the perinatal period were quantified in sheep, a species often used in studies addressing cardiovascular development [13]. They found that during the first 2 weeks of postnatal life, the capillary/cardiomyocyte ratio and capillary density were lower in the left than in the right ventricle, resulting in a greater diffusion distance in the LV. By the fourth week, capillary density and capillary/cardiomyocyte ratio are similar in the two ventricles, indicating an accelerated vascular growth in the LV, which exceeds that of the RV. Taken together, these data underscore the importance of the early postnatal period in neovascularization of the myocardium.

Later Postnatal Growth

Subsequent to the rapid and robust capillary growth during the first 4 postnatal weeks in the rat, capillary growth begins to lag behind cardiomyocyte growth (Fig. 3.1), as evidenced by a threefold increase in left ventricular weight accompanied by a 31% decline in capillary length density between week 5 and week 13 [14]. This drop in capillary length density occurs despite the fact that total capillary length during this period more than doubles. Thus, capillary growth does not fully compensate for myocardial growth. However, capillary volume density is relatively stable during this 8-week period with values between 9 and 10%. Human hearts also undergo a rapid capillary growth during the first few years of postnatal life, as documented by increases in capillary/cardiomyocyte ratio [4]. This ratio is stable after the age of 20 years. Postnatal capillary growth in humans reveals that the more than fourfold increase in heart weight between infancy (<1 year) and childhood (9–14 years) is associated

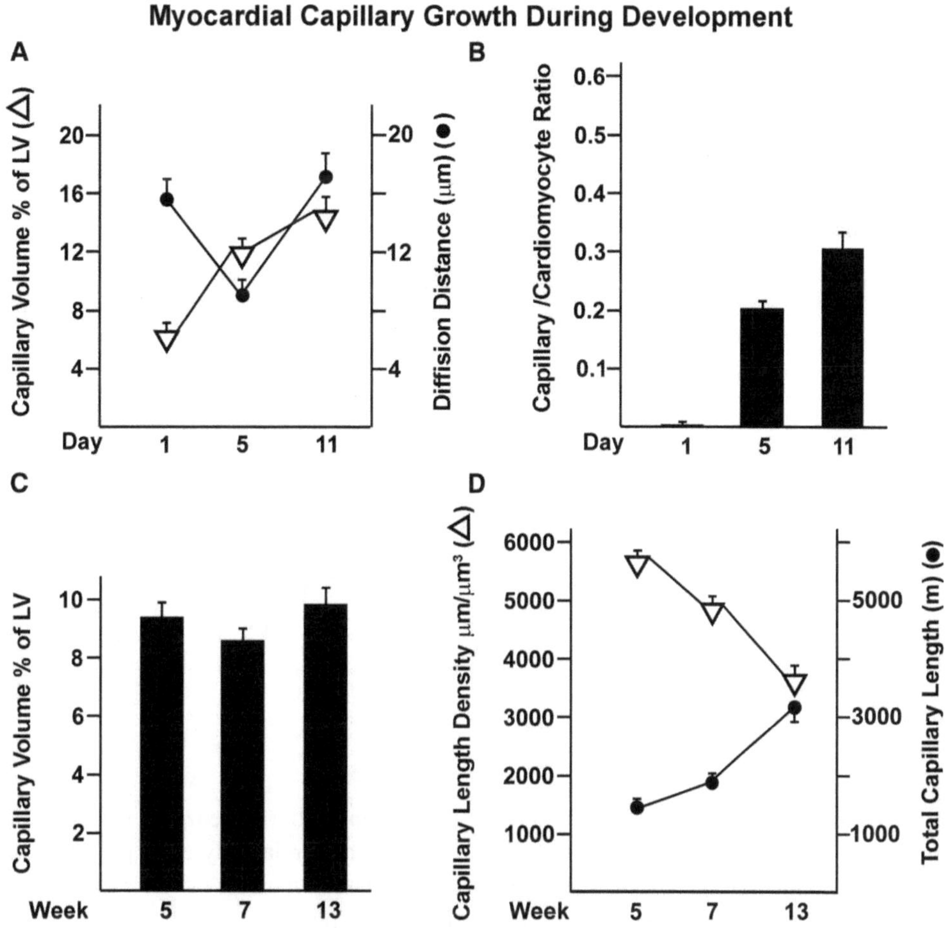

Fig. 3.1 Changes in key capillaries parameters during early postnatal development in rats. (**a**) and (**b**) are data on the first 11 days of postnatal life [9]. Diffusion distance drops during the first 5 days (**a**) due to a proliferation of capillaries that exceeds that of cardiomyocytes (**b**). Between weeks 5 and 13 of postnatal life (data in **c** and **d**) from Mattfeldt and Mall [14]). Capillary volume density is unaltered (**c**) due to continued capillary growth, as indicated by a doubling of total capillary length (**d**). Nevertheless, the large increase in heart mass causes a drop in capillary length density (**d**)

with a 28% decline in capillary density and a 37% increase in capillary domain, as illustrated in Fig. 3.2 [15]. These parameters remain stable into adulthood (ages 15–30 years), despite a further heart weight increase of 43%. Thus, the data indicate that capillary growth continues in the young adult. A comparison of the hearts of children (mean age 5 years) with adults (mean age 50 years) signified a decrease in capillary density of only 11% [4].

Functional capillary density defines the number of capillaries open at a given time point and relates to intercapillary distance. Measurements in beating hearts of rats aged 40–400 days demonstrated an increase in functional intercapillary distance from 12.5 to 19.5 μm [16]. Thus, capillary recruitment was insufficient for maintaining a favorable intercapillary distance. A subsequent study reported values for functional intercapillary distances in rats weighing between 250 and 600 g [17]. However, their data revealed that these values were not significantly altered by increases in heart weight, and that hypoxemia resulted in significant capillary recruitment. However, the concept of capillary recruitment under conditions of hypoxia was not supported by two other studies [18, 19].

Accelerated Myocardial Growth

Pressure overload induced by aortic constriction has been used to study the response of capillaries to accelerated myocardial growth. When pressure overload was induced in 5-day-old rats, capillary growth occurred, but failed to match the twofold increase in LV weight [20]. A narrow window of accelerated capillary growth during early postnatal growth is indicated by a study in which aortic constriction was induced in 2-and 6-day-old rats that were then studied at 60 days; increases in left ventricular weight were 71% and 34% in the rats constricted on days 2 and 6, respectively [21]. Capillary/cardiomyocyte ratios in the rats constricted at 6 days of age were similar to the controls, but this parameter was

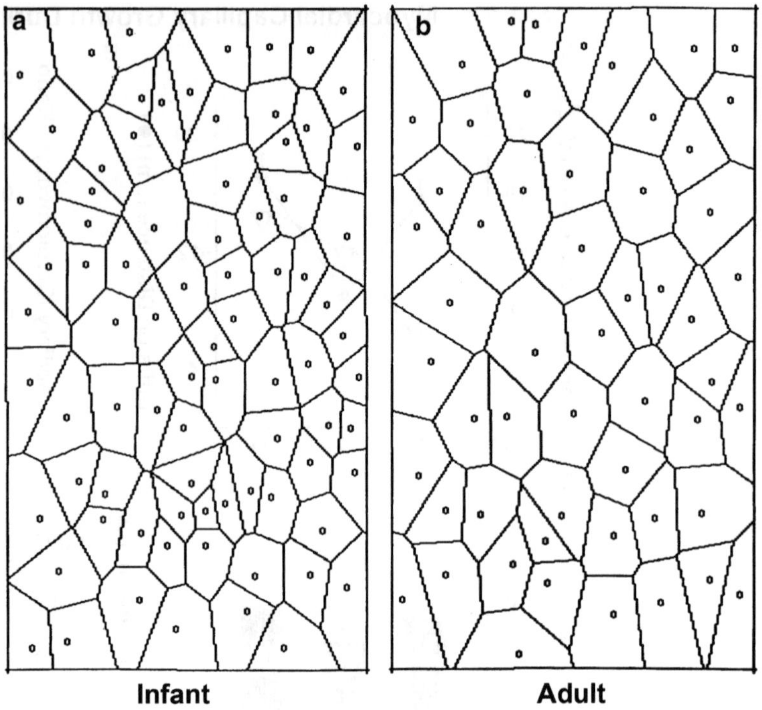

Fig. 3.2 Computer printouts of capillaries (*open circles*) and their domains from an human infant heart (**a**) and an adult heart (**b**). Note the larger capillary domains in the adult; the result from increases in cardiomyocyte cross-sectional areas during postnatal growth (Figure is from Rakusan et al. [15] and was reproduced by permission from Wolters Kluwer)

significantly higher in the rats constricted at age 2 days. Thus, the initiation of the accelerated cardiac growth at an earlier time point caused a capillary growth that was in excess of ventricular growth. These data demonstrate that compensatory capillary growth occurs when pressure overload is initiated during the first week of life and that growth is more marked if initiated earlier during this time period. Similarly, compensatory capillary growth occurs in humans with congenital aortic stenosis [15]. In these individuals, heart weight during infancy was already higher than in nonstenotic controls. Yet capillary density and capillary domain area did not differ from controls in this age group or in adults. Similarly, a 25% biventricular hypertrophy in rats with sideropenic anemia initiated at the time of weaning was characterized by a compensatory capillary and arteriolar growth [22]. Previous observations also noted that capillary density was not altered in infants and children by the presence of pressure or volume overload [23].

Capillary Arteriolar and Venular Domains

Since the arteriolar and venular ends of capillaries differ with regard to pressure and PO_2 values, it follows that the domains of arteriolar capillaries are more favorable for an O_2 supply than those of venular capillaries. Although the ultrastructural differentiation of rat myocardial capillaries is generally complete by the 12th postnatal day [24], the ontogenic development of endothelial cell enzymes of the capillaries continues to develop. In the rat, enzyme heterogeneity occurs later as indicated by a relatively early positive reaction for alkaline phosphatase, but a delay in the expression of dipeptidyl peptidase until postnatal day 20 [25]. Using immunohistochemistry for these enzymes, Batra and Rakusan [26] were able to distinguish myocardial arteriolar (alkaline phosphatase positive) and venular (dipeptidyl peptidase IV positive) capillaries. Their work revealed that by 21 postnatal days, these domains were distinguishable in the rat heart. They found that at all stages between 3 and 34 weeks, venular domains are smaller than their arteriolar counterparts, a finding that is consistent with the lower PO_2 in the former.

The smaller venular capillary domains (reflecting a greater density of venular capillaries) indicate a greater branching or tortuosity at the venular end than at the arteriolar end, a finding that is consistent with the data indicating that capillary growth occurs in response to enhanced metabolism at the venular ends of capillaries [27]. Differentiation of these coronary capillary segments progresses after the first week of postnatal life when a few capillaries are positive for dipeptidyl peptidase [28]; by 21 days, the two components are more clearly visible [26]. Thus, capillary geometry is adjusted to provide smaller diffusion distances for O_2 at the venular ends of the capillaries. Analysis of morphometric data based on the Krogh tissue cylinder model indicates that capillary geometry is able to compensate for the low hemoglobin concentrations that occur during postnatal development [29]. Arteriolar segment length in the rat myocardium continues to increase during postnatal growth, whereas venular

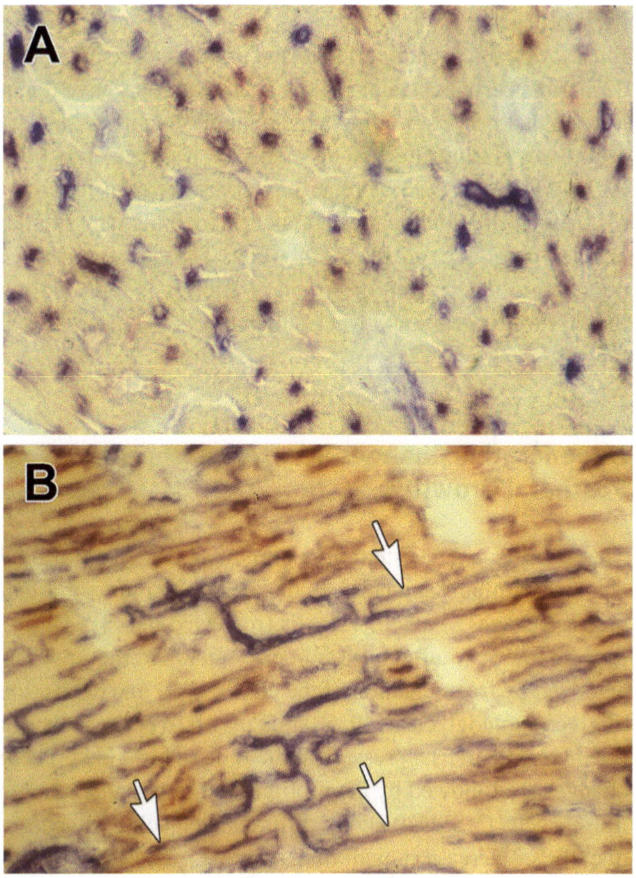

Fig. 3.3 Arteriolar (*blue*) and venular (*red*) capillary segments in a 21-day-old rat. The differentiation of these capillary segments is made possible by immunohistochemistry (see text). Note the staggering of these capillary portions as seen in a cross-sectional field (**a**). In long section (**b**), the transformation from arteriolar to venular capillary can be seen (*arrows*)

segment length plateaus [30]. The venular and arteriolar capillary segments are staggered in relation to a given cardiomyocyte (Fig. 3.3), thus providing at least one arteriolar segment at any given level of cardiomyocyte.

Possible Mechanisms Regulating Postnatal Capillary Growth

Mechanical Factors

As noted in Chaps. 1 and 2, mechanical factors (such as shear stress, stretch, and wall tension) play key roles in microvascular growth. One can appreciate that the increase in metabolism at birth is accompanied by an elevation in blood flow that is associated with increased myocardial capillary growth. Chronic administration of dipyridamole (which increases coronary blood flow by preventing reuptake of adenosine) in young rats doubled the EC uptake of ^{3}H-thymidine, an index of cell proliferation [31]. ECs subjected to increased flow are activated, whereas they are inactivated by decreased flow [32]. Studies in my laboratory have documented that coronary microvascular ECs subjected to stretch (1) upregulate VEGF mRNA and protein; (2) upregulate their VEGFR-2 and Tie-2 expression, and (3) undergo proliferation and migration [33, 34]. These activated (stretched) cells form longer vascular tubes, more branches, and migrate further than non-stretched cells. Thus, one can appreciate how the sudden establishment of coronary flow in the fetus serves as a stimulus for capillary proliferation and vascular growth. This response is likely heightened at the time of birth when flow demand increases, especially in the LV, as rapid growth of the heart increases O_2 demand.

Hypoxia

This is the subject of Chap. 9. The importance of hypoxia during prenatal morphogenesis was discussed in Chap. 2. In explanted mouse heart samples in culture, endothelial sprouts formed under normoxic conditions in samples from 4-week- but not 12-week-old mice [35]. However, under hypoxic conditions, substantial sprouting occurred in the 12 week old group. These findings suggest that late postnatal myocardial angiogenesis is decreased in comparison to an earlier postnatal stage, but is activated in the context of hypoxia.

Mast Cells

A role for mast cells in myocardial capillary growth was suggested by Rakusan and Turek [1] who showed that protamine inhibition, which blocks heparin release from mast cells, limited capillary growth in neonatal rats. A subsequent study, which tested the hypothesis that increases in mast cell numbers occur at the time of increased capillary proliferation, showed that during the first month of postnatal development, mast cell density increased more than tenfold and then declined [36]. Further support for this hypothesis was obtained from rats exposed to high altitude. Mast cell density was significantly increased in the RV even though its mass increased two fold by exposure to chronic hypoxia. Consistent with these data is a study on neonatal rats with cardiac hypertrophy in response to aortic constriction that found that a failure of capillary length to increase in proportion to cardiac mass was associated with a lower mast cell numerical density [20]. Increases in mast cell density are associated with increases in matrix metalloproteinase activity and extracellular matrix degradation [37], factors that are required for angiogenesis. Mast cells also play a role in ventricular remodeling in chronic volume overload [38]. Thus, these cells appear to influence vascularity in both physiological and pathological growth of the heart.

Angiogenic Molecules

Both VEGF and FGF-2 have been found to facilitate capillary growth during the postnatal period [39]. Antibodies to either of these angiogenic factors reduce capillary growth.

Brain derived neurotrophic factor (BDNF) has been shown to be of importance in myocardial capillary development as demonstrated in heterozygous BDNF mice [40]. These mice have impaired EC survival in myocardial capillaries and arteries and die during the early postnatal period due to vascular instability.

Arterial and Arteriolar Growth

Early Rapid Growth of Main Coronary Arteries

Examination of the postnatal coronary arterial tree in the rat demonstrated that the major branches are formed by postnatal day 12 [41], thus subsequent growth involves remodeling to increase diameters and the formation of smaller arteries and arterioles. Measurements of the two main coronary arteries in this species revealed that between 2 and 8 days, the diameter of the left artery increased by 62%, whereas that of the right artery increased by only 38%, a difference that may be attributed to the rapid transition from fetal to adult circulation [42]. During this 6-day period, the length of the two main coronary arteries nearly doubled. Similarly, in humans, the left main coronary artery has a larger diameter than the right; this difference persists throughout development [43]. The major coronary arteries increase in diameter and wall thickness from infancy to adulthood, but wall to lumen ratios tend to decrease. Moreover, the arterial growth tends to be greater in males than in females. A study utilizing human corrosive casts revealed length increases in the left coronary artery and its first- and second-order branches that were relatively proportional to the linear increases in heart mass during postnatal growth [44]. However, the authors failed to find evidence that new first-or second-order branches were formed during the postnatal period.

Arterial Growth and Blood Flow

Blood Flow Volumes and Velocities

Echocardiographic measurements of the left descending coronary artery in healthy children aged 1 month to 16 years were obtained in order to assess the relationship between blood flow, cross-sectional area of the vessel, and age [45]. Not surprisingly, flow volume per heart beat and flow volume per minute increased with age, a finding consistent with the increase in cross-sectional area of the vessel. Left anterior descending artery (LAD) flow volume and LV mass were positively correlated, but myocardial perfusion/LV mass decreased with age. This occurred as a consequence of a decreased flow velocity coupled with an increased heart mass during the neonatal-adolescence growth period. The higher peak flow velocities in the younger children are likely related to higher resting heart rates and therefore greater O_2 demand.

Innervation

Innervation of coronary arteries and arterioles occurs mainly during the early postnatal period. Canine studies have documented that nerve sprouting and an increase in nerve density progresses during the first 6 weeks of postnatal life [46]. Although perivascular adrenergic nerves are seen just prior to birth, formation of their branches to innervate smaller arteries progresses to the sixth week. The development of peptidergic innervation of coronary arteries is rapid during the first week, peaks at 3 weeks, then tapers to adult levels at 6 weeks [47].

Degenerative Changes in Arteries During Postnatal Growth

There exists a consistent literature that describes arterial changes in infants and children that appear to mimic those of the early stages of atherosclerosis (reviewed in [48]). During the first few years after birth, some coronary arteries are characterized by fragmentation of the elastic layer and deposition of glycosaminoglycans [49, 50] that may be a consequence of the increased arterial pressure at the time of birth [51]. These changes are followed by the proliferation of vascular smooth muscle cells (VSMCs) and undifferentiated cells, and consequently an increase in wall thickness [52]. The early degenerative changes also include edema and are considered to be similar to pre-atherosclerotic changes seen in adults [52]. Based on a rather extensive literature regarding this topic, it is clear that the early degenerative changes occur in infants and children and even during the last weeks of gestation [43]. Disagreement regarding these changes concerns interpretation, i.e., physiological vs. pathological [48].

Moon and Rinehart [53] studied 250 individuals dying suddenly from traumatic or "natural" causes. Three histologic alterations were considered as occurring simultaneously: deposits of mucoid substance in the intima and media, areas of degeneration of the internal elastic lamina, and subendothelial fibroblast proliferation. These are the early, prelipid changes characteristic of atherosclerosis. The conclusion that these changes are indeed pathological was suggested by Wilens [54] based on several findings (1) a more common occurrence in vessels prone to atherosclerosis (e.g., coronary), (2) higher incidence in males than females, and (3) absence of these changes in species that do not develop atherosclerosis. Fangman and Hellwig [55] also considered these changes to be pathological because the appearance of thickenings is restricted to areas normally associated with atherosclerosis. A more recent communication documents not only the changes noted above but also smooth muscle infiltration and proliferation in newborn babies and infants [56]. The more common presence of these thickenings at branch points supports the idea that they may be early stages of atherosclerosis.

Possible Mechanisms Underlying Degenerative Changes

In examining the perinatal origins of coronary atherosclerosis, Leistikow and Bolande [57] suggested that this period of development is characterized by a catecholamine release that elevates arterial pressure and subjects the "delicate" coronary arteries to injury. They found that when neonatal piglets were exposed to acute (45 min) noradrenaline-induced hypertension, there occurred an exaggeration of the congenital coronary lesions. Based on this evidence and other findings, they concluded that atherosclerosis is initiated in the fetus and neonate by rheologic (deformation by flow) injury.

The possibility that the degenerative changes are transient was suggested by the finding that the changes were most prominent in 3–4-month-old infants with some decrease in older infants and young adults [50]. In reviewing the literature on the histological changes seen in neonates, Rapola and Personen [52] noted that lesions in coronary arteries in newborns may be the result of short-term noxious factors including metabolic acidosis, infections, and hypoxemia. They then raised the question of the significance of these early lesions in the development of atherosclerosis. Even though the lesions regress, there may remain minor permanent defects that may constitute pre-atherosclerotic lesions. Because these lesions were not always found at necropsy does not mean that they were not present, since most studies did not include all major coronary arteries and their branches. These observations support the hypothesis that these are pathological changes that precede lipid/macrophage deposition. Whether these alterations persist, progress or regress is not presently known, nor is it evident if environmental factors play some role.

Arteriolar Postnatal Growth

Arteriolar postnatal growth in humans involves both an increase in their numbers and development of the smooth muscle layer [58]. Between term and infancy, the density of arterioles <20 μm in diameter increased 2.6-fold and 2.2-fold in the RV and LV, respectively, whereas the density of arterioles in the 20–100-μm range remained fairly constant. In the rat, the total length of the arteriolar + arterial vasculature increased by 47% between postnatal weeks 7 and 22 and by 17% between weeks 22 and 52 [59]. This growth minimized the moderate decrease in arteriolar density.

Postnatal development of porcine coronary arteriolar trees was studied by 3D microvascular—CT reconstruction [60]. Arterioles (about 180–200 μm in diameter) were isolated and then their arterial trees were analyzed with respect to number and tortuosity of branches, cross-sectional areas, and volume of tissue perfused. The results of the study indicated that arteriolar length and the volume of tissue perfused/cross-sectional area of arterioles increased in both ventricles during late fetal development and the first postnatal month. Between one and five postnatal months, arteriolar length and the volume of tissue perfused/cross-sectional area of arterioles continues to increase; however, the increase in the LV is greater than that of the RV. The number of arteriolar generations increases from fetal to 1 month postnatal in both ventricles, but plateaus in the RV, whereas it continues to increase in the LV. In contrast, the degree of tortuosity remains constant in both ventricles. These data indicate that accelerated arteriolar growth in the LV between 1 and 5 months is consistent with the greater myocardial growth in the LV compared to that of the RV. The LV also has a high flow reserve that allows a fivefold or sixfold increase in myocardial perfusion [61].

Factors that Regulate Development of the Coronary Arteriolar and Arterial Hierarchy

As noted in Chap. 2, VEGF, FGFs, PDGF, and TGF-β facilitate growth of the coronary arterial tree during the prenatal period. To determine the roles of VEGF and FGF-2 on the development of the coronary arterial hierarchy, my colleagues and I administered neutralizing antibodies against these growth factors to neonatal rats during the second week of postnatal life [39]. We found that anti-FGF-2 attenuated arteriolar growth, as evidenced by length densities that were 42% lower than those of the non-treated controls. Although anti-VEGF did not alter arteriolar growth, when administered in combination with anti-FGF-2, it caused a marked increase in mean arteriolar diameter without a significant effect on arteriolar length density (Fig. 3.4). Analysis of arteriolar diameter classes revealed that inhibition of both growth factors shifted the length densities of the arteriolar hierarchy, i.e., the proportion of the smallest arterioles (<15 μm) comprised only 23% of arteriolar length density, whereas arterioles 26–50 μm comprised 43% of arteriolar length density. Thus, when both FGF-2 and VEGF were inhibited, the length density of the small, terminal arterioles was only 20% of control, whereas the largest class of arterioles underwent a marked increase in length density. These findings demonstrate that VEGF and FGF-2 interact to define the hierarchy of the coronary arteriolar tree. The early postnatal growth of coronary arterioles is also associated with a peak FGF-2 expression evident during the first 6 days following birth [28].

FGF-1 has also been shown to affect coronary arteriole density and arterial branches [62]. FGF-1 overexpressing mice were found to significantly increase arteriolar density by postnatal week 6 and to affect a 45% enhancement in the number of branches from the left main coronary artery. This growth was associated with a higher myocardial perfusion at various arterial pressures. Because syndecan-4 and its cytoplasmic

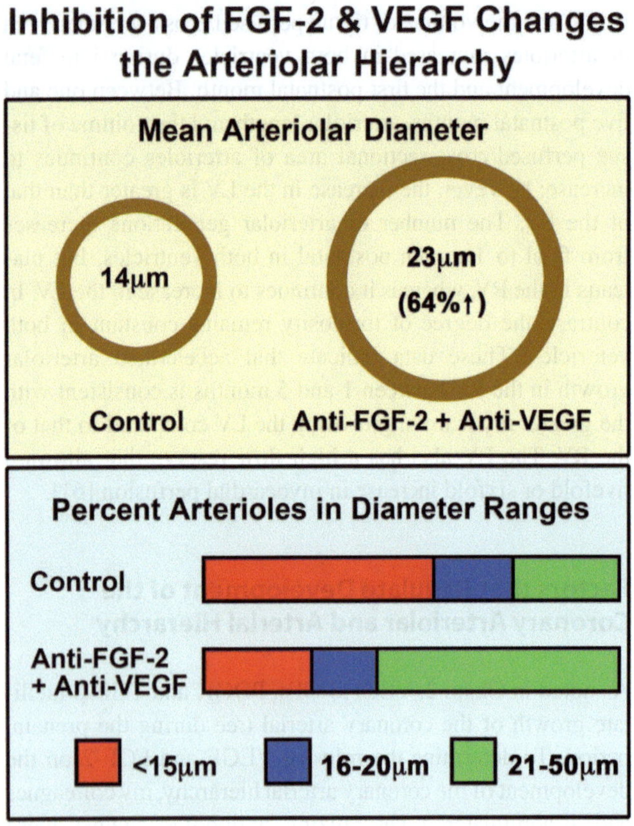

Fig. 3.4 FGF-2 and VEGF regulate the development of postnatal arteriolar hierarchy. When neonatal rats were administered neutralizing antibodies to both growth factors, there occurred decline in the length densities of the smallest arterioles and an increase in the largest arterioles (*bottom panel*). The increase in length density of the largest arterioles resulted in a larger mean arteriolar diameter (*top panel*)

binding partner, synectin, participate in FGF-2 signaling and vascular growth, work in my lab addressed their roles in coronary artery and arteriolar formation by comparing syndecan-4 and synectin null mice with their wild-type counterparts [63]. Micro-computer tomography did not reveal differences in the size and branching patterns of coronary arteries, whereas histological morphometry documented lower length and volume densities in the synectin$^{-/-}$ mice. Syndecan-4 gene disruption caused a decline in arteriolar length density in males, but an increase in this parameter in females. The gender-dependent effect of syndecan-4 may be related to the negative effect of syndecan-4 on estrogen receptors [64]. These data indicate that (1) synectin contributes to the development of coronary arterioles, but not arteries and (2) the effects of syndecan-4 are gender dependent.

Coronary Blood Flow, O_2 Consumption, and Ventricular Function

Significant changes in the workloads and consequently metabolic demand occur at the time of birth. During the fetal period (as documented in lambs), O_2 delivery and myocardial blood flow in the RV exceeds that of the LV [65]. In the neonate, the magnitude of these parameters is reversed, so that O_2 delivery and blood flow increase and decrease in the LV and RV, respectively. These changes correspond to changes in cardiac work and mass in the two chambers, i.e., the LV faces a steep rise in afterload O_2 delivery and blood flow. Changes in intermediary metabolism occur in the neonate as the heart undergoes a transition from lactate and glucose as primary energy substrates to fatty acid utilization as the main energy substrate [66]. This change enables the heart to withstand acute hypoxia or ischemia. It is well established that the fetal heart is more resistant to hypoxia than the adult heart, a finding that is likely an adaptation to its relatively hypoxic environment. Recovery of mechanical function is better in the neonatal heart than in the adult heart during severe oxygen deprivation [67]. Neonatal lambs have been shown to undergo major intracellular changes in myocardial energy metabolism and these changes include the relationship between phosphate metabolites and oxygen consumption [68, 69]. However, there are still unresolved questions regarding the effects of these metabolic changes on coronary vascular growth.

Adaptations to Enhanced Pressure Overload

This topic is also discussed in Chap. 11. The ability of the heart to adapt to pressure overload by increasing coronary vascular growth during early postnatal life is well documented. This compensatory growth includes both the (1) capillaries, enabling normal O_2 diffusion distances and (2) arteries and arterioles, enabling adequate maximal myocardial perfusion and coronary vasodilator reserve. The ability of the neonatal heart to adapt to enhanced afterload was documented in rats that underwent aortic constriction at 1 week of age [70]. At age 3 weeks, minimal coronary vascular resistance was similar in the banded and control rats despite the presence of marked left ventricular hypertrophy, i.e., left ventricular weight/body weight ratio was 80% higher than in the controls. Moreover, coronary flow recovery after 210 min of global ischemia was similar in the control and aortic constricted groups. In contrast, by age 6 weeks, the group with pressure overload displayed an attenuated increase in coronary flow after ischemia and elevated coronary vascular resistance during the reperfusion period. These data indicate that during the first 2 weeks following aortic constriction, coronary vascular cross-sectional area increased significantly, thereby compensating for the increase in ventricular mass. A failure to maintain a compensated state of the coronary vasculature during the subsequent 3 weeks may be due to either (1) a reduced ability for coronary growth or (2) the substantial additional increase in left ventricular mass and arterial pressure. During the first 2 weeks following aortic construction, arterial pressure increased by 34%, whereas between weeks 3 and 6, the increase was 70%. Studies on humans have also noted that an improved diastolic performance and increased LV coronary flow parameters accompany the enhanced LV mass in early postnatal life [71, 72].

The effects of increased pressure overload by aortic banding at 4 weeks of age was studied in 10-week-old lambs [73]. LV peak pressure was 168±10 and 101±5 mmHg in the banded and sham-operated lambs, respectively, but the degree of LV hypertrophy was mild, i.e., 20%. Minimal coronary vascular resistance (per unit LV mass) and capillary density were similar in the banded and sham lambs. These data indicate that compensatory growth of the coronary vasculature is sufficient during increased pressure overload and is associated with a normal maximal perfusion. Other studies have also established that enhanced capillary growth during pressure overload can fully compensate for the marked (twofold to threefold) increase in heart mass in both experimental animals [5, 74] and humans [15, 23]. Data obtained from infants, children, and young adults with congenital aortic stenosis signify that capillary growth compensates for cardiac hypertrophy as indicated by capillary densities and domain areas that are similar in the overloaded and control hearts [15]. This study and others are discussed in more detail in Chap. 11.

Coronary Collaterals

The idea that collaterals are formed in response to various pathological states was a concept that implied that native collaterals are nonexistent or rare. The work of Laurie and Woods [75] put to rest this assumption by providing evidence that coronary anastomoses were present in nearly all of the non-diseased human hearts examined. In individuals aged 5 years or older, 75% had significant anastomoses as determined by the observed filling of radiopaque barium–sulfate–gelatin. Moreover, even some infants had demonstrable anastomoses. One limitation of the study is that collaterals <40 μm in diameter were more difficult to discern, a limitation that probably caused an underestimation of collaterals in the neonates. A comparison of hearts from different age groups revealed that the degree of collateralization was highest in neonates and infants and then declined during childhood and adolescence and increased in adults [76]. The study also found that the incidence and quality of collaterals increased progressively with gestational maturity and body and heart weight. The authors concluded that substantial collaterals are present at the time of birth and that their involution is a reversible process. Thus, native collaterals are well documented, but their further development in later life is a function of adaptations to shear stress in response to hypoxia and ischemia. This adaptation involves a process of remodeling resulting in a substantial (2–20-fold) increase in vessel diameter [77].

Chapter Summary

Early postnatal growth is characterized by a heightened capillary proliferation required to meet the increasing myocardial metabolic demands. This growth serves to limit increases in diffusion distance and thereby maintains adequate tissue PO_2. Arteriolar growth is also impressive during the first few years of postnatal life in humans and the first few months in rodents. The development of the coronary arterial hierarchy occurs by remodeling. The number of major branches is established early. Degenerative changes in the larger arteries suggest that they are similar to the characteristics of the early stages of atherosclerosis. The ability of the neonatal heart to adapt to increased pressure overload surpasses that of the adult, in that coronary flow recovery is normal and vascular growth is substantial. The extent of coronary collaterals is high in neonates and infants, but their development in later life requires ischemic events.

References

1. Rakusan K, Turek Z. Protamine inhibits capillary formation in growing rat hearts. Circ Res. 1985;57:393–8.
2. Shipley RA, Shipley LJ, Wearn JT. The capillary supply in normal and hypertrophied hearts of rabbits. J Exp Med. 1937;65:29–42.
3. Rakusan K, Poupa O. Changes in the diffusion distance in the rat heart muscle during development. Physiol Bohemoslov. 1963;12:220–7.
4. Roberts J, Wearn J. Quantitative changes in the capillary-muscle relationship in human hearts during normal growth and hypertrophy. Am Heart J. 1941;21:617–33.
5. Rakusan K, du Mesnil de Rochemont W, Braasch W, Tschopp H, Bing RJ. Capacity of the terminal vascular bed during normal growth, in cardiomegaly, and in cardiac atrophy. Circ Res. 1967;21:209–15.
6. Rakusan K, Jel'Inek J, Koreck'Y B, Soukupov'A M, Poupa O. Postnatal development of muscle fibres and capillaries in the rat heart. Physiol Bohemoslov. 1965;14:32–7.
7. Voboril Z, Schiebler TH. Development of blood supply in the rat heart. Z Anat Entwicklungsgesch. 1969;129:24–40.
8. Smolich JJ, Berger PJ, Walker AM. Interrelation between ventricular function, myocardial blood flow, and O_2 consumption changes at birth in lambs. Am J Physiol. 1996;270:H741–9.
9. Olivetti G, Anversa P, Loud AV. Morphometric study of early postnatal development in the left and right ventricular myocardium of the rat. II. Tissue composition, capillary growth, and sarcoplasmic alterations. Circ Res. 1980;46:503–12.
10. Muhlfeld C, Singer D, Engelhardt N, Richter J, Schmiedl A. Electron microscopy and microcalorimetry of the postnatal rat heart (*Rattus norvegicus*). Comp Biochem Physiol A Mol Integr Physiol. 2005;141:310–8.
11. van Groningen JP, Wenink AC, Testers LH. Myocardial capillaries: increase in number by splitting of existing vessels. Anat Embryol (Berl). 1991;184:65–70.
12. Legato M. Cellular mechanisms of normal growth in the mammalian heat. I. Qualitative and quantitative features of ventricular architecture in the dog from birth to five months of age. Circ Res. 1979;44:250–62.

13. Smolich JJ, Walker AM, Campbell GR, Adamson TM. Left and right ventricular myocardial morphometry in fetal, neonatal, and adult sheep. Am J Physiol. 1989;257:H1–9.
14. Mattfeldt T, Mall G. Growth of capillaries and myocardial cells in the normal rat heart. J Mol Cell Cardiol. 1987;19:1237–46.
15. Rakusan K, Flanagan MF, Geva T, Southern J, Van Praagh R. Morphometry of human coronary capillaries during normal growth and the effect of age in left ventricular pressure-overload hypertrophy. Circulation. 1992;86:38–46.
16. Henquell L, Odoroff CL, Honig CR. Coronary intercapillary distance during growth: relation to PtO_2 and aerobic capacity. Am J Physiol. 1976;231:1852–9.
17. Korecky B, Hai CM, Rakusan K. Functional capillary density in normal and transplanted rat hearts. Can J Physiol Pharmacol. 1982; 60:23–32.
18. Steinhausen M, Tillmanns H, Thederan H. Microcirculation of the epimyocardial layer of the heart. I. A method for in vivo observation of the microcirculation of superficial ventricular myocardium of the heart and capillary flow pattern under normal and hypoxic conditions. Pflugers Arch. 1978;378:9–14.
19. Eliasen P, Amtorp O. Absence of capillary recruitment during increased coronary blood flow in the working dog heart. Acta Physiol Scand. 1985;124:181–7.
20. Rakusan K, Campbell SE. Spatial relationship between cardiac mast cells and coronary capillaries in neonatal rats with cardiomegaly. Can J Physiol Pharmacol. 1991;69:1750–3.
21. Kolar F, Papousek F, Pelouch V, Ostadal B, Rakusan K. Pressure overload induced in newborn rats: effects on left ventricular growth, morphology, and function. Pediatr Res. 1998;43:521–6.
22. Rakusan K, Cicutti N, Kolar F. Effect of anemia on cardiac function, microvascular structure, and capillary hematocrit in rat hearts. Am J Physiol Heart Circ Physiol. 2001;280:H1407–14.
23. Hort W, Severidt HJ. Capillarization and microscopic changes in the myocardium in congenital heart defects. Virchows Arch Pathol Anat Physiol Klin Med. 1966;341:192–203.
24. Oštádal B, Schiebler T, Rychter Z. Relations between the development of the capillary wall and myoarchitecture of the rat heart. Adv Exp Med Biol. 1975;53:375–88.
25. Lojda Z, Ostadal B, Ruzicova M. Ontogenetic development of membrane-bound proteases and some other enzymes in the endothelial lining of the capillary bed of rat and chicken myocardium. Histochem J. 1985;17:555–7.
26. Batra S, Rakusan K. Capillary network geometry during postnatal growth in rat hearts. Am J Physiol. 1992;262:H635–40.
27. Tomanek RJ, Doty MK, Sandra A. Early coronary angiogenesis in response to thyroxine: growth characteristics and upregulation of basic fibroblast growth factor. Circ Res. 1998;82:587–93.
28. Tomanek RJ, Haung L, Suvarna PR, O'Brien LC, Ratajska A, Sandra A. Coronary vascularization during development in the rat and its relationship to basic fibroblast growth factor. Cardiovasc Res. 1996;31:Spec No:E116–26.
29. Turek Z, Batra S, Rakusan K. Myocardial oxygenation in immature and adult rats. In: Oxygen transport to tissue XV. New York: Plenum Publishing; 1994. p. 253–8.
30. Rakusan K, Cicutti N, Flanagan MF. Changes in the microvascular network during cardiac growth, development, and aging. Cell Mol Biol Res. 1994;40:117–22.
31. Tornling G, Unge G, Skoog L, Ljungqvist A, Carlsson S, Adolfsson J. Proliferative activity of myocardial capillary wall cells in dipyridamole-treated rats. Cardiovasc Res. 1978;12:692–5.
32. Masuda H, Kawamura K, Nanjo H, Sho E, Komatsu M, Sugiyama T, et al. Ultrastructure of endothelial cells under flow alteration. Microsc Res Tech. 2003;60:2–12.
33. Zheng W, Seftor EA, Meininger CJ, Hendrix MJ, Tomanek RJ. Mechanisms of coronary angiogenesis in response to stretch: role of VEGF and TGF-beta. Am J Physiol Heart Circ Physiol. 2001; 280:H909–17.
34. Zheng W, Christensen LP, Tomanek RJ. Differential effects of cyclic and static stretch on coronary microvascular endothelial cell receptors and vasculogenic/angiogenic responses. Am J Physiol Heart Circ Physiol. 2008;295:H794–800.
35. Kiefer FN, Munk VC, Humar R, Dieterle T, Landmann L, Battegay EJ. A versatile in vitro assay for investigating angiogenesis of the heart. Exp Cell Res. 2004;300:272–82.
36. Rakusan K, Sarkar K, Turek Z, Wicker P. Mast cells in the rat heart during normal growth and in cardiac hypertrophy. Circ Res. 1990; 66:511–6.
37. Levick SP, Melendez GC, Plante E, McLarty JL, Brower GL, Janicki JS. Cardiac mast cells: the centrepiece in adverse myocardial remodelling. Cardiovasc Res. 2011;89(1):12–9.
38. Janicki JS, Brower GL, Gardner JD, Forman MF, Stewart Jr JA, Murray DB, et al. Cardiac mast cell regulation of matrix metalloproteinase-related ventricular remodeling in chronic pressure or volume overload. Cardiovasc Res. 2006;69:657–65.
39. Tomanek RJ, Sandra A, Zheng W, Brock T, Bjercke RJ, Holifield JS. Vascular endothelial growth factor and basic fibroblast growth factor differentially modulate early postnatal coronary angiogenesis. Circ Res. 2001;88:1135–41.
40. Donovan MJ, Lin MI, Wiegn P, Ringstedt T, Kraemer R, Hahn R, et al. Brain derived neurotrophic factor is an endothelial cell survival factor required for intramyocardial vessel stabilization. Development. 2000;127:4531–40.
41. Dbaly J. Postnatal development of coronary arteries in the rat. J Anat Entwickl-Gesch. 1973;141:89–101.
42. Ito T, Harada K, Tamura M, Takada G. In situ morphometric analysis of the coronary arterial growth in perinatal rats. Early Hum Dev. 1998;52:21–6.
43. Neufeld HN, Wagenvoort CA, Edwards JE. Coronary arteries in fetuses, infants, juveniles, and young adults. Lab Invest. 1962;11:837–44.
44. Reinecke P, Hort W. [The growth of coronary artery branches in man under physiological conditions. Morphological studies of corrosion casts of the anterior interventricular branch of the coronary artery]. Z Kardiol. 1992;81:110–5.
45. Yasuoka K, Harada K, Tamura M, Takada G. Left anterior descending coronary artery flow and its relation to age in children. J Am Soc Echocardiogr. 2002;15:69–75.
46. Dolezel S, Gerova M, Hartmannova B, Vasku J. Development of the adrenergic innervation in the myocardium and coronary arteries of the dog. Acta Anat (Basel). 1990;139:191–200.
47. Kralios FA, Cluff N, Anderson FL, Hanson GR, Kralios AC. Postnatal development of peptidergic innervation of the canine heart. J Mol Cell Cardiol. 1999;31:215–25.
48. Davies H. Atherogenesis and the coronary arteries of childhood. Int J Cardiol. 1990;28:283–91.
49. Vlodaver Z, Neufeld HN. The musculo-elastic layer in the coronary arteries. A histological and hemodynamic concept. Vasc Dis. 1967; 4:136–45.
50. Moon HD. Coronary arteries in fetuses, infants, and juveniles. Circulation. 1957;16:263–7.
51. Vlodaver Z, Abramovici A, Neufeld HN, Liban E. Coronary arteries in Yemenites. J Atheroscler Res. 1967;7:161–70.
52. Rapola J, Pesonen E. Coronary artery changes in newborn babies. A histological and electron microscopical study. Acta Pathol Microbiol Scand A. 1977;85:286–96.
53. Moon HD, Rinehart JF. Histogenesis of coronary arteriosclerosis. Circulation. 1952;6:481–8.
54. Wilens SL. The nature of diffuse intimal thickening of arteries. Am J Pathol. 1951;27:825–39.
55. Fangman RJ, Hellwig CA. Histology of coronary arteries in newborn infants. Am J Pathol. 1947;23:901.

56. Milei J, Grana DR, Navari C, Azzato F, Guerri-Guttenberg RA, Ambrosio G. Coronary intimal thickening in newborn babies and <or=1-year-old infants. Angiology. 2010;61:350–6.
57. Leistikow EA, Bolande RP. Perinatal origins of coronary atherosclerosis. Pediatr Dev Pathol. 1999;2:3–10.
58. Kurosawa S, Kurosawa H, Becker AE. The coronary arterioles in newborns, infants and children. A morphometric study of normal hearts and hearts with aortic atresia and complete transposition. Int J Cardiol. 1986;10:43–56.
59. Wiest G, Gharehbaghi H, Amann K, Simon T, Mattfeldt T, Mall G. Physiological growth of arteries in the rat heart parallels the growth of capillaries, but not of myocytes. J Mol Cell Cardiol. 1992;24: 1423–31.
60. Ohuchi H, Beighley PE, Dong Y, Zamir M, Ritman EL. Microvascular development in porcine right and left ventricular walls. Pediatr Res. 2007;61:676–80.
61. Zamir M. The physics of coronary blood flow. New York: Springer; 2005.
62. Fernandez B, Buehler A, Wolfram S, Kostin S, Espanion G, Franz WM, et al. Transgenic myocardial overexpression of fibroblast growth factor-1 increases coronary artery density and branching. Circ Res. 2000;87:207–13.
63. Dedkov EI, Thomas MT, Sonka M, Yang F, Chittenden TW, Rhodes JM, et al. Synectin/syndecan-4 regulate coronary arteriolar growth during development. Dev Dyn. 2007;236:2004–10.
64. Baba F, Swartz K, van Buren R, Eickhoff J, Zhang Y, Wolberg W, et al. Syndecan-1 and syndecan-4 are overexpressed in an estrogen receptor-negative, highly proliferative breast carcinoma subtype. Breast Cancer Res Treat. 2006;98:91–8.
65. Fisher DJ, Heymann MA, Rudolph AM. Regional myocardial blood flow and oxygen delivery in fetal, newborn, and adult sheep. Am J Physiol. 1982;243:H729–31.
66. Lopaschuk GD, Collins-Nakai RL, Itoi T. Developmental changes in energy substrate use by the heart. Cardiovasc Res. 1992;26: 1172–80.
67. Jarmakani JM, Nagatomo T, Nakazawa M, Langer GA. Effect of hypoxia on myocardial high-energy phosphates in the neonatal mammalian heart. Am J Physiol. 1978;235:H475–81.
68. Portman MA, Heineman FW, Balaban RS. Developmental changes in the relation between phosphate metabolites and oxygen consumption in the sheep heart in vivo. J Clin Invest. 1989;83: 456–64.
69. Portman MA, Ning XH. Myocardial energy metabolism in the newborn lamb in vivo during pacing-induced changes in oxygen consumption. Pediatr Res. 1995;37:182–8.
70. Yamamoto H, Avkiran M. Left ventricular pressure overload during postnatal development. Effects on coronary vasodilator reserve and tolerance to hypothermic global ischemia. J Thorac Cardiovasc Surg. 1993;105:120–31.
71. Oskarsson G, Pesonen E. Coronary blood flow in healthy neonates: effects of left ventricular function and mass. Pediatr Cardiol. 2004;25:11–6.
72. Kozak-Barany A, Jokinen E, Rantonen T, Saraste M, Tuominen J, Jalonen J, et al. Efficiency of left ventricular diastolic function increases in healthy full-term infants during the first months of life. A prospective follow-up study. Early Hum Dev. 2000;57:49–59.
73. Flanagan MF, Fujii AM, Colan SD, Flanagan RG, Lock JE. Myocardial angiogenesis and coronary perfusion in left ventricular pressure-overload hypertrophy in the young lamb. Evidence for inhibition with chronic protamine administration. Circ Res. 1991;68:1458–70.
74. Flanagan MF, Aoyagi T, Currier JJ, Colan SD, Fujii AM. Effect of young age on coronary adaptations to left ventricular pressure overload hypertrophy in sheep. J Am Coll Cardiol. 1994;24:1786–96.
75. Laurie W, Woods JD. Anastomosis in the coronary circulation. Lancet. 1958;2:812–6.
76. Reiner L, Vrbanovic D, Madrazo A. Interarterial coronary anastomoses in neonatal pigs. Proc Soc Exp Biol Med. 1961;106:732–4.
77. Schaper W. Collateral circulation: past and present. Basic Res Cardiol. 2009;104:5–21.

Structure–Function of the Coronary Hierarchy

4

Introduction

The coronary vasculature is characterized by unique properties that underlie both the performance and adaptability of the coronary circulation. One of its unique features is that transmural perfusion is limited almost entirely to diastole due to the compressive forces that exist during systole. This feature accounts for the fact that epicardial arteries function as capacitance vessels, as documented by Vatner and colleagues [1] and Chilian and Marcus [2]. High metabolic demands and the myocardium's dependence on oxidative metabolism require (1) a relatively high blood flow and (2) short O_2 diffusion distances from capillaries. To accommodate the need for rapid changes in cardiac work, and thus oxygen consumption, the heart must be capable of second-to-second modulation of perfusion. Since vasoreactivity of conduit arteries and the major resistance vessels (small arteries and arterioles) respond differently to vasoactive substances [3], data from each of these vascular beds should not be generalized.

Histology and Cell Biology of Coronary Vessels

In many respects, the morphology of coronary blood vessels is similar to those in other vascular domains. An excellent and detailed description of blood vessel histology and ultrastructure has been provided by Simionescu and Simionescu [4]. Notably, the distinction between arteries and arterioles is somewhat arbitrary and varies from species to species. The most important criterion for the classification "arteriole" is functional, i.e., a major resistance vessel. For example, in humans, arterioles have been defined as having diameters of 200 μm or less, whereas in small mammals even the coronary artery stems have diameters that are only in the range of 100–200 μm. Precapillary vessels, i.e., arteries and arterioles, have in common three tunics (tunicae) (1) intima (endothelium and subendothelium); (2) media (internal elastic lamina and smooth muscle), and (3) adventitia (collagen, elastin, fibroblasts, and nerves). Examples of coronary arteries and arterioles are found in Figs. 4.1 and 4.2. The major histologic differences between various arterial/arteriolar segments of the coronary precapillary vasculature are the (1) thickness of the vessel's wall in relation to its luminal diameter (wall/lumen ratio); (2) amount of collagen in the tunica media, and (3) density of innervation. Morphometric data from dog coronary arterioles revealed a major difference in wall/lumen ratios between the largest arteries and smallest arterioles [5]: 0.04 in large epicardial arteries, 0.09 in arterioles with lumens between 40 and 160 μm, and 0.13–0.28 μm in the smallest arterioles (<20 μm).

The Three Tunics of Arteries and Arterioles (Figs. 4.1 and 4.2)

Tunica Intima: Endothelium and Subendothelium

Endothelial cells (ECs) are linked by gap (communicating) and occluding junctions. The former facilitate direct 2-way communication between ECs and are numerous in arteries and arterioles, absent in capillaries and pericytic venules (venules with pericytes, but no smooth muscle), and rare in muscular venules and veins. The underlying basal lamina is composed mainly of collagens IV, V, and VIII, laminin, heparin sulfate proteoglycans, actin, and sialoglycoproteins. Together, the basal lamina and the ECs constitute the semipermeable barrier of coronary vessels. Contact with cells of the media is made possible by openings in the internal elastic lamina. As noted in the next section, contact with vascular smooth muscle cells (VSMCs) is important for EC-VSMC signaling. Myocardial ECs play many important roles including signal transduction, nitric oxide synthesis, and mechanotransduction.

Tunica Media: Vascular Smooth Muscle

The VSMCs of the coronary vasculature have been described in detail by Forbes [6, 7]. As he points out, the tunica media contains pericytes and primitive (undifferentiated) smooth muscle cells in addition to differentiated

R.J. Tomanek, *Coronary Vasculature: Development, Structure-Function, and Adaptations*,
DOI 10.1007/978-1-4614-4887-7_4, © Springer Science+Business Media New York 2013

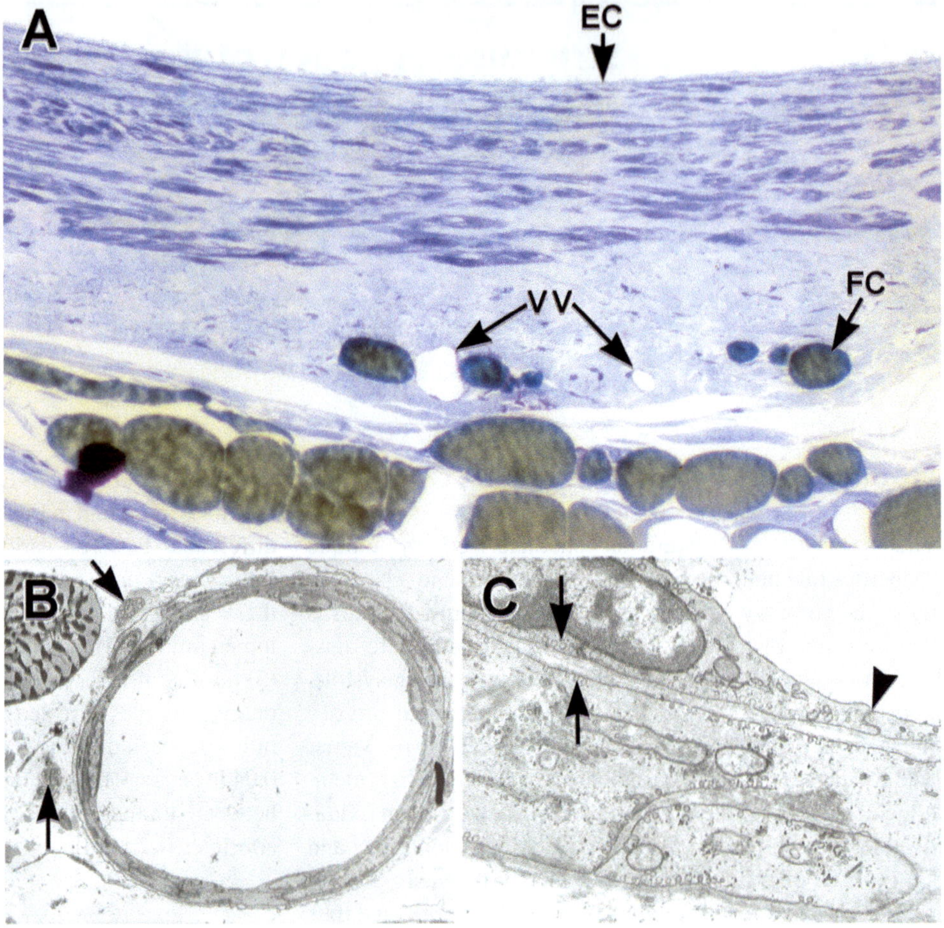

Fig. 4.1 Micrographs of canine coronary artery (**a**) and arterioles (**b** and **c**). (**a**) 1-μm section of an epicardial artery with a media consisting of VSMCs (*blue elongated structures*) and connective tissue (*light blue*) and an adventitia with vasa vasora (VV) and a few fat cells with lipid droplets (FC). Note that the epicardium (bottom of figure) contains numerous fat cells and small vessels. (**b**) Electron micrograph of a small arteriole (about 20 μm in diameter) consisting of an endothelium and one layer of smooth muscle. Note the nerve bundle in the adventitia (*arrows*). A higher power micrograph of a small arteriole (**c**) illustrates the close proximity of an EC and smooth muscle (*bottom* of micrograph), both of which have a basal lamina and numerous plasma membrane vesicles or caveolae (*arrows*). The *arrowhead* indicates a gap junction linking two endothelial cells

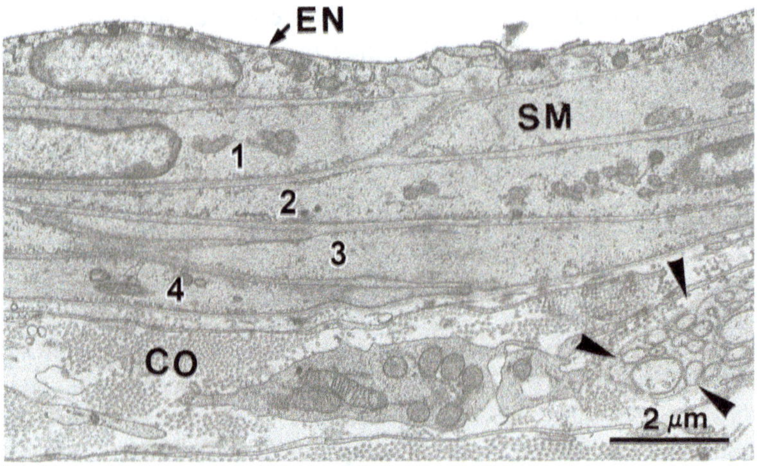

Fig. 4.2 An electron micrograph of a larger canine coronary arteriole containing 3–4 layers of VSMCs (SM) (1, 2, 3, 4), a tunica adventitia with collagen (CO), and nerve axons (*arrow heads*). This micrograph illustrates the close apposition of the smooth muscle cells, their basal laminae, and details of the tunica adventitia. Figure is from Tomanek, 1990 in Coronary circulation. Basic mechanism and clinical relevance (Kajiya et al., eds), Springer-Verlag. p. 8

VSMCs. Collectively, these cells are termed "periendothelial cells" or more commonly perivascular cells. The cells of the coronary tunica media contact one another via (1) simple appositions (where the cell surfaces are separated by 17–30 nm), (2) intermediate junctions, and (3) gap junctions (in some species). VSMC's and EC's contact occurs via gap or gap-like junctions [7], and serves as a structural substrate for EC regulation of smooth muscle reactivity by EC-derived second messengers that respond to EC stimulation on the vessels' luminal surface. VSMCs behave like a syncytium, as was demonstrated when these cells from pig coronary arteries were injected with a fluorescent dye and cultured [8]; the cells were dye coupled, leading to the proposal that these cells may be linked by gap junctions.

In coronary arteries, most VSMCs are arranged circumferentially; the exception being VSMCs adjacent to the endothelium or adventitia; these cells may have a longitudinal polarity [7]. In small arteries or arterioles, such longitudinal strands are not apparent. The tunica media has a variable amount of extracellular matrix; arterioles have the least, whereas large arteries have the most. Boucek and colleagues [9] evaluated the microanatomy of three major coronary arteries—i.e., right, left anterior descending (LAD), and circumflex—of the dog and concluded that each has distinguishing anatomical and physiological properties. They noted some differences in the density of muscle bundles with a spiral course, and in the presence of muscle continuity between a branch and the major artery. The authors noted that the major arteries are subjected to various motions during the cardiac cycle which may relate to differences in structural characteristics. Some specific motions include a left and cephalad rotation of the left coronary artery and a right to left rotation of the right coronary artery during systole. The authors suggested that these arteries and the circumflex are not subjected to equal forces during the heart cycle.

Tunica Adventitia

This outer layer of arteries and veins contains a variety of cell types that enable important functions. Mast cells are the source of histamine and serotonin and are most common in pericytic venules. Macrophages are phagocytic, while eosinophils and plasma cells are sources of local immunological reactions. Collagen and elastin, both secreted by fibroblasts, allow distention and pulsatile changes in luminal diameter, while also protecting against overdistention. The tunica adventitia also contains the sympathetic and parasympathetic nerves. In larger arteries and veins, the tunica adventitia contains the vasa vasora, which provides nutrition to the outer layers of the tunica media. This vascular supply is discussed in detail in a later section of this chapter.

Capillaries and Venules

Capillaries and pericytic venules have similar morphologies, and both consist of ECs and some overlying pericytes. The major difference between the two types of vessels is size: capillaries in the heart are <10 μm in diameter, whereas pericytic venules exceed this limit. A coronary cast reveals the drainage of capillaries into a pericytic venule (Fig. 4.3). As pericytic (non-muscular) venules increase in diameter they acquire more pericytes until the pericytic layer is complete. Muscular venules tend to be >50 μm in diameter and with increasing luminal diameter become muscularized and are classified as muscular venules [10]. The pericytes in

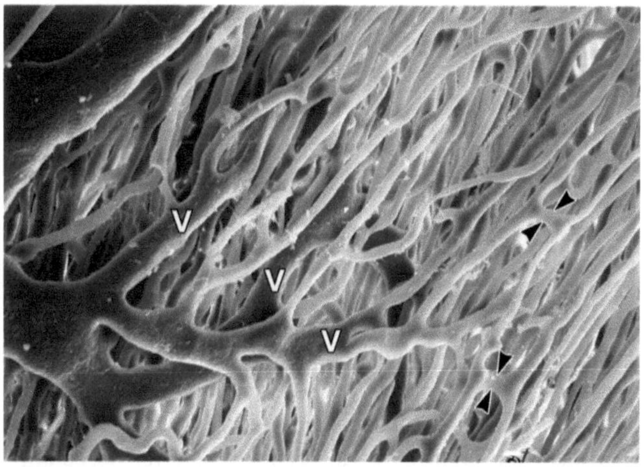

Fig. 4.3 Scanning electron micrograph of a rat coronary corrosion cast. Note the numerous capillaries (*right* and *middle* in micrograph) entering pericytic venules (V). Most of the capillaries run parallel to one another. Intercapillary connections are indicated by *arrow heads*

capillaries and venules appear to interact with their ECs through close cell contacts, as often noted in peg and socket interdigitations of the adjacent cell membranes, as illustrated in Fig. 1.3 [11]. Eleven percent of the EC surface in heart capillaries is covered by pericytes [12]. Possible roles of pericytes in the microvasculature have been reviewed [13]. These cells also play key roles in signaling during vascular development (discussed in Chap. 1) and in maintaining vascular integrity.

Capillaries, as well as venules, are the major vessels for the exchange of substances between blood and tissues. They provide (1) transcellular passage for lipid soluble molecules (e.g., O_2, CO_2); (2) intercellular passage for small water-soluble molecules small pore system), and (3) vesicular channels for macromolecules (large pore system). The latter is facilitated by detachment of caveolae from the cell membrane, movement through the cytoplasm (often by fusion with other caveolae) to form transendothelial channels, which fuse to the cell membrane on the opposite cell surface [7, 14]. An extremely high capillary density in the myocardium is consistent with its high anaerobic metabolic demand. The growth and structural/functional characteristics of myocardial capillaries were addressed in Chap. 3. In the myocardium, diffusion distance for O_2 is minimized by the positioning of capillaries within indentations of the cardiomyocytes. Capillary ECs are linked by tight (occluding) junctions; the remainders of the adjacent cell surfaces are separated by a variable space of 100–300 Å that permits intercellular transport of water-soluble molecules. The numerous vesicles are derivatives of the plasma membrane and function in vesicular transport of macromolecules as demonstrated by Palade [15] a half century ago.

Distribution and Branching of Arteries in Humans (Fig. 4.4)

Coronary casts have been utilized to display the distribution and branching patterns in human as well as animal hearts. The right and left main coronary arteries originate just above the right and left cusps of the aortic valves and pass anteriorly around the pulmonary trunk. It is because they encircle the heart (to the right and left) in a manner of a crown that they were given the name "coronary." The two major branches of the left coronary artery are the circumflex and left anterior descending (also called anterior interventricular branch) and arise near the artery's origin. The left anterior descending artery provides diagonal and interventricular septal branches, whereas the circumflex ends as a posterior left ventricular branch after providing a left marginal branch. The right coronary artery provides several branches anteriorly; these include the atrial, conus, and right marginal. The right coronary artery then passes posteriorly and provides branches to the posterior right and left ventricles and atria; the largest of these branches is the posterior interventricular (posterior descending). A more detailed description of the vessels, seen in Fig. 4.4, is provided in the next section. It is important to recognize that considerable variability exists in the branching patterns of coronary arteries; therefore, anatomical illustrations only reflect frequently observed patterns.

Right and Left Artery Dominance

Coronary dominance patterns in the human heart have been a topic of interest because of their possible relevance to outcomes in coronary artery disease. The term dominant coronary artery (left or right) refers to the artery supplying the greatest area of the heart. Since the left main coronary artery consistently supplies a greater mass of the heart than the right main coronary artery, the term "dominance" refers to the branching patterns rather than to the mass of heart supplied. In the right-dominant pattern, some of the posterior wall of the LV is supplied by branches of the right coronary artery (as seen in Fig. 4.4). Although there are variations in a dominant right pattern, the posterior interventricular branch (also known as posterior descending artery) is a constant feature of right dominance. In the left-dominant pattern, all of the LV posterior wall (and sometimes part of the RV posterior wall) is supplied by branches of the circumflex artery. That most people have right coronary artery dominance was highlighted in a retrospective study of 12,588 patients admitted to the Tehran Heart Center for coronary angiography [16]. Specifically, the percentage of patients with right dominance was 84 and the percentages with left or codominance were 11 and 5, respectively. Although that study did not find any difference between dominant arterial pattern and risk factors for coronary artery disease, evaluation of angiographs revealed that patients with right coronary dominance had a

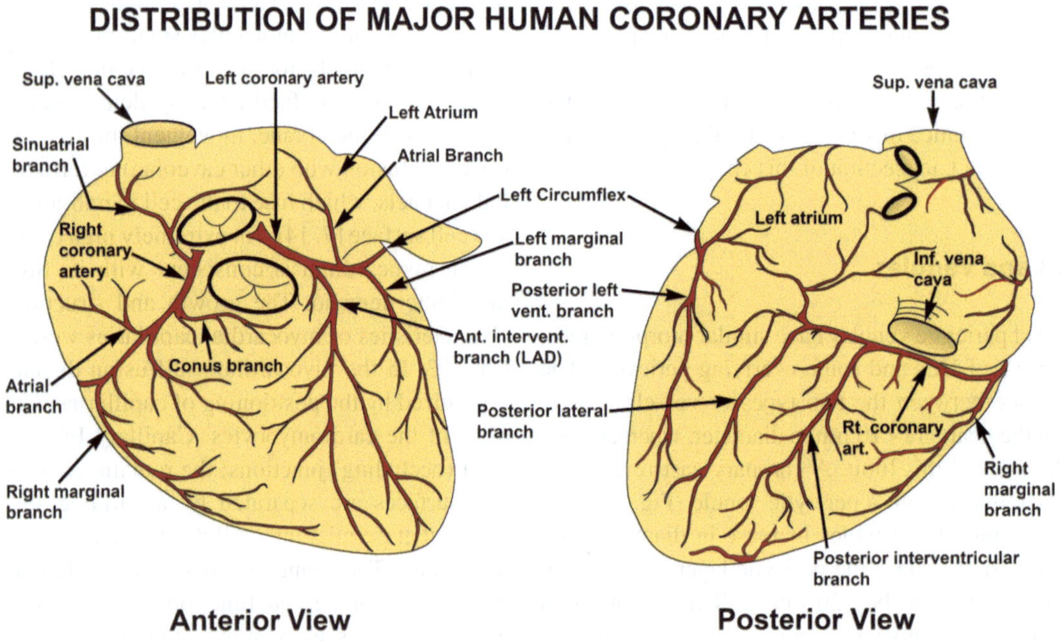

Fig. 4.4 Distribution of major human coronary arteries, most of which are epicardial

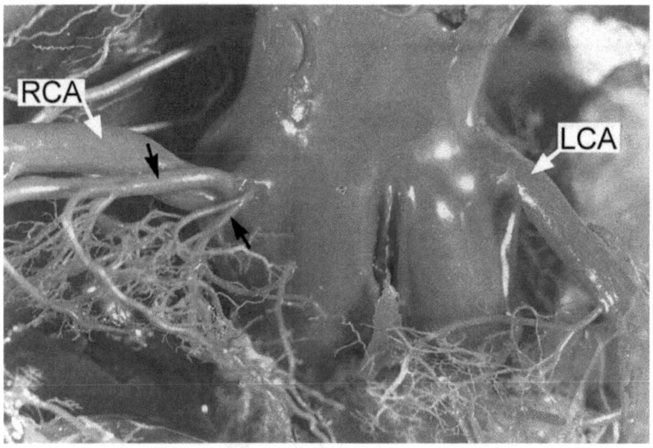

Fig. 4.5 Coronary cast from a human heart revealing the *right* and *left* (RCA, LCA) coronary artery stems as well as a third coronary artery (*arrow*) near the origin of the RCA. The figure is from Zamir, 1990, in Coronary circulation. Basic mechanism and clinical relevance (Kajiya et al., eds) Springer Verlag. p. 16. Reproduced with permission from the publisher

significantly greater incidence of three vessel disease. However, as noted by Allwork [17], in individuals with left coronary artery dominance, the right coronary artery is usually small [18], and thus a proximal occlusion of the left coronary artery would likely cause a large infarction. Among individuals with left coronary artery dominance, the left anterior descending artery (LAD) courses around the heart's apex to supply the inferoapical segment in 87% of cases, whereas among individuals with right coronary artery dominance, this type of LAD course was observed on only 47% of cases [19]. In a study of 225 human hearts, the percentage of males and females with right, left, and codominance patterns was similar [20].

In sum, most individuals have a right coronary artery "dominance" indicated by the origin of the posterior interventricular from this artery. However, the left coronary artery supplies a greater myocardial mass than the right coronary artery.

The Major Coronary Arteries

A great deal of information regarding the anatomy of the coronary arterial trees has been gleaned from casts generated by the injection and corrosion method. Five decades ago, James [21] studied 106 human specimens and provided a detailed analysis of these in a monogram. Since that time, many anatomical studies have provided further details of the coronary arterial hierarchy. The corrosion cast in Fig. 4.5 illustrates the stems of the right and left main coronary arteries. This heart also had a third coronary artery near the origin of the right main artery; one study noted that 47% of human hearts have a third main coronary artery [22].

Left Main Coronary Artery

The left main coronary artery descends in a gentle curve at the base of the pulmonary artery and then divides into the left anterior descending (LAD) and circumflex arteries. The LAD (also called the anterior interventricular branch) enters the anterior interventricular sulcus and continues distally to the hearts' apex, where it supplies branches to the distal posterior LV wall. The left circumflex coronary artery (LCX) bifurcates at right angles from its parent artery and enters the left atrioventricular sulcus. As it courses posteriorly, it provides numerous branches to the lateral LV and ends as a posterior branch in the LV. A variable number of lateral and medial branches arise from the LAD to supply the anterior LV and the interventricular septum. The latter is supplied almost entirely by 4–6 branches of the LAD [23]. However, branches of arteries on the posterior wall also supply the interventricular septum with some collaterals. This dual blood supply is the reason that septal infarcts are rare. Occasionally, the left main coronary artery trifurcates to form the LAD, LCX, and ramus intermedius [24]. The ramus intermedius can supply either the anterior or lateral wall.

Right Main Coronary Artery

This vessel emerges through the right atrioventricular groove, extending to the right and generating several branches on the anterior surface of the right ventricle. These include the conus branch, which courses near the pulmonary trunk, and the right marginal branch, which courses toward the heart's apex. The right main coronary artery then courses posteriorly along the atrial-ventricular border, generates the posterior interventricular branch, and ends along the posterior left atrioventricular junction. At that point it gives rise to the right poster lateral branch. As noted earlier, in some instances (Fig. 4.5), there are two arterial orifices at the right aortic sinus; the second smaller ostium (less than 1 mm in diameter) gives rise to a conal artery or an artery of the sinus mode [21, 23]. Notably, the sinus node artery is the largest atrial artery and supplies blood to both atria and to the sinus node. In most cases, the AV node artery is derived from the right coronary artery; however, in about 10% of human hearts, it is a branch of the left circumflex artery [23].

Diameters of the Main Coronary Arteries

This topic was addressed in a study in which postmortem measurements were made of 514 human hearts from both males and females who were 3–100 years of age at the time of death [25]. The data indicate that the left coronary artery is usually larger than the right, and that the diameter of neither is significantly influenced by heart mass. A considerable variation in artery diameters was noted, as was a trend toward

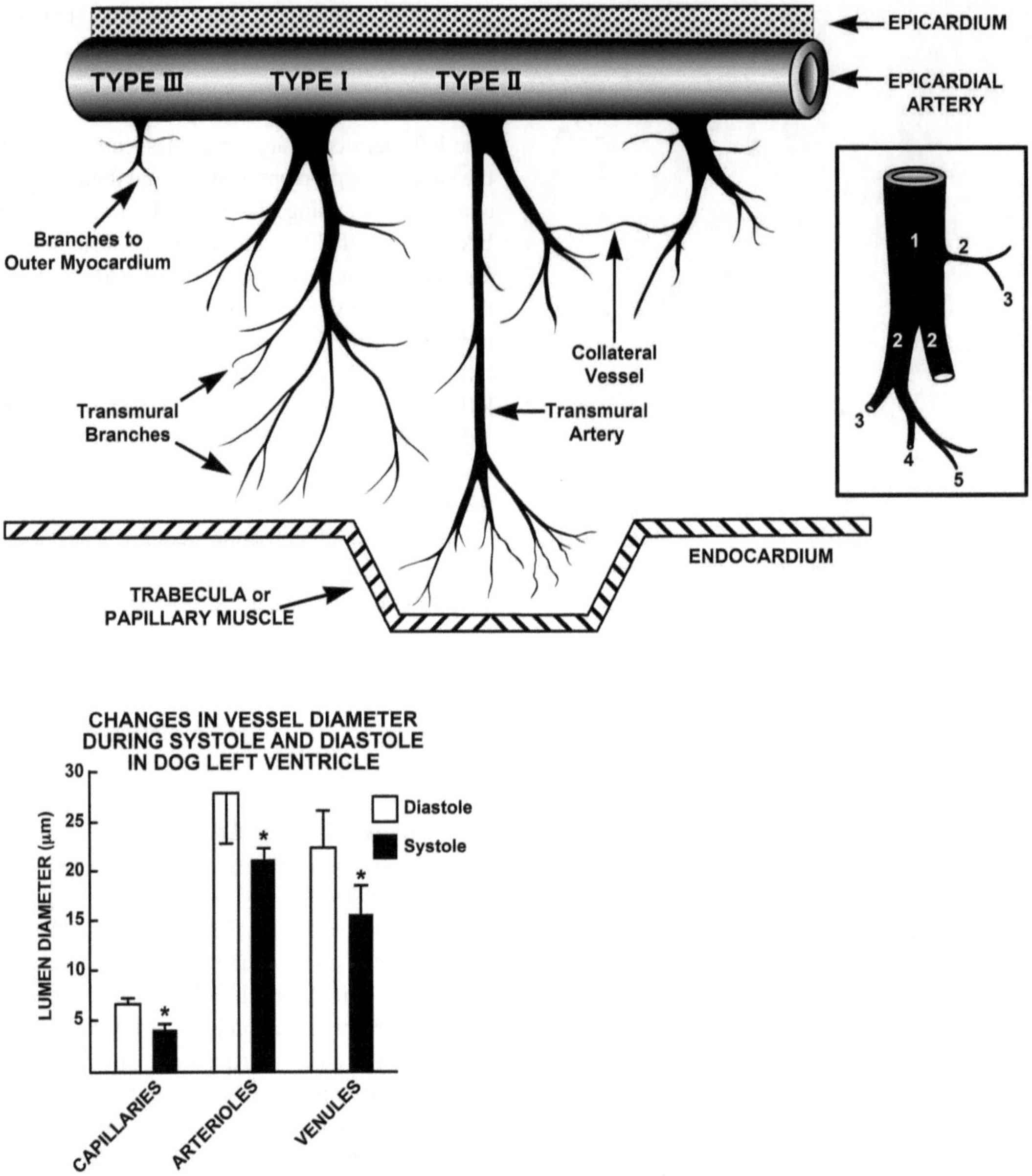

Fig. 4.6 Coronary artery branching patterns. Type I, II, and III patterns are according to classifications provided by Kato [26]. Type I patterns are characterized by numerous intramural branches, whereas Type II distribution is directed mainly to the subendocardial myocardium. Type III consists of short branches that supply the subepicardial myocardium. Diameters of branch generations (2, 3, 4, 5), noted in the inset on *right* side of the figure, indicate that they vary as documented in numerous coronary casts and angiograms. The bar graph illustrates the effects of systole and diastole on coronary vessel diameters documented by Tillmann et al. [27]

an increase in diameter with age. This study failed to find a relationship between the size of the coronary sinus and the diameters of coronary arteries.

Arteries Supplying the Atria

The left atrium receives arterial branches from the left circumflex and right coronary arteries (posterior surface). Branches from the right coronary artery supply the right atrium, including the sinoatrial and atrioventricular nodes.

Branching Patterns

Large coronary arteries are generally epicardial, whereas most transmural arteries are smaller. Septal arteries may be large in humans, a characteristic of dog septal arteries. Intercoronary anastomoses occur in both the superficial and deeper layers of the myocardium. Figure 4.6 is a summary of branching patterns based on the observations of Kato [26], who described three basic arterial distributions in the human left ventricle. The Type I pattern has numerous branches as the artery courses transmurally with the branches becoming smaller as they approach the endocardium. The Type II pattern is characterized by fewer branches as exemplified by the transmural artery as it courses toward the endocardium; its branches terminate in the trabeculae and papillary muscles, an arrangement that favors blood flow to the subendocardium. The Type III pattern is characterized by epicardial vessels with small branches that provide blood flow to the superficial myocardial layer (Fig. 4.6). Thus, Type II and III patterns favor flow to the endomyocardium and epimyocardium, respectively.

The three branching patterns of human hearts, noted above, were compared to those in dogs, pigs, and humans by using postmortem coronary arteriography, soft X-ray postmortem arteriography, and the clearing method [28]. Canine hearts have more numerous Type III vessel patterns than do human hearts and exhibit numerous distinct anastomoses in the epicardial layer. In all canine hearts, the left coronary artery is dominant and the papillary muscles are supplied by only one coronary artery branch; this is in contrast to the vascular supply to papillary muscles in man, which include branches from the LAD and circumflex. Pig hearts are somewhat unique in that they have anastomotic channels to the papillary muscles that are 3.4-fold and 27-fold more numerous than those of man and dog, respectively. These differences may explain why experimental data regarding myocardial ischemia and infarction show some interspecies discord. Pigs are generally considered suitable for studies on the coronary circulation because their coronary artery anatomy and distribution are similar to that of humans [29], with only small differences having been noted between the two species [30]. There are more fundamental differences between the coronary artery patterns in man and dog than between man and pig [29, 31]. Nevertheless, despite these differences in the distributions of the larger distributing coronary arteries in man, dog, and also various rodents, myocardial perfusion is not markedly influenced by these differences. It is more likely that anastomotic channels and vascular density are important.

Arterial Hierarchy

The coronary arterial tree has been characterized using a variety of imaging techniques. As noted earlier, many studies—in both humans and experimental animals—have utilized coronary casts to establish the details of branching patterns and vessel diameters. A classification of coronary arteries in humans into distributing and delivering vessels indicates that the latter have more branches and shorter segments than the former [32]. The relationship between the diameters of the coronary artery stems and the virtual diameter of the heart was shown to be nearly linearly related in 36 species of mammals ranging from mouse to giraffe [33]. This relationship held for hearts that weighed <1 g to >1,000 g. The histological characteristics of large and small coronary arteries are rather similar. As seen in Fig. 4.7, all of these vessels have a distinct internal elastic lamina, and differ mainly with respect to the number of VSMC layers and the amount of elastin in the adventitia.

Morphometric analysis of the pig coronary arterial tree has been used to propose a mathematical model that includes the order number, diameter, length, connectivity matrix, and fractions of vessels of a given order [34], and to provide a complete 3-D reconstruction of the entire porcine coronary vasculature [35]. A structure–function relationship of the coronary circulation based on morphometric measurements and flow simulation has been suggested [36]. Although such data provide some interesting insights into the designs of the

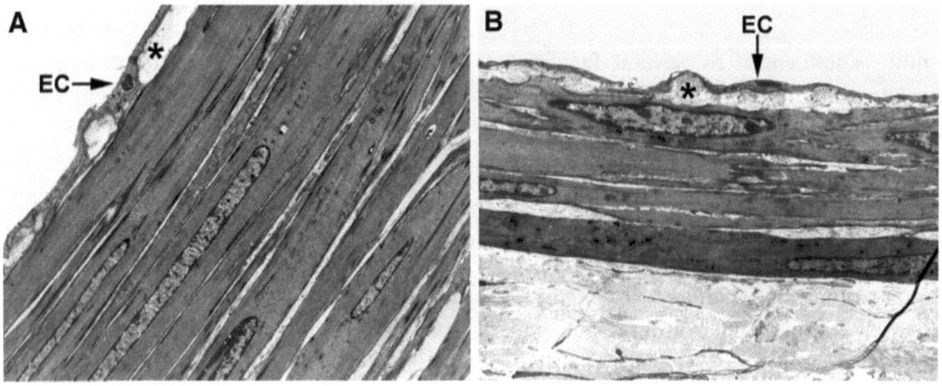

Fig. 4.7 Electron micrographs of the walls of a coronary artery (**a**) and arteriole (**b**) from canine hearts, illustrating closely packed smooth muscle cells, thin endothelial cells (EC), and an internal elastic membrane (*asterisks*). Variability in the amount of extracellular material in the tunica media is common and can be appreciated by comparing the two arteries. The tunica adventitia, with a rich compliment of collagen, is at the bottom of (**b**)

coronary hierarchy, the interpretations need to be limited, since physiological influences are not included in the various assumptions. Predicting branching patterns for coronary arteries based on diameters of various generations of branches is difficult, since—as evident in Fig. 4.6—both small and large branches may be derived from the same parent artery. Thus, the diameter of a second-order branch may be similar to that of a fourth- or fifth-order branch.

Innervation and Adrenergic Receptors

The heart and the coronary vasculature are innervated by sympathetic and parasympathetic nerves that converge on the cardiac plexus, which is located between the concavity of the aortic arch and the tracheal bifurcation. The bilateral sympathetic neural input is from several ganglia: the superior, middle, and inferior cervical, and the first four thoracic ganglia. Right and left vagal nerves provide the parasympathetic axons. In dogs, terminal varicosities of the autonomic nerves are found in the adventitia, but do not extend into the media of large arteries [37]. A study on the development of canine adrenergic innervation has suggested that coronary vessels and the cardiomotor system differ with respect to (1) pathways, (2) shape of termini, and (3) developmental time course [38]. In vivo studies of the coronary responses to sympathetic and parasympathetic activation are complicated by the fact that the myocardium also responds to this activation. Therefore, in vivo analyses require that myocardial metabolism be controlled during measurements, including arterial pressure and heart rate. The effects of autonomic nerves on the vasoactivity of coronary arteries and arterioles are summarized in Table 4.1

Table 4.1 Direct effects of autonomic nerves on vasoactivity of coronary arteries and arterioles

Stimulus	Mediators	Vessel response
Large arteries		
Sympathetic nerves	α_1-AR-VSM (high density)	Constriction (moderate)
Norepinephrine	α_2-AR-VSM (low density)	Constriction (minor)
	β_1-AR-Endothelium (high density)	Dilation
	β_2-AR-Endothelium (low density)	Dilation
Parasympathetic nerves	Muscarinic receptor	Dilation (tonic)
Acetylcholine	Endothelial nitric oxide	
Arterioles		
Sympathetic nerves	α_1-AR VSM (low density)	Constriction*
Norepinephrine	α_2-AR-VSM (high density)	Constriction
	β_1-AR Endothelium (low density)	Dilation
	β_2-AR Endothelium (high density)	Dilation
	β_3-AR Endothelium (high density)	Dilation

AR, adrenergic receptor; VSM, vascular smooth muscle
*The constriction may be indirect, via stimulation of α_1-adrenergic receptors on cardiomyocytes, resulting in the production of a yet unidentified vasoconstrictor.

Regulation of Coronary Flow

Distribution of Coronary Resistance

Coronary blood flow is influenced by several factors (1) physical (perfusion pressure, blood viscosity, and extravascular resistance); (2) neural; (3) myogenic, and (4) metabolic. Because the coronary vascular tree includes vessels with a wide range of diameters and locations within the chamber wall, a variety of regulatory mechanisms exist. Adenosine dilates coronary arterioles, but has little effect on larger conduit and intermediate-size vessels. Therefore, the site of vascular resistance varies depending on the vasomotor stimulus, and can change nonuniformly during maximal vasodilation. As previously demonstrated by direct pressure measurements in a beating cat heart, about 70% of the resistance in coronary circulation resides in small arteries and arterioles during baseline conditions [39]. During maximal vasodilation, total resistance decreases markedly and the drop is most striking in the arterioles, i.e., the vessels which contribute the most to resistance. Under basal conditions, in the cat heart, 55% of the resistance was in arterioles <100 μm in diameter, whereas about 25% of the resistance was proximal to arterial segments >200 μm in diameter. Dipyridamole-induced maximal vasodilation caused a redistribution of resistance: the percent resistance increased 68% in arteries, decreased 60% in arterioles, and increased 13-fold in veins [40]. Thus, the greatest contributors to the increased blood flow during maximal vasodilation in the heart are arterioles. Consistent with these findings are data on hyperemic responses in dog hearts that revealed that arterioles with diameters <100 μm contributed the most to the enhanced flow [41].

Within the left ventricle, the flow is normally slightly higher in the inner than the outer myocardial layers due, in part, to the higher metabolic rate. When coronary pressure is reduced, epimyocardial blood flow is maintained to a greater extent than endomyocardial flow due to a greater autoregulatory range in the epimyocardium [42]. Vasodilation induced by adenosine causes a preferential increase in endomyocardial flow, thereby restoring the endomyocardial/epimyocardial flow ratio. Endomyocardial coronary arterioles have been shown to be more sensitive to adenosine than their epimyocardial counterparts [43].

Metabolic Regulation

Matching coronary blood flow to myocardial consumption involves feedback mechanisms that constitute "metabolic regulation." This concept is based on the existence of a metabolic sensor, namely oxygen, which is coupled to effector mechanisms that in turn control vascular tone. However, other mechanisms for coronary flow regulation need to be considered [44]. The fact that blocking a putative mediator does not completely abolish coronary vasodilation (see reviews by [45, 46]) has made it clear that there are many mediators of metabolic regulation. Perhaps the simplest metabolic sensors are O_2 and CO_2, since arterial hypoxemia and hypercarbia have long been known to cause vasodilation. However, these gases do not account for the total vasodilatory response [45]. When coronary perfusion is elevated, O_2 consumption may also increase, a response known as Gregg's phenomenon. In this circumstance, the increased O_2 consumption has been suggested to be a consequence of cardiomyocytes stretching and coronary vessel distension (reviewed in [47]).

Adenosine as a Messenger

This vasodilatory metabolite, a product of ATP hydrolysis, produces coronary vasodilation, thereby increasing blood flow. Although adenosine is a powerful vasodilator, blocking its receptor does not significantly inhibit blood flow [48–50]. Although adenosine and its receptors do not contribute significantly to basal coronary tone or functional hyperemia [51, 52], the debate concerning these points has not been completely resolved. For example, Edlund et al. [53] found that inhibiting the adenosine receptor decreased basal flow and increased coronary resistance. A role for adenosine during myocardial ischemia has been documented [54]. When exogenous adenosine and adenosine receptors are blocked in dogs with coronary stenosis, coronary vasodilation during exercise is significantly reduced [54, 55]. Although a role for adenosine in exercise-dependent hyperemia was demonstrated by Duncker and colleagues [56], they found that its role was not essential. In addition to its influence on vascular tone, adenosine has also been found to modulate vessel growth by its direct and indirect effects on ECs and VSMCs [57–62]. The role of adenosine in increasing blood flow in the ischemic myocardium is addressed in Chap. 10.

Adenosine interacts with 4 G-protein coupled receptor subtypes (A_1, A_{2A}, A_{2B}, and A_3) that mediate not only coronary flow but also heart rate, cardiomyocyte contraction, cell growth, and tissue remodeling (reviewed in [63]). Smooth muscle and the endothelium both express A_{2A} and A_{2B} receptors, and the receptor activation leading to coronary vasodilation is species specific. In porcine coronary arteries, A_{2A} receptor signaling is the main determinant of endothelial-independent vasodilation, whereas A_{2B} receptor signaling plays a minor role [64]. The effects of adenosine on coronary responses are complicated by the fact that the A_1 receptor activation triggers coronary constriction and inhibits A_2-dependent dilation [65, 66]. With regard to the A_3 receptor, the evidence of its role in coronary vasomotion is contradictory (reviewed in [63]). This receptor may have indirect effects on vascular responses because it is present on other cell types, e.g., mast cells.

Nitric Oxide and Prostaglandins

Nitric Oxide (NO) and prostacyclin are the two most prominent physiological endothelium-derived dilator agonists. Although resting myocardial blood flow is not significantly altered when these vasodilators are inhibited (reviewed in [45]), NO acts as a tonic vasodilator at rest and during increased metabolism. When NO synthesis was blocked, there occurred a decrease in coronary venous oxygen tension at a given O_2 consumption [67–69]. NO-induced vasodilation occurs in all coronary arteries, but especially in large coronary arteries, as evidenced by increases in epicardial artery diameters (reviewed in [45]). Vasodilation of epicardial coronary arteries induced by exercise is accompanied by enhanced NO production and release; these responses are blocked by nitro-L-arginine [68]. The effect of NO on large coronary arteries may be the result of elevated shear stress, e.g., as occurs during exercise. Shear stress is the most physiologically relevant mechanism of endothelium-dependent dilation.

Alfonso et al. [70] demonstrated that prostaglandins (arachidonic acid metabolites of cyclooxygenase) appear in the coronary circulation during hypoxia. These investigators blocked prostaglandin synthesis in vagotomized dogs and found a significant attenuation of the rise in coronary flow during hypoxia. However, support for a role for prostaglandins in metabolic coronary regulation is lacking. In this regard, Dai and Bach [71] demonstrated that the progressive increase in coronary blood flow during exercise was not blunted when cyclooxygenase was inhibited by indomethacin administration. Moreover, aortic pressures and venous PO_2 were unchanged after indomethacin, either during rest or during exercise. However, prostaglandins, specifically prostacyclins, have been shown to play a role in hypoxic-induced coronary dilation, a topic addressed in Chap. 9.

K_{ATP} Channels

Glibenclamide-induced blockage of K_{ATP} channels does not affect myocardial O_2 consumption, but reduces coronary blood flow [45]. The reduction in coronary blood flow is consistent with a large body of evidence that K_{ATP} channels cause hyperpolarization and relaxation of vascular smooth muscle [51], and thus play a role in basal coronary tone. However, since glibenclamide was not effective in attenuating coronary blood flow enhancement during exercise [72], local metabolic vasodilation in response to increased myocardial O_2 consumption is not solely dependent on K_{ATP} sensitive channels.

Reactive Oxygen Species

The production of H_2O_2 is linked to myocardial O_2 consumption [73] and is a consequence of $\cdot O_2^-$ production resulting from electrons leaking from mitochondrial complexes I and III [44]. The vasodilator coronary response to H_2O_2 is well known and considered to be robust. In human coronary arterioles, shear stress was shown to induce endothelial release of H_2O_2, a finding that links it with flow-induced dilation [74].

Myogenic Control

Flow regulation in response to changes in transmural pressure is based on a theory first proposed by Bayliss [75] more than a century ago. He suggested that an increase in pressure or stretch is countered by vasoconstriction, whereas a decrease in pressure leads to dilation. These responses help maintain a circumferential stress and serve to blunt transmission of significant pressure changes to the more fragile downstream vasculature. As reviewed by Liu and Gutterman [76], myogenic responses are most marked in the microcirculation and are present in both experimental animals and humans. Studies by Kuo and colleagues documented myogenic responses in the coronary vessels of pigs [77–80], and demonstrated that changes in pressure cause myogenic responses in porcine arterioles with diameters of 80–100 μm [77, 78]. These investigators found that both epicardial and subepicardial arterioles dilated and constricted in response to decreased and increased intraluminal pressures, respectively [77]. Both spontaneous myogenic tone (at constant pressure) and active myogenic constriction (change in tone to stop changes in pressure) were preserved after endothelial denudation [78]. However, dilation induced either by flow or bradykinin was abolished when the endothelium was removed. These findings suggest that local mechanisms may compete for the regulation of vessel caliber. Indeed, a series of elegant experiments from the Chilian laboratory [79] documented the interplay between shear-induced dilation and pressure-related myogenic tone and showed that flow-induced dilation and myogenic responsiveness occur in coronary porcine venules, as well [80]. Like animal models, human coronary arterioles also exhibit prominent myogenic reactivity with an inverse relationship between vessel diameter and myogenic responsiveness [81]. Myogenic responses are dependent on the vessel's diameter since dilation in response to a drop in pressure is limited mainly to vessels smaller than 150 μm [82, 83], whereas vessels with diameters greater than 150 μm do not undergo a significant vasodilation [77].

A number of mechanisms have been proposed to underlie myogenic constriction, as reviewed by Liu and Gutterman [76]. These include membrane depolarization in response to cation channel stretch activation and molecular signaling cascades. For example, myogenic tone was decreased in human coronary arterioles when MEK 1/2 was inhibited, thus preventing the phosphorylation of ERK 1/2 [84]. Although Reactive Oxygen Species (ROS) modulation of a myogenic response has also been suggested, the work in support of this possibly was carried out on noncoronary vessels, thus the relevance of these findings to the heart has not been established.

Myogenic responses probably do not play a major role in coronary flow (see review by [46]), although they do in some other vascular beds. Experiments by Dole and Nuno [85] documented the role of oxygen tension in the coronary sinus as a determinant of coronary flow. They showed that autoregulation was closely coupled to prevailing venous O_2 consumption, and concluded that variations in the autoregulation index were largely explained by differences in the prevailing venous O_2 concentration. Accordingly, the myogenic response may play only a minor role in autoregulation.

Effects of Flow and Shear Stress on Coronary Vasodilation

Endothelium-dependent dilation of epicardial arteries occurs in response to increased flow [86, 87]. Flow-induced vasodilation is a response to shear stress. This stress is sensed by ECs, which then release NO or other vasodilators. Data supporting this concept come from both in vivo and in vitro studies. Kuo et al. [78] demonstrated flow-induced dilation in isolated arterioles, and also established that the flow-induced dilation is dependent on NO synthesis and an intact endothelium. This group of investigators also documented a range of diameter increases in response to increased flow according to the following hierarchy: large arterioles > intermediate arterioles > small arterioles [78]. Thus, the vasodilatory responses are heterogeneous and depend on the level of the arterial hierarchy. One caveat that needs to be mentioned is that the regulation of shear stress in vivo in the coronary microcirculation does not appear to be as well controlled as that observed in in vitro experiments. The reasons for these differences remain to be identified.

Extravascular Resistance

Subendocardial Vulnerability

The vulnerability of the endomyocardium to infarction is a consequence of the high degree of extravascular resistance in this region of the myocardium. The compressive forces of the myocardium increase transmurally from the epicardium toward the endocardium [88]. The effects of myocardial contraction on the intramural coronary vessels are considered to constitute three resistance categories [89] (1) viscous resistance in the dilated coronary bed; (2) autoregulatory resistance, a consequence of vascular smooth muscle tone; and (3) powerful compressive resistance due to cardiomyocyte contraction. The first two of these are present during both systole and diastole and the third is present only during systole. Perfusion of the endomyocardium is greater during diastole than during systole because resistance during autoregulation is greater in the epimyocardium than in the endomyocardium, and compensates for the compressive forces that occur during systole. Thus, blood flow distribution is usually distributed uniformly during basal conditions. However, perfusion of the endomyocardium is preferentially reduced when partial obstruction of coronary arteries occurs, as demonstrated by the classic experiments of Griggs [90]. Subsequently, the transmural distribution of coronary blood flow was studied by Downey and Kirk [91], who showed that systolic flow in the inner fourth of the myocardium was only 25% of that in the outer fourth of the myocardium. In contrast, the total perfusion (systolic and diastolic) was found to favor the inner myocardium. When the heart is arrested and blood is perfused at a constant pressure, flow to the inner myocardium doubles, but flow in the outer myocardium is unchanged [92]. Peak coronary blood flow in the left ventricle occurs during early diastole, declines during late diastole, and then falls to virtually zero during isovolumetric contraction, when aortic pressure remains low. Coronary flow then increases during mid-systole as arterial pressure increases, but is less than 50% of that which occurs during early diastole.

Phasic Coronary Blood Flow

The "vascular waterfall" has been used to explain how extravascular forces impair coronary blood flow during systole, i.e., differences in the systolic and diastolic phases in coronary blood flow [93]. This model posits that when tissue pressure (i.e., extravascular pressure) exceeds venous pressure, flow is proportional along the gradient between arterial intraluminal pressure and tissue pressure. It predicts that, in the beating heart, the pressure–flow curve will break at the highest tissue pressure in the system. Due to the fact that the deepest vessels in the ventricular wall are subject to the highest pressure from the contracting myocardium, they are the most likely to experience a partial collapse. In the beating heart, coronary blood flow at a given pressure is significantly less than that in the arrested heart, as demonstrated in dogs [93]. The topic of pressure–flow relations in the coronary circulation and the concept of vascular waterfalls have been extensively reviewed [94]. The observation that coronary artery pressure is still high, e.g., even 15–20 mmHg during maximal vasodilation, suggests a high back pressure due to high extravascular pressure.

Flow and Vessel Diameters During Systole

The fact that coronary inflow and outflow occur primarily during diastole and systole, respectively, has been confirmed by many studies since Rebatel first made this suggestion in 1872 (reviewed in [27]). To determine the point where the phase shift of the flow change occurs, Tillmanns and colleagues [27] studied beating dog and turtle hearts using an intramuscular transilluminating system. As illustrated in Fig. 4.6, lumen diameters of arterioles, capillaries, and venules in the dog ventricle decrease significantly during systole due to extravascular compression. Similar changes were noted in turtle hearts. Since the data were derived from the superficial layers of the hearts, the vascular compression in deeper myocardial layers would be expected to have been even greater. As noted earlier, Downey and colleagues [91, 93] established that systole inhibits blood flow more in the endomyocardium than in the epimyocardium. These authors then suggested that the point where the flow pattern changes is the site of transition from arterioles to capillaries. Their experiments utilized turtles because of lower heart rates and less phasic motion, and based flow measurements on red cell velocity. They found that during systole, arteriolar flow was reduced by 57%, whereas flow increased 2.5-fold in capillaries and 2.1-fold in venules.

Neural Control and Coronary Responses (see Table 4.1)

Reviews of neural control of the coronary circulation [95, 96] provide some insights into the direct and indirect effects of autonomic nerve activation on vasoreactivity and coronary flow. Although the direct sympathetic effects on coronary arteries is vasoconstriction, simultaneous activation of these receptors in cardiomyocytes results in increased contractility and metabolism and causes local vascular dilation. When epinephrine or norepinephrine is administered along with a β-blocker there is a uniform transmural coronary vasoconstriction illustrating that the effects of α-adrenergic stimulation are direct [96].

β-Adrenergic Receptors

Stress situations, such as excitement, exercise and pain, result in β-adrenoceptor-mediated increases in heart rate and ventricular function, and consequently enhanced myocardial perfusion. The increase in coronary flow is a consequence of metabolic induced coronary vasodilation (reviewed in [45, 47, 97]). A direct β-adrenergic coronary vasodilation, independent of metabolic factors, has been demonstrated in many laboratories (reviewed in [98]). Many studies have demonstrated a direct β-adrenergic coronary dilation that is independent of metabolic factors [99–104]. The involvement of both β_1 and β_2 receptors in direct coronary vasodilation of epicardial coronary arteries has been demonstrated in dogs [102, 105] and calves [104].

The differences in the vasodilatory responses of large coronary arteries and small arteries and arterioles have been examined with respect to adrenergic receptor subtypes [95, 104, 106, 107]. Large bovine coronary arteries contain more β_1- than β_2-adrenergic receptors, but activation of either subtype elicits vasodilation [104]. However, as documented in an in vitro study, β_1 receptors predominate in the vasodilatory response of large canine coronary arteries [105]. Studies on the canine coronary vasculature have shown that in contrast to the preferential density of β_1-adrenoceptors in large arteries, arterioles contain more β_2-adrenoceptors [108, 109]. Selective blocking of these receptors during prolonged diastoles, when chronotropic and inotrophic influences are absent, blocked vasodilation of resistance vessels [110].

α-Adrenergic Receptors

The ability of α-adrenergic activation to trigger the vasoconstriction of large (epicardial) coronary arteries has long been recognized [111]. However, a reduction in coronary flow is not observed in the beating heart under this circumstance because the metabolic effects of increased heart rate and elevated coronary driving pressure increase metabolism and evoke vasodilation of resistance vessels, and consequently an increase in coronary flow. Vasoconstriction of large coronary arteries occurs in response to either sympathetic nerve activation or infusion of norepinephrine [112]. However, the α-receptor vasoconstrictor response is modest [113] and less than that of small coronary vessels. Resting coronary blood flow in dogs has been shown to be unaffected by sympathetically mediated α-adrenergic vasoconstriction of epicardial arteries [114]. Although the α_1 subtype has generally been considered the main α-adrenergic receptor in large coronary arteries in dogs [113], both the α_1 and α_2 subtypes have been found to elicit vasoconstriction not only in dogs [1, 113, 115, 116] but also in calves [117]. This response is observed when β-adrenergic effects are blocked by propanolol. When the vasoconstrictor effects of norepinephrine, mediated by α-adrenoreceptors, are negated by blockade of these receptors with phenoxybenzamine, norepinephrine activates β_1- and β_2-adrenoceptors to cause vasodilation independent of chronotropic and inotropic effects [118]. Thus, norepinephrine plays a dual role mediating both α-adrenergic vasoconstriction and β-adrenergic vasodilation. The later process is termed "feed forward" control of coronary blood flow. The fact that not all adrenergic receptors on coronary vessels are located in neurovascular junctions explains why humoral activation of adrenergic receptors can produce different effects from neural release of the same transmitters.

The idea that α-adrenergic coronary vasoconstriction has a beneficial effect on coronary blood flow to the inner left ventricular myocardium lacks sufficient evidence (reviewed in [119]). There is evidence that during β-blockade, cardiac sympathetic nerve stimulation increases coronary resistance [112, 113]. In his review, Heusch [119] concludes that under physiological conditions, a favorable effect of α-adrenergic coronary vasoconstriction on transmural blood flow is minimal, at best.

Finally, a very different concept from the traditional one discussed in the preceding section (where the vascular responses are due to activation of α-adrenoreceptors located on VSMCs) is supported by in vitro and in vivo data from several studies [120–122]. This hypothesis states that the activation of the α-adrenoreceptor occurs on cardiomyocytes, which in turn activate a yet unidentified constrictor signal on coronary vessels. This hypothesis is supported by results showing that isolated coronary arterioles do not respond directly to α-adrenergic agonists, but that such stimulation of isolated cardiomyocytes results in the production of a factor that induces endothelin-induced constriction of coronary arterioles. In this scheme, the production of the constrictor factor wanes as metabolic rate increases.

> Regardless of the precise mechanism by which α-adrenergic constriction occurs in the coronary circulation, typically its effects are modest compared to the robust effects of metabolism and of ischemia.

Adrenergic Receptors in Humans

Data from studies of human coronary vessels have, in general, been consistent with those from experimental animals. Data obtained from explanted human hearts (from patients undergoing heart transplants) indicate that acetylcholine selectively dilates coronary resistance vessels, but only moderately (19%) reduces epicardial artery cross-sectional area [123]. An examination of the effects of α-adrenergic signaling revealed that epicardial artery diameters were not significantly altered by α-receptor blockade, suggesting that α-adrenergic receptor tone is minimal in these vessels [124]. That study also showed that the increase in coronary vascular resistance during β-blockade is a function of β_2 receptors, consistent with animal studies documenting a high density of β_2 receptors in resistance vessels. A subsequent study on explanted human hearts revealed that the norepinephrine-induced coronary dilation was blocked by a β_2 antagonist and that the dilation occurred in isolated small arteries and arterioles [125]. The discovery that the endothelium of human arterioles/small arteries (diameters: 70–170 μm) is the site of β_3-adrenergic receptors was also coupled with evidence that these receptors mediate adrenergic vasodilation that is dependent on both NO and vessel hyperpolarization [126].

Three molecular subtypes of α_1-adrenoceptors (α_1A, α_1B and α_1D) are known to exist, each of which is activated by norepinephrine and epinephrine [127]. A study on 25 human hearts provided documentation that the α_1D subtype constitutes 80% of α-adrenergic mRNA and protein [128]. This study also revealed that whereas α_1D predominates in coronary arteries, the α_1A is most abundant in the myocardium. This finding in humans is consistent with data from mice, where α_1D is also the major α-adrenergic subtype in coronary arteries [129].

Parasympathetic Control

Parasympathetic activation causes bradycardia, lowers blood pressure, and decreases O_2 consumption. Such changes evoke vasoconstriction (reviewed by [95]). These indirect effects of parasympathetic activation have been circumvented in canine experiments in which a constant heart rate was maintained by pacing, and such studies have demonstrated that parasympathetic activation increases coronary flow. Moreover, the finding that this response is blocked by atropine indicates that it is acetylcholine mediated [130]. Vagally mediated, nitric oxide dependent, coronary vasodilation also occurs when arterial-, chemo-, baroreceptors, or ventricular receptors are activated (reviewed in [107]). Experiments utilizing two-dimensional intravascular ultrasound demonstrated that muscarinic receptor activation by vagus nerve activity results in tonic vasodilation of the left-circumflex artery in dogs [131]. In healthy humans, intracoronary injections of acetylcholine dilate epicardial arteries, whereas they evoke vasoconstriction in patients with atherosclerosis [132, 133]. This paradoxical effect suggests that endothelial function is impaired in atherosclerotic arteries [134].

Bovine and porcine coronary arteries have been reported to constrict in response to acetylcholine [135, 136]. However, in baboons intracoronary injections of acetylcholine elicited vasoconstriction at high doses and vasodilation at low doses [137]. Feigl [95] noted that two factors may have contributed to the disparate data (1) the direct vasoconstrictive effects of acetylcholine on VSMCs and (2) the vasodilatory effects of EC-derived NO. Thus, the response is likely dependent on the relative strengths of these two influences.

Flow Regulation: Multiple Pathways and Mechanisms
Myocardial blood flow is regulated by a multitude of factors, both intrinsic and extrinsic. First, metabolic regulation plays a prominent role in flow regulation and includes several mediators. Second, myogenic responses are most marked in the microcirculation. Adrenergic regulation of both dilation and constriction is well established. Finally, the importance of extravascular resistance plays a major role in limiting flow to the inner (subendocardial) layers of the ventricular myocardium.

Coronary Venous System

The distribution of major coronary veins is illustrated in Fig. 4.8. Cardiac veins return blood from various regions of the heart and can be classified into two major groups, i.e., the greater cardiac venous system that drains into the coronary system and the remaining venous tributaries that open into the left atrium. The greater cardiac venous system receives venous blood from nearly the entire heart and drains into the posterior right atrium, at the atrioventricular groove, via the coronary sinus. The coronary sinus is an extension of the great cardiac vein, which receives blood from the anterior portion of the left ventricle. Its course parallels that of the left anterior descending artery. The major veins joining the coronary sinus include the (1) posterior vein of the left

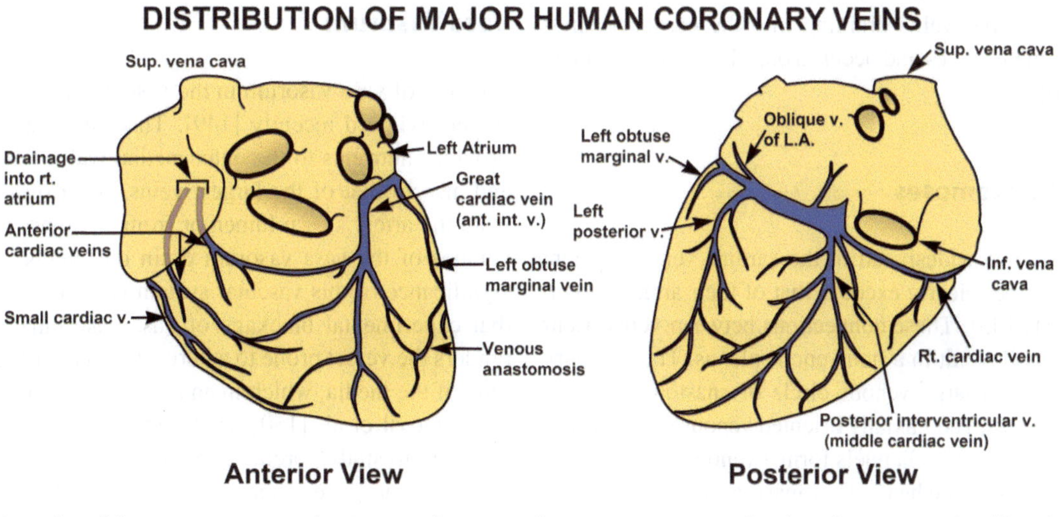

Fig. 4.8 Major veins of the coronary system. Anastomoses between veins are more common that those between arteries. Note their presence, especially near the apex of the heart

ventricle; (2) middle cardiac vein, which lies in the posterior interventricular groove; and (3) small cardiac vein, which receives blood from anterior cardiac veins that course posteriorly from the anterior right ventricle. This vein joins the middle cardiac vein at its junction with the coronary sinus. Drainage patterns of arterial flow determined in isolated canine hearts indicate that the coronary sinus receives 49% of the flow, whereas anterior cardiac veins drain 24% of the flow [138]. Most of the left atrial veins drain into the coronary sinus; these include the oblique vein of Marshall [139]. The remaining venous tributaries open directly into the left atrium [140]. Two types of veins are found in the right atrium. The first includes small veins that drain the atrium and open directly into the atrial cavity, and also larger intramural veins that receive blood from anterior cardiac veins and some septal veins. Left atrial veins empty not only into the atrial cavity but also into the (1) coronary sinus, (2) right atrium, and (3) mediastinal veins [141]. The second source of drainage is the smaller cardiac venous system, which consists of multiple direct channels of small diameter that return blood from the heart chambers into their lumens. For a review of cardiac veins, see von Ludinghausen [141] and Loukas et al. [140].

Coronary Venous Valves

The coronary sinus has a valve known as the Thebesian valve that has been ascribed the function of preventing regurgitation into the coronary sinus during atrial systole. It lies at the junction of the coronary sinus and the right atrium. Though present in the majority (>70%) of human hearts, its morphology is variable [142] and it often does not provide a sufficient surface area to cover the ostium. Accordingly, its role as a barrier to backflow into the coronary sinus is not established. The great cardiac vein usually contains a valve (valve of Vieussens, named after the French anatomist) at its junction with the coronary sinus. This valve is incomplete in many cases. Other veins draining into the coronary sinus have incomplete valves and occur in only 1/3 to 1/6 of human hearts [140].

Venous Anastomoses

Anastomoses are widespread in the cardiac venous system and their number clearly exceeds that of their arterial counterparts [141, 143]. These connections between veins occur at all levels and result in a rich venous plexus. The coronary sulcus contains a large venous circle of anastomotic veins that is joined by several axially oriented venous stems. These interconnected venous channels form a venous basket on the posterior surface of the heart. This anastomotic system forms "two large triangles having their apexes on either side of the apex of the heart" [143]. Connections between the great cardiac vein and the middle cardiac vein are well developed at the apex of the heart.

Smaller (Thebesian) Cardiac Venous System

Small and thin channels, highly variable in number and length, form a subendocardial system that opens into each of the four heart chambers [144]. Experiments carried out in isolated canine hearts demonstrated that 5% and 24% of coronary flow drains directly into the left and right ventricles, respectively [138]. Four categories are usually described [140]. Veno-sinusoidal channels drain sinusoids (expanded capillaries), whereas veno-luminal vessels connect venous networks with ventricular and atrial lumens. Most Thebesian veins, as documented in sheep, are veno-luminal [145]. Arteriolar connections to chamber lumens include direct connections (arterio-luminal) or arteriolar connections through a sinusoidal system (arterio-sinusoidal). The sinusoidal system consists of a network of capillary-like vessels, but their diameters vary along their length [144]. Their expanded portions are 40–75 μm in diameter. Pratt, [146], suggested that this vascular system provides retro-flow and nutrition to the myocardium. Since that time, coronary venous retroperfusion has been suggested as a possible treatment for acute myocardial ischemia. Experiments have shown that synchronized retroperfusion of arterial blood through the great cardiac vein reduces myocardial necrosis in dogs with coronary artery occlusion [147]. In patients undergoing angioplasty of the left anterior descending coronary artery, synchronized retroperfusion was performed by pumping blood from the femoral artery into the great cardiac vein and was found to delay the onset of angina and to reduce its severity [148].

Vasa Vasorum

The role of vasa vasorum in the vasculature has been extensively reviewed recently [149]. This microvascular system provides nutrients to the outer medial wall of large arteries, and also to that of the largest veins. Arterioles arise either from the artery's own lumen or from an adjacent artery; the venules of the vasa vasorum drain into veins. The clinical significance of this vascular system is evident from the fact that experimental blockage of vasa vasorum arterioles (1) renders the vessel prone to atherosclerosis or (2) causes thinning of the media, which in an artery may result in an aneurysm. Gossl et al. [150] used three-dimensional micro-CT scanning to study porcine coronary vessels. They quantified the sizes and generations of branches of the vasa vasorum and noted that these parameters are similar to those of other vascular beds. The general structure of vasa vasorum >40 μm in diameter in the coronary arteries was found to be "tree-like." Most of the vessels comprising vasa vasorum are located in the adventitia, as seen in Fig. 4.1, but smaller branches penetrate the outer tunica media. A study in monkeys found that the coronary arteries receive only a minimal flow from vasa vasorum [151].

Barger et al. [152] showed that the vasa vasorum contributes significantly to the neovascularization of coronary arteries in atherosclerotic regions. These authors suggested that vascular proliferation is the normal response to injury and to the lower O_2 tension that occurs in the plaque. If this is true, proliferation of the vasa vasorum is a response to plaque formation. The significance of the vasa vasorum in plaque formation is clear since this vasculature provides 28 times more nutrition to the vascular wall than that derived from the lumen of the artery [153]. One study documented a nearly tenfold increase in blood flow to the intima–media via the vasa vasorum in atherosclerotic monkeys compared to that in monkeys with normal coronary arteries [154]. That study found that when atherosclerosis regressed, blood flow in the intima–media returned to normal, and the dilatory response to adenosine was blunted. One concern regarding expansion of the vasa vasorum is that these vessels are prone to rupture, as increased permeability and fragility characterize pathological neovascularization [155]. Indeed, the evidence supporting the notion that hemorrhage from the vasa vasorum contributes to unstable atherosclerotic lesions is compelling (reviewed in [156]). Moreover, the enhanced permeability of new vasa vasorum branches is likely to introduce inflammatory agents and macrophages. For example, VEGF is an inflammatory factor in atherosclerosis as it increases vessel permeability. A study of hypercholesterolemic swine found that neovascularization of the vasa vasorum is an early event as it documented a significant increase in vasa vasora density in the coronary arteries of these swine prior to the development of vascular lesions [157].

As noted in a review regarding neovascularization in human atherosclerosis, the vasa vasorum plays a vital role in plaque nutrition [158]. These vessels react to adenosine and endothelin-1, acetylcholine, ATP, and to a number of other vasoactive substances. However, vasa vasorum appears relatively unresponsive to norepinephrine, angiotensin II, and thromboxane A_2, which accounts for their protection against ischemia during sustained sympathetic activity. The vasa vasorum plays a role in plaque maintenance as evidenced by its plaque prevention or regression when angiogenesis is inhibited. A disoriented vasa vasorum neovascularization occurs in porcine coronary arteries when the animals become hypercholesterolemic [157]. This finding suggests that this neovascular response may contribute to the early atherosclerotic remodeling process.

Capillaries

Capillary growth and the significance of various capillary arteriolar and venular parameters (capillary domains, diffusion distance and recruitment) were addressed in Chap. 3. Adaptations of the capillary bed to various conditions are addressed in Chaps. 7 (aging), 8 (exercise), 9 (hypoxia), 10 (ischemia), and 11 (cardiac hypertrophy).

As evidenced by data from humans and experimental animals, capillary density is exceptionally high in the heart because of the high myocardial O_2 demand (Fig. 4.9). Reliable measurements of capillary density, especially those based on thin tissue sections, indicate that the number of capillaries per mm^2, ranges from 2,700 to more than 4,000 in rats, mice, sheep, rabbits, and dogs [159–166]. In the human heart, numerical capillary density is >2,200/mm^2 [167]. Accurate assessment of this parameter depends on obtaining true cross-sectional fields of cardiomyocytes, ability to

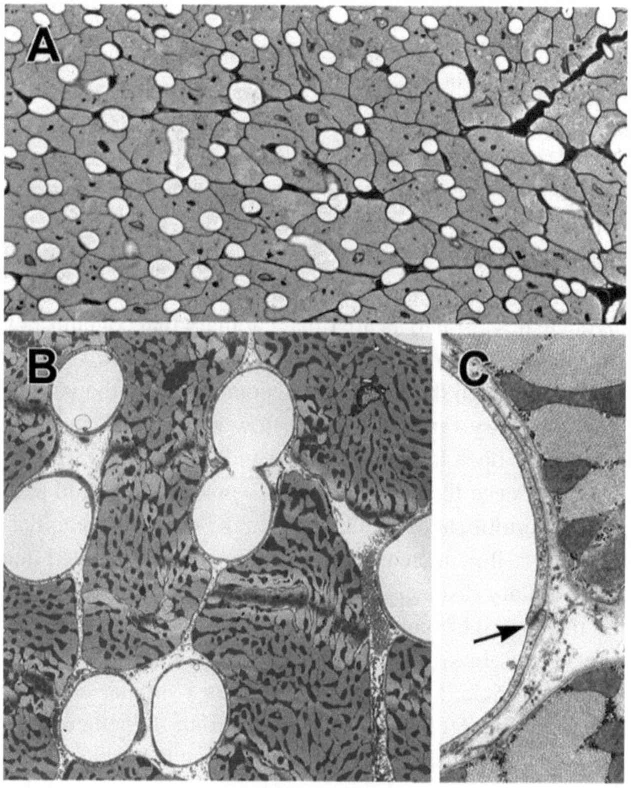

Fig. 4.9 Myocardial capillaries (rat); (**a**) is a 1-μm plastic section stained with silver to outline cardiomyocytes and capillaries. (**b** and **c**) are electron micrographs. Note that diffusion distances are minimized by the arrangement of cardiomyocytes, resulting in capillary indentations into the cells. As indicated in Chap. 3, capillary domains are variable due to their heterogeneity of spacing. The high resolution micrograph (**c**) shows an occluding junction (*arrow*), typical of myocardial capillaries. The extracellular matrix between adjacent cardiomyocytes and the capillary consists of basal laminae and fine reticular fibers

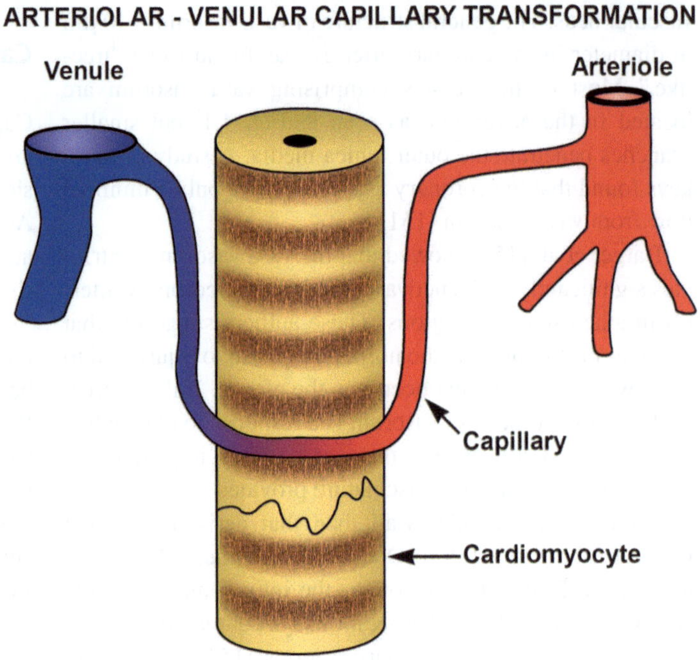

Fig. 4.10 The transformation of a capillary from its arteriolar to venular end is illustrated. Note the color transformation from *red* to blue, indicating a decrease in blood O_2. Capillary segments are situated so that cardiomyocytes are associated with at least one arteriolar capillary segment to receive adequate O_2

identify all capillaries in the field, and fixation and tissue processing that minimize cell separation. As described in Chap. 3, adequate O_2 cardiomyocyte availability is assured by the staggering of arterial and venous capillary segments. This anatomical arrangement provides each cardiomyocyte with an arteriolar capillary segment (Fig. 4.10). As noted in Chap. 3, the arteriolar and venular capillary segments are distributed in a staggered configuration so that each cardiomyocyte lies close to an arteriolar capillary that contains pO_2 values higher than those in venular capillaries.

Flow through the capillaries depends on both the volume of precapillary (artery/arteriole) flow and whether a given capillary is open to flow. Henquell and associates [168] provided evidence that increases in O_2 demand are met, in part, by the recruitment of capillaries, i.e., the number of capillaries open to flow increases with O_2 demand. They noted that intercapillary distance in the rat was slightly shorter in the left than the right ventricle. However, the calculated capillary reserve was less (about 27%) in the left than in the right (59%) ventricle, a finding that indicates a smaller capillary reserve in the left than in the right ventricle. Whether capillary recruitment is sufficient to compensate for the higher O_2 demand has not been demonstrated.

Collateral Circulation

This section concerning the collateral circulation is limited to the nature of the vessels and some concepts regarding their development. Details regarding the collateral circulation are components of other chapters as they pertain to aging (Chap. 7), exercise (Chap. 8), and ischemia, and infarction (Chap. 10); Chap. 5 covers the history of anastomotic channel research in the heart and the debates concerning the significance of these structures.

Coronary collaterals provide an alternative pathway of blood flow to the ischemic myocardium, which may serve to prevent myocardial infarction. As seen in Fig. 4.11, and also Fig. 10.2, the most extensive collateral vasculature is found in the canine epicardium. Native collaterals vary in size, but are usually <50 μm in most species. Large collaterals are generally restricted to the epicardium, whereas smaller collaterals are included transmurally. Human hearts may have collaterals 180 μm in diameter or even larger (see reviews by [169]). The deep anastomoses are often rather numerous and may include vessels with diameters in the 100–200 μm range, whereas in diseased hearts, coronary anastomoses with diameters >200 μm are common [170]. The interarteriolar anastomoses are subjected to remodeling when one of their parent arteries undergoes gradual occlusion. This process is often considered as a form of arteriogenesis and is discussed in the following section. A well-developed coronary collateral circulation has been shown to limit infarct size and to enhance survival (reviewed in [171]).

Remodeling of a Native Collateral

Fulton and van Royen [170] have documented that patients with obstructed arteries develop functional coronary collaterals by remodeling preexisting collateral arterioles. A number of studies have documented a role for the differential

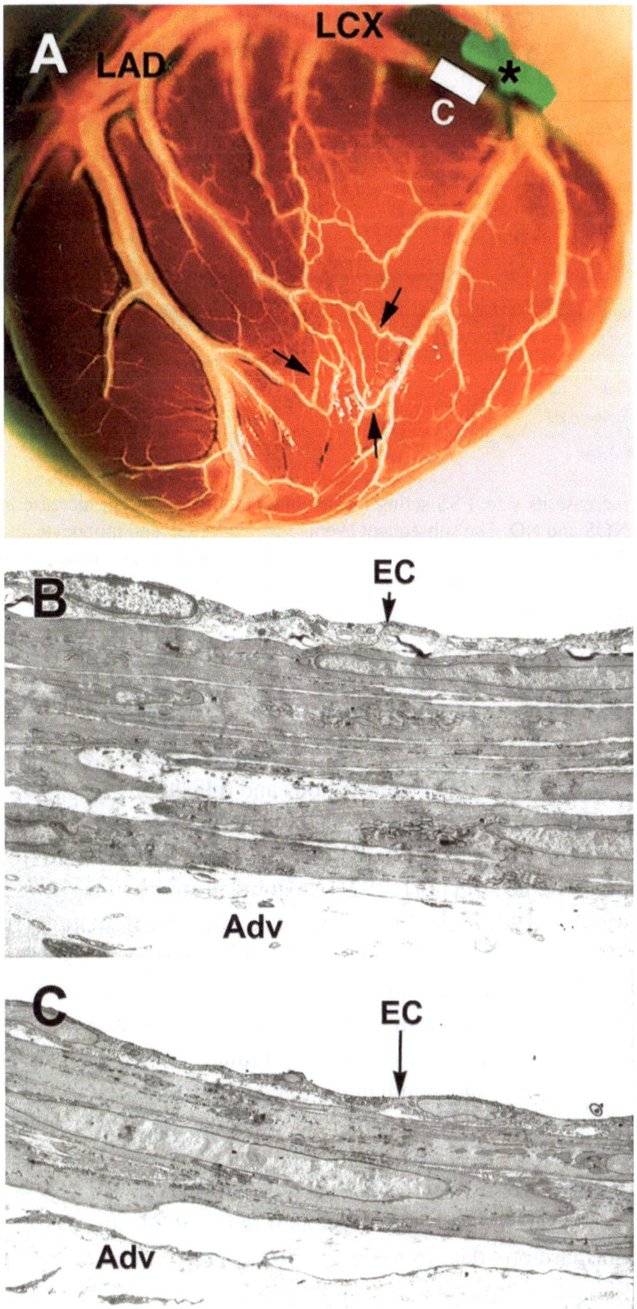

Fig. 4.11 Coronary canine collaterals. (**a**) Developing epicardial collateral vessels (*arrows*) in the left ventricle. The vessels were perfused with gelatin and bismuth SO_4 (image is from Cai et al. Am. J. Physiol. 284:H31, 2003, with permission). (**b** and **c**) are micrographs (Tomanek lab) illustrating canine collaterals of different diameters. Note that the structure of the walls is similar to non-collateral vessels shown in Figs. 4.2 and 4.7. Collaterals can be of various diameters as seen here. The collateral in (**b**) contains 5–6 VSMC layers, whereas the one in (**c**) has 2 VSMC layers. The light areas between the endothelial cells and the VSMC layers consist of elastin (internal elastic lamina). *EC* endothelial cell; *Adv* adventitia

pressure gradient between the two arteries and the consequential increase in the collateral vessel flow as a stimulus for the remodeling process. The collateral vessel remodels outward, thus increasing its diameter and enabling a greater flow. The primary stimulus for the remodeling process is an increase in pulsatile fluid shear stress (FSS), which evokes the cascade of molecular and cellular events summarized in Fig. 4.12. The details of these events have been reviewed [172]. In brief, all NOS isoforms are expressed, which increases NO production and VEGF secretion by ECs. This, in turn, triggers ECs and VSMCs to synthesize MCP-1, a molecule that both attracts and activates monocytes and T-cells. Collateral growth in the rat has been shown to require VEGF [173, 174]. Moreover, coronary artery occlusion in dogs upregulates FGFs 1 and 2 and PDGF-AB in both ECs and VSMCs in coronary collaterals [175]. These growth factors are required for the development of the tunica media. Despite the evidence that pressure gradients stimulate collateral growth, they are not a requisite for growth of smaller collaterals as demonstrated by Chilian and colleagues [176] who partially embolized the circumflex perfusion territory with 25-μm-diameter microspheres in dogs. They found that pressure gradients were not present, but that collateral growth occurred, which implies that ischemia alone is able to stimulate collateral growth.

The stimulation of collateral growth, even in the absence of ischemia, was found to occur in response to granulocyte colony stimulating factor-induced ROS production in cardiomyocytes [177]. Thus, this cytokine mimics some effects of ischemia. Signal transduction cascades in coronary collateral development include outside-in signaling from the ECM and is mediated by integrins [178]. The MAPK/ERK-signal transduction pathway activates the early growth response-1 (Erg-1) transcription factor that is critical for the progression of the cell cycle. This pathway involves FGF-1 and is enhanced by TGF-β1 [179, 180]. The Rho-kinase pathway also plays a role in collateral growth [181, 182]. Rho-kinase controls actin dynamics by its effects on a protein (cofilin) that is expressed in ECs and VSMCs [182].

Inflammatory Cells Play a Key Role in Collateral Remodeling

Monocyte attachment to the endothelium during the early stage of collateral vessel development was documented as early as 1976 [183] and supported the view that collateral vascular remodeling is an inflammatory process. These findings were based on scanning and transmission electronic microscopy to delineate changes in the collateral vessels over time and revealed that the tortuosity of these vessels underlies their non-laminar flow. The studies in Wolfgang Schaper's lab (reviewed in [172]) revealed that the expression of the adhesion molecules ICAM-1 and VCAM-1 is markedly enhanced during collateral development and that these proteins anchor the monocytes to the endothelium. Thus, these data demonstrated roles for several pathways regulating Erg-1 transcription and consequently collateral growth [178].

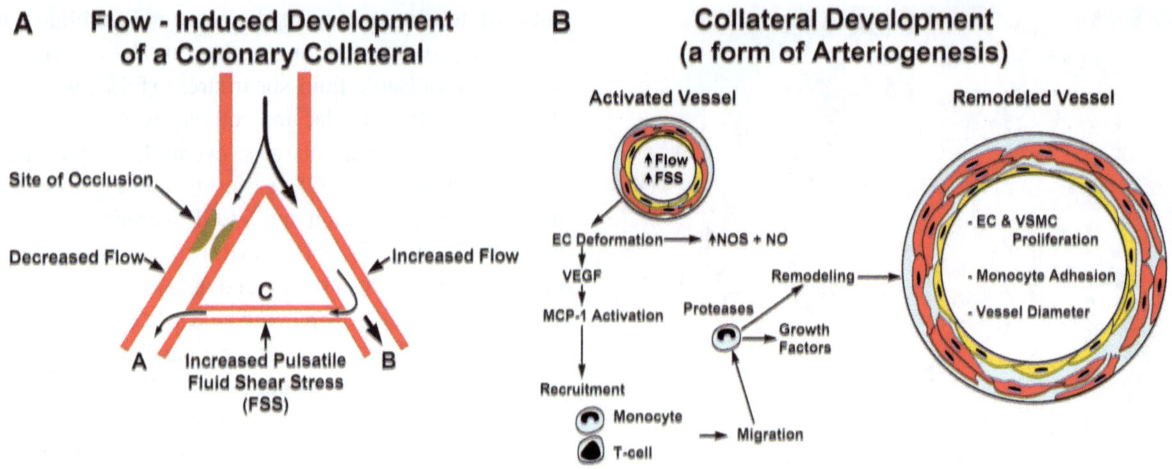

Fig. 4.12 Flow-induced development of coronary collaterals. Occlusion of an artery results in increased flow to an adjacent artery that is connected to the occluded vessel (**a**). The increased flow is transmitted to the collateral which then experiences increased pulsatile fluid shear stress. Pulsatile fluid shear stress (FSS) then stimulates collateral growth (arteriogenesis). As summarized in B, the collateral remodels to increase its size. FSS acting on the endothelium causes an increase in NOS and NO. The subsequent events involve VEGF and monocyte and T cell recruitment, which leads to remodeling of the vessel resulting in both increased diameter and wall thickness. The diagram is based on the review by Schaper [172]. See the text for details

A role for bone marrow-derived cells in collateral remodeling has been suggested. Some investigators have reported that these cells incorporate into the vessel wall [184, 185], whereas others have suggested that their effect is paracrine [186].

Stages of Collateral Remodeling (Reviewed by [172])

The earliest response of a collateral vessel subjected to increased FSS entails an increase in vascular permeability, recruitment of bone marrow cells, and changes in the phenotypes of ECs and VSMCs that prepare them to proliferate. The changes are followed by digestion of extracellular matrix components, which facilitates cell migration, and EC proliferation, followed by proliferation of VSMCs. Next, VSMCs arrange themselves in layers, establish cell–cell contacts, and secrete collagen and elastin to form a new vascular scaffold and a larger vessel. Finally, smaller adjacent collateral vessels regress when flow is not enhanced.

Cardiac Lymphatic Vessels

Until recently, the function of cardiac lymphatic vessels did not receive much attention because of technical problems in studying lymph flow. However, the development of animal models has provided an opportunity to study both normal and impaired lymphatic circulation [187, 188]. Lymphatic vessels exist in the subepicardium, midmyocardium, and subendocardium, as well as in the atrioventricular and semilunar valves [189–192]. The lymphatic capillary plexus is drained through collecting lymphatic vessels into the subclavian vein. Cardiac lymphatic flow is likely due to passive pumping arising from cardiac contractions and relaxations.

The fact that the ventricular contractions are stronger than those of the atria may explain why lymphedema is more frequent in the atria [191, 192]. Anatomical studies have shown that a single longitudinal lymphatic pathway runs parallel to the right conduction bundle [193]. This finding suggests that impaired cardiac lymph flow could contribute to conduction disturbances and arrhythmia; clinical studies have shown lymphedema to be linked to arrhythmias [194]. Blood vessel injury, i.e., subendothelial, interstitial, and intracellular edema, has been shown to occur when cardiac lymph flow is blocked [195]. The presence of lymphatic capillaries surrounding coronary blood vessels suggests that they are important in the collection and removal of fluid [196]. Furthermore, data from dogs with coronary artery occlusion indicate that cardiac lymph flow is decreased [197]. Taken together, these studies suggest that the cardiac lymphatic system helps maintain normal heart function.

References

1. Vatner SF, Pagani M, Manders WT, Pasipoularides AD. Alpha adrenergic vasoconstriction and nitroglycerin vasodilation of large coronary arteries in the conscious dog. J Clin Invest. 1980;65: 5–14.
2. Chilian WM, Marcus ML. Phasic coronary blood flow velocity in intramural and epicardial coronary arteries. Circ Res. 1982;50: 775–81.
3. Forman R, Kirk ES. Comparative effects of vasodilator drugs on large and small coronary resistance vessels in the dog. Cardiovasc Res. 1980;14:601–6.

4. Simionescu N, Simionescu M. The cardiovascular system. In: Cell and tissue biology: a textbook of histology. Baltimore: Urban and Schwarzenberg, Inc; 1988. p. 355–400.
5. Tomanek RJ, Palmer PJ, Peiffer GL, Schreiber KL, Eastham CL, Marcus ML. Morphometry of canine coronary arteries, arterioles, and capillaries during hypertension and left ventricular hypertrophy. Circ Res. 1986;58:38–46.
6. Forbes MS. Ultrastructure of vascular smooth-muscle cells in mammalian heart. In: Kalsner S, editor. The coronary artery. London: Croan Helm; 1982. p. 3–58.
7. Forbes MS. Vascular-smooth muscle cells and other perioendothelial cells of mammalian heart. In: Sperelakis N, editor. Physiology and pathophysiology of the heart. The Netherlands: Kluwer Academic Publishers; 1989. p. 711–54.
8. Beny JL, Connat JL. An electron-microscopic study of smooth muscle cell dye coupling in the pig coronary arteries. Role of gap junctions. Circ Res. 1992;70:49–55.
9. Boucek RJ, Takashita R, Fojaco R. Relation between microanatomy and functional properties of the coronary arteries. Anat Rec. 1963;147:199–207.
10. Rhodin JA. Ultrastructure of mammalian venous capillaries, venules, and small collecting veins. J Ultrastruct Res. 1968;25:452–500.
11. Sims DE. The pericyte—a review. Tissue Cell. 1986;18:153–74.
12. Tilton RG, Kilo C, Williamson JR. Pericyte-endothelial relationships in cardiac and skeletal muscle capillaries. Microvasc Res. 1979;18:325–35.
13. Hirschi KK, D'Amore PA. Pericytes in the microvasculature. Cardiovasc Res. 1996;32:687–98.
14. Simionescu N, Siminoescu M, Palade GE. Permeability of muscle capillaries to small heme-peptides. Evidence for the existence of patent transendothelial channels. J Cell Biol. 1975;64:586–607.
15. Palade GE. Blood capillaries of the heart and other organs. Circulation. 1961;24:368–88.
16. Vasheghani-Farahani A, Kassaian SE, Yaminisharif A, Davoodi G, Salarifar M, Amirzadegan A, et al. The association between coronary arterial dominancy and extent of coronary artery disease in angiography and paraclinical studies. Clin Anat. 2008;21:519–23.
17. Allwork SP. The applied anatomy of the arterial blood supply to the heart in man. J Anat. 1987;153:1–16.
18. Raphael MJ, Hawtin DR, Allwork SP. The angiographic anatomy of the coronary arteries. Br J Surg. 1980;67:181–7.
19. Ilia R, Rosenshtein G, Weinstein J, Cafri C, Abu-Ful A, Gueron M. Left anterior descending artery length in left and right coronary artery dominance. Coron Artery Dis. 2001;12:77–8.
20. Schlesinger M. Significant variations in the anatomic pattern of the coronary vessels. In: Blood, heart and circulation symposium. American Association for the Advancement of Science, Washington, DC; 1940. p. 61–72.
21. James T. Anatomy of the coronary arteries. New York: Medical Division of Harper and Brothers; 1961.
22. Bardoli G. Diseases of the coronary arteries. In: Cardiovascular pathology. New York: Churchill Livingstone; 1983.
23. James TN. Anatomy of the coronary arteries in health and disease. Circulation. 1965;32:1020–33.
24. Kini S, Bis KG, Weaver L. Normal and variant coronary arterial and venous anatomy on high-resolution CT angiography. AJR Am J Roentgenol. 2007;188:1665–74.
25. Rabe D. Diameter determination of the coronary arteries and coronary sinus. Basic Res Cardiol. 1973;68:356–79.
26. Kato T. A comparative study of the coronary arterial structure in the left ventricular free wall in infarcted and non-infarcted human hearts. Jpn Circ J. 1976;40:989–1003.
27. Tillmanns H, Ikeda S, Hansen H, Sarma JS, Fauvel JM, Bing RJ. Microcirculation in the ventricle of the dog and turtle. Circ Res. 1974;34:561–9.
28. Kato T, Yasue T, Shoji Y, Shimabukuro S, Ito Y, Goto S, et al. Angiographic difference in coronary artery of man, dog, pig, and monkey. Acta Pathol Jpn. 1987;37:361–73.
29. Lumb G, Singletary HP. Blood supply to the atrioventricular node and bundle of His: a comparative study in pig, dog, and man. Am J Pathol. 1962;41:65–75.
30. Sahni D, Kaur GD, Jit H, Jit I. Anatomy & distribution of coronary arteries in pig in comparison with man. Indian J Med Res. 2008;127:564–70.
31. Lumb G, Shacklett RS, Dawkins WA. The cardiac conduction tissue and its blood supply in the dog. Am J Pathol. 1959;35:467–87.
32. Zamir M. Distributing and delivering vessels of the human heart. J Gen Physiol. 1988;91:725–35.
33. Thuroff JW, Hort W, Lichti H. Diameter of coronary arteries in 36 species of mammalian from mouse to giraffe. Basic Res Cardiol. 1984;79:199–206.
34. Kassab GS, Imoto K, White FC, Rider CA, Fung YC, Bloor CM. Coronary arterial tree remodeling in right ventricular hypertrophy. Am J Physiol. 1993;265:H366–75.
35. Kaimovitz B, Lanir Y, Kassab GS. A full 3-D reconstruction of the entire porcine coronary vasculature. Am J Physiol Heart Circ Physiol. 2010;299:H1064–76.
36. Kassab GS. Functional hierarchy of coronary circulation: direct evidence of a structure-function relation. Am J Physiol Heart Circ Physiol. 2005;289:H2559–65.
37. Kristek F, Gerova M. Autonomic nerve terminals in relation to contractile and non-contractile structures in the conduit coronary artery of the dog. Acta Anat (Basel). 1987;129:149–54.
38. Dolezel S, Gerova M, Hartmannova B, Vasku J. Development of the adrenergic innervation in the myocardium and coronary arteries of the dog. Acta Anat (Basel). 1990;139:191–200.
39. Chilian WM, Eastham CL, Marcus ML. Microvascular distribution of coronary vascular resistance in beating left ventricle. Am J Physiol. 1986;251:H779–88.
40. Chilian WM, Layne SM, Klausner EC, Eastham CL, Marcus ML. Redistribution of coronary microvascular resistance produced by dipyridamole. Am J Physiol. 1989;256:H383–90.
41. Kanatsuka H, Sekiguchi N, Sato K, Akai K, Wang Y, Komaru T, et al. Microvascular sites and mechanisms responsible for reactive hyperemia in the coronary circulation of the beating canine heart. Circ Res. 1992;71:912–22.
42. Zhang C, Hein TW, Kuo L. Transmural difference in coronary arteriolar dilation to adenosine: effect of luminal pressure and K(ATP) channels. Am J Physiol Heart Circ Physiol. 2000;279:H2612–9.
43. Quillen JE, Harrison DG. Vasomotor properties of porcine endocardial and epicardial microvessels. Am J Physiol. 1992;262:H1143–8.
44. Deussen A, Ohanyan V, Jannasch A, Yin L, Chilian W. Mechanisms of metabolic coronary flow regulation. J Mol Cell Cardiol. 2012; 52:794–801.
45. Tune JD, Gorman MW, Feigl EO. Matching coronary blood flow to myocardial oxygen consumption. J Appl Physiol. 2004;97:404–15.
46. Zhang C, Rogers PA, Merkus D, Muller-Delp JM, Tiefenbacher CP, Potter B, et al. Regulation of coronary microvascular resistance in health and disease. In: Tuma RR, Duran WN, Ley K, editors. Microcirculation. San Diego: Elsevier; 2008. p. 521–49.
47. Feigl EO. Coronary physiology. Physiol Rev. 1983;63:1–205.
48. Jones CE, Hurst TW, Randall JR. Effect of aminophylline on coronary functional hyperemia and myocardial adenosine. Am J Physiol. 1982;243:H480–7.
49. Tune JD, Richmond KN, Gorman MW, Olsson RA, Feigl EO. Adenosine is not responsible for local metabolic control of coronary blood flow in dogs during exercise. Am J Physiol Heart Circ Physiol. 2000;278:H74–84.
50. Yada T, Richmond KN, Van Bibber R, Kroll K, Feigl EO. Role of adenosine in local metabolic coronary vasodilation. Am J Physiol. 1999;276:H1425–33.

51. Deussen A, Brand M, Pexa A, Weichsel J. Metabolic coronary flow regulation—current concepts. Basic Res Cardiol. 2006;101: 453–64.
52. Duncker DJ, Bache RJ. Regulation of coronary blood flow during exercise. Physiol Rev. 2008;88:1009–86.
53. Edlund A, Sollevi A. Theophylline increases coronary vascular tone in humans: evidence for a role of endogenous adenosine in flow regulation. Acta Physiol Scand. 1995;155:303–11.
54. Laxson DD, Homans DC, Bache RJ. Inhibition of adenosine-mediated coronary vasodilation exacerbates myocardial ischemia during exercise. Am J Physiol. 1993;265:H1471–7.
55. Duncker DJ, Laxson DD, Lindstrom P, Bache RJ. Endogenous adenosine and coronary vasoconstriction in hypoperfused myocardium during exercise. Cardiovasc Res. 1993;27:1592–7.
56. Duncker DJ, Stubenitsky R, Verdouw PD. Role of adenosine in the regulation of coronary blood flow in swine at rest and during treadmill exercise. Am J Physiol. 1998;275:H1663–72.
57. Ziada AM, Hudlicka O, Tyler KR, Wright AJ. The effect of long-term vasodilatation on capillary growth and performance in rabbit heart and skeletal muscle. Cardiovasc Res. 1984;18:724–32.
58. Mall G, Schikora I, Mattfeldt T, Bodle R. Dipyridamole-induced neoformation of capillaries in the rat heart. Quantitative stereological study on papillary muscles. Lab Invest. 1987;57:86–93.
59. Symons JD, Firoozmand E, Longhurst JC. Repeated dipyridamole administration enhances collateral-dependent flow and regional function during exercise. A role for adenosine. Circ Res. 1993;73:503–13.
60. Dubey RK, Gillespie DG, Jackson EK. A(2B) adenosine receptors stimulate growth of porcine and rat arterial endothelial cells. Hypertension. 2002;39:530–5.
61. Auchampach JA. Adenosine receptors and angiogenesis. Circ Res. 2007;101:1075–7.
62. Adair TH. Growth regulation of the vascular system: an emerging role for adenosine. Am J Physiol Regul Integr Comp Physiol. 2005;289:R283–96.
63. Headrick JP, Peart JN, Reichelt ME, Haseler LJ. Adenosine and its receptors in the heart: regulation, retaliation and adaptation. Biochim Biophys Acta. 2011;1808(5):1413–28.
64. Teng B, Qin W, Ansari HR, Mustafa SJ. Involvement of p38-mitogen-activated protein kinase in adenosine receptor-mediated relaxation of coronary artery. Am J Physiol Heart Circ Physiol. 2005;288:H2574–80.
65. Tawfik HE, Schnermann J, Oldenburg PJ, Mustafa SJ. Role of A1 adenosine receptors in regulation of vascular tone. Am J Physiol Heart Circ Physiol. 2005;288:H1411–6.
66. Sato A, Terata K, Miura H, Toyama K, Loberiza Jr FR, Hatoum OA, et al. Mechanism of vasodilation to adenosine in coronary arterioles from patients with heart disease. Am J Physiol Heart Circ Physiol. 2005;288:H1633–40.
67. Altman JD, Kinn J, Duncker DJ, Bache RJ. Effect of inhibition of nitric oxide formation on coronary blood flow during exercise in the dog. Cardiovasc Res. 1994;28:119–24.
68. Bernstein RD, Ochoa FY, Xu X, Forfia P, Shen W, Thompson CI, et al. Function and production of nitric oxide in the coronary circulation of the conscious dog during exercise. Circ Res. 1996;79:840–8.
69. Smith Jr TP, Canty Jr JM. Modulation of coronary autoregulatory responses by nitric oxide. Evidence for flow-dependent resistance adjustments in conscious dogs. Circ Res. 1993;73:232–40.
70. Afonso S, Bandow GT, Rowe GG. Indomethacin and the prostaglandin hypothesis of coronary blood flow regulation. J Physiol. 1974;241:299–308.
71. Dai XZ, Bache RJ. Effect of indomethacin on coronary blood flow during graded treadmill exercise in the dog. Am J Physiol. 1984;247:H452–8.
72. Richmond KN, Tune JD, Gorman MW, Feigl EO. Role of K(ATP) (+) channels and adenosine in the control of coronary blood flow during exercise. J Appl Physiol. 2000;89:529–36.
73. Saitoh S, Zhang C, Tune JD, Potter B, Kiyooka T, Rogers PA, et al. Hydrogen peroxide: a feed-forward dilator that couples myocardial metabolism to coronary blood flow. Arterioscler Thromb Vasc Biol. 2006;26:2614–21.
74. Miura H, Bosnjak JJ, Ning G, Saito T, Miura M, Gutterman DD. Role for hydrogen peroxide in flow-induced dilation of human coronary arterioles. Circ Res. 2003;92:e31–40.
75. Bayliss WM. On the local reactions of the arterial wall to changes of internal pressure. J Physiol. 1902;28:220–31.
76. Liu Y, Gutterman DD. Vascular control in humans: focus on the coronary microcirculation. Basic Res Cardiol. 2009;104:211–27.
77. Kuo L, Davis MJ, Chilian WM. Myogenic activity in isolated subepicardial and subendocardial coronary arterioles. Am J Physiol. 1988;255:H1558–62.
78. Kuo L, Davis MJ, Chilian WM. Endothelium-dependent, flow-induced dilation of isolated coronary arterioles. Am J Physiol. 1990;259:H1063–70.
79. Kuo L, Chilian WM, Davis MJ. Interaction of pressure- and flow-induced responses in porcine coronary resistance vessels. Am J Physiol. 1991;261:H1706–15.
80. Kuo L, Arko F, Chilian WM, Davis MJ. Coronary venular responses to flow and pressure. Circ Res. 1993;72:607–15.
81. Miller Jr FJ, Dellsperger KC, Gutterman DD. Myogenic constriction of human coronary arterioles. Am J Physiol. 1997;273: H257–64.
82. Chilian WM, Layne SM. Coronary microvascular responses to reductions in perfusion pressure. Evidence for persistent arteriolar vasomotor tone during coronary hypoperfusion. Circ Res. 1990; 66:1227–38.
83. Kanatsuka H, Lamping KG, Eastham CL, Marcus ML. Heterogeneous changes in epimyocardial microvascular size during graded coronary stenosis. Evidence of the microvascular site for autoregulation. Circ Res. 1990;66:389–96.
84. Khan BF, Renton S, Hussain ST. Aortic aneurysm replacement with Dacron graft in a 34 year old man. How long will the graft last? Postgrad Med J. 2003;79:348–9.
85. Dole WP, Nuno DW. Myocardial oxygen tension determines the degree and pressure range of coronary autoregulation. Circ Res. 1986;59:202–15.
86. Muller JM, Davis MJ, Chilian WM. Integrated regulation of pressure and flow in the coronary microcirculation. Cardiovasc Res. 1996;32:668–78.
87. Zhang H, Sunnarborg SW, McNaughton KK, Johns TG, Lee DC, Faber JE. Heparin-binding epidermal growth factor-like growth factor signaling in flow-induced arterial remodeling. Circ Res. 2008;102:1275–85.
88. Losano G, Gattullo D, Pagliaro P. Properties of the myocardium affecting the coronary circulation. Cardioscience. 1995;6:13–7.
89. Klocke FJ. Coronary blood flow in man. Prog Cardiovasc Dis. 1976;19:117–66.
90. Griggs Jr DM, Nakamura Y. Effect of coronary constriction on myocardial distribution of iodoantipyrine-131-I. Am J Physiol. 1968;215:1082–6.
91. Downey JM, Kirk ES. Distribution of the coronary blood flow across the canine heart wall during systole. Circ Res. 1974;34:251–7.
92. Russell RE, Chagrasulis RW, Downey JM. Inhibitory effect of cardiac contraction on coronary collateral blood flow. Am J Physiol. 1977;233:H541–6.
93. Downey JM, Kirk ES. Inhibition of coronary blood flow by a vascular waterfall mechanism. Circ Res. 1975;36:753–60.
94. Hoffman JI, Spaan JA. Pressure-flow relations in coronary circulation. Physiol Rev. 1990;70:331–90.

95. Feigl EO. Neural control of coronary blood flow. J Vasc Res. 1998;35:85–92.
96. Feigl EO. Neural control of the coronary circulation. In: Neurocardiology. Mount Kisco, NY: Futura Publishing Company; 1988. p. 123–31.
97. Bassenge E, Heusch G. Endothelial and neuro-humoral control of coronary blood flow in health and disease. Rev Physiol Biochem Pharmacol. 1990;116:77–165.
98. Baumgart D, Heusch G. Neuronal control of coronary blood flow. Basic Res Cardiol. 1995;90:142–59.
99. Klocke FJ, Kaiser GA, Ross Jr J, Braunwald E. An intrinsic adrenergic vasodilator mechanism in the coronary vascular bed of the dog. Circ Res. 1965;16:376–82.
100. Hamilton FN, Feigl EO. Coronary vascular sympathetic beta-receptor innervation. Am J Physiol. 1976;230:1569–76.
101. McRaven DR, Mark AL, Abboud FM, Mayer HE. Responses of coronary vessels to adrenergic stimuli. J Clin Invest. 1971;50: 773–8.
102. Vatner SF, Hintze TH, Macho P. Regulation of large coronary arteries by beta-adrenergic mechanisms in the conscious dog. Circ Res. 1982;51:56–66.
103. von Restorff W, Bassenge E. Transient effects of norepinephrine on myocardial oxygen balance. Pflugers Arch. 1977;370:131–7.
104. Vatner DE, Knight DR, Homcy CJ, Vatner SF, Young MA. Subtypes of beta-adrenergic receptors in bovine coronary arteries. Circ Res. 1986;59:463–73.
105. Nakane T, Tsujimoto G, Hashimoto K, Chiba S. Beta adrenoceptors in the canine large coronary arteries: beta-1 adrenoceptors predominate in vasodilation. J Pharmacol Exp Ther. 1988;245:936–43.
106. Young MA, Vatner SF. Regulation of large coronary arteries. Circ Res. 1986;59:579–96.
107. Zhao G, Hintze TH, Kaley G. Neural regulation of coronary vascular resistance: role of nitric oxide in reflex cholinergic coronary vasodilation in normal and pathophysiological states. In: Myocardial ischemia: mechanisms, reperfusion, protection. Basal, Switzerland: Burkhauser Verlag; 1996. p. 1–19.
108. Molenaar P, Jones CR, McMartin LR, Summers RJ. Autoradiographic localization and densitometric analysis of beta-1 and beta-2 adrenoceptors in the canine left anterior descending coronary artery. J Pharmacol Exp Ther. 1988;246:384–93.
109. Murphree SS, Saffitz JE. Delineation of the distribution of beta-adrenergic receptor subtypes in canine myocardium. Circ Res. 1988;63:117–25.
110. Trivella MG, Broten TP, Feigl EO. Beta-receptor subtypes in the canine coronary circulation. Am J Physiol. 1990;259:H1575–85.
111. Young MA, Knight DR, Vatner SF. Autonomic control of large coronary arteries and resistance vessels. Prog Cardiovasc Dis. 1987;30:211–34.
112. Kelley KO, Feigl EO. Segmental alpha-receptor-mediated vasoconstriction in the canine coronary circulation. Circ Res. 1978;43: 908–17.
113. Heusch G, Deussen A, Schipke J, Thamer V. Alpha 1- and alpha 2-adrenoceptor-mediated vasoconstriction of large and small canine coronary arteries in vivo. J Cardiovasc Pharmacol. 1984;6: 961–8.
114. Chilian WM, Boatwright RB, Shoji T, Griggs Jr DM. Evidence against significant resting sympathetic coronary vasoconstrictor tone in the conscious dog. Circ Res. 1981;49:866–76.
115. Holtz J, Saeed M, Sommer O, Bassenge E. Norepinephrine constricts the canine coronary bed via postsynaptic alpha 2-adrenoceptors. Eur J Pharmacol. 1982;82:199–202.
116. Woodman OL, Vatner SF. Coronary vasoconstriction mediated by alpha 1- and alpha 2-adrenoceptors in conscious dogs. Am J Physiol. 1987;253:H388–93.
117. Young MA, Vatner DE, Knight DR, Graham RM, Homcy CJ, Vatner SF. Alpha-adrenergic vasoconstriction and receptor subtypes in large coronary arteries of calves. Am J Physiol. 1988;255:H1452–9.
118. Miyashiro JK, Feigl EO. Feedforward control of coronary blood flow via coronary beta-receptor stimulation. Circ Res. 1993; 73:252–63.
119. Heusch GJ. The paradox of α-adrenergic coronary vasoconstriction revisited. J Mol Cell Cardiol. 2011;16–23.
120. Tiefenbacher CP, DeFily DV, Chilian WM. Requisite role of cardiac myocytes in coronary alpha1-adrenergic constriction. Circulation. 1998;98:9–12.
121. Merkus D, Duncker DJ, Chilian WM. Metabolic regulation of coronary vascular tone: role of endothelin-1. Am J Physiol Heart Circ Physiol. 2002;283:H1915–21.
122. Merkus D, Brzezinska AK, Zhang C, Saito S, Chilian WM. Cardiac myocytes control release of endothelin-1 in coronary vasculature. Am J Physiol Heart Circ Physiol. 2005;288:H2088–92.
123. Hodgson JM, Marshall JJ. Direct vasoconstriction and endothelium-dependent vasodilation. Mechanisms of acetylcholine effects on coronary flow and arterial diameter in patients with nonstenotic coronary arteries. Circulation. 1989;79:1043–51.
124. Hodgson JM, Cohen MD, Szentpetery S, Thames MD. Effects of regional alpha- and beta-blockade on resting and hyperemic coronary blood flow in conscious, unstressed humans. Circulation. 1989;79:797–809.
125. Sun D, Huang A, Mital S, Kichuk MR, Marboe CC, Addonizio LJ, et al. Norepinephrine elicits beta2-receptor-mediated dilation of isolated human coronary arterioles. Circulation. 2002;106:550–5.
126. Dessy C, Moniotte S, Ghisdal P, Havaux X, Noirhomme P, Balligand JL. Endothelial beta3-adrenoceptors mediate vasorelaxation of human coronary microarteries through nitric oxide and endothelium-dependent hyperpolarization. Circulation. 2004;110:948–54.
127. Graham RM, Perez DM, Hwa J, Piascik MT. alpha 1-adrenergic receptor subtypes. Molecular structure, function, and signaling. Circ Res. 1996;78:737–49.
128. Jensen BC, Swigart PM, Laden ME, DeMarco T, Hoopes C, Simpson PC. The alpha-1D Is the predominant alpha-1-adrenergic receptor subtype in human epicardial coronary arteries. J Am Coll Cardiol. 2009;54:1137–45.
129. Turnbull L, McCloskey DT, O'Connell TD, Simpson PC, Baker AJ. Alpha 1-adrenergic receptor responses in alpha 1AB-AR knockout mouse hearts suggest the presence of alpha 1D-AR. Am J Physiol Heart Circ Physiol. 2003;284:H1104–9.
130. Feigl EO. Parasympathetic control of coronary blood flow in dogs. Circ Res. 1969;25:509–19.
131. Kovach JA, Gottdiener JS, Verrier RL. Vagal modulation of epicardial coronary artery size in dogs. A two-dimensional intravascular ultrasound study. Circulation. 1995;92:2291–8.
132. Ludmer PL, Selwyn AP, Shook TL, Wayne RR, Mudge GH, Alexander RW, et al. Paradoxical vasoconstriction induced by acetylcholine in atherosclerotic coronary arteries. N Engl J Med. 1986;315:1046–51.
133. Werns SW, Walton JA, Hsia HH, Nabel EG, Sanz ML, Pitt B. Evidence of endothelial dysfunction in angiographically normal coronary arteries of patients with coronary artery disease. Circulation. 1989;79:287–91.
134. Vita JA, Treasure CB, Nabel EG, McLenachan JM, Fish RD, Yeung AC, et al. Coronary vasomotor response to acetylcholine relates to risk factors for coronary artery disease. Circulation. 1990;81:491–7.
135. Young MA, Knight DR, Vatner SF. Parasympathetic coronary vasoconstriction induced by nicotine in conscious calves. Circ Res. 1988;62:891–5.
136. Cowan CL, McKenzie JE. Cholinergic regulation of resting coronary blood flow in domestic swine. Am J Physiol. 1990;259: H109–15.

137. Knight DR, Shen YT, Young MA, Vatner SF. Acetylcholine-induced coronary vasoconstriction and vasodilation in tranquilized baboons. Circ Res. 1991;69:706–13.
138. Hammond GL, Austen WG. Drainage patterns of coronary arterial flow as determined from the isolated heart. Am J Physiol. 1967; 212:1435–40.
139. Piffer CR, Piffer MI, Zorzetto NL. Anatomic data of the human coronary sinus. Anat Anz. 1990;170:21–9.
140. Loukas M, Bilinsky S, Bilinsky E, el-Sedfy A, Anderson RH. Cardiac veins: a review of the literature. Clin Anat. 2009;22:129–45.
141. von Ludinghausen M. The venous drainage of the human myocardium. Adv Anat Embryol Cell Biol. 2003;168:I–VIII, 1–104.
142. Mak GS, Hill AJ, Moisiuc F, Krishnan SC. Variations in Thebesian valve anatomy and coronary sinus ostium: implications for invasive electrophysiology procedures. Europace. 2009;11:1188–92.
143. Gensini GG, Digiorgi S, Coskun O, Palacio A, Kelly AE. Anatomy of the coronary circulation in living man; coronary venography. Circulation. 1965;31:778–84.
144. von Ludinghausen M. The clinical anatomy of coronary arteries. Adv Anat Embryol Cell Biol. 2003;167:III–VIII, 1–111.
145. Ansari A. Anatomy and clinical significance of ventricular Thebesian veins. Clin Anat. 2001;14:102–10.
146. Pratt F. The nutrition of the heart through the vessels of Thebesius and the coronary veins. Am J Physiol. 1898;1:86–103.
147. Drury JK, Yamazaki S, Fishbein MC, Meerbaum S, Corday E. Synchronized diastolic coronary venous retroperfusion: results of a preclinical safety and efficacy study. J Am Coll Cardiol. 1985;6:328–35.
148. Kar S, Drury JK, Hajduczki I, Eigler N, Wakida Y, Litvack F, et al. Synchronized coronary venous retroperfusion for support and salvage of ischemic myocardium during elective and failed angioplasty. J Am Coll Cardiol. 1991;18:271–82.
149. Mulligan-Kehoe MJ. The vasa vasorum in diseased and nondiseased arteries. Am J Physiol Heart Circ Physiol. 2010;298:H295–305.
150. Gossl M, Rosol M, Malyar NM, Fitzpatrick LA, Beighley PE, Zamir M, et al. Functional anatomy and hemodynamic characteristics of vasa vasorum in the walls of porcine coronary arteries. Anat Rec A Discov Mol Cell Evol Biol. 2003;272:526–37.
151. Heistad DD, Armstrong ML, Marcus ML. Hyperemia of the aortic wall in atherosclerotic monkeys. Circ Res. 1981;48:669–75.
152. Barger AC, Beeuwkes 3rd R, Lainey LL, Silverman KJ. Hypothesis: vasa vasorum and neovascularization of human coronary arteries. A possible role in the pathophysiology of atherosclerosis. N Engl J Med. 1984;310:175–7.
153. Kumamoto M, Nakashima Y, Sueishi K. Intimal neovascularization in human coronary atherosclerosis: its origin and pathophysiological significance. Hum Pathol. 1995;26:450–6.
154. Williams JK, Armstrong ML, Heistad DD. Vasa vasorum in atherosclerotic coronary arteries: responses to vasoactive stimuli and regression of atherosclerosis. Circ Res. 1988;62:515–23.
155. Bates DO, Harper SJ. Regulation of vascular permeability by vascular endothelial growth factors. Vasc Pharmacol. 2002;39:225–37.
156. Ritman EL, Lerman A. The dynamic vasa vasorum. Cardiovasc Res. 2007;75:649–58.
157. Kwon HM, Sangiorgi G, Ritman EL, McKenna C, Holmes Jr DR, Schwartz RS, et al. Enhanced coronary vasa vasorum neovascularization in experimental hypercholesterolemia. J Clin Invest. 1998; 101:1551–6.
158. Moreno PR, Purushothaman KR, Sirol M, Levy AP, Fuster V. Neovascularization in human atherosclerosis. Circulation. 2006; 113:2245–52.
159. Bassingthwaighte JB, Yipintsoi T, Harvey RB. Microvasculature of the dog left ventricular myocardium. Microvasc Res. 1974;7: 229–49.
160. Rakusan K, Cicutti N, Flanagan MF. Changes in the microvascular network during cardiac growth, development, and aging. Cell Mol Biol Res. 1994;40:117–22.
161. Rakusan K, Heron MI, Kolar F, Korecky B. Transplantation-induced atrophy of normal and hypertrophic rat hearts: effect on cardiac myocytes and capillaries. J Mol Cell Cardiol. 1997; 29:1045–54.
162. Tomanek RJ, Barlow PA, Connell PM, Chen Y, Torry RJ. Effects of hypothyroidism and hypertension on myocardial perfusion and vascularity in rabbits. Am J Physiol. 1993;265:H1638–44.
163. Tomanek RJ, Aydelotte MR, Torry RJ. Remodeling of coronary vessels during aging in purebred beagles. Circ Res. 1991;69: 1068–74.
164. Tomanek RJ, Busch TL. Coordinated capillary and myocardial growth in response to thyroxine treatment. Anat Rec. 1998;251:44–9.
165. Torry RJ, O'Brien DM, Connell PM, Tomanek RJ. Dipyridamole-induced capillary growth in normal and hypertrophic hearts. Am J Physiol. 1992;262:H980–6.
166. Smolich JJ, Walker AM, Campbell GR, Adamson TM. Left and right ventricular myocardial morphometry in fetal, neonatal, and adult sheep. Am J Physiol. 1989;257:H1–9.
167. Rakusan K, Flanagan MF, Geva T, Southern J, Van Praagh R. Morphometry of human coronary capillaries during normal growth and the effect of age in left ventricular pressure-overload hypertrophy. Circulation. 1992;86:38–46.
168. Henquell L, Odoroff CL, Honig CR. Coronary intercapillary distance during growth: relation to PtO_2 and aerobic capacity. Am J Physiol. 1976;231:1852–9.
169. Bloor CM, Liebow AA. Coronary collateral circulation. Am J Cardiol. 1965;16:238–52.
170. Fulton WF, VanRoyean N. The coronary collateral circulation in man. In: Schaper W, Schaper J, editors. Arteriogenesis. Boston: Kluwer Academic Publishers; 2004. p. 297–331.
171. Traupe T, Gloekler S, de Marchi SF, Werner GS, Seiler C. Assessment of the human coronary collateral circulation. Circulation. 2010;122:1210–20.
172. Schaper W. Collateral circulation: past and present. Basic Res Cardiol. 2009;104:5–21.
173. Toyota E, Warltier DC, Brock T, Ritman E, Kolz C, O'Malley P, et al. Vascular endothelial growth factor is required for coronary collateral growth in the rat. Circulation. 2005;112:2108–13.
174. Matsunaga T, Warltier DC, Weihrauch DW, Moniz M, Tessmer J, Chilian WM. Ischemia-induced coronary collateral growth is dependent on vascular endothelial growth factor and nitric oxide. Circulation. 2000;102:3098–103.
175. Wu S, Wu X, Zhu W, Cai WJ, Schaper J, Schaper W. Immunohistochemical study of the growth factors, aFGF, bFGF, PDGF-AB, VEGF-A and its receptor (Flk-1) during arteriogenesis. Mol Cell Biochem. 2010;343:223–9.
176. Chilian WM, Mass HJ, Williams SE, Layne SM, Smith EE, Scheel KW. Microvascular occlusions promote coronary collateral growth. Am J Physiol. 1990;258:H1103–11.
177. Carrao AC, Chilian WM, Yun J, Kolz C, Rocic P, Lehmann K, et al. Stimulation of coronary collateral growth by granulocyte stimulating factor: role of reactive oxygen species. Arterioscler Thromb Vasc Biol. 2009;29:1817–22.
178. Deindl E. Arteriogenesis: a focus on signal transduction cascades and transcription factors. Thromb Haemost. 2007;98:940–3.
179. Thannickal VJ, Aldweib KD, Rajan T, Fanburg BL. Upregulated expression of fibroblast growth factor (FGF) receptors by transforming growth factor-beta1 (TGF-beta1) mediates enhanced mitogenic responses to FGFs in cultured human lung fibroblasts. Biochem Biophys Res Commun. 1998;251:437–41.
180. Deindl E, Hoefer IE, Fernandez B, Barancik M, Heil M, Strniskova M, et al. Involvement of the fibroblast growth factor system in adaptive and chemokine-induced arteriogenesis. Circ Res. 2003;92:561–8.
181. Eitenmuller I, Volger O, Kluge A, Troidl K, Barancik M, Cai WJ, et al. The range of adaptation by collateral vessels after femoral artery occlusion. Circ Res. 2006;99:656–62.

182. Boengler K, Pipp F, Broich K, Fernandez B, Schaper W, Deindl E. Identification of differentially expressed genes like cofilin2 in growing collateral arteries. Biochem Biophys Res Commun. 2003;300:751–6.
183. Schaper J, Konig R, Franz D, Schaper D. The endothelial surface of growing coronary collateral arteries. Intimal margination and diapedesis of monocytes. A combined SEM and TEM study. Virchows Arch A Pathol Anat Histol. 1976;370:193–205.
184. Takahashi T, Kalka C, Masuda H, Chen D, Silver M, Kearney M, et al. Ischemia- and cytokine-induced mobilization of bone marrow-derived endothelial progenitor cells for neovascularization. Nat Med. 1999;5:434–8.
185. Kalka C, Masuda H, Takahashi T, Kalka-Moll WM, Silver M, Kearney M, et al. Transplantation of ex vivo expanded endothelial progenitor cells for therapeutic neovascularization. Proc Natl Acad Sci USA. 2000;97:3422–7.
186. Ziegelhoeffer T, Fernandez B, Kostin S, Heil M, Voswinckel R, Helisch A, et al. Bone marrow-derived cells do not incorporate into the adult growing vasculature. Circ Res. 2004;94:230–8.
187. Cui Y. Confocal imaging: blood and lymphatic capillaries. Scientific World J. 2006;6:12–5.
188. Cui Y, Urschel JD, Petrelli NJ. The effect of cardiopulmonary lymphatic obstruction on heart and lung function. Thorac Cardiovasc Surg. 2001;49:35–40.
189. Patek AJ, Haig C. The occurrence of abnormal dark adaptation and its relation to vitamin a metabolism in patients with cirrhosis of the liver. J Clin Invest. 1939;18:609–16.
190. Miller AJ, Pick R, Katz LN. The importance of the lymphatics of the mammalian heart: experimental observations and some speculations. Circulation. 1964;29(SUPPL):485–7.
191. Cui Y. Impact of lymphatic vessels on the heart. Thorac Cardiovasc Surg. 2010;58:1–7.
192. Cui Y. The role of lymphatic vessels in the heart. Pathophysiology. 2010;17:307–14.
193. Uhley HN, Leeds SE, Sung MA. The subendocardial lymphatics of the canine heart. A possible role of the lymphatics in the genesis of conduction disturbances and arrhythmias. Am J Cardiol. 1972;29:367–71.
194. Stoll C, Alembik Y, Dott B, Kieffer P. Lymphedema combined with brachydactyly and tachycardia. Genet Couns. 1998;9:33–7.
195. Solti F, Lengyel E, Jellinek H, Schneider F, Juhasz-Nagy A, Kekesi V. Coronary arteriopathy after lymphatic blockade: an experimental study in dogs. Lymphology. 1994;27:173–80.
196. Schraufnagel DE. Forms of lung lymphatics: a scanning electron microscopic study of casts. Anat Rec. 1992;233:547–54.
197. Szlavy L, Koster K, de Courten A, Hollenberg NK. Early disappearance of lymphatics draining ischemic myocardium in the dog. Angiology. 1987;38:73–84.

Historical Perspectives

5

Introduction

A historical review of the discoveries regarding the coronary vasculature and circulation indicates that progress in this field was hampered by technical difficulties and often also by a resistant scientific community. Although most of the earliest attempts to advance physiology and medicine were based on speculation and philosophy rather than experimentation, some understanding of anatomy was present as early as two millennia ago, as indicated by drawings of hearts and other organs. Galen (A.D. 131–201) was the most proliferative writer concerning medical matters of his time, and his ideas influenced medical education and practice for several centuries [1]. He noted the left and right coronary arteries and used the term "coronary" in describing them. His teachings were considered infallible for more than a century, and consequently any contradictions to his views were dismissed as erroneous. It was the great anatomist Vesalius (1514–1564) who introduced histology and cellular biology to the medical community and he challenged the assumptions of Galen, based on his dissections and descriptions of the coronary vasculature [2]. But it was not until the nineteenth and twentieth centuries that scholars were outspoken in declaring that the errors of Galen had delayed progress in medical science [3]. As noted in this chapter, the understanding of the anatomy and physiology of the coronary system was hampered by the politics of the times and often the stubbornness and arrogance of the ruling physicians and scientists.

The overall goal of Chap. 5 is to note some of the major contributions that enhanced our understanding of the coronary system or provided technical advancements, and to highlight those individuals who made key observations and discoveries. The chapter is intended to provide historical perspectives rather than to be an exhaustive review of the topic. More detailed reviews where historical landmarks of our understanding of coronary vessels and circulation can be found include Willius and Dry [1], Herrick [2], Aciero [4], Gregg [5], and Sarton [6]. This chapter focuses mainly on the observations, discoveries, and developments up to 1965.

Historical Figures of the Renaissance

Although there were a number of individuals who made contributions during this era, I have selected six who, in my opinion, enabled the greatest advances in the field (Table. 5.1).

Leonardo da Vinci (1452–1519)

This Renaissance man was both artist and scientist and has been described as "a defender of reason, an enemy of superstition, but an idealist" [6]. He is perhaps best known as a "physiologic anatomist" because he left numerous notes commenting on the functions of structures that he drew. His accurate drawings of the coronary arteries and their branches, and also the entire cardiovascular system, are classics. He was the first to demonstrate that the coronary arteries originate from the coronary sinuses [7]. da Vinci's understanding of the coronary vasculature and general circulation demonstrates that he was ahead of his time as revealed in his own words: "The heart is not the beginning of life, but it is a vessel made of dense muscle, vivified and nourished by the artery and vein, as are the other muscles" (quotation from [8]). Though this message is seemingly obvious today, it was quite novel for his time. Because his contributions were in the form of unpublished notes and illustrations, they were not recognized during his lifetime, but only centuries later [6]. In reviewing the various descriptions of da Vinci, one can easily conclude that he was a genius who did not attempt to leave a legacy of his own importance.

Andreas Vesalius (1514–1564)

An anatomist, Vesalius performed his own dissections and published *De Humani Corporis Fabrica* (The Fabric of the Human Body), a work that is considered a masterpiece and gave rise to modern anatomy [6]. This book included detailed

R.J. Tomanek, *Coronary Vasculature: Development, Structure-Function, and Adaptations*,
DOI 10.1007/978-1-4614-4887-7_5,

Table 5.1 Some historical milestones (pre-1970)

Year (AD)	Milestone
1543	Andreas Vesalius described the coronary vasculature and also performed first resuscitation of arrested heart
1661	Capillary anastomoses and circulation between arteries and veins described by Malpighi
1669	Lower described intercoronary anastomoses and also performed blood transfusions in animals
1698	Pierre Chirac demonstrated that cardiac arrest occurred in response to coronary ligation
1703	Lorenzo Bellini of Pisa provided descriptions of coronary ossification
1708	Adam Thebesius injected materials into the coronary arteries and described their passage into the ventricles (the Thebesian vessels were named after him)
1715	The course of the coronary arteries, the valve of the large coronary vein, and the coronary sinus were detailed by Raymond Vieussens
1726	Francesco Albertini related pain in the arms and shoulders to heart disease and emphasized dyspnea as symptom
1759	First detailed description of the classical symptoms of angina pectoris, recorded by Edward Hyde as observed in his father
1761	John Baptist Morgagni described ossification of left coronary artery and coronary sclerosis
1772	William Heberden provided the classical description of angina pectoris, but the work was published only posthumously in 1802
1850	Sir Richard Quain described the decreased blood supply and ossified coronary arteries in regions of myocardial necrosis
1854	Earliest demonstration of vasomotor nerves and their mechanism and subsequent documentation of vasoconstriction by sympathetic nerves by Claude Bernard
1867	Use of nitrites in treatment of angina pectoris
1872	Rebatel used experimental approaches to study the mechanics and regulation of coronary blood flow
1879	Nitroglycerin introduced by William Murrell for the treatment of angina pectoris
1881	Cohnheim and associates established coronary disease as the cause of infarction, myofibrosis, and sclerosis
1894	William Porter noted that since cardiac fibrillations and sudden death did not always occur after coronary occlusion, coronary arteries were not end arteries
1895	Langendorff demonstrated control of coronary flow using his isolated heart preparation
1898	Porter detailed histopathological features of myocardial infarction and physiological changes and their relationship to coronary artery ligation
1903	Einthoven adapted the string galvanometer for recording the heart's action currents
1910	First experimental coronary bypass (an anastomosis between aorta and left main coronary artery) by Alexis Carrel. In 1912, Carrel was awarded the Nobel Prize in Physiology and Medicine for his work on "vascular suture and transplantation of blood vessels and organs"
1912	First record of truly representative and detailed account of coronary thrombosis by James Herric
1919	Detailed account of capillary circulation and O_2 diffusion by August Krogh. Krogh was awarded the Nobel Prize in 1920.
1920	Harold E.B. Pardee correlated T-wave changes of the electrocardiogram with sudden obstruction of the coronary arteries
1920s–1940s	Studies of Anrep, Wearn, Wiggers, and Gregg detailed the factors governing coronary flow and its distribution and the underlying anatomic considerations
1931	Werner Forssmann performed the first angiography. He later (1956) shared a Nobel Prize with André Frédéric and Dickinson Woodruff Richards for work on cardiac catheterization
1940	H.L. Blumgart and colleagues published an extensive study documenting the relationship between pathological findings and angina, thrombosis and myocardial infarction
1948	The work of Acel Keys and the Framingham study was a landmark in promoting coronary disease by treating risk factors
	Nitrous oxide used by Eckenhoff and colleagues to measure coronary blood flow
1950	H.L. Blumgart and colleagues established the value of porcine hearts for studies of collateral vessel formation and function
1962	β-blockers used to treat angina were introduced to improve myocardial blood flow
1963	Robert Berne published the adenosine hypothesis as a regulator of coronary blood flow
1963	Thomas Fogarty and colleagues devised a balloon catheter that was used for arterial embolectomy
1964	First saphenous vein aortocoronary bypass surgery was done by Garrett et al
1966	Kolessov performed the first human coronary arterial anastomosis by constructing an internal mammary-coronary artery bypass
1967	W. Schaper and R. Vandesteene documented quantitatively the progression of growth and remodeling of coronary collaterals in response to ischemia and demonstrated their role in prevention of myocardial infarction
1968	Neutze and colleagues documented the usefulness of radioactive microspheres for the assessment of myocardial blood flow

illustrations of the coronary vessels, as well as the first description of the large coronary vein and the coronary sinus. Vesalius also supported the view that coronary vessels communicate with the chambers of the heart. A rather spectacular demonstration attributed to Vesalius was his resuscitation of an arrested heart using bellows. Beyond these advances in our understanding of the coronary vasculature, Vesalius made many other contributions, e.g., (1) described the diagnostic features of pericardial effusion and the significance of pericardial adhesions, (2) described mitral stenosis, and (3) provided the first diagnosis of a thoracic aneurysm in a patient [1]. The anatomical details that emerged from his numerous dissections cast doubts on Galen's dictums, which had many adherents. Vesalius proudly stated, "I could have done nothing more worthwhile than to give a new description of the whole human body, of which nobody understood the anatomy" [9].

William Harvey (1578–1657)

The work of Harvey was the first scientific inquiry based on experimental facts. He convincingly demonstrated that blood flows in a circle from the heart via arteries and returns by way of veins. Harvey also predicted the existence of capillary circulation and he described the anatomy and basic physiology of the systemic and pulmonary circulations. His work repudiated the non-scientific assumptions that had been held for many centuries beginning with Galen. Harvey dissected hearts from more than 80 species and addressed the key questions concerning the motion of the heart and the propulsion of blood [10]. His discoveries were based on his reasoning, as well as some mathematical calculations. For example, from stroke volume and pulse rate, he concluded that if blood did not circulate, the human body would have to produce at least 1,800 L of new blood each day [11].

Marcello Malpighi (1628–1694)

Malpighi was the first to describe the capillary circulation in a letter sent to a friend in 1661. He noted a capillary anastomosis between arteries and veins, thus proving Harvey's prediction made some 30 years earlier. Malpighi's observations were made possible by the invention of the compound microscope around 1590 [1].

Richard Lower (1631–1691)

A keen physiologist and clinician, Lower made several key contributions. Among these was the demonstration that coronary collaterals exist between arteries, based on his observation that ink injected into one artery appeared in an adjacent artery. Lower successfully transfused blood into animals and suggested that this procedure might be useful in humans. After injecting venous blood into the lungs and noting the subsequent bright red color, he concluded that blood absorbed air during its passage through the lungs. Moreover, he made notable observations regarding cardiac mechanics and described the changes that occur during systole.

Raymond Vieussens (1641–1716)

Vieussens' 1715 publication, "*Traité nouveau de la structure et des caused du mouvements natural de Coeur,*" cited by Willius and Dry [1], contains many of his observations regarding coronary anatomy. For example, he noted that the coronary vasculature is connected to the heart chambers, developed the concept of myocardial anoxia, and described the course of the coronary arteries (see Fig. 5.1). In addition to his contributions regarding coronary anatomy, Vieussens described valvular defects, mitral stenosis, and the significance of pericardial adhesions and pathological changes of the heart.

Progress in Specific Areas

Vessels of Thebesius: Nutrition of the Heart

This topic received attention mainly during a 200-year period beginning with the first experimental evidence (based on serial sections of the heart), provided by Raymone Vieussens in 1706 (noted in [12]), that coronary arteries communicate with the heart's chambers. Two years later, Adam Christian Thebesius [13] published a more detailed description of this special coronary circulation, which now carries his name. After injecting water into the coronary sinus, he observed channels that opened into the heart's chamber. Thebesius also injected air and colored liquids (mixed with wax and glue) into the coronary veins, thereby delineating their distribution and connections. In 1715, Vieussens published further experimental data revealing the passage of tracers from the coronaries through the endocardium. Subsequently, many investigators confirmed these observations, although a few continued to deny the existence of Thebesian vessels (reviewed in [14]) (Fig. 5.2).

A particularly significant contribution to the understanding of Thebesian vessels was made by Pratt [12], who was able to maintain a heartbeat in a cat heart for an hour by perfusing blood through these channels. This work demonstrated, for the first time, the nutritional value of this system of vessels, which enables them to maintain heart function. Pratt went on to suggest that Thebesian vessels could contribute to cardiac recovery from fibrillary contractions and also recovery from simple arrest in the absence of fibrillations. Finally, Wearn [14] discovered the presence of direct communications between coronary veins and the vessels of Thebesius. His work was based on measuring effluent from both human and feline hearts that had been injected with dyes. These hearts were fixed by perfusion and subjected to histological analysis of serial sections. A key discovery from these experiments was that in some hearts, blockage of coronary arteries did not result in death at an earlier time point. Accordingly,

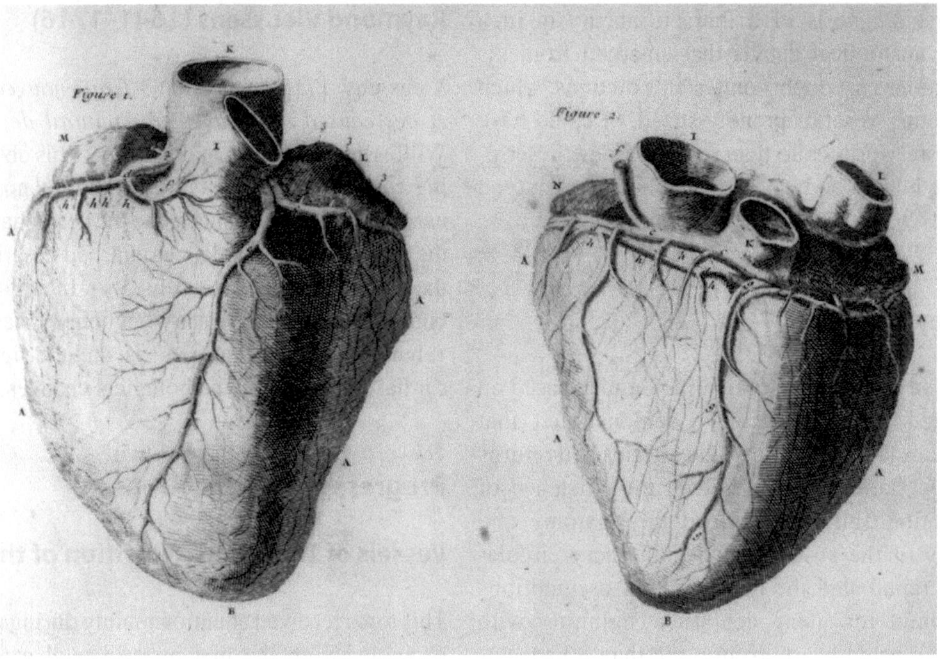

Fig. 5.1 Drawings of the coronary arteries (*left: anterior view; right: posterior view*) from the book by R. Vieussens: *Traite Nouveau de la Structure et dex Causes du Mouvement Naterel du Coer*. Toulouse, 1715 (figure is from the National Library of Medicine)

Wearn concluded that the Thebesian vessels were able to serve as an alternative blood supply in these individuals. This hypothesis was further supported by his experiments demonstrating myocardial integrity after gradual closure of the coronary arteries. Subsequently, Wearn and his colleagues injected celloidin into the coronaries, thus blocking flow into these channels, and found that flow through the Thebesian vessels did not necessitate passage through the capillary bed [15]. These experiments established the presence of arterioluminal, as well as arteriosinusoidal vessels.

Coronary Anastomoses

Early Studies

As noted earlier, Richard Lower is credited with providing the first experimental demonstration of anastomoses between coronary arteries by injecting arteries and tracing the injectate into adjacent arteries [16]. Since that time, such communications have been repeatedly documented, as summarized in a review [17]. Although Lower's work was generally accepted, there were some who denied or questioned the existence of intercoronary anastomoses even two centuries later. The concept that coronary arteries are "end" or "terminal" arteries was based on the fact that occlusion of an artery resulted in an infarction. Thus, the physiological significance of coronary artery anastomoses was considered unimportant by many in the scientific community. Yet in 1880, Langer (cited by [18]) gave a good description of the flow of a resin between right and left coronary arteries in human hearts and stressed their clinical importance. A few years later, Pratt [12] stated that the term "terminal" artery simply implies that the "resistance in the anastomosing branches is greater than the blood pressure in the arteries leading to these branches." Thus, these anastomotic channels were not considered to be of functional significance. A detailed study by Jamin and Merkel [19] described anastomotic channels of small diameter in several regions of the human heart. That study indicated that these channels were more numerous than indicated by earlier studies that were not able to resolve small vessels due to technical limitations.

Coronary Blood Flow

Establishing the Concepts

Perhaps the earliest published report presenting a valid view of coronary blood flow is that of Scaramucci, which appeared in 1869 (discussed by [4]). He noted that (1) transmural blood flow is preempted during systole and (2) large coronary surface arteries serve as a reservoir during systole and recoil during diastole. This concept did not receive sufficient attention, as his monograph collected dust in archives for many years. Eighteen years later, Stroem advanced the theory that coronary arteries received blood only during diastole since the opening of the aortic cusps prevents flow into the ostia during systole (cited in [4]). Here we have an example of misdirection in understanding key concepts because of the limited availability of relevant information.

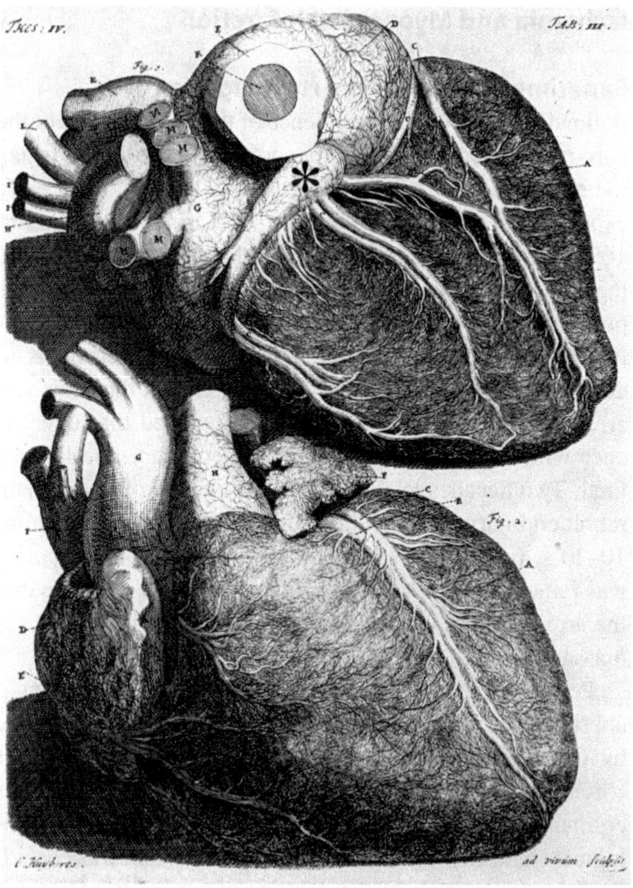

Fig. 5.2 Detailed drawings of the coronary vasculature based on human hearts preserved and then injected with wax. Drainage of the venous system into the coronary sinus (*asterisks*) is seen in the post prior view (*top of figure*). An anterior view of the heart (*bottom*) illustrates the left anterior coronary artery and vein. These drawings are from Frederik Ruysch: *Thesaurus Anatomicus Quartus (Tab III)*. Amsterdam, 1704

Although the rich network of cardiac nerves was detailed a century earlier (Fig. 5.3) was not described in detail until 1926 by Woolard, who found both sympathetic and parasympathetic innervation of the large coronary artery branches and that the vagus was the major supplier of the smaller branches [20]. Although neural control of blood vessels (vasoconstrictive role of sympathetic nerves) was not understood until the discovery by Claude Bernard in the mid-nineteenth century [1], the responses of the coronary arteries were still not well understood as late as the 1930s [21]. This limited understanding was due, in part, to the fact that other coronary and metabolic influences masked the direct effects of nerves on coronary vessels.

The relationship between coronary blood flow and myocardial contraction was problematic for investigators during the mid-nineteenth century. Eventually, Rebetel [22] noted that during systole, a large blood flow occurred in the large coronary arteries, whereas no flow was observed in the capillaries. Because capillary flow occurred during diastole only, he concluded that compression of these vessels during systole limits flow, thus validating Saramucci's conclusions (some 200 years earlier) regarding myocardial perfusion. One problem that remained to be resolved at that time was the visualization of the capillary bed. In 1899, Meigs was able to fill parts of the capillary bed with Berlin blue and then a complete filling was accomplished by Wearn [23] 3 decades later. Wearn's micrographs illustrated numerous intercapillary connections, capillary connections to venules, and the orientation of capillaries with respect to cardiomyocytes. In this classic histology paper, Wearn found capillary density to be about 4,000/mm^2, a figure that is consistent with current data.

Measurement of Coronary Blood Flow

Langendorff [24] was the first to measure coronary blood flow. In his 1899 paper (based on an isolated cat heart), he predicted that blood flow is phasic based on his notations of the time of contraction and the rhythmical variations in perfusion pressure. Langendorff measured coronary venous outflow and found that it increased during systole. He also measured coronary inflow and arterial pressure and noted that the velocity stream has two peaks, one during systole and one during diastole. Langendorff was the first to accurately describe systolic and diastolic characteristics by observing inflow into large coronary arteries during systole and restriction of outflow from these vessels due to the forces of muscle contraction.

Further progress in understanding blood flow came in 1913, when Markwalder and Starling [25] used a heart-lung preparation to estimate blood flow in the heart. They reported a value of about 60 mL/100 g of tissue, which is lower than that occurring in vivo. A year later, Morawitz and Zahn [26] made an important contribution by measuring the rate of coronary flow by collecting venous blood from the coronary sinus after direct catheterization. They reported the three factors that increase coronary blood flow (1) increased arterial pressure, (2) sympathetic nerve stimulation or a release of adrenaline, and (3) metabolites when O_2 supply is decreased. A decade later, Nakagawa [27], who employed a heart-lung preparation, described "automatic regulation" or coronary circulation. Five years later, Anrep and colleagues [28] developed a more precise method of measuring coronary flow by using a hot wire anemometer to document inflow and outflow in a denervated heart-lung preparation (Fig. 5.3). Several important developments occurred during the next few years. Velocity curves in coronary arteries were recorded by Hochreim and colleagues, who used a newly developed optical velocity recorder, or tachograph, developed by Broemser in 1928 (cited by [5]). Rössler and Pascual [29] used the hot-wire anemometer to study coronary circulation in isolated perfused hearts to study the effects of various drugs on coronary flow. This approach enabled them to delineate how the drugs influence our heart rate and how they may mask, accentuate, or reverse the drugs' direct effect on flow.

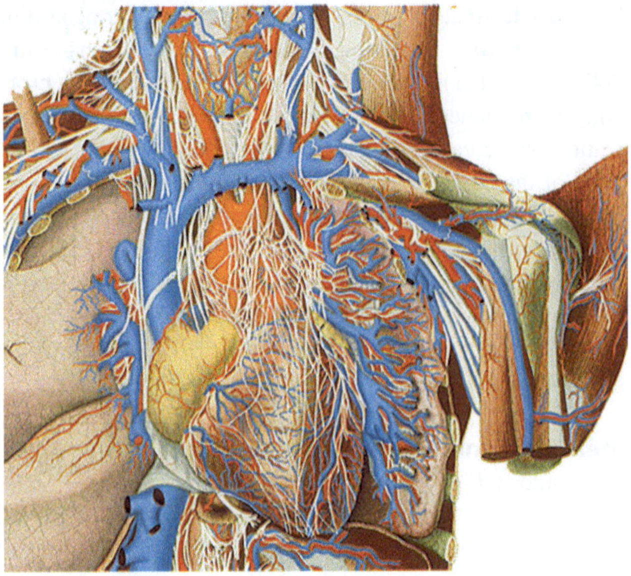

Fig. 5.3 A drawing by Antonio Serantoni (artist and engraver) illustrating the coronary vessels and cardiac nerves from the work of Paolo Mascagni (1752–1815). This is a portion of *Viscera Tab II*, published in Anatomia Universa in 1823. The figure is courtesy of University of Iowa, Hardin Health Sciences Library

The employment of a flow meter (Fig. 5.4) made it possible to record flow in the branches of a coronary artery [30]. This involved using a sensitive optimal manometer to record the small pressure drop in an air chamber as fluid (Locke's solution) entered the coronary artery. The system was modified by Gregg, who used the animal's own blood to more accurately mimic the natural conditions of perfusion [5]. In 1948, Eckenhoff utilized nitrous oxide to measure coronary blood flow. This method is based on the difference in the amount of a substance taken up in an organ, divided by the difference in the concentration in arterial versus venous blood, i.e., the Fick principle. In 1959, Marston generated the first recording of phasic coronary blood flow using a noncannulating electromagnetic flow probe invoking Faraday's induction law, i.e., a conductor moving in a magnetic field produces electrical current.

Radioactive microspheres were first employed in the 1960s to measure blood flow. This method is based on the assumption that microspheres (usually 15–25 μm in diameter) lodged in tissue segments are uniformly mixed. The number of microspheres is calculated by determining the radioactivity in the samples and in the blood, and thus the determination of the flow distribution. This method was used by Rudolph and Heymann [31] to measure the distribution of blood flow in fetuses in utero, and subsequently by Buckberg and associates [32] to measure coronary blood flow in lambs, sheep, and dogs. Their study addressed a number of technical issues and set the stage for the wide use of this approach over the next 4 decades. A more detailed discussion of the methods used to measure coronary blood flow can be found in the monogram by Marcus [33].

Ischemia and Myocardial Infarction

Experimental Coronary Artery Ligation

Following Harvey's clear evidence of the nutritive role of the coronary circulation, a basis for coronary heart disease began to be recognized, though not necessarily accepted. The early experiments on coronary ligation by Chirac, published in 1698, did not come to light until Marshall Hall suggested that the topic of experimental coronary ligation should be pursued [4]. Heeding this admonition, Erichsen [34] published the results of his coronary ligation experiments in dogs and reported that 23.5 min after ligation, the heart was arrested. Based on this finding, he concluded that interference with the passage of blood in the coronary arteries was fatal. Two decades later, Bezold [35] clamped the left main rabbit coronary artery and noted a decline in heart rate after 10–20 s, followed by restoration of heart rate if the clamp was removed. Of particular significance was his finding that the arrested heart can be restored by (1) electric shocks, (2) massage, and (3) vagal stimulation.

Perturbation of the coronary arteries was an experimental approach that was also utilized during the nineteenth century by Cohnheim and Weigert, both of whom were pupils of Virchow [4]. The former described cardiac function after coronary artery ligation, whereas the latter described histological changes in the infarcted myocardium and was considered the "expounder of the doctrine of coronary infarction" [36]. Cohnheim reported on the collapse of arterial pressure as a cause of ventricular fibrillation and noted that death could occur within 1 min of coronary artery occlusion. He also commented on the significance of coronary thrombi and emboli, and in 1882, he discovered that coronary occlusion does not always result in death—a finding that suggested an alternate blood flow. These observations contributed to the debate concerning coronary anastomoses, which gained momentum in the twentieth century.

Thrombi and Coronary Sclerosis

The doctrine of cardiac infarction is credited to Weigert, who, in 1880, made some astute observations regarding this topic (cited by [36]). He described coronary artery occlusions with relation to thrombosis and atheromatosis, and most importantly, he noted that anastomotic channels may slow the degenerative changes in cardiomyocytes. Although coronary thrombosis was first described in 1850 by Cruieilhier (cited by [36]), it was not until 30 years later that its role in ischemia and infarction was appreciated. Often overlooked is Mathew Baillie's 1788 observation that death from a "cardiac polyp" was actually caused by a thrombus (cited by [1]). The early 1880s were an important time period for establishing concepts regarding ischemia and infarction (noted by [36]). Most importantly, Cohnheim and Huber affirmed coronary artery disease as the cause of infarction and coronary sclerosis. They noted that secondary changes at the border of an infarct are the product of nonpurulent inflammation, and that thrombosis contributes to coronary sclerosis. These observations brought to the forefront the role of thrombi in myocardial ischemia and infarction.

Carl Weigert [37] was the first to distinguish the effects of gradual coronary occlusion from those of abrupt occlusion by noting the slow atrophy and degeneration of cardiomyocytes in the former which contrasted with the rather rapid cardiomyocyte loss in the latter. Many studies during the early twentieth century noted that neither acute nor gradual coronary artery stenosis always results in a myocardial infarction. Ultimately, 60 years later, experiments by H.B. Burchell [38] demonstrated that coronary arteries enlarge under these conditions, a finding that provided a possible explanation for the lack of infarction in these hearts.

It was not until 1916 that a histologic study on experimental infarction in dogs documented the sequence of events that occur when a coronary artery is abruptly occluded [39]. This study detailed the now-classic changes that occur in cardiomyocytes in the context of hemorrhage and edema during the first 48 h following occlusion. Moreover, the study described the changes seen up to 70 days after occlusion, including those in the border zone. One particularly astute observation was that the final area of the infarct is smaller than the area seen affected during the first 48 h after ligation.

Angina Pectoris

The classic description of angina was provided by Heberden in 1772 [40]. He noted that the symptoms appear upon walking, or more likely, climbing a hill (most often observed in males over the age of 50), and include tightness in the chest, shortness of breath, and pain in the chest and arms. However, Heberden considered angina to reflect spasmodic episodes and not inflammatory conditions, even though pathological changes in the coronary arteries were described by Morgagni as early as 1761 (cited by [4]). Morgagni, the founder of pathological anatomy, described arterial plaques and dissecting aneurysms and, most importantly, recognized angina pectoris as being related to the ossification of arteries [41]. However, this association was not emphasized by others until the next century. Notably, 2 decades later, a physician by the name of Hunter provided a self-described diagnosis of angina, noting the roles of both emotion and exertion—including their presence during sleep—in the onset of the symptoms and the disease progression. He died suddenly and the findings at autopsy indeed revealed coronary artery ossification.

From Cause to Effect

A link between ischemia and angina pectoris was proposed by Alan Burns in 1809 in his book addressing diseases of the heart (referenced by [40]). Based on his observations regarding the impediment of flow by a tourniquet on a limb over a period of time, he reasoned that calcification or ossification of a coronary artery would impede the flow of blood, cause an energy and expenditure imbalance, and result in angina. In 1842, two papers were published that delineated such a connection between angina and coronary occlusion. One study [34] revealed (1) that cardiac arrest occurred after coronary ligation and (2) that enhanced coronary flow increased the heartbeat. The other paper emphasized that ossification of coronary arteries was related to angina and death [42]. A few years later, Vogel [43] suggested that cholesterol is the main constituent of atherosclerotic plaques. However, even in the twentieth century, doubt about the angina-ischemia relationship lingered because some patients who died during episodes of angina did not demonstrate evidence of coronary artery disease; conversely, autopsy reports of some patients who had no history of angina revealed extensive coronary artery disease [44].

Although the relationship between angina pectoris and myocardial infarction was accepted by almost everyone in the medical community in the mid-nineteenth century [2], the role of sclerosed coronary arteries was often overlooked as a cause of angina and infarction. Even the eminent pathologist Virchow stressed the importance of inflammation and myocardial fibrosis, rather than coronary occlusion, as underlying causes. As late as 1868, von Dusch held the view that angina pectoris was a rare condition and that inflammation of the cardiac plexus was the cause, in most cases. The debate concerning the theories regarding the cause of angina pectoris during the 1920s was considerable until data from electrocardiograms, based on both patients and dogs, documented the ischemia-angina relationship [45, 46]. A link between oxygen and angina was provided by evidence that individuals with angina experienced pain when they breathed oxygen-poor air [47, 48].

Coronary Artery Spasm

Spasm of coronary arteries had already been suggested as an alternate cause of angina in 1879 by John Fothergill, as noted in a review of the topic [49]. Fothergill held the view, apparently shared by others, that vasomotor spasms caused an increase in blood pressure and cardiac distention and consequently caused angina. Spasm of the heart, rather than the arteries, had previously been proposed as a cause of angina by Latham [50]. However, during the early twentieth century, the notion that spasm might be a cause of angina gained some adherents, based on the observation that some autopsies revealed normal coronary arteries in individuals who died suddenly. The first notable consideration of angina as an arterial disease that could be caused by either arterial blockage or spasms was by the eminent physician, William Osler [51]. McAlpin [49] notes that the debate concerning a role for arterial/arteriolar spasms continued into the mid-twentieth century, and that even in the 1960s, there was a "great reluctance" to even use the term "coronary arterial spasm."

One key problem in resolving this issue was a lack of precise invasive methods that did not of themselves elicit coronary spasms. It was only in the 1960s and 1970s that, based on data from both humans and dogs, led to coronary artery spasms becoming widely recognized as a cause of angina. It was also found that spasms may be superimposed on athermanous coronary artery stenosis.

Origin of Pain

In a review of the early experiments on the origin of pain that characterizes angina, Lie [44] noted the key experiments of Sutton and Lueth in the late 1920s. These investigators externalized the ends of a loose ligature that surrounded a coronary artery of a conscious dog and were able to tighten and loosen the ligature by means of a flanged glass tube; they observed that pain occurred with occlusion and ceased with release of the occlusion. Moreover, pain was not elicited when the epicardium and cardiac muscle were ligated. Thus, these experiments suggested that coronary occlusion is the trigger for pain. They excluded the possibility that the pain was due to nerve compression by paralyzing the adventitial nerves. However, given that the occlusion of these vessels did not produce pain, the experiments only verified that the artery's nerves transmit the pain. Subsequently, Sutton and Lueth showed that blocking blood flow by introducing a knob into the lumen of a coronary artery elicited pain in the absence of nerve compression. That pain was not elicited when the lumen of the aorta was damaged indicated that angina pain originated in the coronary arteries rather than in the aorta. When Katz et al. [52] repeated these experiments, he found that the results were inconsistent. Based on this finding, he concluded that ischemia is but one mechanism that causes angina.

Lie [44] noted that attention to the question of the origin of pain in angina began to wane in the 1930s as investigators focused more on the causes and consequences of coronary artery narrowing. By that time, there was a general consensus that myocardial ischemia caused pain, but no clear proof of the messenger of the pain. Carl Wiggers [53] discussed the functional consequences of coronary occlusion in his presentation at the American College of Physicians in 1944 and suggested that "anoxia plus accumulation of the products of anaerobic metabolism" are the "immediate" result of two dangerous effects produced by ischemia. First, ectopic heart beats are triggered because of the "functional state" at or near border zones. The ectopic heart beats lead to ventricular fibrillation and may then cause acute or progressive heart failure. Second, pain could be elicited by the chemical products of metabolism or anoxia, as well as by mechanical stretching of the ischemic region. Wiggers [54] concluded that although pain is transmitted via sympathetic nerves, it could originate within the myocardium or the arteries, or from stretch of the ischemic region (acting as a mechanical excitant).

Atherosclerosis

Although Aristotle and his contemporaries reported the occurrence of bone tissue in the heart in 364 B.C., their observation did not receive any attention for quite some time [41]. It was only centuries later that others, such as Benivieni (1507), provided descriptions of lesions similar to those now termed atherosclerosis. In *Chronology of Atherosclerosis* [41], one can find details of the works that led to our understanding of atherosclerosis before 1960. It was Morgagni who, in 1761, gave special attention to the coronary arteries, along with other vessels. Most importantly, he associated chest pain with ossification of the arteries, and he challenged the view that plaques were caused by aging. Vogel [43] made a seminal contribution by bringing to light the fact that cholesterol was the major constituent of atherosclerotic plaques. Smith [41] indicates in his review that some of the important developments in the early twentieth century included Mönckeberg's findings in 1903 that medial calcinosis is separate and distinct from intimal forms of arteriosclerosis. By 1904, the term "atherosclerosis" was adopted because it incorporated two pathological characteristics of arteries: "athero" and "sclero," meaning mushy and hardening, respectively, derived from Greek. Two years later, Klotz [55] suggested that the term "arteriosclerosis" be used broadly to include (1) atherosclerosis, (2) atheromatosis, (3) Mönckeberg's sclerosis, and (4) hyperplasic arteriosclerosis.

Experimental atherosclerosis in animals was an important development of the 1930s, and the etiological factors and developmental steps were enumerated by Anitschkow [56]. He clearly described the changes associated with feeding rabbits a high cholesterol diet and the regression of these changes when this diet was discontinued. His work triggered many studies on this topic, which were reviewed by Katz and Stamler [57] 20 years later. In sum, during the first 6 decades of the twentieth century, profound advances were made regarding our understanding of atherosclerosis [41]. These advances are closely linked with progress in preventing and treating coronary ischemia and infarction.

The Twentieth Century

Progress in the twentieth century, especially after World War II, was enabled by technological achievements. One of the most important clinical advances was the advent of pharmacological treatments of myocardial ischemia. Langley [58] stated that recent progress was such "that prognosis could be favorable for 75 % of persons who survive an initial acute myocardial infarction," a clear contrast to expectations for survival by most in the nineteenth century. The advances in coronary research and treatment that contributed to this revolution have

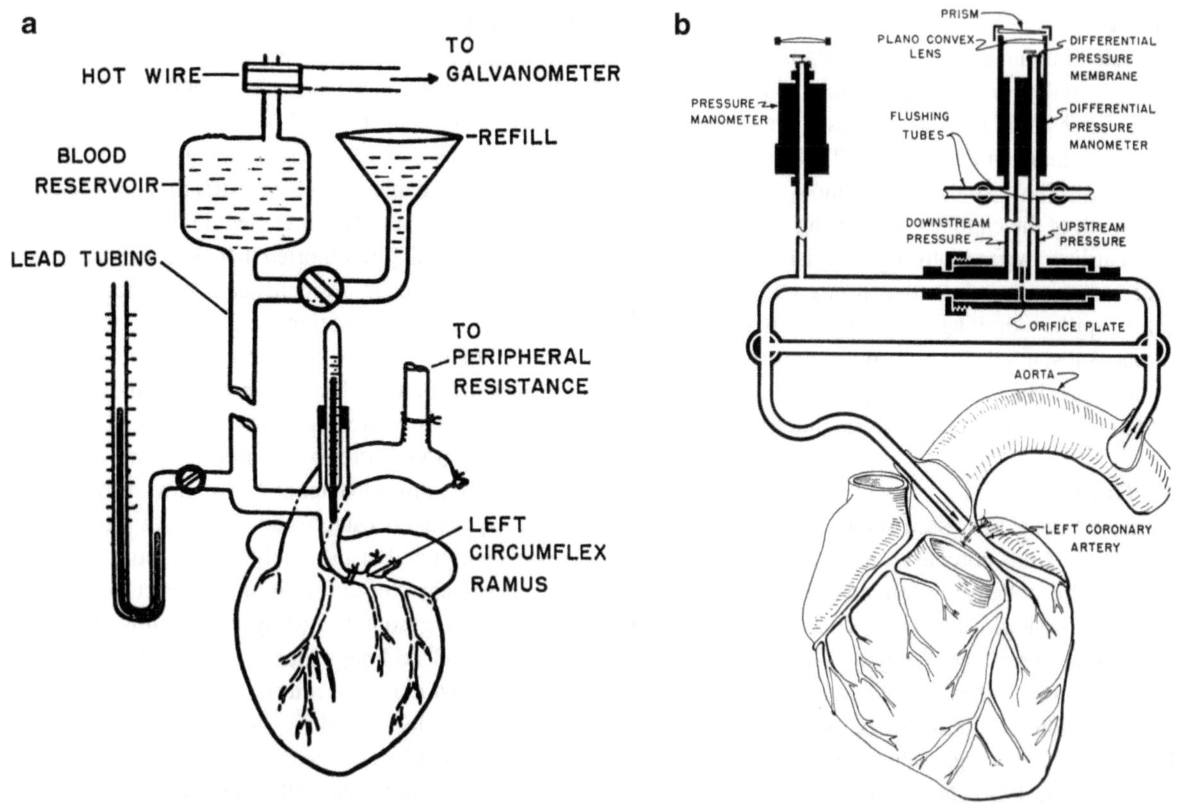

Fig. 5.4 Diagrams illustrating apparati for measuring coronary blood flow. (**a**) The principle of an anemometer for measuring flow variations in the left circumflex artery used by Anrep and colleagues in 1927 [28]. (**b**) Diagram of an orifice meter and differential manometer used in this preparation to measure coronary flow. The cannula was inserted into the brachiocephalic artery, passed through the aorta and tied in the left coronary artery at its origin. This apparatus was used by Gregg and Green in 1940 to determine the effects of different variables on coronary blood flow. The figures are from Gregg, D. *Coronary Circulation in Health and Disease*. Philadelphia: Lea and Febiger, 1950

already been noted under specific topics in this chapter. By the 1960s, our understanding of coronary blood flow regulation had progressed significantly (see review by [59]). The roles of local factors and the concept of metabolic and neural influences were recognized, as were mechanical factors. The hope at that time was that integrated investigations using physiological and biochemical approaches would be pursued in "unanesthetized dogs under a variety of physiological conditions" [59]. The goal of this section is to highlight the work of several leaders who made significant contributions and to comment on advances in several areas.

Four Giants of the First 50 Years

C.J. Wiggers

Our understanding of the coronary circulation, as well as cardiovascular physiology, in general, was greatly enhanced by the work of Carl Wiggers. His laboratory conducted experiments on the innervation of the coronary vessels [60], systolic and diastolic coronary flow and pulse pressures [30, 61], collateral flow [21], and the relationship between ischemia and myocardial fibrillation [53, 62]. These studies were published during the first 4 decades of the twentieth century, a period when many basic concepts of the coronary vasculature were still being debated. In addition to his own discoveries, Wiggers [21] provided insightful interpretations regarding our understanding of coronary circulation in the context of a review. Prior to that review, he had authored a book on circulation that included clinical aspects of the subject [63].

G.V. Anrep

Like his contemporary Carl Wiggers, Anrep made seminal observations regarding the coronary circulation and its measurement [64–66]. He and his colleagues cannulated the right, left anterior descending and left circumflex arteries and documented their flow variations using their anemometer (Fig. 5.4). Studies from Anrep's laboratory compared innervated to denervated hearts in a heart-lung preparation (that they developed) and revealed that vasomotor changes regulate coronary flow [67, 68]. A year later, measurements of phasic changes in coronary flow documented that venous flow increases during systole and decreases during diastole [69].

Joseph Wearn

Using isolated human cat and rabbit hearts, Wearn and colleagues injected the coronary vasculature with dyes and were able to visualize capillaries, as well as other components of the microvasculature, including the Thebesian vessels [14, 15, 23, 70–72]. These studies were among the first to quantify the growth of the capillary bed during childhood and the effect of cardiac hypertrophy on capillary density. Wearn demonstrated connections between arteries and Thebesian veins and capillary drainage into Thebesian veins. He also noted that substantial arterial flow moves through the Thebesian veins. His studies on myocardial capillaries were the first to employ quantitative (morphometric) methods.

Donald Gregg

The work of Gregg addressed many issues critical to our understanding of the coronary circulation and its components. He and his colleagues defined the venous drainage of the heart [73], a topic that had previously received little attention. Like Anrep and Wiggers, Gregg studied phasic variations of coronary flow [74–76], an area of research pioneered in his studies with Carl Wiggers [76]. Gregg also provided valuable insights regarding coronary blood flow during ischemia [77]. In 1950, he published the book *Coronary Circulation in Health and Disease,* which detailed progress in the field, critically evaluated the data available at the time, as well as the interpretations thereof, and stressed the importance of both basic and clinical studies relevant to heart disease.

Advances: 1900–1950

Anatomy of Coronary Vessels

Despite the advent of microscopy in the seventeenth century, few studies had addressed the histology of the human coronary vasculature by the early twentieth century. One investigator who did provide some valuable insights into the subject was Wolkoff, who described the normal coronary histology in humans [78] and animals [79], as well as the histological changes characteristic of atherosclerosis [80]. Another was Gross [81], who published a detailed study of normal human coronary arteries and arterioles and compared the changes that occur from birth to middle age. He compared the major coronary arteries and provided detailed descriptions of these vessels, as well as arterioles. Two major monograms, published in the 1920s, reviewed experimental data and provided anatomical details of the coronary vasculature. The first was by Gross [82] and the second by the eminent anatomist Spalteholz [83]. Thus, the first 3 decades of the twentieth century included significant publications that detailed the anatomy and histology of coronary vessels.

Coronary Anastomoses

During the early twentieth century, the functional significance of intercoronary anastomoses was established by many studies (reviewed in [84, 85]). Some key experiments by Spalteholz [83] and Gross [82] were based on injection techniques that enabled these investigators to visualize small anastomoses that were not evident in the experiments of others. Moritz et al. [86] reported that extra cardiac anastomoses of coronary arteries are enhanced by pericardial adhesions based on their observation that the area of infarction was smaller than the region perfused by the occluded artery. Consistent with this observation was the finding that the very rich collaterals between coronary arteries of dogs prevented gross infarction. Moreover, canine coronary collaterals were found to permit substantial blood flow [66, 87]. Overall, these experiments established significant retrograde flow in vessels peripheral to an acutely ligated coronary artery. Proof that these anastomoses are in fact interarterial channels was provided by gasometric analysis revealing the presence of arterial blood. Although the occurrence of anastomotic channels between coronary arteries became accepted, the functional importance of these connections was still debated during the first half of the twentieth century.

The contention that collaterals in normal human hearts serve a physiologically useful purpose was proven by Prinzmetal et al. [88, 89] who used several approaches in their experiments, e.g., fluorescein and radioactive tracers to demonstrate flow in these channels. Moreover, Eckstein et al. [87] had previously demonstrated the time course of collateral development following coronary artery occlusion. A decade later, Herman Blumgart and colleagues [84] provided evidence that an 87% reduction in coronary artery diameter is incompatible with survival. They also provided data regarding the development of coronary collaterals and suggested that the occasional improvement in patients with angina may be due to the gradual development of an anastomotic circulation.

Angina, Thrombosis, Infarction

Monroe Schlesinger [90] injected coronary arteries postmortem with colored radiopaque lead phosphate in agar and then dissected the entire coronary tree. This technique opened the door to accurately locating both specific areas of arterial narrowing and the presence of collaterals. Two years later, [91], he published a classic, 91-page paper with Blumgard and Davis [92] detailing 125 autopsy cases on patients who presented with angina pectoris, coronary thrombosis, or congestive heart failure. This work revealed that (1) a history of angina is usually associated with one or more occlusions (although occlusion may exist in the absence of a history of angina), (2) larger collaterals are most common in hearts with stenotic or occlusive disease, and (3) hearts in people diagnosed with congestive heart failure most often contain diffuse fibrosis.

Coronary Blood Flow

In 1927, Blumgart and Yens measured the velocity of blood flow in humans by radium injection. This method was useful because it revealed that patients with cardiac decompensation or chronic myocarditis had circulation times in excess to those of patients with no signs of heart disease. Blumgart used the method to evaluate blood velocity in patients with various diseases. Among the deviations he found in patients with cardiovascular disease were (1) conspicuous slowing of pulmonary blood flow, (2) relationship between deceased pulmonary blood flow and cardiovascular disease, and (3) relationship between vital capacity of lungs and pulmonary circulation [93].

The experiments of Markwalder and Starling [25] regarding control of the coronary circulation led to several important conclusions which have stood the test of time. These included the role of epinephrine as a vasodilator, the dependence of flow on pressure, and the observation that flow through the coronary sinus reflects flow through the entire heart. Although some of these observations had been reported earlier, Markwalder and Starling provided numerous data from single experiments. Subsequent experiments by Hausler [94] on isolated hearts demonstrated the interactions of changes in the coronary vessels and changes in heart rate and contractility. His experiments demonstrated that coronary flow is regulated by agents acting either directly on the coronary vessel or indirectly by their effect on the myocardium. This was a critical discovery that was later used to explain possible conflicting data from experiments using various pharmacological agents. The use of nitrous oxide to determine blood flow was adapted to the coronary circulation by Bing and colleagues [95], who made many key observations on coronary blood flow and O_2 in normal individuals and those with cardiovascular disease. They provided baseline values for coronary flow and oxygen extraction and noted changes in patients with congestive heart failure, essential hypertension, hypothyroidism, aortic stenosis, coronary occlusion, and anemia. Coronary blood flow measurements in intact dogs were conducted by Eckenhoff and colleagues [96–98]. These studies documented oxygen as the major metabolic factor controlling coronary blood flow and that perfusion pressure also plays a role. Meanwhile, Foltz et al. [99] correlated coronary blood flow with dynamic functions of the heart, e.g., cardiac work, heart rate, and cardiac output, and concluded that "there is no one factor which exclusively controls or dominates the regulation of the coronary circulation."

Data on human hearts also brought to light important clinical observations during the first half of the twentieth century. A study by Dock [100] provided data indicating that the capacity of the coronary vasculature is compromised by age and cardiac hypertrophy (see Chaps. 7 and 11, respectively, for more details on this topic). Moreover, it was shown that the age-related decline in coronary capacity is exacerbated by the presence of cardiac hypertrophy. Compromised blood flow in perfused, isolated hearts from diseased patients was shown to be related to heart failure [101], a finding that brought some attention to the potential role of coronary circulation in compromised heart function.

Cardiac Arteriography

Although intracardiac catheterization in animals had been accomplished during the early twentieth century, Werner Forssmann , in 1929, catheterized himself and had X-rays taken showing the catheter in the right ventricle (described by Baim and Bing [102]). He continued his work on animals, as well as on himself, using contrast material. In 1931, 2 years after his initial experiment, Forssmann presented his findings to the illustrious Surgical Congress, but was allowed only 4 min to speak. He then collaborated with Andre Cournand and Dickenson Richards and in 1956 shared the Nobel Prize with them. Coronary angiography received attention in the 1940s because of the work in Sweden by Radner [103] and Broden et al. [104]. Radner [103] attempted angiography of the coronary arteries in patients and concluded that injections of the contrast fluid into the aorta revealed only minimal images of the main coronary arteries. Moreover, he reported that the procedure caused complications in 2 of 5 patients. However, in 1950, Pearl and colleagues described a method of visualizing the coronary arteries of dogs via a roentgenkymograph by injecting a contrast agent via a catheter passed from the carotid or femoral arteries to the aortic sinus. This method produced good arteriograms without causing adverse complications and thus opened the door to new advances in the field of cardiac arteriography.

Advances: 1951–1970

Coronary Arteries, Collaterals and Myocardial Infarction

Thomas James was clearly a major contributor to our understanding of this topic as evidenced by his numerous publications during these 2 decades. Many of his studies were based on coronary casts from patients who died of various noncardiac causes. James et al. [105] was able to visualize the blood supply to the interventricular septum and showed it to be derived mainly from the diagonally penetrating arteries from the left anterior descending coronary artery. This study also revealed that the interventricular septum contains numerous anastomoses between the left and right coronary arteries. He [106] studied the patterns of arteries of the ventricular free walls in 82 human hearts and demonstrated the variabilities that are relevant to electrocardiographic and clinical syndromes. Similarly, the atrial coronary arteries were studied in 43 human hearts [105]. In sum, the numerous specimens studied by James give him some unique insights into the collaterals, including the types of collaterals, their role in the coronary circulation, and their location within the heart [107]. The relationship between the coronary circulation and the conduction system and their relationship to acute myocardial infarction were presented in considerable detail [108]. This review included structure–function correlates, coronary casts from normal and infarcted human hearts, comparisons of various sites of infarction, and numerous clinical insights into acute myocardial infarction.

Although our understanding of coronary collaterals was still limited by the mid-twentieth century, there was general agreement that after acute coronary constriction, some myocardial tissue can be salvaged by the collateral circulation [18]. In particular, it was noted that survivors of myocardial infarction have a variable number of enlarged collaterals that enable the ischemic myocardium to regain its contractile ability. Whether native collaterals are of significance was challenged by many, including Carl Wiggers (1952), who noted that none of the experiments by his group could document significant collateral flow. His position that an ischemic stimulus was necessary for functional collateral flow was supported by experimental animal studies demonstrating collateral growth in response to coronary occlusion [109]. Vineberg [110] implanted the mammary artery into the myocardium and reported that over 50% of the implants produced communications with the coronary vessels. Enhancement of collateral vessels as a means of providing an alternative blood supply was tested by some, then novel, approaches. These attempts to stimulate collateral growth included mechanical abrasion, chemical irritation, and coronary sinus obstruction [111–113]. The Beck approach [111] of artificially inducing inflammation of the pericardium initially showed attenuation of the symptoms [114]. However, many patients developed chronic constrictive pericarditis, a complication that led to the procedure's replacement by other surgical interventions [115]. An important outcome of these various experiments and clinical applications was the realization that collaterals could contribute sufficient blood flow to an ischemic region, as shown in canine experiments [113].

Collateral vessel development as a protective adaptation was demonstrated by a gradual (4–6 days) reduction of flow in a porcine coronary artery [116, 117]. Other studies [84, 118] also documented collateral vessel development in dogs and pigs. The use of ameroid occluders provided a model of gradual occlusion of a coronary vessel that mimics the situation in humans. The ameroid constrictor was first utilized in the 1950s by Litvak et al. [119] and characterized during the next decade by Schaper [120]. This approach provided a standardized means of inducing ischemia that is still widely utilized. These animal experiments provided encouragement that collateral development could occur in man. In this regard, the anatomical study of human hearts based on coronary casts provided strong evidence that (1) collaterals are present in even non-diseased hearts and (2) the collateral vessels are more developed in the context of coronary artery narrowing [121].

A detailed exploration of human coronary collaterals was undertaken by Fulton (1965). He was able to discern anastomoses as small as 20 μm in diameter at various depths in all four heart chambers. Moreover he documented extra cardiac communications, i.e., mediastinal and pericardial. The monogram by Wolfgang Schaper [120] provided a wealth of knowledge on coronary collaterals and further deepened interest in their development. Schaper et al. [118] stated that "the only defense against the obstructive disease of the coronary arteries is the development of a collateral circulation." He stressed the use of animal experimentation because of the limitations in humans and documented the value of both porcine and canine models for studies of coronary collaterals. Of particular importance is the finding that both capillary and precapillary anastomoses develop into a functional circulatory network in both species. Schaper and Vendesteene [122] provided the first quantitative evidence regarding the stages of transformation of a small myocardial arteriole into a functional collateral vessel in response to gradually developed ischemia. This canine study revealed that the development of collaterals could prevent infarction even after the coronary artery became totally occluded. Ten years earlier, Richard Eckstein [123] demonstrated that the increase in collateral vascular growth in response to a moderate constriction of the left circumflex artery in dogs is enhanced by exercise training for 6–8 weeks. This contribution was especially noteworthy because exercise in the absence of coronary artery narrowing has not been found to enhance collateral growth, a topic addressed in Chap. 8.

Coronary Endarterectomy and Bypass Surgery

Animal research conducted by May and Bailey led to the development of coronary endarterectomy in patients by Bailey et al. [124]. This procedure required passing a current-like tip into the coronary artery and removing strips of the intima from the sites of atherosclerotic plaques. The two patients who underwent this procedure demonstrated improved blood flow. In 1963, another group reported their experiences with 10 patients with extensive coronary atherosclerosis and incapacitating angina pectoris [125]. Five of the 10 patients survived the surgery. Implantation of the mammary artery into a tunnel within the myocardium (the "Vineberg" procedure) was first reported in 1950 [126], but was gradually abandoned. The feasibility of a coronary bypass in humans may well have been sparked by Carrel's creation of the first successful artificial anastomosis between the aorta and the left coronary artery [127]. This was accomplished by diverting blood during the operation by intubation and lateral diversion and utilizing intratracheal intubation to maintain respiration. The first and second saphenous vein aortocoronary bypass surgeries were performed in 1964 and 1967 (reviewed in [128]). Animal experiments in the 1950s and 1960s led to the first arterial anastomosis to a coronary artery in 1966 [129]. Kolessov created an internal mammary-coronary artery anastomosis that precipitated an upsurge of bypass surgeries [115].

During the next decade, large numbers of patients underwent the Kolessov procedure; the low mortality, reduced angina, and exercise tolerance resulted in great enthusiasm for this surgical intervention. At the end of that decade, a review of the topic concluded that "the coronary bypass operation appears to be an appropriate method of treatment for patients with coronary occlusive disease and either chronic or unstable angina pectoris refractory to conventional medical therapy, but who are without severe impairment of left ventricular function" [130]. Advances in microsurgery techniques and excellent angiography made bypass grafts very successful by the early 1970s. In less than a decade, mortality from bypass grafting went from more than 50% to less than 5% [131]. Moreover, the need for stress risk factor control was emphasized in both symptomatic and asymptomatic patients, which presumably had an impact on mortality rates.

Myocardial Blood Flow

In 1957, Berne et al. were able to show that since coronary vasodilation occurs only when arterial O_2 levels fall below 5.5 vol.%, the vasodilation during hypoxemia is related to myocardial hypoxia. These data underscored the correlation between myocardial O_2 consumption and coronary blood flow. Six years later, Berne suggested that cardiac nucleotides may play a role in regulating coronary blood flow [132]. He noted that during hypoxia, adenine nucleotide derivatives appear in the sinus of the dog heart, and suggest that adenosine was a regulator of coronary blood flow. The use of radioactive inert gases (^{85}Kr and ^{133}Xe) in the 1950s and 1960s provided advantages over the measurement of retrograde flow [133]. By injecting inert gases beyond the site of coronary occlusion, the clearance of the gas provided a somewhat better estimate of collateral flow. However, the employment of radioactive microspheres in the 1960s provided the advantage of being able to measure regional myocardial perfusion [133]. In 1968, Neutze and colleagues reported regional blood flows and resistances in various organs using 50-μm-diameter radioactive microspheres. This study on rabbits and one on dogs published 1 year later [134] were the first to measure myocardial perfusion in the heart. Using microspheres (ranging in size from 14 to 61 μm), they were able to measure flows in both the epimyocardium and endomyocardium of dogs. In both studies, the flows were determined in unanesthetized animals. These studies validated a technique that has become the gold standard for assessing myocardial perfusion.

During the 1950s and 1960s, numerous studies addressed the regulation of coronary blood flow, but a clear consensus was still lacking on many issues. Feinburg and Katz [135] demonstrated that epinephrine and norepinephrine in the dog heart increased coronary blood flow and coronary venous O_2 content, despite wide fluctuations in heart rate and mean aortic pressure. However, it eventually became clear later that the increased blood flow in response to epinephrine was secondary to the increased work of the myocardium [136, 137]. Similarly, although the stellate ganglia were found to be implicated in vasoconstriction, [136], Feigl [137] demonstrated that stimulation of the stellate ganglion sometimes resulted in very small increases in coronary blood flow and he noted that the increase was always associated with some small increase in heart rate or pulse pressure. Other studies conducted during this period revealed the increase in coronary blood flow after sympathetic nerve stimulation to be a consequence of increased O_2 consumption, myocardial contraction, and metabolites [59]. During the mid-1960s, the increase in coronary flow in response to vagal stimulation was believed to be secondary to mechanical factors [138, 139]. However, in 1969, Feigl was able to account for the known determinants of coronary blood flow and therefore demonstrate that direct vagal parasympathetic stimulation causes vasodilation in the coronary vasculature.

The role of adenosine in coronary vasodilation received support from a study that documented its increase during severe hypoxia [140], a finding that has since been confirmed many times. The role of metabolites in coronary vasodilation also gained support and became prominent as underlying autoregulation (reviewed in [59]). However, as stated by Berne in 1964, the complete picture of how coronary blood flow is regulated "must await results of an integrated investigation of physiological and biochemical studies on the unanesthetized animal."

In 1962, the Katz group challenged the long-held assumption that the amount of coronary sinus drainage represents a fixed percentage of the total venous outflow of the heart [141]. Using an open-chest dog preparation, these investigators established that the drainage from the LV to the coronary sinus channels is variable according to (1) the level of stress imposed on the heart and (2) the influence of inotropic agents. Moreover, they suggested that healthy and diseased hearts may differ with regard to the percentage of blood draining into the coronary sinus versus that entering the extracoronary sinus channels. These experiments revealed notable deviations from the mean 60% of coronary flow into the coronary sinus during tachycardia.

Coronary Arteriography

The 1950s were characterized by considerable progress in cardiology. With respect to advances in coronary catheterization, highlights included (1) the increase in the frequency of cardiac surgeries and catheterization of the left and right side of the heart, (2) establishment of many catheterization laboratories, and (3) development of many new diagnostic tools. The latter included hydrogen and oxygen electrodes, catheter tip manometers, flow meters, and dye indicators. It was coronary arteriography that helped open the doors to various surgical interventions that were realized in the following decade.

The development of cardiac catheterization permitted precise cardiac diagnoses in less than an hour and, by 1999, over a million of these procedures had been performed in the USA [102]. A key study was that of Di Guglielmo and Guttadauro [142], who used arteriography to analyze variations in the coronary arteries. Selective coronary catheterization became a widely used procedure in the late 1950s [143]. It was by accident that the first selective coronary arteriogram was obtained in 1958 [102]. Sones and his colleagues were withdrawing their catheter from the left ventricle when it entered the right coronary artery and they were able to clearly visualize the artery and its distal branch. The contrast material that was injected did not cause adverse effects, a finding that contradicted to the prevalent view during the 1950s. Data from animal experiments, e.g., Pearl et al. [144], paved the way for the development of a method of coronary angiography in 1956 by Levy and colleagues [145] that could be used in humans.

Over the next decade, coronary arteriography patients benefitted from improved techniques derived from clinical studies. In 1967, Hultgren et al. published data from 55 patients with angina and positive exercise stress tests. The study showed that occlusive disease, detected by arteriography of at least two major coronary arteries, was present in all of these patients. That same year, a review of the clinical aspects of coronary arteriography noted that selective arteriography could visualize vessels with luminal diameters in the 100–200-μm range [146]. However, one of the problems noted with the technique was that because it was anatomical rather than physiological, it was not always possible to correlate the data with those from electrocardiograms. Thus, the functional capacity of the coronary system was not necessarily consistent with the arteriographic data. Despite these reservations, arteriography during the 1960s became useful and led to enthusiasm for further advancements of the technique.

Microscopy and Tracer Methods

Advances in microscopy opened doors to new opportunities for cellular and subcellular studies. For example, development of phase-contrast and ultraviolet microscopes allowed more in-depth exploration of the coronary circulation. Of particular importance was the advent of electron microscopy. This technique facilitated discoveries regarding the intracellular and extracellular structure of the vasculature. Moore and Ruska [147] were the first to provide detailed descriptions of the fine structure of mammalian of coronary capillaries and arterioles. They noted endothelial vesicles and EC junctions and discussed vesicular transport. A year later, Parker [148] provided an anatomical basis for various coronary artery functions by pointing out cellular junctions, caveolae and vesicles, and other characteristics. Soon thereafter, the intercellular and neuromuscular relationships in coronary arterioles [149] and details of their endothelium [150] were also provided. Moreover, another study provided details concerning intercellular junctions, and the vesicular system of capillary endothelium and its relationship to myocardial pericytes [151]. The use of electron microscopy opened the door to studies using small molecular tracers to study permeability [152] and enabled a detailed look at coronary atherosclerosis [153, 154]. During the 1960s, electron microscopy was used extensively to document cardiomyocyte alterations resulting from hypoxia and ischemia, and these observations provided a structural basis for underlying physiological and pathological mechanisms. These studies were reviewed by Ferrans and Roberts [155] and are topics discussed in Chaps. 9 and 10.

Development of the Coronary Vasculature

The lack of understanding regarding the formation of the coronary vasculature in the embryo prior to 1989 seems beyond comprehension considering the advances that have been made since that time (this is the topic of Chap. 2). A brief description regarding coronary vessel development appears in a book chapter in 1962 [156]. The authors, like those of subsequent papers and books published during the next 2 decades, believed that the main coronary arteries sprouted from the aorta. Indeed, this assumption was finally put to rest by Bogers et al. [157], who provided evidence that the coronary ostia and stems are formed by an ingrowth of an endothelial strand into the aorta. The 1960s did experience the first descriptions of coronary vessel development by a Czech group of investigators. These included the development and branching of coronary arteries in the chick [158] and rat [159]. Then in 1971, the sequences of vascularization in these species was documented [160–162]. Notwithstanding these accomplishments, progress in our understanding of coronary vessel development during a good part of the twentieth century lagged significantly behind the advances in embryology of the heart during this period.

The Coronary System: Progress Delayed

Several factors loom as impediments to scientific progress in the field of coronary vasculature and circulation up to the mid-nineteenth century. First, the dissemination of discoveries and ideas was a slow process, often limited to a monogram, letters to friends, or notebooks. Another problem was that the status of some physicians or scientists was so great that challenges to their ideas or teachings were disregarded. The best example of false concepts taught for centuries are the teachings of Galen (138–201 AD), who erroneously conceived the anatomy of physiology of the cardiovascular system.

The rarity with which new ideas were accepted is evident from the lag between the discovery of important concepts and their incorporation into teaching, or into clinical practice. For example, in the mid-eighteenth century, Jenner and Parry linked coronary ossification to angina—yet in 1868, a century later, von Dusch spoke of angina as a rare condition resulting in few deaths (cited by [163]). At that time, many still considered pericarditis as the cause of myocardial infarction. A second notable example is the reluctance to acknowledge the presence of collaterals in the heart despite their documentation by tracers. A third example is the delay in accepting Herrick's classic work on coronary thrombosis published in 1912. Herrick [164] stressed the link between clinical observation and autopsy findings. When presented at a scientific meeting in 1912, his paper failed to stimulate much discussion. He later stated that it was not until 1918 that "physicians in America and later in Europe woke up" regarding his diagnosis later known as "heart attack" [165]. Finally, although the heart was receiving considerable attention in the mid-nineteenth century, the coronary circulation was not. Even by 1838, the Cyclopedia of Anatomy and Physiology (Reid 1838), which contained many detailed descriptions of the heart, devoted only 1.5 pages to the coronary vasculature and circulation.

References

1. Willius FA, Dry TJ. A History of the Heart and the Circulation. Philadelphia: Saunders; 1948.
2. Herrick JB. A Short History of Cardiology. Springfield: Chas. C. Thomas; 1942.
3. Graubard M. Circulation and Respiration: The Evolution of an Idea. New York: Harcourt, Brace and World; 1964.
4. Acierno L. The History of Cardiology. London: Parthenon Publishing Corporation; 1994.
5. Gregg D. Coronary Circulation in Health and Disease. Philadelphia: Lea and Febiger; 1950.
6. Sarton G. Men of Science in the Renaissance. Bloomington: Indiana University Press; 1957.
7. Leibowitz J. The History of Coronary Heart Disease. Berkley and Los Angeles: University of California Press; 1970.
8. McMurrich JP. Leonardo da Vinci. Baltimore: The Anatomist; 1930.
9. Simmons JG. The Scientific 100. New York: Fall River Press; 1996.
10. Silverman ME, Wooley CF. A history of the heart. Hurst's: the heart, vol. I. New York: McGraw-Hill; 2008.
11. Duffin J. History of Medicine. A Scandalously Short Introduction. Toronto: University of Toronto Press; 1999.
12. Pratt F. The nutrition of the heart through the vessels of Thebesius and the coronary veins. Am J Physiol. 1898;1:86–103.
13. Thebesius A. De circulo sanquinis in corde. Leiden;1708.
14. Wearn JT. The Role of the Thebesian Vessels in the Circulation of the Heart. J Exp Med. 1928;47:293–315.
15. Wearn JT. Nature of vascular communications between the coronary arteries and chambers of the heart. American Heart Journal. 1933;9:143.
16. Lower R. Tractus de corte, item de motu et colore sanquinis et chylioum eum transitu. Amstelodami;1669.
17. Blumgart HL. Coronary disease: clinical-pathologic correlations and physiology. Bull N Y Acad Med. 1951;27:693–710.
18. Mautz FR. Anatomical and physiological considerations in the development of a collateral circulation to the myocardium. Diseases of the chest. 1957;31:265–85.
19. Jamin F, Merkel H. Die Koronditerien des menschlichen Herzen unter normalen und pathologischen Verhaltnissen;1907.
20. Woollard HH. The Innervation of the Heart. J Anat. 1926; 60:345–73.
21. Wiggers CJ. The physiology of the coronary circulation. In: Levy RL, editor. Disease of the Coronary Arteries and Cardiac Pain. New York: MacMillan and Company; 1936. p. 57–108.
22. Rebetel F. Recherches Experimentales sur la Circulation daus les Arteres Coronaries. Paris: These (E 288); 1872.
23. Wearn JT. The Extent of the Capillary Bed of the Heart. J Exp Med. 1928;47:273–90.
24. Langendorff O. Zur kenntnissdes Blutlaufs in den kranzgefassendes hersen. Pflugers Archiv Physiol. 1899;78:423–40.
25. Markwalder J, Starling EH. A note on some factors which determine the blood flow through the coronary circulation. J Physiol. 1913;47:275–85.
26. Morawitz P, Zahn A. Untersuchungen uber den Coronarkreis lauf. Dtsch Arch Klin Med. 1914;116:364–408.
27. Nakagawa T. On the coronary circulation in the heart-lung preparation. J Physiol. 1922;56:340–7.
28. Anrep GV, Cruickshank E, Downing A, Suba Rau A. The coronary circulation in relation to the cardiac cycle. Heart. 1927; 14:111–33.
29. Rossler R, Pascual W. The coronary circulation in the isolated perfused heart. J Physiol. 1932;74:1–16.
30. Wiggers C, Cotton F. Studies on the coronary circulation. II. The systolic and diastolic flow through the coronary vessels. Am J Physiol. 1933;106:597.
31. Rudolph AM, Heymann MA. The circulation of the fetus in utero. Methods for studying distribution of blood flow, cardiac output and organ blood flow. Circ Res. 1967;21:163–84.
32. Buckberg GD, Luck JC, Payne DB, Hoffman JI, Archie JP, Fixler DE. Some sources of error in measuring regional blood flow with radioactive microspheres. J Appl Physiol. 1971;31:598–604.
33. Marcus ML. The cornary circulation in health and disease. New York: McGraw-Hill; 1983.
34. Erichsen J. On the influence of the coronary circulation on the action of the heart. Lond Mag Gazette. 1842;2:561–5.
35. Bezold A. Von den Veraderungen des Herzschlages nach verschliessung der coronarterian. Untersuchungen aus dem phsiologischen laboratorium in Wuzburg. 1867;256–87.
36. Benson R. The present status of coronary arterial disease. Arch Pathol and Lab Med. 1926;2:876–916.

37. Weigert C. Uber die pathologischen Gerinnungs-vorgange. Virchows Arch Path Anat. 1880;79:87–123.
38. Burchell HB. Adjustments in coronary circulation after experimental coronary occlusion with particular reference to vascularization of pericardial adhesions. Arch Int Med. 1940;65:240.
39. Karsner HT, Dwyer JE. Studies in infarction: IV. Experimental bland infarction of the myocardium, myocardial regeneration and cicatrization. J Med Res. 1916;34:21–40.3.
40. Opie LH. Angina pectoris: the evolution of concepts. J Cardiovasc Pharmacol Ther. 2004;9 Suppl 1:S3–9.
41. Smith T. A chronology of atherosclerosis. Am J Pharm. 1960;132:390–405.
42. Hall M. On the mutual relations between anatomy, physiology, pathology and therapeutics, and the practice of medicine; Being the Gulstonian Lectures for 1842. London;1842.
43. Vogel J. The pathological anatomy of the human body. Philadelphia: Lea and Blanchard; 1847.
44. Lie RK. The angina pectoris controversy during the 1920s. Acta Physiol Scand Suppl. 1991;599:135–47.
45. Smith F. The ligation of coronary arteries with electrocardiographic study. Arch Int Med. 1918;22:8–27.
46. Pardee H. An electrocardiographic sign of coronary artery obstruction. Archives of Internal Medicine. 1920;26:244–57.
47. Dietrich S, Schwiegk H. Angina pectoris und des herzuskels. Zietschrift fur Klinische Medzin. 1933;125:195–242.
48. Rotschild MA, Kissin M. Induced general anoxemia causing S-T deviation in the electrocardiogram. Am Heart Assoc J. 1933;8:745–54.
49. McAlpin R. Coronary arterial spasm: a historical perspective. J History of Med and Allied Sci. 1980;35:288–311.
50. Latham PM. Lectures on Subjects Connected with Clinical Medicine. London: Logman; 1846.
51. Osler W. The Lumleian lectures on angina pectoris II. Lancet. 1910;175(4517):839–44.
52. Katz LN, Lindner E, Landt H. On the Nature of the Substance(S) Producing Pain in Contracting Skeletal Muscle: Its Bearing on the Problems of Angina Pectoris and Intermittent Claudication. J Clin Invest. 1935;14:807–21.
53. Wiggers CJ. The functional consequences of coronary occlusion. Ann Int Med. 1945;23:158–69.
54. Wiggers CJ. The functional consequences of acute coronary occlusion. J Ark Med Soc. 1946;43:48.
55. Klotz O. Experimental production of arteriosclerosis. Br Med J. 1906;2:1767.
56. Anitschkow N. Experimental Atherosclerosis in Animals. New York: MacMillan; 1933.
57. Katz LN, Stamler J. Experimental Atherosclerosis. Springfield: C.C. Thomas; 1953.
58. Langley RW. The changing outlook in coronary disease. Calif Med. 1949;71:31.
59. Berne RM. Regulation of Coronary Blood Flow. Physiological reviews. 1964;44:1–29.
60. Wiggers CJ. The innervation of the coronary vessels. Am J Physiol. 1909;24:391.
61. Wiggers CJ, Cotton F. Studies on the coronary circulation. I. The coronary pressure pulses and their interpretation. Am J Physiol. 1933;106:9.
62. Wiggers CJ, Wegria R, Pinera B. The effects of myocardial ischemia on fibrillation threshold—the mechanism of spontaneous fibrillation following coronary occlusion. Am J Physiol. 1940;131:309–16.
63. Wiggers CJ. Modern Aspects of the Circulation in Health and Disease. Philadelphia: Lea and Febiger; 1923.
64. Anrep GV, Blalock A, Hammouda M. The distribution of the blood in the coronary vessels. J Physiol. 1929;67:87.
65. Anrep GV, Downing AC. A method for the quantitative measurement of quick hcnages in the outflow of liquids. J Sci Instrum. 1925–1926;3:221.
66. Anrep GV, Hausler H. The coronary circulation: I. The effect of changes of the blood-pressure and of the output of the heart. J Physiol. 1928;65:357–73.
67. Anrep GV, Segall HN. The central and reflex regulation of the heart rate. J Physiol. 1926;61:215–31.
68. Anrep GV, Segall HN. The regulation of the coronary circulation. Heart. 1926;13:239.
69. Anrep GV, King B. The significance of the diastolic and systolic blood-pressures for the maintenance of the coronary circulation. J Physiol. 1927–1928;64:341.
70. Shipley RA, Shipley LJ, Wearn JT. The Capillary Supply in Normal and Hypertrophied Hearts of Rabbits. J Exp Med. 1937;65:29–42.
71. Roberts J, Wearn J, Badal J. The capillary muscle ratio in normal and hypertrophied human hearts. Proc Soc Exp Biol and Med. 1938;38:322.
72. Wearn JT. Alterations in the heart accompanying growth and hypertrophy. Bull Johns Hopkins Hosp. 1941;68:363.
73. Gregg DE, Shipley RE. Studies of the venous drainage of the heart. The American journal of physiology. 1947;151:13–25.
74. Gregg DE. Phasic changes in flow through different coronary branches, blood, heart and circulation. AAAS. 1940;13:81.
75. Gregg DE, Shipley RE. Augmentation of left coronary inflow with elevation of left ventricular pressure and observations on the mechanism for increased coronary inflow iwth increased cardiac load. Am J Physiol. 1944;142:44.
76. Gregg DE, Green HD, Wiggers CJ. Phasic variations in peripheral coronary resistance and their determinants. Am J Physiol. 1935;112:362.
77. Gregg DE, Green HD. Effects of viscosity, ischemia, cardiac output and aortic pressure on coronary blood flow measured under a constant perfusion pressure. Am J Physiol. 1940;130:108.
78. Wolkoff K. Uber die histologische Struktur der Coronararterien des Menschlichen Herzens. Virchows Arch F Path Anat. 1923;241:42–58.
79. Wolkoff K. Uber die Alters Veranderungen der Arterien bei Tieren. Virchows Arch F Path Anat. 1924;252:208–28.
80. Wolkoff K. Uber die Atherosklerose der Coronaraterien des Herzen. Beitr Z Path Anat UZ Allg Pathol. 1929;82:555–96.
81. Gross L, Epstein EZ, Kugel MA. Histology of the coronary arteries and their branches in the human heart. Am J Path. 1933;10:253–73.
82. Gross L. The blood supply to the heart in its anatomical and clinical aspects. New York: Hoeber; 1921.
83. Spalteholz K. Die Arterien der Herwand. Anatomische untersuchungen an Menschen und Tierherzen: S. Hirzel; 1924.
84. Blumgart HL, Zoll PM, et al. The experimental production of intercoronary arterial anastomoses and their functional significance. Circulation. 1950;1:10–27, pl.
85. Bloor CM, Liebow AA. Coronary Collateral Circulation. Am J Cardiol. 1965;16:238–52.
86. Moritz AR, Hudson CL, Orgain ES. Augmentation of the Extracardiac Anastomoses of the Coronary Arteries through Pericardial Adhesions. J Exp Med. 1932;56:927–31.
87. Eckstein RW, Gregg D, Prichard W. The magnitude and time of development of the collateral circulation in occluded carotid and coronary arteries. Am J Physiol. 1941;132:351.
88. Prinzmetal M. A quantitative method for determining collateral coronary circulation. Preliminary report on normal human hearts. J Mt Sinai Hosp. 1942;8:933–9.
89. Prinzmetal M, Simkin B, et al. Studies on the coronary circulation; the collateral circulation of the normal human heart by

coronary perfusion with radioactive erythrocytes and glass spheres. Am Heart J. 1947;33:420–42.
90. Schlesinger MJ. An injection plus dissection study of coronary artery occlusions and anastomoses. Am Heart J. 1938;15:528–68.
91. Schlesinger M. Significant variations in the anatomic pattern of the coronary vessels. Am Assoc Adv Sci Blood Heart Circ. 1940;61–72.
92. Blumgart HL. Studies on the relation of the clinical manifestations of angina pectoris, coronary thrombosis and myocardial infarction to the pathological findings. Am Heart J. 1940;19:1–91.
93. Blumgart HL, Yens OC. STUDIES ON THE VELOCITY OF BLOOD FLOW: I. The Method Utilized. The Journal of clinical investigation. 1927;4:1–13.
94. Hausler H. The coronary circulation: III. The dependence of changes in the coronary blood flow on cardiac and local vascular factors. The Journal of physiology. 1929;68:324–32.
95. Bing RJ, Hammond MM, et al. The measurement of coronary blood flow, oxygen consumption, and efficiency of the left ventricle in man. American Heart Journal. 1949;38:1–24.
96. Eckenhoff JE, Hafkenschiel JH, Landmesser CM. The coronary circulation in the dog. The American journal of physiology. 1947;148:582–96.
97. Eckenhoff JE, Hafkenschiel JH, et al. Cardiac oxygen metabolism and control of the coronary circulation. The American journal of physiology. 1947;149:634–49.
98. Eckenhoff JE. The physiology of the coronary circulation. Anesthesiology. 1950;11:168–77.
99. Foltz EL, Page RG, Sheldon WF, Wong SK, Tuddenham WJ, Weiss AJ. Factors in variation and regulation of coronary blood flow in intact anesthetized dogs. The American journal of physiology. 1950;162:521–37.
100. Dock W. The Capacity of the Coronary Bed in Cardiac Hypertrophy. The Journal of experimental medicine. 1941;74:177–86.
101. Kountz WB, Smith JR. The Flow of Blood in the Coronary Arteries in Pathological Hearts. The Journal of clinical investigation. 1938;17:147–52.
102. Baim D, Bing RJ. Cardiac catheterization. Cardiology: the evolution of the science and the art. New Brunswick: Rutgers University Press; 1999. p. 1–29.
103. Radner S. An attempt at the roentgenologic visualization of coronary blood vessels in man. Acta radiol. 1945;26:497–502.
104. Broden B, Jonsson G, Karnell J. Thoracic aortography; observations on technical problems connected with the method and various risks involved in its use. Acta Radiol. 1949;32:498–508, illust.
105. James TN, Burch GE. The atrial coronary arteries in man. Circulation. 1958;17:90–8.
106. James TN. The arteries of the free ventricular walls in man. The Anatomical record. 1960;136:371–84.
107. James TN. The delivery and distribution of coronary collateral circulation. Chest. 1970;58:183–203.
108. James TN. The coronary circulation and conduction system in acute myocardial infarction. Progress in cardiovascular diseases. 1968;10:410–49.
109. Paul MH, Norman LR, Zoll PM, Blumgart HL. Stimulation of inter-arterial coronary anastomoses by experimental acute coronary occlusion. Circulation. 1957;16:608–14.
110. Vineberg A, Munro DD, Cohen H, Buller W. Four years' clinical experience with internal mammary artery implantation in the treatment of human coronary artery insufficiency including additional experimental studies. J Thorac Surg. 1955;29:1–32. discussion, -6.
111. Beck CS, Leighninger DS. Operations for coronary artery disease. Journal of the American Medical Association. 1954;156: 1226–33.
112. Beck CS, Leighninger DS. Scientific basis for the surgical treatment of coronary artery disease. Journal of the American Medical Association. 1955;159:1264–71.
113. Leighninger DS. A laboratory and clinical evaluation of operations for coronary artery disease. J Thorac Surg. 1955;30: 397–410.
114. Feil H. Clinical Appraisal of the Beck Operation. Ann Surg. 1943;118:807–15.
115. Frick MH. Coronary bypass surgery. An overview. Ann Clin Res. 1978;10:235–41.
116. Lumb G, Hardy LB. Collateral Circulation in the Heart. North Carolina medical journal. 1963;24:456–60.
117. Kong Y, Chen JT, Zeft HJ, Whalen RE, McIntosh HD. Natural history of experimental coronary occlusion in pigs: a serial cineangiographic study. American Heart Journal. 1969;77:45–54.
118. Schaper W, Jageneau A, Xhonneux R. The development of collateral circulation in the pig and dog heart. Cardiologia. 1967;51:321–35.
119. Litvak J, Siderides LE, Vineberg AM. The experimental production of coronary artery insufficiency and occlusion. American Heart Journal. 1957;53:505–18.
120. Schaper W. The Collateral Circulation of the Heart. Amsterdam/ London: Elsevier North-Holland Publishing Company; 1971.
121. Baroldi G, Mantero O, Scomazzoni G. The collaterals of the coronary arteries in normal and pathologic hearts. Circulation research. 1956;4:223–9.
122. Schaper W, Vandesteene R. The rate of growth of interarterial anastomoses in chronic coronary artery occlusion. Life sciences. 1967;6:1673–80.
123. Eckstein RW. Effect of exercise and coronary artery narrowing on coronary collateral circulation. Circ Res. 1957;5:230–5.
124. Bailey CP, May A, Lemmon WM. Survival after coronary endarterectomy in man. Journal of the American Medical Association. 1957;164:641–6.
125. Mulder DG, Kattus Jr AA, Fonkalsrud EW, Longmire Jr WP. The Surgical Treatment of Acquired Aortic Stenosis. The Journal of thoracic and cardiovascular surgery. 1963;46:468–81.
126. Vineberg AM, Niloff PH. The value of surgical treatment of coronary artery occlusion by implantation of the internal mammary artery into the ventricular myocardium; an experimental study. Surg Gynecol Obstet. 1950;91:551–61.
127. Carrel A. VIII. On the Experimental Surgery of the Thoracic Aorta and Heart. Ann Surg. 1910;52:83–95.
128. McIntosh HD, Garcia JA. The first decade of aortocoronary bypass grafting, 1967–1977. A review. Circulation. 1978;57:405–31.
129. Kolessov VI. Mammary artery-coronary artery anastomosis as method of treatment for angina pectoris. The Journal of thoracic and cardiovascular surgery. 1967;54:535–44.
130. Kouchoukos NT, Kirklin JW. Coronary bypass operations for ischemic heart disease. Mod Concepts Cardiovasc Dis. 1972; 41:47–51.
131. Spencer FC, Glassman E. Surgical procedures for coronary artery disease. Annu Rev Med. 1972;23:229–44.
132. Berne RM, Blackmon JR, Gardner TH. Hypoxemia and coronary blood flow. The Journal of clinical investigation. 1957;36:1101–6.
133. Gregg DE. The natural history of coronary collateral development. Circulation research. 1974;35:335–44.
134. Domenech RJ, Hoffman JI, Noble MI, Saunders KB, Henson JR, Subijanto S. Total and regional coronary blood flow measured by radioactive microspheres in conscious and anesthetized dogs. Circulation research. 1969;25:581–96.
135. Feinberg H, Katz LN. Effect of catecholamines, l-epinephrine and l-norepinephrine on coronary flow and oxygen metabolism of the myocardium. The American journal of physiology. 1958; 193:151–6.

136. Berne RM, Degeest H, Levy MN. Influence of the Cardiac Nerves on Coronary Resistance. The American journal of physiology. 1965;208:763–9.
137. Feigl EO. Sympathetic control of coronary circulation. Circulation research. 1967;20:262–71.
138. Daggett WM, Nugent GC, Carr PW, Powers PC, Harada Y. Influence of vagal stimulation on ventricular contractility, O2 consumption, and coronary flow. The American journal of physiology. 1967;212:8–18.
139. Ross G. Blood flow in the right coronary artery of the dog. Cardiovascular research. 1967;1:138–44.
140. Katori M, Berne RM. Release of adenosine from anoxic hearts. Relationship to coronary flow. Circulation research. 1966; 19:420–5.
141. Lafontant RR, Feinberg H, Katz LN. Partition of coronary flow and cardiac oxygen extraction between coronary sinus and other coronary drainage channels. Circulation research. 1962;11:686–98.
142. Di Guglielmo L, Guttadauro M. Anatomic variations in the coronary arteries; an arteriographic study in living subjects. Acta radiol. 1954;41:393–416.
143. Sones Jr FM, Shirey EK. Cine coronary arteriography. Mod Concepts Cardiovasc Dis. 1962;31:735–8.
144. Pearl F, Friedman M, Gray N, Friedman B. Coronary arteriography in the intact dog. Circulation. 1950;1:1188–92.
145. Levy LM, Hannon DW, Sprafka JL, Baronofsky ID. A method for coronary arteriography. Ann Surg. 1956;143:412–5.
146. Likoff W, Segal BL, Kasparian H. Clinical aspects of coronary arteriography. The American journal of cardiology. 1967;19:497–501.
147. Moore DH, Ruska H. The fine structure of capillaries and small arteries. J Biophys Biochem Cytol. 1957;3:457–62.
148. Parker F. An electron microscope study of coronary arteries. The American journal of anatomy. 1958;103:247–73.
149. Lever JD, Ahmed M, Irvine G. Neuromuscular and intercellular relationships in the coronary arterioles. A morphological and quantitative study by light and electron microscopy. Journal of anatomy. 1965;99:829–40.
150. Ahmed MM. The fine structure of endothelium in coronary arterioles. Acta anatomica. 1968;69:327–42.
151. Bruns RR, Palade GE. Studies on blood capillaries. I. General organization of blood capillaries in muscle. The Journal of cell biology. 1968;37:244–76.
152. Karnovsky MJ. The ultrastructural basis of capillary permeability studied with peroxidase as a tracer. The Journal of cell biology. 1967;35:213–36.
153. Togawa K. Electron microscopical studies on the coronary atherosclerosis. II. Age-related changes in the coronary artery in infancy. Kumamoto Med J. 1965;18:184–99.
154. Meessen H. Contribution on the morphology of coronary sclerosis. Advances in cardiology. 1970;4:3–19.
155. Ferrans VJ, Roberts WC. Myocardial ultrastructure in acute and chronic hypoxia. Cardiology. 1971;56:144–60.
156. Licata R. Coronary circulation: embryology. New York: New York Academ. Press; 1962.
157. Bogers AJ, Gittenberger-de Groot AC, Poelmann RE, Peault BM, Huysmans HA. Development of the origin of the coronary arteries, a matter of ingrowth or outgrowth? Anat Embryol (Berl). 1989;180:437–41.
158. Dbaly J. The development of branching of the coronary arteries in the chick. Morfologie (Czk). 1964;12:401–14.
159. Dbaly J, Ostadal B, Rychter Z. Development of the coronary arteries in rat embryos. Acta Anat. 1968;71:209–22.
160. Rychter Z, Jelinek R. Progress of vascularization of the ventricular myocardium in the chick embryo. Physiol Bohemoslov. 1971;20:131–8.
161. Rychter Z, Jelinek R, Marhan O. Progress of vascularization of the ventricular myocardium in the rat embryo. Physiol Bohemoslov. 1971;20:527–32.
162. Rychter Z, Ostadal B. Mechanism of the development of coronary arteries in chick embryo. Folia Morphol (Praha). 1971;19: 113–24.
163. Herrick JB. Historical Note. Diseases of the Coronary Arteries and Pain. New York: MacMillan Company; 1936. p. 17–27.
164. Herrick JB. Clinical features of sudden obstruction of the coronary arteries. JAMA. 1912;59:2015.
165. Herrick J. Memories of Eighty Years. Chicago: University of Chicago Press; 1949. p. 196–200.

Coronary Anomalies

6

Abbreviations

ACAOS	Anomalous coronary artery originating from opposite sinus of Valsalva
CCHD	Cyanotic congenital heart disease
LAD	Left anterior descending artery
LCA	Left coronary artery
LV	Left ventricle
MB	Myocardial bridging (bridge)
RCA	Right coronary artery
RV	Right ventricle
SCD	Sudden cardiac death

Introduction

Significance of Coronary Anomalies

Frequency of Occurrence

Although the literature contains a plethora of descriptions regarding coronary anomalies, our understanding of the mechanisms that underlie their origins remains poor. Congenital coronary anomalies are usually cited as occurring in about 1% of the population [1, 2]. However, in his review of 1,950 angiograms, Angelini [3] found that 5.64% of the individuals had coronary anomalies, but cautioned that this population may have included some individuals with suspected cases of coronary anomalies. He [4] called attention to the complex problem of defining coronary anomalies, which are usually defined only anatomically, without regard to clinical relevance. Of data from 12,457 patients who underwent coronary angiography, most (89%) of the anomalies were those of origin and distribution [2]. In some cases, what could be classified as an anomaly is more appropriately termed "an anatomical variation." Such examples include the left circumflex artery arising from a separate ostium at the left sinus of Valsalva, a finding that constitutes 36% of coronary "anomalies" [5] or a third coronary ostium giving rise to the conal artery (this occurs in nearly 50% of the population, as noted in Chap. 4). Recognizing the functional significance of each anomaly is the most important parameter to be evaluated.

Lethal Coronary Anomalies

Although most anomalies are not risk factors, there are those that are lethal, i.e., the so-called malignant anomalies [6] (1) right coronary artery (RCA) originates from left cusp of Valsalva and artery courses between the aorta and pulmonary trunk and (2) left coronary artery (LCA) originates from the right cusp of Valsalva and courses between the aorta and pulmonary trunk. The assumption that a given coronary artery anomaly noted at necropsy is the cause of a patient's angina, syncope, myocardial infarction, or sudden death may not always be true. As Angelini [4] cautions, patient to patient variability is such that a given anomaly, as shown by exercise stress tests, does not necessarily predispose every patient to myocardial ischemia. In some cases, additional factors, e.g., coronary spasms, compression, or clotting, may play a role in combination with the anomaly itself or may even be independent of the anomaly. However, the potential for sudden death in certain anomalies is now appreciated. Of particular note is the origin of a coronary artery from the opposite sinus that has a transmural course through the aortic wall. Such anomalies are not usually discovered during a stress test. However, this type of anomaly, as noted in this chapter, can be the major source of sudden death in athletes.

Chapter Objectives

The first part of this chapter reviews the types of coronary anomalies, including intrinsic anomalies, and their association with congenital heart malformations. The second part addresses the possible alterations in mechanisms that regulate the formation of the coronary vasculature and the role of coronary artery anomalies in sudden death. The remainder of the chapter focuses on the link between coronary abnormalities and congenital and early childhood diseases. For more

R.J. Tomanek, *Coronary Vasculature: Development, Structure-Function, and Adaptations*,
DOI 10.1007/978-1-4614-4887-7_6, © Springer Science+Business Media New York 2013

details regarding coronary anomalies, I recommend these monograms: Neufeld and Schneeweiss [7], Angelini [3] and [8], and reviews by Angelini [4, 9] and [10].

Classification of Coronary Anomalies in Human Hearts

A commonly used classification of coronary anomalies is based on anatomical considerations. One simple classification is (1) abnormalities in origin and distribution and (2) intracoronary communications and fistulae [11]. Another system classification uses three categories (1) anomalies of origin and course, (2) anomalies of intrinsic coronary arterial anatomy, and (3) anomalies of termination [9, 12], and includes anomalous anastomotic vessels as a fourth category. Anomalies of origin and course include the bulk of anomalies cited in the literature. Examples of intrinsic coronary arterial anatomy include coronary aneurysms, coronary artery atresia, ostial dimple or stenosis, and bridging (intramural passage of a portion of an epicardial artery). Anomalies of termination are rarer, but include a variety of coronary artery terminations, e.g., coronary sinus, or one of the chambers of the heart. Ogden [13] classified congenital coronary anomalies as minor, major, or secondary. Perloff [8] distinguishes between anomalies unassociated with congenital heart disease and those associated with congenital heart disease as two major headings. Within the first category, he includes various anomalies, whereas his second category considers specific congenital heart diseases, such as tetralogy of Fallot, and complete transposition of the great arteries (TGA). He also adds a third classification: "Acquired anomalies of coronary arteries secondary to congenital heart disease."

Anomalies of Aortic or Pulmonary Origin

Anomalous origins of coronary arteries often occur in hearts that are free of congenital heart malformation. Many anomalies of origin are not problematic as they do not limit myocardial perfusion, whereas others occurring in conjunction with complex congenital heart disease or as isolated abnormalities are clinically relevant [11]. As already noted, one problematic type of anomaly is origin of a coronary artery from the opposite sinus of Valsalva, especially if the anomalous artery has an intramural course for the aorta [9, 10]. Another serious coronary anomaly is coronary artery origin from the pulmonary trunk, which results in myocardial ischemia and often heart failure [11]. This anomaly, if untreated, has an estimated mortality of 35% to more than 85% [14]. Coronary arterial fistulae in about 50% of patients result in congestive heart failure, rupture, coronary steal, or infective endocarditis. Even individuals without symptoms may be at

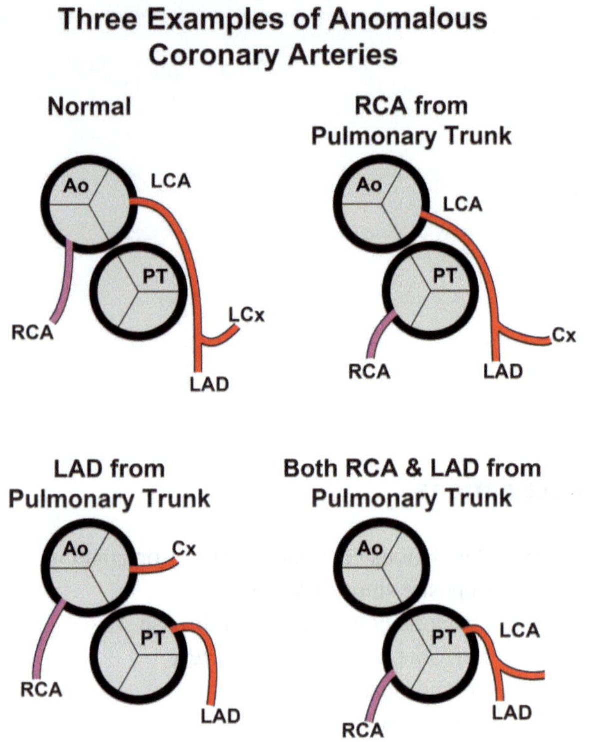

Fig. 6.1 Three types of coronary anomalies of origin are illustrated. *Ao* aorta; *PT* pulmonary trunk; *LCA* left coronary artery; *LAD* left anterior descending artery; *Cx* circumflex artery

risk, as evidenced by data from the American Heart Association, indicating that 19% of deaths in athletes occur in individuals with coronary anomalies [15]. These and other anomalies are discussed below, and examples of coronary anomalies of origin are provided in Fig. 6.1.

Anomalous Origin from the Opposite Sinus of Valsalva

Anomalous Origin from the Opposite Sinus of Valsalva (ACAOS) that involves the anomalous to course between the aortic root and the pulmonary trunk is associated with the highest risk of mortality [9, 16]. Not surprisingly, an anomalous artery originating from the opposite sinus of Valsalva (ACAOS) has been linked to sudden death, a topic addressed later in this chapter. Figure 6.2 illustrates two examples of this type of anomaly. One proposed mechanism of sudden occlusion of the anomalous left main coronary artery is compression or kinking of the vessel during vigorous activity (reviewed in [17]). A second possibility concerns the short oblique course of the anomalous artery, which presumably could collapse during exercise and systolic expansion of the great vessels [15]. Even if the LCA originates from the right sinus of Valsalva without an intramural course in the aortic wall, the patient may experience disabling angina and

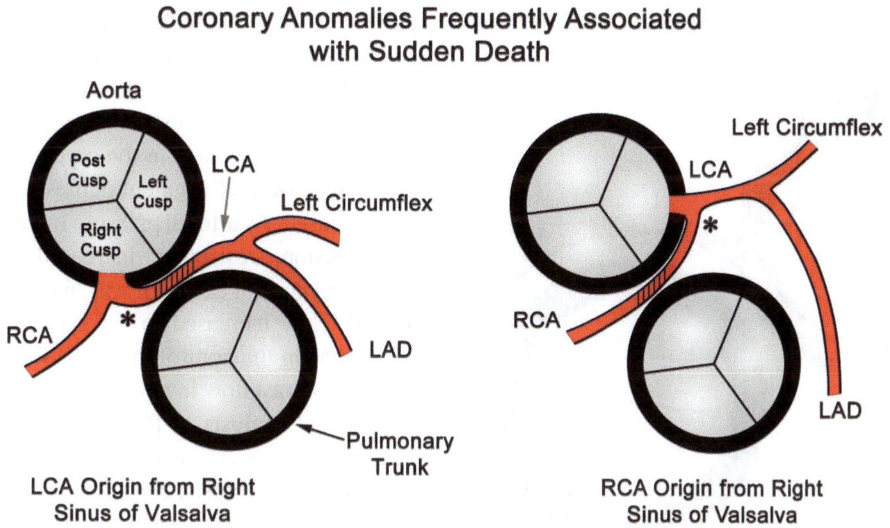

Fig. 6.2 Coronary anomalies of origin often associated with sudden death involve passage of the anomalous artery between the aorta and pulmonary trunk. The *asterisks* indicates an anomalous origin of the left coronary artery (LCA) in the left figure and an anomalous origin of the right coronary artery (RCA) in the right figure. The cross-hatched area of the anomalous arteries indicates sites were compression during systole may occur

syncope [18]. ACAOS is of particular clinical significance if it involves the LCA.

Intramural Course Through the Aortic Wall

If the anomalous coronary artery is intramural within the aorta, i.e., the artery passes some distance within the wall of the aorta before emerging (Fig. 6.3), patients more frequently have angina or syncope [19]. The length of the intramural portion of the coronary artery correlates with the patient's symptoms. These findings lead to the conclusion that both the course of the coronary artery (passage between the great vessels) and its intramural path within the aorta contribute to myocardial ischemia. Angelini [20] concluded that both right and left ACAOS are characterized by an intramural segment in the aortic wall and that it is this intramural segment that is narrowed by systolic compression, especially during exercise. A prospective study of 577 patients, referred for control of stents or screening of risk factors, found that 21% had coronary artery anomalies [10]. Of the six patients who presented with an ACAOS, four had ostial stenosis ≥60 % and the course of the anomalous was retroaortic in three and intra-arterial in three. None of the proximal anomalous coronary arteries displayed evidence of atherosclerosis. Thus, as proposed by Angelini and colleagues [9], the stenosis could be due to coronary hypoplasia. To address the effect of the precise point of the right ACAOS from the left sinus of Valsalva, two groups of 87 patients with this anomaly were studied [21]. Group 1 had a high intramural course (Fig. 6.3), i.e., the right coronary ostium in the aorta was located above the pulmonary valve, whereas group 2 consisted of patients in whom the coronary ostium was below the level of the pulmonary valve. Patients in group 1 had a much greater prevalence of typical angina (43%) compared to the patients in group 2 (6%). Major adverse cardiac events were also markedly higher in patients with the high intramural course. These data support the hypothesis that if the position of the intra-arterial course is in the region where systolic compression is greatest, the chances of myocardial ischemia and major cardiac events are more likely.

Two Case Reports of Intramural Course

The significant risk with an intramural course is underscored by a case report of a 56-year-old female who had a "normal" origin of the left main coronary artery from the left sinus of Valsalva, but its origin was tangential and its course intramural [22]. The effect was described as an inferior tilt with its intramural course displaying various degrees of lateral compression during three angiograms conducted over a 5 year period. These episodes of compression correlated with her symptoms of angina and dyspnea. The patient's symptoms were completely relieved following surgical repair that included osteoplasty. This case illustrates the effect of an intramural course on myocardial ischemia. Angelini [20] has concluded that "only the intramural course of the ectopic artery seems to be related to proximal coronary obstruction in L-ACAOS." Another case on an intramural course of ACAOS was associated with sudden cardiac arrest in a 24 year old man [23]. Multidetector computed tomography revealed that his RCA originated from the left sinus of Valsalva with an intramural course in the aorta and a severe compression between the aorta and pulmonary artery. A histological specimen from a proximal sample of the anomalous

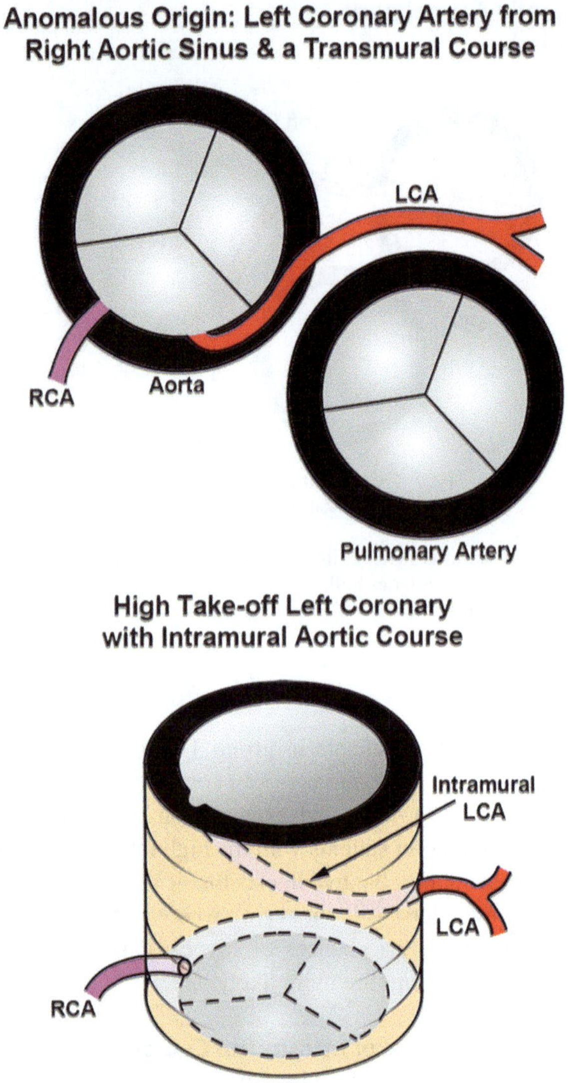

Fig. 6.3 An additional complication with an anomalous origin from the wrong sinus of Valsalva occurs if the artery takes an intramural course within the aortic wall as seen in the top illustration. Here the left coronary artery (LCA) passes posteriorly through the aortic wall before emerging. This situation places additional compression on the artery during systole and constitutes the highest risk for myocardial ischemia of all coronary anomalies. A high takeoff and intramural course, seen in the bottom figure, is even more likely to cause an ischemic event because the high takeoff places the intramural portion of the anomalous artery closer to the pulmonary artery and exposes it to additional compression. In this bottom illustration the LCA ostium begins above the right sinus of Valsalva

coronary artery, obtained at the time of surgery, showed that the intramural segment had intimal fibrous thickening, fragmentation of elastin and smooth muscle degeneration.

Experimental Data

To elucidate potential pathophysiological mechanisms of sudden death from ACAOS, and Bartoli [24] evaluated regional blood flow and hemodynamics in a juvenile calf with a left ACAOS. At baseline, blood flow was greater in the LCA than in the RCA. However when heart rate and metabolic demand were increased with dobutamine, the increase blood flow to the LCA was 20% lower than that in the RCA and was lower in the myocardium perfused by the LCA. Moreover, ST-segment depression was worse as heart rate increased. As arterial pressure increased with phenylephrine infusion, resistance increased more than fivefold, whereas in control calves, it was unchanged. Although mean diastolic flow increased to the same level in the calf with ACAOS as in the control group, systolic flow decreased by 20%. In contrast flow increased by 50% in the control group. Histological analysis of the left ventricle (LV) indicated a high incidence of apoptosis, hypertrophy of surviving cardiomyocytes and fibrosis, increased capillary density, and collaterals; in contrast, the RV was normal. The authors concluded that this anomaly was associated with ischemia and myocardial damage.

Origin from Pulmonary Artery

Infant Mortality and Sudden Death

Early infant mortality and sudden death in adults are common outcomes of untreated patients with an anomalous coronary artery originating in the pulmonary artery [25, 26]. In most cases, it is the LCA that has a pulmonary origin [3]. In their review of 147 cases of this anomaly, Wesselhoeft and colleagues [26] noted that they present in one of four ways (1) in infancy with angina or cardiomyopathy; (2) or later with mitral insufficiency; (3) continuous murmur, or (4) they die as adults. Although this anomaly is considered to be rare, the number of cases has increased for two reasons. First, greater detection of this anomaly has been a consequence of the utilization of noninvasive methods [25]. Second, there is now a recognition that this anomaly is often misdiagnosed as some form of coronary heart disease or cardiomyopathy, as indicated by a study of 23 patients [27]. The seriousness of this anomaly is indicated by the fact that symptomatic infants present with congestive heart failure and features of severe dilated cardiomyopathy; early diagnosis reveals a limited collateral circulation from the RCA and left ventricular ischemia and infarction [28]. Three examples of anomalous origins from the pulmonary artery are provided in Fig. 6.1.

Symptoms and Adaptations

The observation that symptoms often do not develop until 2 months after a normal birth led to the description in 1933 of a clinical syndrome by Bland, White, and Garland which bears their name [29]. A review of 60 patients with an anomalous coronary artery indicated that the onset of symptoms occurred prior to the second or third week following birth in only 7 of these patients [26]. Most of the patients died during the first year. The first distinction between patients who died during the first year and those who survive to adulthood was proposed by Kaunitz [30]. He noted that the onset of symptoms often coincided with the closure of the ductus arteriosus at 2 months, and that in surviving adults, the RCA was dilated and provided significant collateral vessels to the anomalous LCA. However, the direction of blood flow in the anomalous artery cannot be assumed, since flow may be either from or into the pulmonary artery [31], and therefore coronary steal may or may not occur [32]. Which of these directions of flow occurs depends on the pressure in the artery originating from the pulmonary trunk. If the pressure is low, a coronary steal will occur, resulting in ischemia and some degree of collateral growth. For example, a 45-year-old patient with angina and incapacitation presented with a left coronary pressure of 35/10 mmHg [33]. Following ligation of the anomalous coronary artery at its pulmonary origin, the pressure rose to 105/30 mmHg and her symptoms disappeared. Figure 6.4 illustrates the changes in flow through the coronary arteries during the closure of the ductus arteriosus and the development of coronary anastomoses.

In summary, anomalous coronary artery origins from the aorta and origin from the pulmonary artery have serious consequences in most cases. Both are often associated with sudden death, especially during exercise. If a coronary artery originating from the opposite sinus of Valsalva has a transmural course through the aorta, the risk of infarct and mortality is especially high. Origin of a coronary artery from the pulmonary artery is related to angina, cardiomyopathy, and infant mortality.

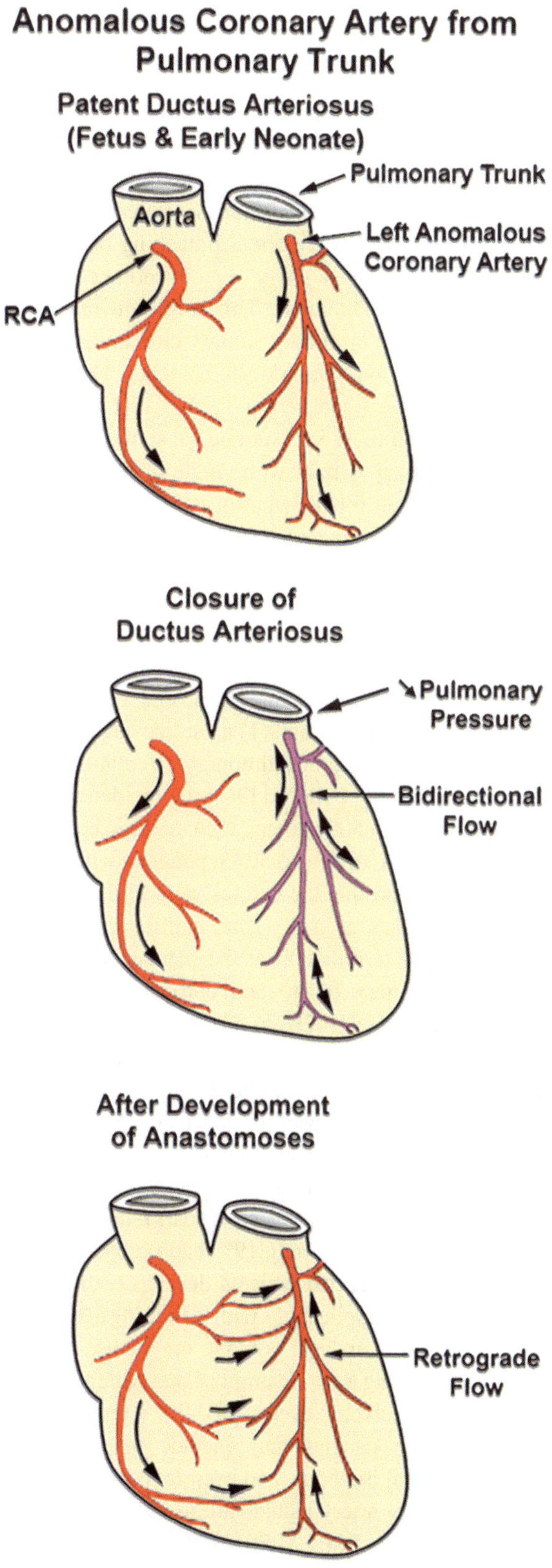

Fig. 6.4 Anomalous left coronary artery from the pulmonary trunk is shown in the fetus and early neonate (*top*), after closure of the ductus arteriosus (*middle*) and subsequent to the development of anastomoses (*bottom*). Myocardial perfusion is not problematic prior to the closure of the ductus arteriosus since blood from the left and right outflow tracts is mixed. With closure of the ductus, pulmonary pressure decreases and flow in the anomalous left coronary artery is bidirectional. This situation evokes growth of collateral vessels between the right and left coronary arteries. If pressure in the right coronary artery is sufficiently high, the left coronary artery will experience retrograde flow. If the pressure is inadequate, a coronary steal will occur and the left coronary artery perfusion region will experience ischemia

Single Coronary Ostium

When one coronary ostium fails to form, leaving a single coronary artery to emerge from the ostium, the latter gives rise to normally formed branches which are distributed over the entire heart if the anomaly is not associated with congenital heart disease [8]. Since normal branching patterns exist, the term "single coronary artery" is a misnomer [34], but is frequently used in the literature. This developmental anomaly does not necessarily limit the coronary circulation if there is an absence of any hypoplasia of its branches. However, this anomaly may have associated anomalies that are linked to perfusion abnormalities. For example, an analysis of 19 cases of a single coronary ostium with single or multiple fistulas demonstrated all but 6 had symptoms such as cyanosis, fatigability, angina, dyspnea, and palpations [35].

Coronary Fistulas

A coronary fistula, defined as "a sizable communication between a coronary artery and (1) a cardiac cavity or (2) any segment of the systemic or pulmonary circulation" is more common than initially believed [36]; the incidence has been reported to be one in 500 patients who undergo cardiac catheterization [37]. A review of 243 patients with coronary artery fistulas found that the fistulas were unilateral in 80% of the patients, bilateral in 18%, and multilateral in 2% [38]. The frequency of termination of the fistulas was highest in the pulmonary artery (44%) and coronary sinus or right atrium (28%), but only 13% in the RV and 8% in the left ventricle (LV) or left atrium.

Coronary arterial fistulas in childhood are associated with low morbidity [37, 39]. Review of data from 187 patients with coronary artery fistulas indicates that of those aged ≥20 years, 63% had preoperative symptoms or complications including myocardial infarction and congestive heart failure, whereas in patients <20 years of age, only 19% had preoperative symptoms [39]. Thus, untreated patients develop both symptoms and fistula-related complications with increasing age. Coronary fistulas, owing to their large volume, may cause a coronary steal by the draining of a disproportional volume of blood flow, leading to ischemic events [40–44]. Clinical presentations in pediatric patients may include fatigue, dyspnea, angina, myocardial ischemia, and even myocardial infarction [45, 46]. Coronary artery fistulas are usually congenital and not gender specific [44]. Multivessel coronary-ventricular fistulae have been shown to cause endomyocardial ischemia as a consequence of coronary steal [47]. Fistulous communications have also been found in both right and left hypoplastic ventricles, such as in the setting of pulmonary atresia, when the interventricular septum is intact [48].

Coronary Anomalies Involving the Coronary Sinus

Although a variety of congenital abnormalities—including atresia, hypoplasia, left to right shunt and "unroofed" coronary sinus—involve the coronary sinus, they have received little attention. However, already in 1966, there was a recognition that some, although not most, of these anatomical anomalies are functionally significant [49]. One needs to appreciate the process of venous development appropriately described as a "progression and regression of the three major paired venous systems," i.e., vitelline, umbilical, and common cardinal [50]. Hypoplasia of the coronary sinus occurs when blood is diverted into the dilated Thebesian veins, and atresia of the coronary sinus ostium causes drainage into the persistent left superior vena cava [51]. In two reported cases of this type of drainage, two bilateral superior vena cavas were found, with the left draining into the right via an innominate venous connection. In 37 reported cases of coronary sinus orifice atresia, the alternative outflow was also found to have occurred via the left superior vena cava in 16, an unroofed coronary sinus in 9, venous channels leading to the right or left atrium in 9, and a combination of these in 3 [52]. Although a persistent left superior vena cava usually is found to be an isolated anomaly, it can also be associated with any of the malformations of the heart and great vessels [53].

Intrinsic Coronary Anomalies

Myocardial Bridging

Description

As illustrated in Fig. 6.5, if an epicardial artery or segment develops in a transmural direction within the myocardium, it lies within a "myocardial bridge" (reviewed in [54, 55]). A review of five autopsy studies [56] notes that of 1,976 hearts, 13.4% displayed myocardial bridging (MB). The pathological significance of this anomalous course has been noted; however, it is also considered to be an anatomical variant [57]. Nevertheless, the potential for ischemic episodes is indicated by the fact that flow through an artery surrounded by myocardium could be limited, especially during tachycardia. Coronary hemodynamics in MB is characterized by phasic vessel compression, persistent diastolic vessel diameter reduction retrograde flow, and in some cases, a reduction in coronary reserve [58]. The latter has been shown to be improved by stent placement in individuals with this anomaly [58]. A retrospective study on 42 patients with myocardial bridging (MB), but without a history of myocardial infarction and with no substantial evidence of atherosclerosis, found stress-induced perfusion abnormalities in 40% of

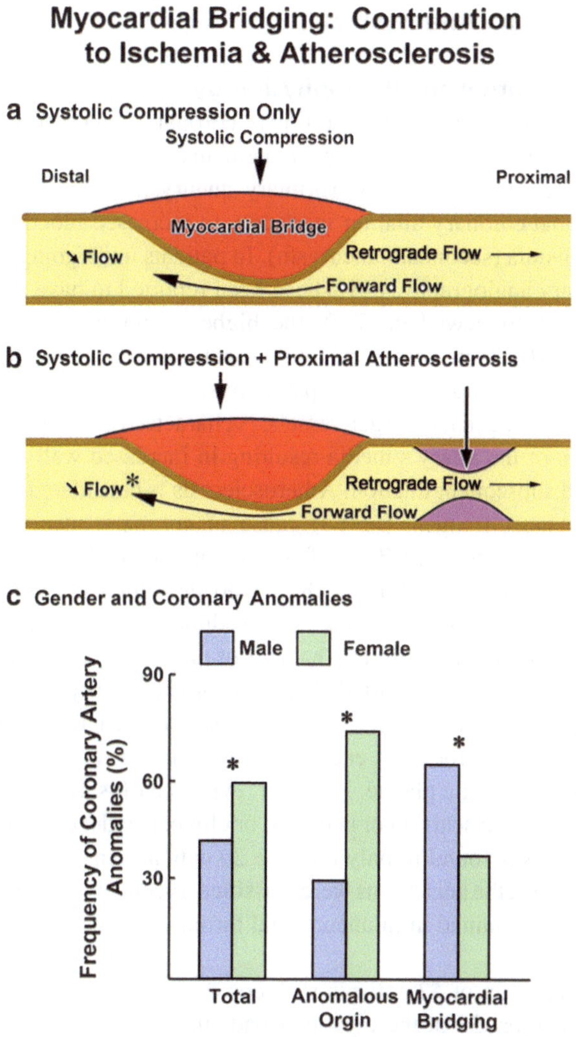

Fig. 6.5 Myocardial bridging (development of an epicardial artery or a segment of the artery within the myocardial wall) is associated with systolic compression and therefore limitations in coronary flow, as seen in (**a**). Myocardial bridging can also result in atherosclerotic plaques (**b**) proximal to the myocardial bridge, which further attenuates flow through the artery. *Asterisks* note that flow is reduced further when systolic compression is accompanied by the presence of atherosclerosis proximal to the myocardial bridge. (**c**) Data from Aydar et al. [63] indicate that myocardial bridging is more frequent in males than in females. In contrast, coronary anomalies in general and anomalous origin of a coronary artery are more frequent in females. $*p \leq 0.01$

the patients [59]. Both the incidence and severity of the ischemia were related to the degree of artery constriction. MB is common in hypertrophic cardiomyopathy, with a frequency up to 41% of the patients [60–62]. Myocardial bridging, studied in 124 cases, was found to be nearly twice as common in males than females, [63]. Since as seen in Fig. 6.5, coronary anomalies in general, as well as anomalies of origin, are significantly more frequent in females than males. Thus, the significantly higher prevalence of MB in males stands in contrast to that of other anomalies.

Mechanisms

The two mechanisms by which MB causes coronary disease are each affected by the length, thickness, and location of the myocardial bridge [64, 65]. One mechanism is direct MB compression on the artery, usually the LAD, during systole, which delays arterial relaxation during diastole, causing a reduction in blood flow. The second mechanism is development or enhancement of coronary atherosclerosis, causing stenosis proximal to the MB, a consequence of endothelial injury provoked by systolic retrograde flow in the proximal segment of the artery [58, 66]. The combination of MB compression and proximal stenosis cause a greater reduction in flow. A number of studies have reported a relationship between coronary artery disease and MB (reviewed in [64]). Between 1968 and 2000, 183 cases of MB without significant atherosclerosis have been described in the literature [64]. These patients exhibit angina and myocardial ischemia, despite a lack of any significant coronary artery lesion; these findings suggest that these symptoms are a consequence of MB compression. Patients with myocardial infarction and MB were found to have a greater intima/media ratio in the proximal segments of the LAD than patients with MB, but no myocardial infarction [65]. The data indicate that when the arterial segment proximal to the MB develops atherosclerosis, the chances of myocardial infarction are increased. The presence of atherosclerosis in the proximal portion of a bridged artery is more common than its presence in the distal portion (reviewed in [55]). Neonatal intima formation is an early event since all patients by the third postnatal month have some demonstrable intimal mass [67]. The development of MB in early postnatal life may accelerate the atherosclerotic process by altering the hemodynamics upstream from the MB. As noted later in this chapter, MB is often found in young (<35 years) individuals who died suddenly [68].

Conclusions

Demonstration of significant myocardial bridging has been made via recent advances (e.g., intracoronary Doppler and intravascular ultrasound) and have allowed the characterization of morphological and hemodynamic alterations [69]. These include (1) phasic, systolic vessel compression; (2) persistent reduction in diastolic lumen; (3) increased blood flow velocities; (4) retrograde systolic flow; and (5) decreased coronary flow reserve. Most of the patients with myocardial bridging present with symptoms and signs of ischemia [69]. The symptoms are aggravated by factors such as tachycardia and increases in systolic arterial pressure.

Coronary Artery Atresia

The site of an atretic coronary artery is usually marked by an ostial dimple, a remnant of atresia, which, if congenital, consists of fibrous tissue [43]. Ostial dimples are common in hearts with only one coronary artery. True left main coronary atresia (LMCA) is defined as (1) an absence of the left coronary ostium, (2) the proximal left main artery trunk ends blindly, and (3) blood flows from the RCA to the left via small collateral arteries and retrograde in at least one of the left-sided arteries [70]. In contrast to a single coronary ostium, in which flow is centrifugal flowing toward smaller arteries, in atresia, the left main coronary artery blood flows from the collateral arteries retrograde in at least part of this circulatory unit. A review of seven pediatric cases of LMCA atresia in 1997 [70] reported that heart failure, angina, and dyspnea were common symptoms. In most cases, the anomalous collateral circulation may be inadequate, and therefore, not surprisingly, patients develop myocardial ischemia and eventually heart failure [71]. Coronary ostial occlusion, resulting from coronary atresia, is often found in the context of pulmonary valve atresia [43]. Because the symptoms of atherosclerotic coronary artery disease and coronary artery atresia are similar, the later may be interpreted as the former [72]. Accordingly, the occurrence of coronary atresia may have a higher incidence than that reported in the literature.

Coronary Hypoplasia

Coronary hypoplasia is a term denoting an incomplete congenital development of a coronary artery characterized by significantly smaller than normal luminal diameters, which limit flow to their dependent myocardium [73–75]. Hypoplasia of right, left, or circumflex arteries is characterized by their development only to the lateral borders of the heart [73]. A study on inbred Syrian hamsters with one rudimentary, severely underdeveloped and one normal coronary artery concluded that the various branching patterns were similar to those in humans [76]. In this animal model, rudimentary coronary arteries were seen originating from any of the three sinuses of Valsalva and in some cases, were associated with arteries originating from the pulmonary trunk and the aorta.

When either of the two main coronary arteries is hypoplastic, resulting in a narrow lumen, the other main artery compensates by providing additional branches [77]. Hypoplasia of the left main coronary artery can be compensated by additional branches from the right main coronary artery, such as those serving much of the lateral wall of the LV, including the posterior descending artery. When the right main coronary artery is hypoplastic, the posterior descending branch arises from the left circumflex artery. These compensations are usually compatible with a long life.

Coronary Aneurysms

Description and Pathophysiology

As described by Angelini [3], coronary aneurysms, or ectasia, can occur as dilated segments with an associated decrease in blood flow (primary aneurysm) or as diffuse global coronary dilation secondary to increased blood flow or fistula (secondary aneurysm). In patients undergoing coronary angiography, 1–5% have been reported to have aneurysms (reviewed in [78]); the highest reported incidence was 10.1% in young and old patients with ischemic heart disease in India [79]. The pathophysiology of the coronary artery, like that of larger vessels, is characterized by destruction of the artery's media resulting in increased wall stress and subsequent dilation. Atherosclerosis is considered to be the most frequent (>50%) cause of coronary aneurysms, whereas about 20–30% of aneurysms are believed to be congenital [80]. Roberts [81], who described the clinical and morphological features of 20 adults with aneurysms of epicardial arteries, found that half of this group had multiple aneurysms. He reported that 79% of the aneurysms contained thrombi that in each case caused severe narrowing of the lumen. Moreover, each of these aneurysms contained an atherosclerotic plaque. However, evidence of ischemia, i.e., myocardial scarring or necrosis, or clinical evidence of ischemia was found in only 8 of the 20 patients. In 4 of the 20 patients, the aneurysms were classified as congenital because none contained intra-aneurysmal thrombi or atherosclerotic plaque.

A study of 52 patients with coronary arterial aneurysms found that 38 of these patients had atherosclerotic coronary aneurysms, which were often associated with symptoms of ischemia [82]. Congenital, rather than acquired aneurysms are the major type found in patients younger than 33 years [83]. Some of the clinical manifestations in patients with aneurysms, in addition to myocardial infarctions, include exertion-induced angina, compression of adjacent structures (e.g., vena cava or atria), and development of fistulas between the aneurysm and pulmonary artery with possible rupture leading to sudden death [84]. The possibility of spasms in coronary arteries with aneurysms was suggested by Bove and Vlietstra [85], who found that two patients with diffuse aneurysms, but no appreciable stenosis, had augmented vasoconstrictor responses to ergonovine. Analysis of data from 276 patients revealed that coronary aneurysms are an independent predictor of mortality with only 71% of the patients surviving for 5 years [86]. A huge intramural coronary artery aneurysm is especially problematic, causing angina pectoris and a coronary steal [87]. In a case where the aneurysm protruded into the left ventricular chamber, it rapidly filled during diastole and in systole, causing a retrograde flow through the LAD.

Possible Causes of Coronary Aneurysms

Coronary aneurysms most frequently associated with atherosclerosis may be secondary to that disease, whereas those associated with Kawasaki disease and those known to be congenital are of a different etiology [88]. However, in all types the major structural abnormality that underlies an aneurysm is destruction of the media, as noted in a study of 30 patients with this coronary artery lesion [89]. The investigators observed that portions of the vessel with intact media did not develop aneurysms and that myocardial infarction was a prominent feature of the disease. A review of the pathogenesis of coronary aneurysms indicates a role for matrix metalloproteinases, since they appear to be overexpressed in aneurysms [84]. This finding is consistent with the destruction of the artery's tunica media, i.e., degradation of components of the extracellular matrix causes dilation of the vessel. Sorrell et al. [90] proposed that chronic overstimulation of the endothelium by NO or NO donors can predispose a coronary artery to aneurysm. This hypothesis was based on evidence that coronary artery aneurysms are often associated with prolonged exposure to herbicides [91], which contain acetylcholinesterase inhibitors and could cause acetylcholine to increase and evoke vasodilation.

Congenital Coronary Anomalies Associated with Congenital Heart Malformations

Many congenital heart malformations have associated coronary anomalies as noted in both humans [8] and experimental animals [92, 93]. With regard to the latter, malformations of the outflow tract [e.g., double outlet right ventricle (DORV), TGA, and common truncus arteriosus] can be induced by retinoic acid administration [93]. Spontaneous, random mutation in an iv/iv mouse strain, characterized by cardiac heterotaxia, is also associated with coronary anomalies in 84% of these mice [92]. The coronary anomalies associated with congenital heart malformations are described below. Three types of anomalies are illustrated in Fig. 6.6.

Persistent Truncus Arteriosus

Description

Persistent truncus arteriosus (PTA) results from a failure of the truncus arteriosus to divide into an aortic and pulmonary channel, a situation which results in blood flow from both ventricles into a common channel. The increase in pulmonary blood flow leads to congestive heart failure. This malformation has a high mortality as infants with PTA usually die within the first few months of postnatal life [8] and only 35% of medically treated patients survive beyond 6 months of age [94]. The number of truncus cusps is variable. Some examples from studies by Shrivastava and Edwards [95], de la Cruz et al. [96] and Henaine et al. [97] provide the following percentages: tricuspid, 56–70; bicuspid, 7–21; and bicuspid, 10–24.

Coronary Anomalies

According to Sherman [98], who reviewed 503 specimens, coronary abnormalities are more common in PTA than in most other congenital heart defects. They often occur in combination and are potential contributors to operative mortality and sudden death at later times [99]. A survey of 7 studies [94–96, 100–104] reported coronary anomalies in a total of 543 cases; 9.6% of hearts with PTA had only a single coronary ostium. Although the number of valves in the common arterial trunk is variable, as illustrated in Fig. 6.7, the formation of the valves is independent of the coronary orifices [105]. This study reported that of hearts with four leaflets, 77% had coronary artery orifices in adjacent sinuses, a finding that supports independent formation of coronary orifices and valve leaflets. It is the orientation of the valves that is important in this respect. For example, when the cusps

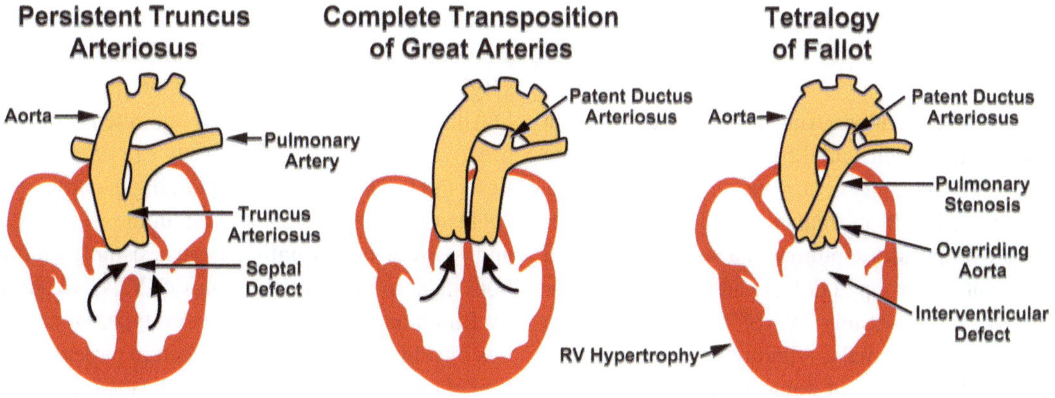

Fig. 6.6 Three common cardiac malformations are illustrated. The coronary artery anomalies associated with these and other types of cardiac malformations are discussed in the text of this chapter

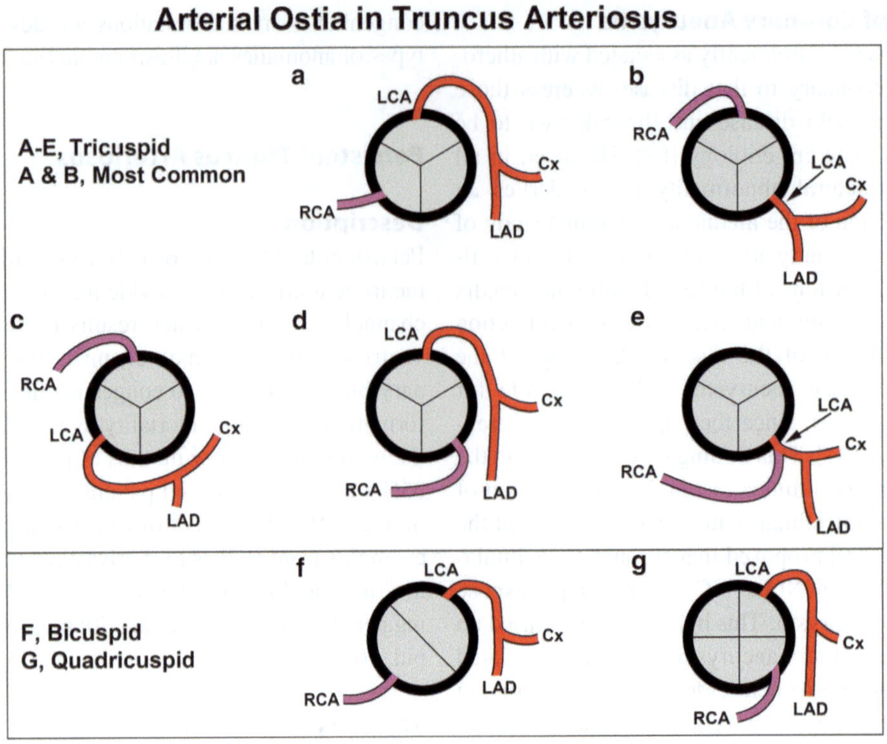

Fig. 6.7 Persistent truncus arteriosus is associated with a variety of coronary artery anomalies of origin, as illustrated here. Specific types of anomalies may be associated with the number of aortic cusps: (**a**–**e**) tricuspid; (**f**) bicuspid; (**g**) quadricuspid. The diagram includes some examples, with no regard to their frequency and is based mainly on studies by de la Cruz et al. [96] and Lenox et al. [99]

are anterior/posterior, the LCA or a single coronary ostium arises from the posterior, cusp, and when the valves are bicuspid and oriented right/left, the right and left coronary arteries arise above the right and left cusps, respectively (reviewed in [8]). The coronary artery origins in PTA hearts, studied by another group of investigators [94], was found to vary as follows: single coronary ostium, 18.5%; high posterior origin of left coronary, 18.5%; stenosis of one coronary artery, 7%. The locations of arterial ostia and the course of the main coronary arteries are illustrated in Fig. 6.7.

Transposition of the Great Arteries

Description

In this anomaly of ventriculoarterial discordance the aorta arises from the right ventricle and the pulmonary artery from the left ventricle. The anomaly occurs because the conotruncal septum fails to follow its normal course. TGA may occur with (1) an intact ventricular septum, (2) a ventricular septal defect, or (3) a ventricular septal defect and a left ventricular obstruction [106]. Approximately 75% of TGA patients have the first type of cardiac anomaly. Although the incidence of complete TGA is about 5–8% of congenital cardiac malformations [107, 108], it accounts for 25% of deaths during the first year of postnatal life that are attributed to congenital heart disease [109]. To support life, a communication between the systemic and pulmonary circulation must exist to allow oxygenated blood from the pulmonary circuit to enter the systemic circulation. This occurs via connections between the two circulatory units, most commonly by a ventricular septal defect, or by an atrial septal defect or a patent ductus arteriosus.

Coronary Anomalies

Dual sinus origin, i.e., origin of a coronary artery from each of two facing sinuses of Valsalva (left and posterior) was the normal pattern (90% of cases of TGA); the right sinus of Valsalva does not face the right ventricular outflow tract [8]. Coronary anomalies in 5 of 32 patients with TGA included a single right or LCA or inverted origin of coronary arteries [110]. A review of 12 cases of corrected transposition of the great vessels discovered a variety of coronary artery anomalies [111]. These included (1) single coronary ostium, (2) LAD arising from RCA and circumflex with its own ostium, and (3) four hearts with eccentric ostia, including one with both ostia in the posterior sinus of Valsalva. As summarized by Burch and Sahn [112], several types of coronary anomalies of origin and patterns are seen in patients with transposition of the great vessels of which the most common (14–22%) is origin of the circumflex artery from the RCA and a posterior course around the pulmonary artery. Origin of the LCA from the posterior sinus of Valsalva and RCA from the left sinus Valsalva is the most frequent coronary anomaly associated with this congenital heart defect. Other anomalies include a single coronary ostium (4–6%), circumflex origin from the posterior sinus, and RCA from left sinus with the LAD as a branch (2–8%), and less frequently, both coronaries arising from the posterior sinus of Valsalva. Of particular significance is the observation that transposition of the great vessels is the condition most often associated with an aortic intramural course of one of the main coronary arteries [113]. Among 103 autopsy specimens of transposed great arteries, Gittenberger-deGroot and colleagues [114] found and described three cases of an aortic intramural course of a coronary artery.

Tetralogy of Fallot

Description

Unequal division of the conus results in anterior displacement of the conotruncal septum, which in turn produces four cardiovascular abnormalities (1) ventricular sepal defect, (2) overriding aorta, (3) pulmonary stenosis, and (4) hypertrophy of the right ventricle. The malalignment of the septum is the major cause of right ventricular outflow obstruction [115]. Tetralogy of Fallot accounts for 7–10% of all congenital cardiac malformations [116].

Coronary Anomalies

The incidence of coronary anomalies associated with Tetralogy of Fallot has been found to be 5.9% of 611 children undergoing transatrial-transpulmonary repair [117] and 12.2% in 607 Turkish children [118]. The latter study found that 60% of the anomalies were accounted for by (1) the LAD originating from the right coronary sinus or the RCA and (2) a single coronary ostium. In 92% of the anomalies the coronary artery crossed the right ventricular outflow tract, a condition that constitutes a danger during cardiac repair [116]. Pulmonary atresia and/or major aortopulmonary collateral arteries may be present in a subgroup of these patients [119].

Double Outlet Ventricle

Description

This term indicates that both great arteries originate (either exclusively or predominantly) from either the right or left ventricle. Since double outlet left ventricle accounts for less than 5% of this category, most data are based on DORV, which includes a wide range of anatomic arrangements; therefore, classification has often been difficult [120]. There is general agreement that the relationships of the great vessels vary from normal to side-by-side pattern (aorta to the right of the pulmonary artery or TGA) [43]. DORV is defined as a type of ventriculoarterial connection in which both great vessels arise entirely or predominantly from the right ventricle [120]. The great arteries are separated from each other by a septum at their outlet.

Coronary Anomalies

It appears that the specific coronary anomalies depend on the relationships, i.e., positions, between the great vessels. A review of this topic [43] notes that when the aorta is positioned anteriorly to the right, the coronary patterns, though varied, mimic the pattern typical of TGA without DORV (RCA from posterior sinus and LCA from left coronary sinus) in 73% of the cases. In cases where the great vessels cross normally, the coronary patterns resemble those of normal hearts.

Univentricular Heart

Description

A univentricular or single ventricle receives blood from both atria and has either two separate valves or one common atrioventricular valve, and in 80% of the cases, the ventricle has left ventricular features [121]. A univentricular heart is defined as a "condition in which both atrioventricular orifices enter or a common atrioventricular sinus enters a common ventricular sinus from which the arterial trunks emerge with their coni" [122]. Univentricular hearts are of two types: with rudimentary chamber (outlet chamber or rudimentary pouch) and without rudimentary chamber (no outlet chamber or rudimentary pouch) [123]. As noted by Perloff [8], alterations in cardiac physiology and clinical manifestations vary according to the presence or absence of pulmonary disease, stenosis, and the morphology and function of the atrioventricular connections.

Coronary Anomalies

The most common pattern of coronary arteries, found in 12 of 17 hearts, was the origin of the LCA from the left posterior aortic sinus and the RCA from right posterior aortic sinus [123]. Of the variations seen in the other 5 hearts, the course of the LCA between the aorta and pulmonary artery noted in one heart appeared to have the potential for ischemic events.

Possible Mechanisms Underlying Various Coronary Anomalies

Anomalous Aortic and Pulmonary Artery Origin

As described in Chap. 2, a plexus of vascular tubes surrounds the aorta and pulmonary trunk and then penetrates the aorta to form the coronary ostia. Although numerous strands initially penetrate the aortic wall in all three of the aortic sinuses, ostia are limited only to the left and right sinuses in the normal heart [124]; ostia are formed via apoptosis, allowing the penetrating ECs to form a channel [125]. The remaining (nonostial) strands then disappear [124]. The fact that anomalous origins occur is not surprising considering the necessity of close temporal and spatial regulation of this event. The mechanisms that direct EC invasion of the aortic wall require several key molecules as noted below. Considering the complex molecular mechanisms necessary for coronary vasculogenesis, angiogenesis, and arteriogenesis signaling, there are many errors that can result in coronary anomalies. However, pinpointing the causes of developmental anomalies necessitates relying mainly on experimental animal models.

Dependence on Growth Factors

The formation of the coronary vasculature is dependent on the spatial and temporal expression of several key growth factors (detailed in Chap. 2). As noted above and emphasized here, formation of the arterial system depends on the development of a network of vascular tubes that penetrate the aortic root at the left and right sinuses of Valsalva. One can then appreciate that failure of this network to form in an appropriate spatial pattern could lead to anomalous origins of the coronary arteries. Formation of the tubular network, as well as formation of the coronary ostia and stems, is dependent on a number of growth factors, including VEGFs and FGFs.

VEGF

Studies on quail embryos, in my laboratory, revealed that inhibition of VEGFs, particularly VEGF-B, precludes or limits ostial formation, resulting in the absence of coronary artery stems or the formation of only a single coronary ostium [126]. Inhibition of VEGF signaling, using a soluble VEGFR-1/VEGFR-2 chimera, not only precluded formation of both coronary ostia in nearly all embryos, but also decreased myocardial development of the compact region. One of the great curiosities regarding the specific sites of coronary ostial formation is the specific spatial signal that dictates the sites, limiting one coronary to the left and the other to the right sinus of Valsalva. In our studies on quail embryos, we determined that the sites of ostial formation were adjacent to high focal densities of VEGFR-2 and VEGFR-3 transcripts [127]. A relationship between VEGFR-2 and apoptosis was found in embryonic mice [128]. When the mothers of the mice were placed on a low protein diet, the peritruncal presence of VEGFR-2 and apoptosis were delayed and resulted in either the absence of coronary artery formation or the formation of only a single coronary ostium. These data indicate that the high density of VEGFR-2 transcripts at the sites of ostial formation facilitate apoptosis of aortic cells, thus permitting the penetration of endothelial cells into the aortic wall.

The absence of a single VEGF splice variant also can affect coronary abnormalities. In mouse embryos that solely express $VEGF_{120}$, a loss of $VEGF_{164}$ and $VEGF_{188}$ causes spatiotemporal changes in VEGF and Notch signaling [129]. Coronary anomalies in 50% or more of the $VEGF_{120/120}$ embryos included small coronary arteries, large veins and lymphatics, and increased microvascular density. An abnormal number of coronary orifices and an abnormal origin of the interventricular artery were other common anomalies reported. The authors noted that the alterations affected both endothelial cell differentiation and the subsequent arteriogenesis. Their findings are consistent with previous in vitro data documenting that $VEGF_{165}$, but not $VEGF_{120}$, stimulates coronary vasculogenesis/angiogenesis in quail embryonic hearts [130].

Coronary Artery Formation Requires Multiple Growth Factors

Our data also revealed that recruitment of VSMCs and their employment in the media of arteries and arterioles require FGFs, PDGF, and VEGF [126, 131]. Moreover, Langlois et al. [132] found that conditional inactivation of TGF-β type II receptor in the epicardium, myocardium, and VSMCs impairs differentiation of the VSMCs in coronary vessels. Ng and colleagues [133] suggested that a loss of glypican-3 function delays the formation of the vascular plexus because it is a co-receptor for FGF-9 and results in a decrease in sonic hedgehog (Shh) mRNA expression and signaling. FGF-9, as detailed in Chap. 2, plays a key role in coronary vessel formation in the embryo. The authors noted that excessive coronary arteries were formed and fewer veins were present. They concluded that this imbalance caused coronary fistulas. Since the transcription factor CHF1/Hey2 is implicated in a variety of developmental abnormalities, Watanabe and colleagues [134] studied CHF1/Hey knockout mice and found a number of coronary abnormalities including dysmorphic large vessels with levels of markers for venous identity, and reduced recruitment of VSMCs into arteries. RT-PCR analysis demonstrated that PDGF and angiopoietin/Tie2 signaling were altered prior to the development of the coronary arteries. Because CHF1/Hey2 is expressed in the myocardium, epicardium, and VSMCs, the authors concluded that defects in any of these tissues could contribute to the coronary abnormalities.

A Role for Hypoxia

Hypoxia, as discussed in Chaps. 1, 2, and 9, activates or facilitates coronary angiogenesis. However, it has been shown that either hypoxia or hyperoxia can cause coronary vessel anomalies. Altered hypoxia-inducible factor-1α gene levels in embryonic chick hearts were found to correlate with coronary vessel anomalies [135]. Incubation of chicken eggs under 15% ambient O_2 (hypoxia) or 75–40% (hyperoxia) resulted in anomalies of the proximal coronary arteries that included right coronary origin from posterior aortic sinus, three coronary ostia, and tortuous course and anastomotic connections. Both hypoxia and hyperoxia increased HIF-1α protein expression and the protein expression of VEGF-A, PDGF-B, and Tie-2. It has been shown that abnormally high levels of HIF-1α, as occur in Cited2$^{-/-}$ mice (Cited2 is a negative regulator of HIF-1α), are associated with cardiac defects in regions that are particularly hypoxic [136]. The myocardial vessels were more permeable and VEGF was elevated. By reducing HIF-1α, the cardiac and coronary defects were partially rescued [137]. These findings indicate that the appropriate level of HIF-1α is necessary for proper coronary ostial and artery formation.

Neural Crest Cells

Neural crest cells are requisite for the formation of coronary ostia, as evidenced by ectopic origins or the formation of only a single coronary ostium when these cells are ablated [138]. Neural crest cells penetrate the aortic wall to guide the ECs that enter the aorta to form the coronary ostia [139]. Ablation of these cells in chick embryos causes conotruncal anomalies [140, 141]. Bis-diamine treatment causes disruption of neural crest cell migration [142] by causing an impairment of the neural cell adhesion molecule, N-CAM [143]. As a consequence, the number of neural crest cells is reduced [144]; this reduction is a likely reason that coronary anomalies occur in conjunction with conotruncal defects. Neural crest cells play a key role in the formation of the coronary ostia and stems, as indicated by experiments in which their ablation caused both abnormal truncal division and coronary anomalies [138]. This study concluded that neural crest cell ablation in and of itself can cause both abnormal truncal division and anomalous coronary arteries. Disruption of the epicardium, the source of vascular cells, and limited vascular structures were also observed in this model [145]. The epicardium did not firmly adhere to the myocardium, which may have contributed to the poor development of the plexus and an attenuated epicardial–mesenchymal transition.

Gap Junction Protein

The gap junction protein connexin 43 (Cx43) has also been shown to play a role in normal coronary development [146–148]. Cx43 may play a role in gene regulation, since its C terminus localizes in the cell's nucleus [149]. That Cx43α1 is essential for coronary artery development was documented by Li et al. [150], who found a variety of coronary anomalies in Cx43α1 knockout mice. Their data revealed increased migration and proliferation of proepicardial cells associated with a loss of coupling, which suggests that the coronary artery anomalies are due to abnormalities that occur prior to the establishment of the system of vascular tubes. In the heterozygous Cx43α1 knockout mice, 22 of 25 mice displayed variable coronary artery patterns, including anomalous origins, multiple accessory arteries, and dual septal–conal branches [148]. These data, based on micro-CT scanning and histology, indicate that a loss of one Cx43α1 allele causes coronary defects in patterning.

Other Contributors to Coronary Anomalies

Another contributor to coronary anomalies is a perlecan mutation. This proteoglycan, present in basal laminae, contains heparin sulfate glycosaminoglycan chains. When perlecan is mutated, 70% of the coronary arteries originate in anomalous locations, e.g., the RCA originates from the posterior aortic sinus [151]. These hearts also developed TGA. Another study documented anomalous coronary artery patterning in mice lacking the Tbx1 gene that encodes a T-box containing transcription factor [152]. The anomalies included altered trajectories, e.g., left coronary crossing over ventrally or dorsally, and anomalous origins of arteries.

Coronary Anomalies and Sudden Death

Sudden cardiac death (SCD) in individuals <35 years of age is rare, but most often is associated with previously undetected cardiovascular abnormalities [68, 153–155]. A postmortem investigation of 1,200 specimens from individuals with congenital heart disease found that 27 of the hearts had anomalous origins of coronary arteries [155]. Sixteen of these individuals died suddenly and most (81.5%) had an anomalous coronary originating from the aorta, whereas only 18.5% had a LCA originating from the pulmonary artery. The sudden death was frequently the first manifestation of the disease and in 50% of the cases, death occurred during physical effort. Taylor and colleagues [156] reviewed the records of 242 patients with coronary artery anomalies and found that 78 deaths occurred suddenly. Consistent with other studies, left or RCA origin from the opposite sinus was the most common anomaly. Young patients (≤35 years) were four times as likely to die suddenly, and during exercise, than patients older than 35 years. In children, congenital coronary anomalies rather than coronary disease is the major cause

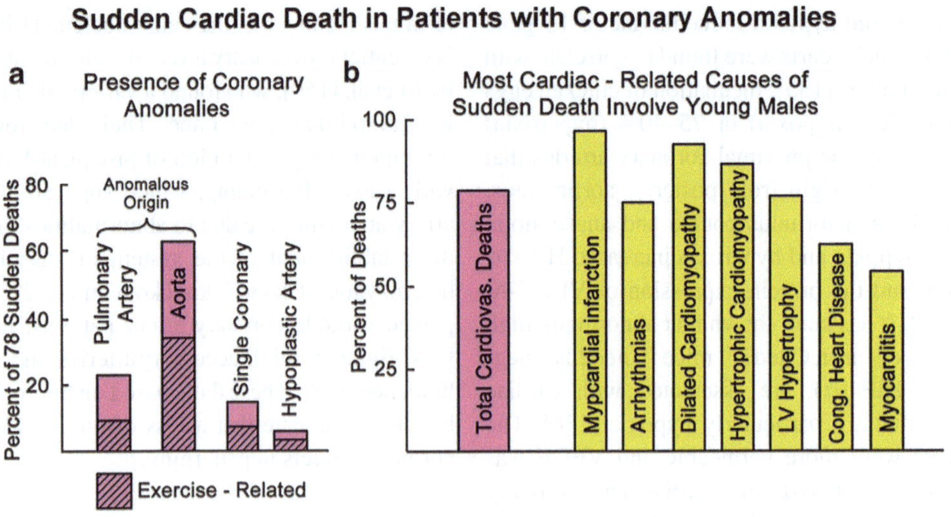

Fig. 6.8 (**a**) If patients with coronary anomalies die suddenly of a cardiac-related death, the cause is most often associated with an anomalous origin from the aorta, followed by anomalous origin from the pulmonary artery (the latter is rarer than the former). Sudden deaths related to coronary anomalies are 6 times more frequent in individuals aged 30 years or less than those over the age of 30. A high percentage of these deaths in the young occur during exercise. These data are from Taylor et al. [156]. (**b**) Sudden cardiac-related deaths occur more frequently in males than in females, especially those from myocardial infarction and cardiomyopathies. The bar graph indicates percentage of deaths from various causes that occurred in males. Note that the overall frequency of cardiac-related deaths is 3 times higher in young males than in young females. These data are based on 241 cardiac deaths in a study by Puranik et al. [189]

of SCD [155, 157–159]. Figure 6.8 includes (a) the types of coronary anomalies associated with SCD and the age group most affected and (b) the gender differences in the related causes of sudden death.

In an investigation of 9 sudden coronary deaths in 7 boys and 2 girls ranging from 14 days to 16 years of age (mean = 8 years), an anomalous course of coronary arteries was documented in 7 of the 9 deaths [159]. Five of the anomalies consisted of a left or right artery from the wrong coronary sinus; the others were coronary artery dysplasia, common coronary artery from the pulmonary trunk, arteritis, and slit-like malformed ostium. Analysis of 7,857 pediatric autopsy cases (mean age 2.2 years) revealed a 0.5% incidence of anomalous coronary arteries; 43% of these were anomalous origin from the aorta and 40% were origins from the pulmonary trunk [160]. The latter were associated with an earlier death (1.4 years), 100% incidence of cardiomegaly and a 92% incidence of myocardial scarring. SCD in individuals <1 year was associated with coronary anomalies in 10 of 20 cases, whereas coronary anomalies in a group aged 1–21 years who experienced SCD occurred in only 12 of 50 cases [157]. These data indicate (1) a high incidence of coronary anomalies in persons <21 years of age and (2) that this anomaly is associated with twice the rate of SCD in those persons <1 year of age. The anomalies were of a high risk type: origin from wrong sinus, ostial stenosis, abnormal angle of origin, and ostial "flap" or "ridge." Of the coronary anomalies in patients <21 years of age ($n = 70$), the acute angle of origin combined with ectopic origin was the most common finding.

Physical Exertion and the Risk of Sudden Cardiac Death

The relationship between a sport-related activity and SCD in young adults was evaluated in a study of 690 SCDs in individuals aged 14–40 years [161]. Of the 34 individuals who died during or shortly after a sport-related death, 9 had atherosclerosis, 8 had hypertrophic cardiomyopathy, and 4 had an anomalous coronary artery. The average age of the group with atherosclerosis was greater (32 years) than that of hypertrophic cardiomyopathy (24 years) and anomalous coronary artery (21 years). These findings indicate that SCD from hypertrophic cardiomyopathy and anomalous coronary artery tends to occur more often in the young. The North Italian registry of sudden death in the young (<35 years) includes 300 cases of SD; the mortality rate of athletes was 2.9 compared to only 0.9 in nonathletes and indicates the increased risk of SD in sports activity [162, 163]. These data, from individuals who lived in the Veneto region of Italy, are validated by autopsy findings, ECG, and clinical findings. Importantly, the study indicates that sport per se was not the cause of the enhanced mortality, but rather that it triggered SD in athletes who were affected by cardiovascular conditions (e.g., coronary anomalies, cardiomyopathy, and premature coronary artery disease) that predisposed them to ventricular arrhythmias during physical exercise. Moreover, the screening of athletes reduced the number of individuals with cardiomyopathy in the athlete group; accordingly the cardiomyopathy was not a major cause in SD.

Among 6.3 million military recruits (aged 18–35 years), there were 126 sudden, nontraumatic deaths, of which 36% and 61% were associated with cardiomyopathy and coronary artery pathology, respectively [153]. Of the latter group, 54% had an anomalous coronary artery and 26% demonstrated evidence of coronary atherosclerosis. In each case, the coronary anomaly consisted of the LCA arising from right sinus of Valsalva and coursing between the aorta and the pulmonary trunk. This study, which included data derived over a 25-year period, found that 86% of the nontraumatic sudden deaths were related to exercise stress. A subsequent study based on 902 subjects included demographic and autopsy data from the Department of Defense Cardiovascular Death Registry; the data showed that SCD was associated with an anomalous coronary artery in 4% of individuals aged ≤35 years and only in 0.2% of those aged >35 years [164]. In the younger group, SCD related to a coronary artery anomaly occurred in 8% of subjects during exertion and in only <1% of subjects during nonexertion conditions. In the subjects age >35 years, SCD associated with death occurred only in 1 subject and was not exertion related. Although SCD in these young men and women was relatively rare, there are two important insights gained from the data (1) the anomalous origin of the LCA and its passage between the aorta and pulmonary trunk constitute a major risk for SCD and (2) exercise stress is most commonly the context in which sudden death occurred. As noted earlier in this chapter, of all of the coronary artery anomalies associated with sudden coronary death, the anomalous origin of an artery from the opposite sinus has been most frequently associated with ischemia and ventricular arrhythmias, particularly when the anomalous coronary artery courses between the great arteries (reviewed in [28, 154]). Anomalous origin of the left or the RCA from the opposite sinus is both considered a high risk for SCD, especially during exercise.

SCD in Athletes

Although the cardiovascular benefits of exercise training are well established, vigorous exertion may trigger SCD in both sedentary individuals and in athletes. In an analysis of 160 cases of SCD in high school and college athletes between 1983 and 1993 that were not related to trauma, most were found to be associated with cardiomyopathy and coronary anomalies [165]. The data also revealed that male athletes are at a much greater risk than females, even after adjusting for participation frequency. However, the data were not adjusted for the intensity of the various sports, which may be a factor that influenced the results. As reviewed by Corrado and colleagues [163] and Link and Estes [166], the incidence of SCD among athletes is greater than in nonathletes and is not surprising because of the strenuous effects required in sports such as soccer, distance running, and basketball. In US athletes, hypertrophic cardiomyopathy is the most frequent finding in SCD, followed by congenitally abnormal coronary arteries, whereas in nonathletes, coronary artery disease and anomalous coronary arteries are most frequent findings [167]. A retrospective SCD study by Basso et al. [16] included 27 athletes aged 9–32 years with wrong coronary sinus anomalies who died during or after intense exertion on the athletic field. Since none of the anomalous coronary arteries were significantly narrowed by atherosclerosis, atherosclerotic narrowing of major coronary arteries was not a factor affecting the results. Ten of the athletes experienced symptoms considered to be of cardiovascular origin, e.g., syncope, palpitations, chest pain, and dizziness on effort. On the basis of these findings, the authors concluded that a history of exertional syncope, palpitations, or chest pain requires exclusion of this anomaly by 2d echocardiography or direct visualization by CMR or CT and eventually coronary angiography. In six hearts that were available for histological examination, all showed evidence of acute ischemia, i.e., contraction band necrosis and early neutrophil infiltration. Three hearts had anomalous LCA and three had anomalous RCA arteries from the wrong sinus of Valsalva, and each was characterized by both an acute angle takeoff and a slit-like ostial lumen.

Mechanisms of SCD Due to Anomalous Coronary Arteries

Several causes of hypoperfusion of anomalous coronary arteries resulting in SCD have been proposed [16]. Anomalous origin of either the right and left main coronary artery with passage between the great arteries is considered to be perhaps the most clinically significant anomaly [168]. Of 73 cases of wrong sinous origin, 10 were fatal. This anomaly is likely to be subjected to compressive systolic forces when passing between the two great arteries [169, 170], especially when the anomalous artery has an intramural course. Another possible incidence of hypoperfusion is an acute angle of origin that includes an extended, slit-like intramural passage through the aortic wall, which becomes further narrowed by dilation of the aorta [171, 172].

Coronary Abnormalities in Congenital Diseases

Cyanotic Congenital Heart Disease

Pulmonary Hypertension

The presence of systemic-to-pulmonary shunts in patients with congenital heart disease causes pulmonary arterial hypertension [173]. If this condition of increased flow and pressure in the pulmonary arteries persists, obstructive arteriopathy may develop, causing increased pulmonary vascular resistance. When pulmonary resistance exceeds that of the systemic resistance, flow in the shunt will be reversed, i.e., the systemic-to-pulmonary shunt becomes a pulmonary-to-systemic shunt, causing a central cyanosis. This shunt reversal constitutes the classic picture of Eisenmenger syndrome.

Coronary Artery Alterations

Typically, the epicardial coronary arteries in Cyanotic Congenital Heart Disease (CCHD) are dilated, tortuous, and in some cases, ecstatic [174]. Epicardial arteries exhibit a loss of smooth muscle, increases in collagen, and duplication of the internal elastic lamina [175]. Although basal coronary flow is markedly increased, hyperemic flow is normal [176]. The ability of these vessels to dilate is likely due to the thinner tunica media and a lack of atherosclerosis in adults with CCHD [177]. Characteristically, these patients have hypocholesterolemia and erythrocytosis. As noted by the authors of this study, hypoxemia, NO upregulation, hyperbilirubinemia, and low platelet counts, in addition to hypocholesterolemia, are contributing variables to the low incidence of coronary atherosclerosis in CCHD.

Microvascular Remodeling

To explain the adequate hyperemic response in the coronary vasculature in patients with CCHD, we hypothesized that microvascular remodeling occurred [178]. Necropsy heart specimens from patients with Eisenmenger's syndrome were compared to structurally normal and abnormal hypertrophied hearts, as well as to normal hearts. Arteriolar length density was lower in the hearts from Eisenmenger patients compared to the other groups, but arteriolar diameter was 34% greater compared to structurally normal, but hypertrophied hearts. These findings indicate that preservation of coronary flow reserve in CCHD is due to remodeling of the major resistance vessels, i.e., increased arteriolar diameters, which compensate for the lower arteriolar length density.

Noncompaction of the Ventricular Myocardium

Cardiac Abnormalities Due to Noncompaction

During early embryonic development, as described in Chap. 2, the myocardium has a narrow band of compact myocardium adjacent to the epicardium; the remainder of the myocardium is composed of trabeculae with intervening sinusoid continuous with the ventricle's lumen. Ventricular growth is characterized by an expansion of the compact region and development of vascular channels within this growing tissue. Ventricular noncompaction may be an isolated abnormality or may be associated with other congenital anomalies, including obstruction of the right or left outflow tracts and CCHD [179, 180]. Arrhythmias, heart failure, and embolism are the three major clinical manifestations of noncompaction. In a study of 24 patients with noncompaction, 33% had heart failure, 20% had rhythm abnormalities, and 20% had cardiomegaly [181]. Mortality in patients with noncompaction is high, as indicated by a 6-year follow-up study of ten patients, eight of whom died during this period of time [182].

Perfusion and Flow Reserve Deficits

Communication between the coronary arteries and sinusoids was noted in human [183] and avian [184] hearts with noncompaction. The consequences of noncompaction include perfusion defects and ischemic lesions [185–187]. Isolated ventricular noncompaction in children (age 10–14) was documented to be deficient in myocardial perfusion and coronary flow reserve [186]. Another study verified a decreased coronary flow reserve in 12 patients (mean age, 49 years) with noncompaction [187]. However, the data revealed that the flow reserve was not confined to noncompacted segments, but was presented in most segments with wall motion abnormalities. Experiments in my laboratory on embryonic quail hearts have established a relationship between growth factor inhibition and noncompaction [131, 188]. Neutralizing antibodies to VEGFs, FGF-2, and PDGF each had effects on the formation of coronary arteries and also limited the compaction process in the ventricles. VEGF-B inhibition had the most profound effect; as in most cases, it negated the formation of the main coronary arteries and virtually prevented compaction.

References

1. Davis JA, Cecchin F, Jones TK, Portman MA. Major coronary artery anomalies in a pediatric population: incidence and clinical importance. J Am Coll Cardiol. 2001;37:593–7.
2. Yildiz A, Okcun B, Peker T, Arslan C, Olcay A, Bulent Vatan M. Prevalence of coronary artery anomalies in 12,457 adult patients who underwent coronary angiography. Clin Cardiol. 2010;33:E60–4.
3. Angelini P, Villason S, Chan Jr A, Diez JG. Normal and anomalous coronary arteries in humans. In: Coronary artery anomalies: a comprehensive approach. Philadelphia: Lippincott, Williams and Wilkins; 1999. p. 27–150.
4. Angelini P. Coronary artery anomalies—current clinical issues: definitions, classification, incidence, clinical relevance, and treatment guidelines. Tex Heart Inst J. 2002;29:271–8.
5. Cieslinski G, Rapprich B, Kober G. Coronary anomalies: incidence and importance. Clin Cardiol. 1993;16:711–5.

6. Rahalkar AM, Rahalkar MD. Pictorial essay: coronary artery variants and anomalies. Indian J Radiol Imaging. 2009;19:49–53.
7. Neufeld HN, Schneeweiss A. Coronary artery disease in infants and children. Philadelphia: Lea and Febiger; 1983. pp. 1–30.
8. Perloff JK. The clinical recognition of congenital heart disease. Philadelphia: Sauders; 2003.
9. Angelini P. Coronary artery anomalies: an entity in search of an identity. Circulation. 2007;115:1296–305.
10. Rodriguez-Granillo GA, Rosales MA, Pugliese F, Fernandez-Pereira C, Rodriguez AE. Prevalence and characteristics of major and minor coronary artery anomalies in an adult population assessed by computed tomography coronary angiography. EuroIntervention. 2009;4:641–7.
11. Rapp AH, Hillis LD. Clinical consequences of anomalous coronary arteries. Coron Artery Dis. 2001;12:617–20.
12. Kayalar N, Burkhart HM, Dearani JA, Cetta F, Schaff HV. Congenital coronary anomalies and surgical treatment. Congenit Heart Dis. 2009;4:239–51.
13. Ogden JA. Congenital anomalies of the coronary arteries. Am J Cardiol. 1970;25:474–9.
14. Lee AC, Foster E, Yeghiazarians Y. Anomalous origin of the left coronary artery from the pulmonary artery: a case series and brief review. Congenit Heart Dis. 2006;1:111–5.
15. Maron BJ, Thompson PD, Puffer JC, McGrew CA, Strong WB, Douglas PS, et al. Cardiovascular preparticipation screening of competitive athletes. A statement for health professionals from the Sudden Death Committee (clinical cardiology) and Congenital Cardiac Defects Committee (cardiovascular disease in the young), American Heart Association. Circulation. 1996;94:850–6.
16. Basso C, Maron BJ, Corrado D, Thiene G. Clinical profile of congenital coronary artery anomalies with origin from the wrong aortic sinus leading to sudden death in young competitive athletes. J Am Coll Cardiol. 2000;35:1493–501.
17. Cheitlin MD, MacGregor J. Congenital anomalies of coronary arteries: role in the pathogenesis of sudden cardiac death. Herz. 2009;34:268–79.
18. Safi AM, Rachko M, Tang A, Ketosugbo A, Kwan T, Afflu E. Anomalous origin of the left main coronary artery from the right sinus of Valsalva: disabling angina and syncope with noninterarterial courses case report of two patients. Heart Dis. 2001;3:24–7.
19. Kaushal S, Backer CL, Popescu AR, Walker BL, Russell HM, Koenig PR, et al. Intramural coronary length correlates with symptoms in patients with anomalous aortic origin of the coronary artery. Ann Thorac Surg. 2011;92:986–91, discussion 91–2.
20. Angelini P. Anomalous origin of the left coronary artery from the opposite sinus of valsalva: typical and atypical features. Tex Heart Inst J. 2009;36:313–5.
21. Lee HJ, Hong YJ, Kim HY, Lee J, Hur J, Choi BW, et al. Anomalous origin of the right coronary artery from the left coronary sinus with an interarterial course: subtypes and clinical importance. Radiology. 2012;262:101–8.
22. Angelini P, Walmsley R, Cheong BY, Ott DA. Left main coronary artery originating from the proper sinus but with acute angulation and an intramural course, leading to critical stenosis. Tex Heart Inst J. 2010;37:221–5.
23. Jo Y, Uranaka Y, Iwaki H, Matsumoto J, Koura T, Negishi K. Sudden cardiac arrest: associated with anomalous origin of the right coronary artery from the left main coronary artery. Tex Heart Inst J. 2011;38:539–43.
24. Bartoli CR, Wead WB, Giridharan GA, Prabhu SD, Koenig SC, Dowling RD. Mechanism of myocardial ischemia with an anomalous left coronary artery from the right sinus of Valsalva. J Thorac Cardiovasc Surg. 2012;144(2):402–8.
25. Yau JM, Singh R, Halpern EJ, Fischman D. Anomalous origin of the left coronary artery from the pulmonary artery in adults: a comprehensive review of 151 adult cases and a new diagnosis in a 53-year-old woman. Clin Cardiol. 2011;34:204–10.
26. Wesselhoeft H, Fawcett JS, Johnson AL. Anomalous origin of the left coronary artery from the pulmonary trunk. Its clinical spectrum, pathology, and pathophysiology, based on a review of 140 cases with seven further cases. Circulation. 1968;38:403–25.
27. Zheng JY, Han L, Ding WH, Jin M, Zhang GZ, Xiao YY, et al. Clinical features and long-term prognosis of patients with anomalous origin of the left coronary artery from the pulmonary artery. Chin Med J (Engl). 2010;123:2888–94.
28. Frommelt PC, Frommelt MA. Congenital coronary artery anomalies. Pediatr Clin North Am. 2004;51:1273–88.
29. Moodie DS, Fyfe D, Gill CC, Cook SA, Lytle BW, Taylor PC, et al. Anomalous origin of the left coronary artery from the pulmonary artery (Bland-White-Garland syndrome) in adult patients: long-term follow-up after surgery. Am Heart J. 1983;106:381–8.
30. Kaunitz PE. Origin of left coronary artery from pulmonary artery; review of the literature and report of two cases. Am Heart J. 1947;33:182–206.
31. Edwards JE. The direction of blood flow in coronary arteries arising from the pulmonary trunk. Circulation. 1964;29:163–6.
32. Rowe GG. Inequalities of myocardial perfusion in coronary artery disease ("coronary steal"). Circulation. 1970;42:193–4.
33. Baue AE, Baum S, Blakemore WS, Zinsser HF. A later stage of anomalous coronary circulation with origin of the left coronary artery from the pulmonary artery. Coronary artery steal. Circulation. 1967;36:878–85.
34. Angelini P. Congenital coronary artery ostial disease: a spectrum of anatomic variants with different pathophysiologies and prognoses. Tex Heart Inst J. 2012;39:55–9.
35. Ishii Y, Suzuki T, Kobayashi T, Arakawa H. Single coronary artery with right ventricular fistula: case report and literature review. Congenit Heart Dis. 2010;5:56–9.
36. Steinberg I, Holswade GR. Coronary arteriovenous fistula. Am J Roentgenol Radium Ther Nucl Med. 1972;116:82–90.
37. Holzer R, Johnson R, Ciotti G, Pozzi M, Kitchiner D. Review of an institutional experience of coronary arterial fistulas in childhood set in context of review of the literature. Cardiol Young. 2004;14:380–5.
38. Said SA. Current characteristics of congenital coronary artery fistulas in adults: a decade of global experience. World J Cardiol. 2011;3:267–77.
39. Liberthson RR, Sagar K, Berkoben JP, Weintraub RM, Levine FH. Congenital coronary arteriovenous fistula. Report of 13 patients, review of the literature and delineation of management. Circulation. 1979;59:849–54.
40. Gupta NC, Beauvais J. Physiologic assessment of coronary artery fistula. Clin Nucl Med. 1991;16:40–2.
41. Skimming JW, Walls JT. Congenital coronary artery fistula suggesting a "steal phenomenon" in a neonate. Pediatr Cardiol. 1993;14:174–5.
42. Mukai H, Minemawari Y, Hanawa N, Mita T, Motoe M, Nakata T. Coronary stenosis and steal phenomenon in coronary-pulmonary fistula–assessment with stress thallium tomography after coronary angioplasty and fistulectomy. Jpn Circ J. 1993;57:1021–6.
43. Angelini P, de la Cruz MV. The relationship between coronary arteries and congenital heart disease. In: Coronary artery anomalies: a comprehensive approach. Philadelphia: Lippincott, Williams and Wilkins; 1999.
44. Raju MG, Goyal SK, Punnam SR, Shah DO, Smith GF, Abela GS. Coronary artery fistula: a case series with review of the literature. J Cardiol. 2009;53:467–72.
45. Balanescu S, Sangiorgi G, Castelvecchio S, Medda M, Inglese L. Coronary artery fistulas: clinical consequences and methods of closure. A literature review. Ital Heart J. 2001;2:669–76.
46. Wang NK, Hsieh LY, Shen CT, Lin YM. Coronary arteriovenous fistula in pediatric patients: a 17-year institutional experience. J Formos Med Assoc. 2002;101:177–82.

47. Weaver JC, McCrohon JA, Rees D, Prasan AM. Multivessel coronary-ventricular fistulae and ischaemia on cardiac MRI. Int J Cardiol. 2010;139:e36–8.
48. Anderson RH, Spicer D. Fistulous communications with the coronary arteries in the setting of hypoplastic ventricles. Cardiol Young. 2010;20 Suppl 3:86–91.
49. Mantini E, Grondin CM, Lillehei CW, Edwards JE. Congenital anomalies involving the coronary sinus. Circulation. 1966;33:317–27.
50. Chou MC, Wu MT, Chen CH, Lee MH, Tzeng WS. Multidetector CT findings of a congenital coronary sinus anomaly: a report of two cases. Korean J Radiol. 2008;9(Suppl):S1–6.
51. Gerlis LM, Gibbs JL, Williams GJ, Thomas GD. Coronary sinus orifice atresia and persistent left superior vena cava. A report of two cases, one associated with atypical coronary artery thrombosis. Br Heart J. 1984;52:648–53.
52. Watson GH. Atresia of the coronary sinus orifice. Pediatr Cardiol. 1985;6:99–101.
53. von Ludinghausen M, Lechleuthner A. Atresia of the right atrial ostium of the coronary sinus. Acta Anat (Basel). 1988;131:81–3.
54. Alegria JR, Herrmann J, Holmes Jr DR, Lerman A, Rihal CS. Myocardial bridging. Eur Heart J. 2005;26:1159–68.
55. Loukas M, Von Kriegenbergh K, Gilkes M, Tubbs RS, Walker C, Malaiyandi D, et al. Myocardial bridges: a review. Clin Anat. 2011;24:675–83.
56. Nakanishi R, Rajani R, Ishikawa Y, Ishii T, Berman DS. Myocardial bridging on coronary CTA: an innocent bystander or a culprit in myocardial infarction? J Cardiovasc Comput Tomogr. 2012;6:3–13.
57. Sharma J, Hellenbrand W, Kleinman C, Mosca R. Symptomatic myocardial bridges in children: a case report with review of literature. Cardiol Young. 2011;21:490–4.
58. Klues HG, Schwarz ER, vom Dahl J, Reffelmann T, Reul H, Potthast K, et al. Disturbed intracoronary hemodynamics in myocardial bridging: early normalization by intracoronary stent placement. Circulation. 1997;96:2905–13.
59. Gawor R, Kusmierek J, Plachcinska A, Bienkiewicz M, Drozdz J, Piotrowski G, et al. Myocardial perfusion GSPECT imaging in patients with myocardial bridging. J Nucl Cardiol. 2011; 18:1059–65.
60. Kitazume H, Kramer JR, Krauthamer D, El Tobgi S, Proudfit WL, Sones FM. Myocardial bridges in obstructive hypertrophic cardiomyopathy. Am Heart J. 1983;106:131–5.
61. Navarro-Lopez F, Soler J, Magrina J, Esplugues E, Pare JC, Sanz G, et al. Systolic compression of coronary artery in hypertrophic cardiomyopathy. Int J Cardiol. 1986;12:309–20.
62. Basso C, Thiene G, Mackey-Bojack S, Frigo AC, Corrado D, Maron BJ. Myocardial bridging, a frequent component of the hypertrophic cardiomyopathy phenotype, lacks systematic association with sudden cardiac death. Eur Heart J. 2009;30:1627–34.
63. Aydar Y, Yazici HU, Birdane A, Nasifov M, Nadir A, Ulus T, et al. Gender differences in the types and frequency of coronary artery anomalies. Tohoku J Exp Med. 2011;225:239–47.
64. Ishikawa Y, Kawawa Y, Kohda E, Shimada K, Ishii T. Significance of the anatomical properties of a myocardial bridge in coronary heart disease. Circ J. 2011;75:1559–66.
65. Ishikawa Y, Akasaka Y, Suzuki K, Fujiwara M, Ogawa T, Yamazaki K, et al. Anatomic properties of myocardial bridge predisposing to myocardial infarction. Circulation. 2009;120:376–83.
66. Ge J, Jeremias A, Rupp A, Abels M, Baumgart D, Liu F, et al. New signs characteristic of myocardial bridging demonstrated by intracoronary ultrasound and Doppler. Eur Heart J. 1999;20:1707–16.
67. Ikari Y, McManus BM, Kenyon J, Schwartz SM. Neonatal intima formation in the human coronary artery. Arterioscler Thromb Vasc Biol. 1999;19:2036–40.
68. Corrado D, Thiene G, Cocco P, Frescura C. Non-atherosclerotic coronary artery disease and sudden death in the young. Br Heart J. 1992;68:601–7.
69. Bourassa MG, Butnaru A, Lesperance J, Tardif JC. Symptomatic myocardial bridges: overview of ischemic mechanisms and current diagnostic and treatment strategies. J Am Coll Cardiol. 2003;41:351–9.
70. Musiani A, Cernigliaro C, Sansa M, Maselli D, De Gasperis C. Left main coronary artery atresia: literature review and therapeutical considerations. Eur J Cardiothorac Surg. 1997;11:505–14.
71. Elian D, Hegesh J, Agranat O, Guetta V, Har-Zahav Y, Rath S, et al. Left main coronary artery atresia: extremely rare coronary anomaly in an asymptomatic adult and an adolescent soccer player. Cardiol Rev. 2003;11:160–2.
72. Karadag B, Ayan F, Ismailoglu Z, Goksedef D, Ataev Y, Vural VA. Extraordinary cause of ischemic chest pain in a young man: congenital ostial atresia of the right coronary artery. J Cardiol. 2009;54:335–8.
73. Casta A. Hypoplasia of the left coronary artery complicated by reversible myocardial ischemia in a newborn. Am Heart J. 1987; 114:1238–41.
74. Rigatelli G, Docali G, Rossi P, Bovolon D, Rossi D, Bandello A, et al. Congenital coronary artery anomalies angiographic classification revisited. Int J Cardiovasc Imaging. 2003;19:361–6.
75. Celik T, Iyisoy A, Kursaklioglu H, Kose S, Kilic S, Amasyali B, et al. Does coronary artery size really matter? Echocardiography. 2005;22:479–86.
76. Duran AC, Arque JM, Fernandez B, Fernandez MC, Fernandez-Gallego T, Rodriguez C, et al. Rudimentary coronary artery in Syrian hamsters (Mesocricetus auratus). Anat Histol Embryol. 2009;38:270–4.
77. Vlodaver Z, Neufeld HN, Edwards JE. Coronary arterial variations in the normal heart and in congenital heart disease. New York: Academic Press; 1975.
78. Manginas A, Cokkinos DV. Coronary artery ectasias: imaging, functional assessment and clinical implications. Eur Heart J. 2006;27:1026–31.
79. Sharma SN, Kaul U, Sharma S, Wasir HS, Manchanda SC, Bahl VK, et al. Coronary arteriographic profile in young and old Indian patients with ischaemic heart disease: a comparative study. Indian Heart J. 1990;42:365–9.
80. Cohen P, O'Gara PT. Coronary artery aneurysms: a review of the natural history, pathophysiology, and management. Cardiol Rev. 2008;16:301–4.
81. Roberts WC. Natural history, clinical consequences, and morphologic features of coronary arterial aneurysms in adults. Am J Cardiol. 2011;108:814–21.
82. Virmani R, Robinowitz M, Atkinson JB, Forman MB, Silver MD, McAllister HA. Acquired coronary arterial aneurysms: an autopsy study of 52 patients. Hum Pathol. 1986;17:575–83.
83. Lenihan DJ, Zeman HS, Collins GJ. Left main coronary artery aneurysm in association with severe atherosclerosis: a case report and review of the literature. Cathet Cardiovasc Diagn. 1991;23:28–31.
84. Chrissoheris MP, Donohue TJ, Young RS, Ghantous A. Coronary artery aneurysms. Cardiology in review. 2008;16:116–23.
85. Bove AA, Vlietstra RE. Spasm in ectatic coronary arteries. Mayo Clin Proc. 1985;60:822–6.
86. Baman TS, Cole JH, Devireddy CM, Sperling LS. Risk factors and outcomes in patients with coronary artery aneurysms. Am J Cardiol. 2004;93:1549–51.
87. Bjork VO, Bjork L. Intramural coronary artery aneurysm. A coronary artery steal syndrome. Journal of Thoracic and. Cardiovasc Surg. 1967;54:50–3.
88. Syed M, Lesch M. Coronary artery aneurysm: a review. Prog Cardiovasc Dis. 1997;40:77–84.

89. Markis JE, Joffe CD, Cohn PF, Feen DJ, Herman MV, Gorlin R. Clinical significance of coronary arterial ectasia. Am J Cardiol. 1976;37:217–22.
90. Sorrell VL, Davis MJ, Bove AA. Current knowledge and significance of coronary artery ectasia: a chronologic review of the literature, recommendations for treatment, possible etiologies, and future considerations. Clin Cardiol. 1998;21:157–60.
91. England JF. Herbicides and coronary ectasia. Med J Aust. 1981;1:140.
92. Icardo JM, Colvee E. Origin and course of the coronary arteries in normal mice and in iv/iv mice. J Anat. 2001;199:473–82.
93. Ratajska A, Ciszek B, Zajaczkowska A, Jablonska A, Juszynski M. Angioarchitecture of the venous and capillary system in heart defects induced by retinoic acid in mice. Birth Defects Res A Clin Mol Teratol. 2009;85:599–610.
94. Butto F, Lucas Jr RV, Edwards JE. Persistent truncus arteriosus: pathologic anatomy in 54 cases. Pediatr Cardiol. 1986;7:95–101.
95. Shrivastava S, Edwards JE. Coronary arterial origin in persistent truncus arteriosus. Circulation. 1977;55:551–4.
96. de la Cruz MV, Cayre R, Angelini P, Noriega-Ramos N, Sadowinski S. Coronary arteries in truncus arteriosus. Am J Cardiol. 1990;66:1482–6.
97. Henaine R, Azarnoush K, Belli E, Capderou A, Roussin R, Planche C, et al. Fate of the truncal valve in truncus arteriosus. Ann Thorac Surg. 2008;85:172–8.
98. Sherman FE. An atlas of congenital heart disease. Philadelphia: Lea and Febiger; 1963.
99. Lenox CC, Debich DE, Zuberbuhler JR. The role of coronary artery abnormalities in the prognosis of truncus arteriosus. J Thorac Cardiovasc Surg. 1992;104:1728–42.
100. Anderson KR, McGoon DC, Lie JT. Surgical significance of the coronary arterial anatomy in truncus arteriosus communis. Am J Cardiol. 1978;41:76–81.
101. Crupi G, Macartney FJ, Anderson RH. Persistent truncus arteriosus. A study of 66 autopsy cases with special reference to definition and morphogenesis. Am J Cardiol. 1977;40:569–78.
102. Calder L, Van Praagh R, Van Praagh S, Sears WP, Corwin R, Levy A, et al. Truncus arteriosus communis. Clinical, angiocardiographic, and pathologic findings in 100 patients. Am Heart J. 1976;92:23–38.
103. Bharati S, McAllister Jr HA, Rosenquist GC, Miller RA, Tatooles CJ, Lev M. The surgical anatomy of truncus arteriosus communis. J Thorac Cardiovasc Surg. 1974;67:501–10.
104. Bogers AJ, Bartelings MM, Bokenkamp R, Stijnen T, van Suylen RJ, Poelmann RE, et al. Common arterial trunk, uncommon coronary arterial anatomy. J Thorac Cardiovasc Surg. 1993; 106:1133–7.
105. Suzuki A, Ho SY, Anderson RH, Deanfield JE. Coronary arterial and sinusal anatomy in hearts with a common arterial trunk. Ann Thorac Surg. 1989;48:792–7.
106. Jaggers JJ, Cameron DE, Herlong JR, Ungerleider RM. Congenital Heart Surgery Nomenclature and Database Project: transposition of the great arteries. Ann Thorac Surg. 2000;69:S205–35.
107. Gutgesell HP, Garson A, McNamara DG. Prognosis for the newborn with transposition of the great arteries. Am J Cardiol. 1979;44:96–100.
108. Levin DL, Paul MH, Muster AJ, Newfeld EA, Waldman JD. d-Transposition of the great vessels in the neonate. A clinical diagnosis. Arch Intern Med. 1977;137:1421–5.
109. Liebman J, Cullum L, Belloc NB. Natural history of transpositon of the great arteries. Anatomy and birth and death characteristics. Circulation. 1969;40:237–62.
110. Pasquini L, Sanders SP, Parness IA, Colan SD. Diagnosis of coronary artery anatomy by two-dimensional echocardiography in patients with transposition of the great arteries. Circulation. 1987;75:557–64.
111. Ismat FA, Baldwin HS, Karl TR, Weinberg PM. Coronary anatomy in congenitally corrected transposition of the great arteries. Int J Cardiol. 2002;86:207–16.
112. Burch GH, Sahn DJ. Congenital coronary artery anomalies: the pediatric perspective. Coron Artery Dis. 2001;12:605–16.
113. Zwadlo C, Meyer GP, Schieffer B, Westhoff-Bleck M. Anomalous intramural course of coronary arteries in congenital heart disease-three case reports and review of the literature. Congenit Heart Dis. 2012;7(2):139–44.
114. Gittenberger-de Groot AC, Sauer U, Quaegebeur J. Aortic intramural coronary artery in three hearts with transposition of the great arteries. J Thorac Cardiovasc Surg. 1986;91:566–71.
115. Soto B, Pacifico AD, Ceballos R, Bargeron Jr LM. Tetralogy of Fallot: an angiographic-pathologic correlative study. Circulation. 1981;64:558–66.
116. Bailliard F, Anderson RH. Tetralogy of Fallot. Orphanet J Rare Dis. 2009;4:2.
117. Brizard CP, Mas C, Sohn YS, Cochrane AD, Karl TR. Transatrial-transpulmonary tetralogy of Fallot repair is effective in the presence of anomalous coronary arteries. J Thorac Cardiovasc Surg. 1998;116:770–9.
118. Kervancioglu M, Tokel K, Varan B, Yildirim SV. Frequency, origins and courses of anomalous coronary arteries in 607 Turkish children with tetralogy of Fallot. Cardiol J. 2011;18:546–51.
119. Piran S, Bassett AS, Grewal J, Swaby JA, Morel C, Oechslin EN, et al. Patterns of cardiac and extracardiac anomalies in adults with tetralogy of fallot. Am Heart J. 2011;161:131–7.
120. Walters 3rd HL, Mavroudis C, Tchervenkov CI, Jacobs JP, Lacour-Gayet F, Jacobs ML. Congenital Heart Surgery Nomenclature and Database Project: double outlet right ventricle. Ann Thorac Surg. 2000;69:S249–63.
121. Anderson RH, Macartney FJ, Tynan M, Becker AE, Freedom RM, Godman MJ, et al. Univentricular atrioventricular connection: the single ventricle trap unsprung. Pediatr Cardiol. 1983; 4:273–80.
122. Lev M, Liberthson RR, Kirkpatrick JR, Eckner FA, Arcilla RA. Single (primitive) ventricle. Circulation. 1969;39:577–91.
123. Keeton BR, Lie JT, McGoon DC, Danielson GK, Ritter DG, Wallace RB. Anatomy of coronary arteries in univentricular hearts and its surgical implications. Am J Cardiol. 1979;43:569–80.
124. Ando K, Nakajima Y, Yamagishi T, Yamamoto S, Nakamura H. Development of proximal coronary arteries in quail embryonic heart: multiple capillaries penetrating the aortic sinus fuse to form main coronary trunk. Circ Res. 2004;94:346–52.
125. Velkey JM, Bernanke DH. Apoptosis during coronary artery orifice development in the chick embryo. Anat Rec. 2001;262: 310–7.
126. Tomanek RJ, Ishii Y, Holifield JS, Sjogren CL, Hansen HK, Mikawa T. VEGF family members regulate myocardial tubulogenesis and coronary artery formation in the embryo. Circ Res. 2006;98:947–53.
127. Tomanek RJ, Schatteman GC. Angiogenesis: new insights and therapeutic potential. Anat Rec. 2000;261:126–35.
128. Silva-Junior GO, Aguila MB, Mandarim-de-Lacerda CA. Insights into coronary artery development in model of maternal protein restriction in mice. Anat Rec (Hoboken). 2011;294:1757–64.
129. van den Akker NM, Caolo V, Wisse LJ, Peters PP, Poelmann RE, Carmeliet P, et al. Developmental coronary maturation is disturbed by aberrant cardiac vascular endothelial growth factor expression and Notch signalling. Cardiovasc Res. 2008;78:366–75.
130. Yue X, Tomanek RJ. Effects of VEGF(165) and VEGF(121) on vasculogenesis and angiogenesis in cultured embryonic quail hearts. Am J Physiol Heart Circ Physiol. 2001;280:H2240–7.
131. Tomanek RJ, Hansen HK, Christensen LP. Temporally expressed PDGF and FGF-2 regulate embryonic coronary artery formation and growth. Arterioscler Thromb Vasc Biol. 2008;28:1237–43.

132. Langlois D, Hneino M, Bouazza L, Parlakian A, Sasaki T, Bricca G, et al. Conditional inactivation of TGF-beta type II receptor in smooth muscle cells and epicardium causes lethal aortic and cardiac defects. Transgenic Res. 2010;19:1069–82.
133. Ng A, Wong M, Viviano B, Erlich JM, Alba G, Pflederer C, et al. Loss of glypican-3 function causes growth factor-dependent defects in cardiac and coronary vascular development. Dev Biol. 2009;335:208–15.
134. Watanabe T, Koibuchi N, Chin MT. Transcription factor CHF1/Hey2 regulates coronary vascular maturation. Mech Dev. 2010;127:418–27.
135. Wikenheiser J, Wolfram JA, Gargesha M, Yang K, Karunamuni G, Wilson DL, et al. Altered hypoxia-inducible factor-1 alpha expression levels correlate with coronary vessel anomalies. Dev Dyn. 2009;238:2688–700.
136. Yin Z, Haynie J, Yang X, Han B, Kiatchoosakun S, Restivo J, et al. The essential role of Cited2, a negative regulator for HIF-1alpha, in heart development and neurulation. Proc Natl Acad Sci USA. 2002;99:10488–93.
137. Xu B, Doughman Y, Turakhia M, Jiang W, Landsettle CE, Agani FH, et al. Partial rescue of defects in Cited2-deficient embryos by HIF-1alpha heterozygosity. Dev Biol. 2007;301:130–40.
138. Hood LC, Rosenquist TH. Coronary artery development in the chick: origin and deployment of smooth muscle cells, and the effects of neural crest ablation. Anat Rec. 1992;234:291–300.
139. Waldo KL, Kumiski DH, Kirby ML. Association of the cardiac neural crest with development of the coronary arteries in the chick embryo. Anat Rec. 1994;239:315–31.
140. Kirby ML, Turnage 3rd KL, Hays BM. Characterization of conotruncal malformations following ablation of "cardiac" neural crest. Anat Rec. 1985;213:87–93.
141. Nishibatake M, Kirby ML, Van Mierop LH. Pathogenesis of persistent truncus arteriosus and dextroposed aorta in the chick embryo after neural crest ablation. Circulation. 1987;75:255–64.
142. Fujino H, Nakagawa M, Okagawa H, Shimada M. Immunochemical distribution of N-CAM in normal and bis-diamine treated rats. Circulation. 1996;94(8):2823.
143. Okagawa H, Nakagawa M, Simada M. Immunolocalization of N-CAM in the heart of the early developing rat embryo. Anat Rec. 1995;243:261–71.
144. Nishijima S, Nakagawa M, Fujino H, Hanato T, Okamoto N, Shimada M. Teratogenic effects of bis-diamine on early embryonic rat heart: an in vitro study. Teratology. 2000;62:115–22.
145. Hanato T, Nakagawa M, Okamoto N, Nishijima S, Fujino H, Shimada M, et al. Developmental defects of coronary vasculature in rat embryos administered bis-diamine. Birth Defects Res B Dev Reprod Toxicol. 2011;92:10–6.
146. Walker DL, Vacha SJ, Kirby ML, Lo CW. Connexin43 deficiency causes dysregulation of coronary vasculogenesis. Dev Biol. 2005;284:479–98.
147. Liu S, Liu F, Schneider AE, St Amand T, Epstein JA, Gutstein DE. Distinct cardiac malformations caused by absence of connexin 43 in the neural crest and in the non-crest neural tube. Development. 2006;133:2063–73.
148. Clauss SB, Walker DL, Kirby ML, Schimel D, Lo CW. Patterning of coronary arteries in wildtype and connexin43 knockout mice. Dev Dyn. 2006;235:2786–94.
149. Dang X, Doble BW, Kardami E. The carboxy-tail of connexin-43 localizes to the nucleus and inhibits cell growth. Mol Cell Biochem. 2003;242:35–8.
150. Li WE, Waldo K, Linask KL, Chen T, Wessels A, Parmacek MS, et al. An essential role for connexin43 gap junctions in mouse coronary artery development. Development. 2002;129:2031–42.
151. Gonzalez-Iriarte M, Carmona R, Perez-Pomares JM, Macias D, Costell M, Munoz-Chapuli R. Development of the coronary arteries in a murine model of transposition of great arteries. J Mol Cell Cardiol. 2003;35:795–802.
152. Theveniau-Ruissy M, Dandonneau M, Mesbah K, Ghez O, Mattei MG, Miquerol L, et al. The del22q11.2 candidate gene Tbx1 controls regional outflow tract identity and coronary artery patterning. Circ Res. 2008;103:142–8.
153. Eckart RE, Scoville SL, Campbell CL, Shry EA, Stajduhar KC, Potter RN, et al. Sudden death in young adults: a 25-year review of autopsies in military recruits. Ann Intern Med. 2004; 141:829–34.
154. Frommelt PC. Congenital coronary artery abnormalities predisposing to sudden cardiac death. Pacing Clin Electrophysiol. 2009;32 Suppl 2:S63–6.
155. Frescura C, Basso C, Thiene G, Corrado D, Pennelli T, Angelini A, et al. Anomalous origin of coronary arteries and risk of sudden death: a study based on an autopsy population of congenital heart disease. Hum Pathol. 1998;29:689–95.
156. Taylor AJ, Rogan KM, Virmani R. Sudden cardiac death associated with isolated congenital coronary artery anomalies. J Am Coll Cardiol. 1992;20:640–7.
157. Steinberger J, Lucas Jr RV, Edwards JE, Titus JL. Causes of sudden unexpected cardiac death in the first two decades of life. Am J Cardiol. 1996;77:992–5.
158. Virmani R, Burke AP, Farb A. Sudden cardiac death. Cardiovasc Pathol. 2001;10:275–82.
159. Tavora F, Li L, Burke A. Sudden coronary death in children. Cardiovasc Pathol. 2010;19:336–9.
160. Lipsett J, Cohle SD, Berry PJ, Russell G, Byard RW. Anomalous coronary arteries: a multicenter pediatric autopsy study. Pediatr Pathol. 1994;14:287–300.
161. Burke AP, Farb A, Virmani R, Goodin J, Smialek JE. Sports-related and non-sports-related sudden cardiac death in young adults. Am Heart J. 1991;121:568–75.
162. Corrado D, Basso C, Rizzoli G, Schiavon M, Thiene G. Does sports activity enhance the risk of sudden death in adolescents and young adults? J Am Coll Cardiol. 2003;42:1959–63.
163. Corrado D, Basso C, Schiavon M, Thiene G. Does sports activity enhance the risk of sudden cardiac death? J Cardiovasc Med (Hagerstown). 2006;7:228–33.
164. Eckart RE, Shry EA, Burke AP, McNear JA, Appel DA, Castillo-Rojas LM, et al. Sudden death in young adults: an autopsy-based series of a population undergoing active surveillance. J Am Coll Cardiol. 2011;58:1254–61.
165. Van Camp SP, Bloor CM, Mueller FO, Cantu RC, Olson HG. Nontraumatic sports death in high school and college athletes. Med Sci Sports Exerc. 1995;27:641–7.
166. Link MS, Mark Estes 3rd NA. Sudden cardiac death in athletes. Prog Cardiovasc Dis. 2008;51:44–57.
167. Cross BJ, Estes 3rd NA, Link MS. Sudden cardiac death in young athletes and nonathletes. Curr Opin Crit Care. 2011;17:328–34.
168. Kragel AH, Roberts WC. Anomalous origin of either the right or left main coronary artery from the aorta with subsequent coursing between aorta and pulmonary trunk: analysis of 32 necropsy cases. Am J Cardiol. 1988;62:771–7.
169. Cheitlin MD, De Castro CM, McAllister HA. Sudden death as a complication of anomalous left coronary origin from the anterior sinus of Valsalva. A not-so-minor congenital anomaly. Circulation. 1974;50:780–7.
170. Roberts WC, Siegel RJ, Zipes DP. Origin of the right coronary artery from the left sinus of valsalva and its functional consequences: analysis of 10 necropsy patients. Am J Cardiol. 1982; 49:863–8.
171. Baltaxe HA, Wixson D. The incidence of congenital anomalies of the coronary arteries in the adult population. Radiology. 1977;122:47–52.

172. Barth 3rd CW, Bray M, Roberts WC. Sudden death in infancy associated with origin of both left main and right coronary arteries from a common ostium above the left sinus of Valsalva. Am J Cardiol. 1986;57:365–6.
173. Galie N, Manes A, Palazzini M, Negro L, Marinelli A, Gambetti S, et al. Management of pulmonary arterial hypertension associated with congenital systemic-to-pulmonary shunts and Eisenmenger's syndrome. Drugs. 2008;68:1049–66.
174. Bjork L. Ectasia of the coronary arteries. Radiology. 1966;87:33–4.
175. Chugh R, Perloff JK, Fishbein M, Child JS. Extramural coronary arteries in adults with cyanotic congenital heart disease. Am J Cardiol. 2004;94:1355–7.
176. Brunken RC, Perloff JK, Czernin J, Campisi R, Purcell S, Miner PD, et al. Myocardial perfusion reserve in adults with cyanotic congenital heart disease. Am J Physiol Heart Circ Physiol. 2005;289:H1798–806.
177. Fyfe A, Perloff JK, Niwa K, Child JS, Miner PD. Cyanotic congenital heart disease and coronary artery atherogenesis. Am J Cardiol. 2005;96:283–90.
178. Dedkov EI, Perloff JK, Tomanek RJ, Fishbein MC, Gutterman DD. The coronary microcirculation in cyanotic congenital heart disease. Circulation. 2006;114:196–200.
179. Weiford BC, Subbarao VD, Mulhern KM. Noncompaction of the ventricular myocardium. Circulation. 2004;109:2965–71.
180. Bartram U, Bauer J, Schranz D. Primary noncompaction of the ventricular myocardium from the morphogenetic standpoint. Pediatr Cardiol. 2007;28:325–32.
181. Ergul Y, Nisli K, Demirel A, Varkal MA, Oner N, Dursun M, et al. Left ventricular non-compaction in children and adolescents: clinical features, treatment and follow-up. Cardiol J. 2011;18:176–84.
182. Ritter M, Oechslin E, Sutsch G, Attenhofer C, Schneider J, Jenni R. Isolated noncompaction of the myocardium in adults. Mayo Clin Proc. 1997;72:26–31.
183. Lauer RM, Fink HP, Petry EL, Dunn MI, Diehl AM. Angiographic demonstration of intramyocardial sinusoids in pulmonary-valve atresia with intact ventricular septum and hypoplastic right ventricle. N Engl J Med. 1964;271:68–72.
184. Dusek J, Ostadal B, Duskova M. Postnatal persistence of spongy myocardium with embryonic blood supply. Arch Pathol. 1975;99:312–7.
185. Soler R, Rodriguez E, Monserrat L, Alvarez N. MRI of subendocardial perfusion deficits in isolated left ventricular noncompaction. J Comput Assist Tomogr. 2002;26:373–5.
186. Junga G, Kneifel S, Von Smekal A, Steinert H, Bauersfeld U. Myocardial ischaemia in children with isolated ventricular noncompaction. Eur Heart J. 1999;20:910–6.
187. Jenni R, Wyss CA, Oechslin EN, Kaufmann PA. Isolated ventricular noncompaction is associated with coronary microcirculatory dysfunction. J Am Coll Cardiol. 2002;39:450–4.
188. Tomanek RJ, Hansen HK, Dedkov EI. Vascular patterning of the quail coronary system during development. Anat Rec A Discov Mol Cell Evol Biol. 2006;288:989–99.
189. Puranik R, Chow CK, Duflou JA, Kilborn MJ, McGuire MA. Sudden death in the young. Heart Rhythm. 2005;2:1277–82.

Aging

7

Abbreviations

EC	Endothelial cells
eNOS	Endothelial nitric oxide synthase
FGF	Fibroblast growth factor
LAD	Left anterior descending artery
NO	Nitric oxide
VEGF	Vascular endothelial growth factor
VSMC	Vascular smooth muscle

Introduction

Aging is associated with both structural and functional changes in the cardiovascular system. Some of the alterations are inevitable, i.e., they constitute biological aging ("senescence"), whereas others are disease related and more likely to occur in older individuals ("senile"). Senescence is characterized by ultrastructural changes in cardiomyocytes such as lipofuscin accumulations, autophagic vacuoles, mitochondrial degeneration, and dilated vesicles (reviewed in [1]). Blood vessel changes in the elderly and in senescent animals include endothelial dysfunction [2, 3], impaired nitric oxide (NO) availability, arterial stiffness [4], intimal and medial thickening [5], arteriosclerosis and increased systemic vascular resistance [6], and impaired angiogenesis [7] and impaired vascular repair [8]. Aging also enhances the probability of certain cardiovascular diseases, e.g., hypertension and coronary artery disease [5, 9]. Alterations in aged arteries are similar to those that develop in younger animals in response to experimentally induced hypertension and atherosclerosis [5]. These findings underscore the concept that aging is a major risk factor for cardiovascular diseases [5]. The first part of this chapter briefly addresses vascular aging changes that occur in a variety of vascular beds. The rest of the chapter focuses on the effects of aging on (1) the coronary vasculature and myocardial perfusion and (2) myocardial ischemia and infarction.

Vascular Aging and Disease

An extensive review of vascular structural and functional changes was provided by Marin [10] in which he includes data from both experimental animals and humans and discusses the relationship of aging to hypertension and atherosclerosis. It is well established that age is a risk factor for hypertension, coronary disease, stroke, and heart failure, which suggests a link between these diseases and age [5]. For example, stiffness of large arteries, a characteristic of aging, also occurs in hypertension and in patients with heart failure [11]. The classic experiments of Wolinsky [12] demonstrated that the changes in the aortic wall in rats in response to elevated arterial pressure are similar, though more severe, to those of aging. Although both aging and hypertension contribute to arterial stiffness, aging contributes most to systolic stiffness, which causes a widened pulse pressure [13]. The idea that aging is a component of the "cardiovascular continuum" (that has been used to explain the development of cardiovascular diseases that result in heart failure) is consistent with the fact that aging may not only cause vascular changes but also impair myocardial supply/demand resulting in myocardial ischemia [14]. Moreover, there is considerable evidence indicating that aging plays a pathological role in atherosclerosis, which is a cause of myocardial ischemia and infarction [15].

Cellular Senescence

Cellular senescence is a stress response that results in "a permanent withdrawal from the cell cycle and the appearance of distinct morphological and functional changes associated with an impaired cellular homeostasis" [16]. A first clue of cellular senescence was recognized long ago by the fact that normal cells have a limited ability to proliferate in culture. Since that time the senescent phenotype has been repeatedly demonstrated; its characteristics include growth

R.J. Tomanek, *Coronary Vasculature: Development, Structure-Function, and Adaptations*,
DOI 10.1007/978-1-4614-4887-7_7,

arrest, altered gene expression, and the presence of senescence markers [17]. One key change that occurs with repeated replications in cells is that telomeres, structures that cap and stabilize the ends of chromosomes, shorten and the ends of chromosomes become uncapped, which leads to activation of the DNA damage response pathway (reviewed in [16, 18]). Dysfunctional telomeres trigger the senescence phenotype via the p53 pathway [17]. Telomere shortening during aging has been documented in endothelial cells (ECs) and increased rates of shortening have been found in patients with coronary artery disease, suggesting that telomere shortening plays a role in both senescence and coronary artery disease [19].

Common Vascular Changes During Aging

Aging and Endothelial Dysfunction

The fact that endothelial dysfunction causes many functional impairments is not surprising since this cell layer performs a variety of functions (see reviews [2, 20–22]). Endothelial functions decline with age, and endothelial cells (ECs) are more prone to apoptosis and have a limited regenerative capacity [2]. Vasodilator responses are attenuated in the aged as evidenced by both human and animal studies.

Endothelial dysfunction in the vasculature of senescent individuals is highlighted by the numerous studies that have found that endothelial-independent vasodilation is little affected, whereas endothelial-dependent vasodilation is impaired. Impairment of flow-mediated vasodilation in the brachial arteries of healthy men aged 63 ± 1 years was about 50% lower than that in young (23 ± 1 year) men [23]. ECs obtained from the brachial artery revealed that old subjects had a twofold higher level of nitrotyrosine, a marker of oxidative stress, than their young counterparts. Increased expression of NADPH oxidase and nuclear factor-kappa B were also documented as factors that may contribute to EC oxidative stress during aging. Moreover, aging augments the responses to vasoconstrictors [3]. The situation is exacerbated by cardiovascular risk factors, e.g., hypertension, hypercholesterolemia, and diabetes that contribute to the development of atherosclerosis [24]. Aging vessels accumulate oxidative damage that leads to functional impairment. It is excessive generation of O_2^- that inactivates NO leading to the formation of high levels of peroxynitrite (ONOO–). Csiszar et al. [25] suggested that in addition to this inactivation, aging may be associated with changes in the expression or activity of eNOS and a gradual loss of antioxidant defense mechanisms. Associated with the increased formation of reactive oxidative species is a reduction in NO and the endothelium-derived hyperpolarizing factor [26]. Mesenteric arteries and arterioles from senescent (24 month) rats released less NO in response to shear stress than those from young (6 month) rats [27]. This attenuation was caused by increased superoxide production, reduced superoxide dismutase (SOD) activity, and impaired eNOS activation in response to shear stress. Endothelial dysfunction may be caused, in part, by eNOS uncoupling and a reduction in tetrahydropterin, an essential eNOS cofactor as demonstrated in mesenteric arteries of 2-year-old rats [28]. The importance of NO is twofold (1) it is considered to be the primary endogenous vasodilator and (2) it is also the most important anti-atherosclerotic factor, due to its ability to control oxidation, inflammation, and vascular growth [3]. Flow is one of the most important activators of NO. However, senescent ECs are less sensitive to shear stress, which accounts, in part, for their attenuated NO production [29]. A progressive impairment of both ECs and vascular smooth muscle cells (VSMCs) occurs during the aging process and appears to cause alterations in communication between the two cell types [26]. The ECs undergo a change from an anti-atherosclerotic to a proatherosclerotic phenotype.

Arterial Aging

Aging changes in arteries have long been recognized and particular attention has been given to pulsatile phenomena and arterial stiffness. Aortic stiffness increases with age, resulting in enhanced impedance [30, 31]. Some arterial changes are progressive, beginning already in infancy (noted in Chap. 3), as evidenced by fraying and fracture of elastic lamella in the proximal aorta [32]. It is estimated that the effects of aortic stiffening on "isolated systolic hypertension" affect the majority of individuals by the time they reach the age of 80 years [33, 34]. The increase in arterial stiffness and systolic pressure and a decrease in diastolic pressure (reviewed in [14]) limits coronary flow because myocardial perfusion occurs almost entirely during diastole. As documented by morphometric analysis of large arteries, VSMCs become more irregular in shape and there is a tendency for the extracellular matrix component of the artery to increase [35]. Decreased arterial compliance occurs in other elastic but not muscular arteries, which also remodel to increase wall thickness and are associated with a higher cardiovascular morbidity and mortality [11]. In the carotid artery, these changes have been found to often coexist with calcifications and plaques in the same subject [11]. A comparison of aortae from old (65 ± 6 years) compared to those from young (23 ± 3 years) individuals indicates a proinflammatory profile in the former [36]. In the old subjects, the aortic intimae have been found to (1) be diffusely thickened, (2) contain numerous fetal-like VSMCs, and (3) have high levels of Angiotensin II signaling molecules, and MMT-2 and -9. These changes, which occurred in the absence of lipid infiltration, indicate a

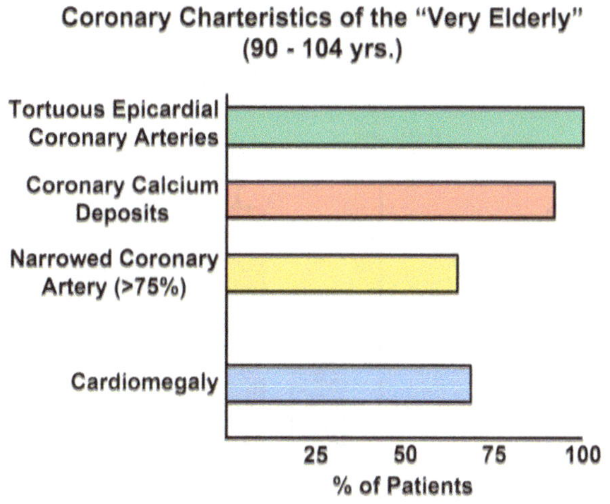

Fig. 7.1 The percent of patients over the age of 90 years who demonstrated various alterations in their coronary arteries is indicated. The most consistent characteristics are tortuous epicardial coronary arteries and the presence of calcium deposits. Data are from Waller and Morgan. Cardiovasc. Clin. 18:361, 1988 [38]

fertile substrate for the development of arterial diseases such as atherosclerosis.

A review by Lakatta et al. [5] points out that age-related changes in one segment of the vascular bed may differ from that of another, as a consequence of differences in the vessel's structure. This may account for the finding that, unlike central (elastic) arteries, muscular arteries do not become stiffer during aging. It is the fragmentation and calcification of elastin and an increase in collagen that greatly contribute to the increased stiffness in the central arteries [4]. Intimal thickening is common in central arteries and is due in part to smooth muscle cell invasion. In aging rats, VSMCs necrosis also has been documented in cerebral arteries [37].

Coronary Artery Characteristics in the "Very Elderly"

Individuals who have lived more than 90 years are more likely to have coronary arteries that have been spared some of the disease processes that often occur in middle age and later. Thus, their vessels may be more representative of the processes of "normal" biological aging. Waller and Morgan [38] considered the aging changes in the hearts of 77 individuals aged 90–103 years based on observations at necropsy; the alterations in the coronary arteries are summarized in Fig. 7.1. All hearts were characterized by tortuous epicardial arteries. In 92% of the hearts, coronary arteries had calcium deposits; and in 64%, coronary artery narrowing exceeding 75% of the cross-sectional area was noted. Cardiac anatomical abnormalities found in 76 of the 77 cases included cardiomegaly in 69% of the individuals.

Microvascular Alterations

Considerable evidence now supports the role of a decline in NO in microvascular aging (reviewed in [39]). There appears to be general agreement that reduced NO bioavailability is a major cause of age-related impairment of vascular reactivity. There is currently an increased interest in the roles of hydrogen peroxide and peroxynitrite in the aging microvasculature. Cerebral microvessels in senescent rats show increases in the production of protein carbonyls, higher glutathione peroxidase, and decreased metalloproteinase (MMP-2) activity [40]. These changes may enhance the propensity of cerebral diseases. A review by Riddle and colleagues [41] cites evidence for microvascular rarefaction and a loss of plasticity in some regions of the brain, which contribute to a decline in cerebral blood flow. Cerebral arterioles in old rats are characterized by atrophy and decreased distensibility. Cerebral perfusion abnormalities in senescent rats may be due a combination of (1) changes in microvascular intrinsic tone, (2) decreased arteriolar density, and (3) arteriole-to-arteriole anastomoses [42]. A decrease in renal cortical microvessels has also been found in senescent mice [43]. Aging of cutaneous microvascular cells involves attenuation of proliferation, which limits growth responses to injury [44].

Structural Changes in Coronary Arteries and Arterioles During Aging

Lumen Diameter, Density, and Wall Thickness

Arteries

My colleagues and I studied the left anterior descending coronary artery (LAD) and its first branch from beagles aged 1 and 11 years [45]. Although lumen diameters were similar in the young and old beagles, medial wall thickness in the old group was more than double that of the young beagles and thus resulted in large increases in wall/lumen ratios. Morphometric analysis revealed that the increased wall thickness was a consequence of an increase in both VSMCs and interstitium. The largest contributor to the enhanced wall thickness was the interstitium, which was characterized by enhancement of collagen; compared to the young beagles, collagen was sevenfold and tenfold higher in the LAD and its first branch, respectively. These changes are illustrated in Fig. 7.2. An increase in collagen in the media of coronary arteries is a structural alteration that contributes to coronary arterial stiffness, which is significantly increased in humans aged 60 and older [46]. Coronary wall thickening, determined by magnetic resonance imaging, has also been shown to be age related [47]. The increase in wall thickness did not alter lumen diameter, indicating an outward vessel remodeling consistent with the beagle study. Lumen diameter, determined at necropsy, was also found to be unchanged in an aged

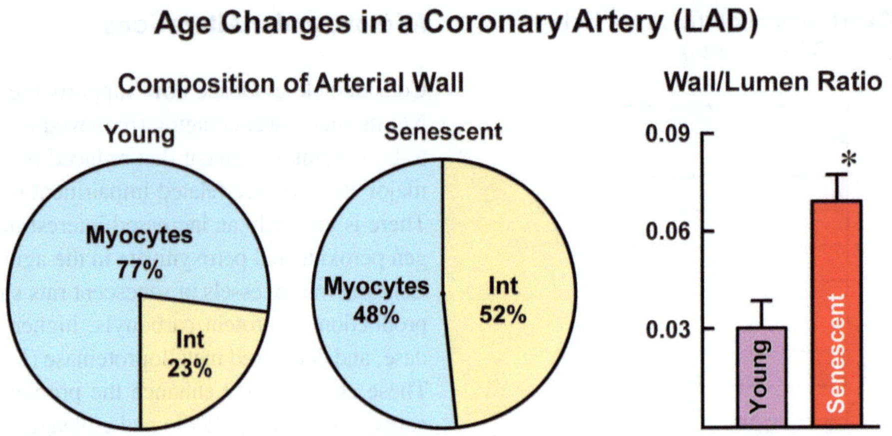

Fig. 7.2 Composition of the left anterior descending coronary artery (LAD) wall in beagles aged 1 year (young) and 11 years (old). The percent of the tunica media occupied by interstitium (primarily connective tissue) in the old is more than double that found in young beagles. Moreover, the thickness of the coronary artery wall in relation to its luminal diameter is increased more than twofold in the old group. Lumen diameters are similar in the two groups. *Asterisks*, statistically significant ($p<0.001$). The data are from Tomanek et al. Circ. Res. 69:1068, 1991 [45]

population [48]. Postmortem analysis of coronary wall structure also revealed thicker tunica medias in the vessels from 55 to 74-year-old subjects compared to an 18–24-year-old group; this increase was largely due to an abundant extracellular matrix and collagen [49]. The authors concluded that the increased wall/lumen ratios were related to a lower circumferential stress and that this factor contributed to a higher frequency of necrotic atheromas.

Arterioles

The study on old beagles [45], cited above, documented that in contrast to arteries, wall/lumen ratios of various lumen size arteriolar classes from <15 to 50 μm were similar to the 1 year beagles in both the midmyocardium and endomyocardium. However, studies in rodents have provided evidence of age-related arteriolar changes. In rats, wall/lumen ratio was increased slightly in most size classes of arterioles between middle age (15 months) and senescence (24 months), with the most significant change occurring in the endomyocardium [124]. Another study also found that arteriolar wall thickness increased between 11 and 16 months in this species, whereas arteriolar density remained stable during this period of life [50]. An analysis of rat coronary arteriolar length densities of two size classes revealed that between 12 and 20 months of age decreases in this parameter occurred in the 6–20 μm but not 21–40 μm range [107]. The decrease was significant in all three layers of the LV: epimyocardium, midmyocardium, and endomyocardium, and appears to be related to an absolute decrease in the number of the 6–20-μm diameter arterioles because their aggregate length was decreased during this period of life. In mice, a decrease in arteriolar density and an increase in wall thickness, coupled with an increase in lumen diameter between 2 and 21 months, were reported [51]. Since the young mice were not yet adults, it is possible that some of the change may have transpired during maturation.

Cellular Changes in the Vascular Wall

Cellular breakdown in the coronary arterial walls of rats was found to increase with aging [52]. Using electron microscopy, the study noted deposits of granules, vesicles, myelin figures and other debris in both the intima and media. The authors suggested that during aging, cells of the tunica media die and phagocytosis becomes inadequate, which leads to deposition of these breakdown products. In addition, the study demonstrated the presence of periadventitial (veil) cells containing phagosomes. One possible contributor to vascular aging may be changes in lifestyle. At least the suggestion that a decline in activity may accelerate arterial aging is indicated by data on captive, caged, Rhesus monkeys aged <20 or 30 years [53]. Coronary arterial sclerosis is characterized by dilation, remarkable wall thinning and muscle atrophy of the tunica media, and an increase in fibrosis. Since atherosclerotic changes are similar to those of aging, Patek and colleagues [54] addressed the susceptibility of old coronary arteries to atherosclerosis. They found that arteries of 24-month-old rats contained some vacuoles and occasional splitting of the internal elastic lamina. However, within 1 week after intravascular injection of carbon, lesions of arterial wall were noted, namely internal elastic lamina rupture and proliferation and smooth muscle reorientation. In 5-month-old rats, similar changes required a minimum of 5 months to develop. These findings indicate that coronary arteries become less resistant to damage with age.

Neural Changes

Compared to young (3 month), senescent (24 month) rats have fewer dopamine D2 receptors in the walls of their coronary arteries [55]. This decline occurred in large, medium, and small coronary arteries. These receptors were found on nerve fibers, mostly in the epicardium and myocardium, and to a lesser degree in the endocardium. Although the consequences of this receptor loss have not been elucidated, dopexamine (a dopamine analog) has been shown to decrease systemic vascular resistance [56]. This finding suggests that a loss of these dopamine receptors could contribute to an attenuated vasodilation in older individuals. A decrease in sympathetic nerve fibers in the coronary arteries of senescent rats has also been established [57], as has a decline in noradrenergic innervation of large, medium, and small coronary arteries [58].

Extracellular Changes

As recently reviewed [59], cardiac fibrosis is an aging characteristic which leads to a progressive increase in ventricular stiffness and impaired diastolic function. The literature is mainly focused on cardiac remodeling, healing, and heart failure with less attention given to the role of fibrosis in coronary vascular function. Nevertheless, perivascular fibrosis involving accumulation of collagen types I and III surrounding coronary arteries and arterioles has been demonstrated in patients with hypertensive heart disease [60, 61]. In patients with arterial hypertension, the loss of coronary vasodilator reserve and periarterial fibrosis was double that in normotensive subjects and correlated with minimal coronary vascular resistance [60]. In hypertensive patients treated with the ACE inhibitor perindopril, perivascular arteriolar collagen was markedly reduced and coronary reserve improved, despite no significant decrease in arteriolar wall area [62]. These data indicate that perivascular fibrosis, independent of wall thickness, contributes to a reduced coronary vasodilatory capacity in patients with hypertension. Similarly, pressure overload via aortic constriction [63], renovascular hypertension [64], and salt-loading in spontaneously hypertensive rats (SHR) [65] cause fibrosis and decreased coronary reserve. These data support the idea that the coronary perivascular fibrosis that occurs during aging is a likely contributor to diminished coronary vasodilator reserve in the elderly.

Functional Changes in Coronary Arteries and Arterioles During Aging

Endothelial Dysfunction

Endothelial dysfunction is common to many types of vessels and vascular beds, as noted earlier in this chapter. Coronary arteries undergo alterations similar to those found in other vascular beds. In isolated porcine coronary arteries, noradrenaline-induced endothelial-dependent relaxation to noradrenaline in the presence of propanolol was lower in aged (3–4 years) than in young (4–6 months) pigs [75]. The independent relaxation to noradrenaline, via α2-adrenoceptor was attenuated by aging. Thus, vascular aging may affect the sympathetic regulation of coronary vascular tone by attenuating endothelium-dependent relaxation via adrenoceptors. Cultured coronary arteries from senescent (26 month) rats had 5 times the number of apoptotic ECs compared to those from young (3 month) rats [66]. Moreover, the arteries from the senescent group had greater expression of tumor necrosis factors (both TNF-α and TNF-β) and caspase 3 activities. When TNF was inhibited or NO was blocked, apoptotic cell death was decreased. These data lend support to the hypothesis that decreased levels of NO in the aged coronary arteries may lead to impaired endothelial function in the elderly. Further support for this conclusion comes from data derived from cultured porcine arterial ECs [67]. Senescence in these cells, produced by multiple passaging for up to 4 weeks, was associated with decreased NO production, with a decline in several signaling pathways, activation of apoptotic pathways, and increased oxidative stress.

Impairment of Vasodilation

Adenosine Release and Coronary Responses

Aging is associated with changes in vasoreactivity that are, for the most part, similar to those seen in other vascular beds. Many studies have documented impaired coronary artery vasoreactivity during aging. Vasodilation in response to adenosine in 12–18-month-old rats was shown to be significantly lower than in rats aged 3–4 months [68]. This reduction in vasodilatory response may be a consequence of maturation as suggested by Jenner [69], who found that adenosine A_3, but not A_{2B}, receptor responses were lower in 1-year-old than in 4-month-old rats. To compare the effects of senescence on responses to adenosine Fischer 344 X Brown Norway hybrid rats, a strain known to show aging effects without the confounding effects of disease was studied [70]. The data revealed that adenosine A_1 and A_2 receptor-mediated effects on coronary flow were similar in aged (24–26 months) and young adult (4–6 months) rats. Adenosine production was compared in the hearts of young and old Fischer 344 rats [71, 72]. Adenosine release after adrenergic stimulation was attenuated in old rats compared to their young counterparts, due in part to a reduced mitochondrial AMP synthesis [72].

Responses to Catecholamines

Data from old (12 years) beagles indicate that the vasodilatory response of coronary arteries induced by isoproterenol is less compared to their young adult (2 years) counterparts, whereas norepinephrine-induced contractions were greater [73]. The attenuated relaxation induced by isoproterenol noted in the senescent group occurred in large and medium-sized arteries, but not in small arteries. Similarly, in older patients (68–86 years), noradrenaline induced significant contraction, but had either no effect or evoked only a weak contraction in coronary arteries in young (aged 23–58 years) patients [74]. In contrast, contraction induced by endothelin-1 did not differ in the two groups. Attenuation of adrenaline-induced vasodilation via the α-2 adrenoceptor in coronary arteries in old, compared to young pigs, has also been reported [75]. Moreover, the data revealed a relationship between the decrease in vasodilation and fatty streaks.

Impaired Acetylcholine-Induced Vasodilation

Coronary vasodilation in patients with normal coronary arteries, but atypical chest pains, was addressed in a study that determined increases in blood flow in response to various doses of acetylcholine [76]. Although the increase in coronary blood flow varied widely among the patients, it correlated negatively with age ($r=-0.86$). Machii et al. [77] tested the hypothesis that the age-related decline in arteriolar relaxation in response to acetylcholine is a consequence of increases in myocardial-derived angiotensin and H_2O_2. They found that the supernatant from isolated, paced cardiomyocytes from senescent rats contained more H_2O_2, less catalase and a lower SOD activity than that from the young rats. When the supernatant was placed on isolated arterioles, acetylcholine-induced relaxation was less in arterioles from the old rats than in those from a young group. In sum, these data demonstrate that aging alters cardiomyocyte metabolic properties, which then impair NO-dependent vasodilation in coronary arterioles.

The vasodilatory dose–response to acetylcholine was evaluated in patients with no history of arterial hypertension or hypercholesterolemia and with angiographically normal coronary arteries [78]. In patients aged 22–60 years, the acetylcholine-induced vasodilator capacity of the coronary microvasculature decreased with advancing age ($r=0.62$). Another study compared two groups of patients aged 9–29 and 31–68 years to determine if the vasodilatory response of coronary arteries was blunted in the older group [79]. Heart rate was maintained constant, while acetylcholine was injected into the left coronary artery. The data indicated that acetylcholine dilated all segments except the proximal segment in the young group, whereas it constricted most segments of the LAD in the older group. However, since the responses to the endothelium-independent vasodilator nitroglycerin were similar in the two age groups, the data suggest that endothelial dysfunction may underlie the constrictor effects to acetylcholine in the older patients.

Impaired Flow-Induced Vasodilation

Investigations on flow-induced signaling have documented impairment with aging, e.g., a decline in flow-induced NO production has been found in senescent rats [80]. Coronary arterioles from senescent rats have a reduced expression of eNOS and Cox-1 and an enhanced expression of iNOS in the endothelium [25]. The study also demonstrated that although increases in flow elicit NO synthesis and release, NO bioavailability is decreased, which can lead to impaired N-mediated vasodilation. In female rats, flow-induced NO, but not H_2O_2, was lower in coronary arterioles of senescent rats compared to those of young adults [81]. Removal of H_2O_2 with catalase reduced flow-induced vasodilation in both age groups, indicating that it, as well as NO, is critical for flow-induced vasodilation. The investigators concluded that the decline in NO-mediated vasodilation is a consequence, at least in part, from impaired ROS and in particular to O_2^-. An important finding in this regard is that the increased biological activity of superoxide rather than the decrease in the enzyme that produces NO accounts for the reduced myocardial O_2 consumption by NO in senescent rats [82]. Accordingly, these findings implicate oxidative stress in age-related changes in both cardiac function and altered regulation of vascular tone. Although reactive oxygen species play a role in flow-mediated dilation [83], excess vascular oxidative stress reduces NO availability and functions as a vascular stressor [84].

Arteriolar vasodilation also occurs via VEGF stimulation, as documented in a study that compared senescent and young rats [85]. The data showed that the flow-dependent vasodilation is NO mediated and that impaired VEGFR-2-mediated PI3-kinase/Akt signaling contributes to the attenuated vasodilation in senescent rats. Flow-stimulated VEGFR-2 phosphorylation in the arterioles from the senescent rats was lower compared to those from their young counterparts. These data are consistent with those from humans that revealed that VEGF-induced vasodilation in patients aged >70 years is decreased compared to patients aged <70 years [86]. Moreover, the mobilization of progenitor cells in the older group was decreased.

Arteries and Arterioles Differ in Vasodilatory Responses

The vasoactive responses of arterioles differ in some respects from those of arteries. One point of consideration is the finding that in coronary arteries, anaerobic metabolism predominates, whereas in arterioles, aerobic metabolism is higher [87, 88]. In aged rats, SDH and NADHD (respiratory chain metabolism marker $NADH_2$-tetrazolium reductase) are decreased in both coronary arteries and arterioles, indicating reduced aerobic metabolism [88]. Coronary arterioles also undergo a decline in SDH. However, ATPase is increased in the arteries, but decreased in arterioles.

Altered Vasoconstrictor Responses

Several studies have documented age-associated enhanced contractility of coronary arteries in senescent rats [89–91]. In Wistar Kyoto rats aged 2 years, serotonin induced a concentration-dependent contraction that was greater than that in their 3-month-old counterparts [90]. These enhanced responses were found to rely on both (1) a serotonin receptor agonist affinity and (2) the efficiency of the excitation–contraction coupling process [89]. Contractile responses to endothelin-1 and KCl, as well as serotonin, were also found to increase in rat coronary arteries between 12 and 72 weeks of age [91]. In small coronary arteries of senescent rats, stretch-induced spontaneous tone was higher than in 3-month-old rats and was further increased after endothelial denudation [92]. Moreover, the arteries of the senescent rats had a greater contractile response to 5-hydroxytryptamine (5-HT) than their young counterparts, a finding that the investigators attributed to an augmented contractile response to Ca^{2+}. These findings are consistent with data from isolated coronary arteries that revealed greater contractile responses to 5-HT in both the proximal and distal segments of the arteries from senescent rats compared to those from young rats [89]. The greater sensitivity to 5-HT in arteries of senescent rats could be accounted for by an increase in 5-HT2 receptor affinity for 5-HT.

The exaggerated responses to endothelin-1 in arteries from senescent rats have been shown to be associated with increased levels of Ca^{2+} sensitive PKC α,β and βII [93]. Consistent with these data, endothelin-1 caused a greater impairment of coronary flow in isolated hearts from senescent than young adult rats [94]. This enhanced vasoconstriction to endothelin-1 was independent of the lower release of NO in the aged group. In contrast to these findings, the concentration-dependent contractions to endothelin-1 of coronary artery rings from dogs aged >9 years were fivefold lower than those from dogs aged <9 years [95]. However, contractility in the coronary artery rings in response to 5-hydroxytryptamine (5-HT) was sixfold higher in the older group. Thus, in this canine model, aging is associated with marked and opposite effects on coronary artery reactivity to these vasoconstrictors. Smooth muscle contractility per se was not altered by aging since contractile responses to KCl were not significantly different between the two groups. Unlike the greater contractility to endothelin-1 in coronary arteries of aged rats noted in most studies, arterioles from senescent rats were found to have a diminished contractility to this constrictor than arterioles from their young counterparts [96]. The attenuated response to endothelin-1 in the senescent rat arterioles was due primarily to augmented release of endothelial vasodilators since NO was higher in the older group and removal of the endothelium or L-NAME treatment enhanced the contractile responses to levels similar to those of the young rats.

Evidence for a possible molecular basis underlying basal and stimulated contraction of coronary vessels is derived from studies that have documented changes in large conductance voltage and Ca^{2+}-activated K^+ (BK_{Ca}) channels. An age-related decrease in channel density was found in the coronary arteries of old rats, and a decrease in channel protein expression was also noted in 61–70-year-old humans compared to those aged 19–56 [97]. Coronary VSMC α subunit protein reduction and a corresponding loss of β1 transcripts of these channels were found in senescent rats and considered to have a major impact on basal, and possibly stimulated, coronary contraction [98]. The authors concluded that the age-related reduction in the large conductance, voltage- and Ca 2^+-activated K^+ channels involves a parallel decrease in alpha and beta 1 functional expression. The alpha and beta BK_{Ca} channel subunits in senescent rat arteries were significantly lower than those in young rats and their contractile responses to iberiotoxin were only 30% of those of their younger counterparts [99]. Basal tone, as well as calcium-dependent tone, was lower in coronary arteries from old compared to young rats. Taken together, these changes increase the risk of coronary artery spasm, myocardial ischemia an infarct in the elderly [100].

Functional Changes in Coronary Arteries and Arterioles: Conclusions

Impairment of vasodilation, largely due to endothelial dysfunction, and enhanced contractile response are age-related factors that limit coronary reserve. Limited angiogenesis, reduced NO availability, and oxidative stress are contributing factors to myocardial perfusion abnormalities. The changes that occur during aging differ with regard to the type of coronary vessel.

Changes in the Capillary Bed During Aging

Capillary Density is Reduced in Senescence

A decline in capillary density with age has been documented in several studies in rats [101–106], mice [51], and dogs [45]. The decline in this parameter is not usually uniform throughout the heart, as it has been shown to occur in the endomyocardium, but not in the epimyocardium [103], and in the apex and mid-LV, but not at the base [105]. Anversa et al. [107] found that following a reduction between 4 and 12 months of age, capillary density in rats increased by 20 months. The increase in total number of capillary profiles across the both ventricular

Fig. 7.3 Aging in myocardial capillaries in beagles includes a reduction in capillary length density, which is significant ($p<0.001$) in the endocardium. In contrast, capillary diameter is increased by 30% and affects an increase in capillary volume density. These changes also show a trend in the midmyocardium. *Asterisks*, statistically significant ($p<0.01$). The data are from Tomanek et al. Circ. Res. 69:1068, 1991 [45]

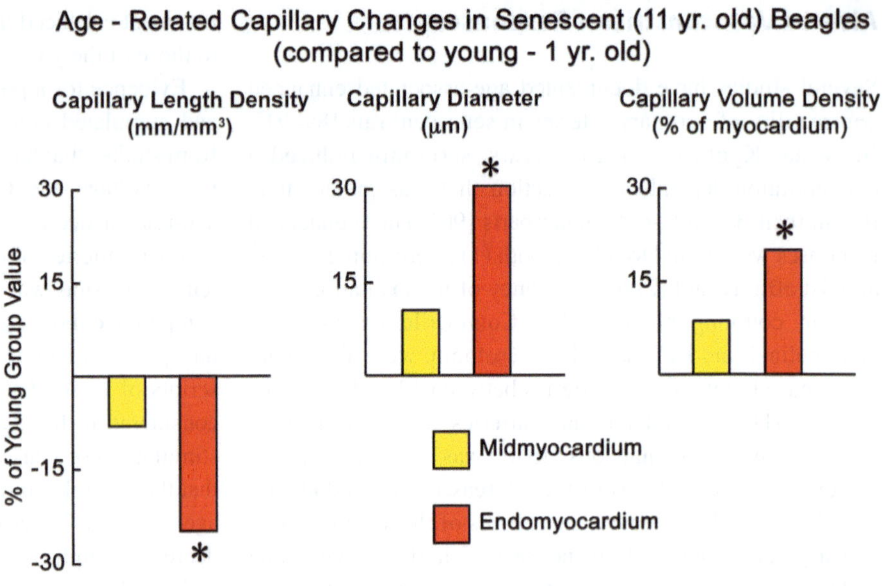

walls in the older age group indicates that capillary growth can occur late in life. Capillary recruitment as occurs during hypoxia is also limited by age as documented in a study on rats using cinemicrophotography of beating hearts [108]. This decline, which occurs between 4 and 12 months, results in a greater diffusion distance during increased O_2 demand. As illustrated in Fig. 7.3, capillary remodeling in the hearts of the old beagles (11 years of age) is indicted by the finding that length density of these vessels was lower in the endomyocardium, whereas volume density was slightly higher [45]. Thus, a significant increase in capillary diameters, in the face of a lower length density, provided an adaptation allowing normalization of capillary volume.

Mechanisms of Impaired Angiogenesis

The decrease in capillary density in the senescent heart is primarily due to impaired angiogenesis, which could be due to a variety of age-related impairments, such as a decrease in signaling events. Capillary growth can be stimulated in the myocardia of senescent rats, as indicated by experiments in which cardiac hypertrophy (an increase in heart weight/body weight ratio of 44 %) was induced by injections of thyroxine in 24-month-old rats [109]. In this model, capillary growth was proportional to the increase in heart mass, as indicated by volume and surface densities, and intercapillary distances that were similar to those of non-hypertrophic hearts. The lower age-related capillary densities noted in many studies may be largely due to down regulation of VEGF and VEGFR-2, as documented by Besse et al. [106]. These investigators found that in 24-month-old rats (1) growth factor and receptor was reduced and (2) intramyocardial protein therapy with $VEGF_{165}$-induced angiogenesis in these senescent rat hearts was similar to that induced in those aged 3 months. In vitro studies on aging of myocardial microvascular cells also provide data that indicate a link between decreased VEGF gene activation and impaired angiogenesis [110, 111]. Compared to microvascular endothelial cells from 3-month-old rats, those from rats aged 24 months displayed impaired angiogenesis, reduced VEGF protein, and reduced transport of HIF-1α to the nucleus and binding to the VEGF gene promoter [110]. Activation of VEGF gene expression by AMPK (activated protein kinase) was shown to enhance angiogenesis by 2.1-fold and VEGF mRNA by 3.7-fold in the microvascular ECs from the senescent rats [111]. The study also revealed that the treatment caused MAPK/Erk ½ phosphorylation, a finding that suggests this event as a likely mechanism for the improved angiogenesis.

In vitro experiments are an alternative approach to study the effects of aging on the responsiveness of ECs. Work by Garfinkel et al. [112] compared EC proliferation and migration in presenescent (<25 cell doublings) and senescent (60 cell doublings) human umbilical vein endothelial cells (HUVECs). They found that tyrosine phosphorylation of FGF-1 substrates Src and cortactin was impaired in senescent HUVECs, and they were unable to migrate in response to FGF-1, thus implicating the attenuation of the FGF-1 signal transduction pathway in the impairment of proliferation and migration of ECs. Consistent with these findings is the discovery that bovine aortic ECs from senescent cell passages also impaired migration and proliferation, which can be normalized by treatment with FGF-2 [113].

-

Taken together, the data indicate that aging is associated with a decreased capillary density due to limitations in the angiogenesis. The proliferative capacity of ECs, however, is not precluded, but rather is due to an inadequate evoking stimulus, e.g., VEGF, HiF-1α, and FGF.

Effects of Aging on Myocardial Perfusion

Data from Humans

Attenuation of coronary vasodilator reserve, as demonstrated by the hyperemic response, has been reported in healthy volunteers aged 70 years and older [114]. The study also found that after the age of 60, both resting flow and systolic pressure are increased. Data from 26 asymptomatic patients denote a lower coronary blood flow evoked by acetylcholine in patients ≥50 years of age than in those <50 years of age, and that papaverine also evoked a smaller increase in blood flow in the older compared to the younger patients [115]. The relationship between increases in coronary flow to acetylcholine and papaverine was inversely correlated with age.

Data from Experimental Animals

Maximal Perfusion and Coronary Reserve

Data from experimental animals have demonstrated that myocardial perfusion is attenuated during the aging process. More than 4 decades ago, Weisfeldt and colleagues [116] showed that maximal coronary flow in isolated hearts was lower in senescent rats (24–27 months) than in their counterparts aged 12 months. Myocardial O_2 consumption during baseline conditions was similar in the two groups, but under severe hypoxia, O_2 extraction was reduced in the senescent group and was associated with an attenuated increase in coronary blood flow/g heart weight. A reduction in maximal myocardial perfusion in both LV and RV, measured with microspheres in rats, was documented in both 12- and 20-month-old rats compared to a group aged 4 months [117]. This perfusion attenuation was noted in both the endomyocardium and epimyocardium, but was more marked in the former. Moreover, coronary reserve was impaired in the oldest group and the impairment was significantly greater in the LV than the RV. We [109, 118] and others [119, 120] also found that coronary reserve was significantly impaired in senescent rats compared to those in young adult rats.

The coronary response to cold stress was compared in young (25 ± 1 years) and older (65 ± 2 years) healthy adults by exposing the subjects to a 20-min bout of whole body cold stress [121]. Cooling increased ventricular wall stress (a determinant of myocardial O_2 consumption) in both groups, but the magnitude of the increase was twofold greater in the older group. However, coronary vasodilation occurred only in the young adults and coronary perfusion time fraction decreased in the old, but not in the young adult group. Similarly, a cold air inhalation for 5 min, combined with an isometric handgrip for 2 min, revealed that old, but not young subjects had an accentuated heart rate–pressure product without a concomitant increase in coronary blood flow velocity [122]. These findings suggest a disassociation between oxygen supply and demand in the hearts of older individuals.

Endothelial Dysfunction and Flow Recovery

Endothelial function has been shown to be a factor in the age-related decline in capacity of coronary flow recovery and the release of NO after prolonged cardioplegic arrest [123]. Coronary blood flow was measured in isolated hearts of rats before and after a 4-h cardioplegic arrest. Recovery of flow (difference between pre- and postischemic values) decreased with age. Responses to 5-hydroxytryptamine (% increase in flow) declined with age, especially between 5 and 15 months. The postischemic values were lowest in the 26 month old group. The decline in flow in response to L-NMMA (an inhibitor of NO production) was less impaired in the 15- and 26-month age groups, indicating that aging was associated with an abnormality in endothelial function. In contrast, flow increases in response to the endothelial-independent vasodilator, glyceryl trinitrate, either before or after ischemia, was not affected by aging.

> In conclusion, many studies have shown that aging is characterized by myocardial perfusion abnormalities, due at least in part to endothelial dysfunction. Both maximal myocardial perfusion and coronary vasodilator reserve are attenuated during aging.

Hypertension, Atherosclerosis, and Aging

Hypertension

Hypertension, as noted earlier in this chapter, has been reported to mimic some of the changes seen in the aging heart and its vasculature. For example, residual bodies (lipofuscin granules), characteristic of aging cells, accumulated more markedly in cardiomyocytes of SHR than in the normotensive controls during the life span [103]. We tested the hypothesis that late onset hypertension evokes both myocardial and vascular remodeling and limits the size of the coronary vasculature [118, 124, 125]. Renal hypertension (one kidney with a figure 8 wrap) was induced in middle-aged (12 month) and old (21 month) rats and the rats were studied 3 months later. Both groups of hypertensive rats exhibited (1) loss of cardiomyocytes, with hypertrophy of surviving cardiomyocytes and (2) increases in wall to lumen ratios of the smallest arterioles (<15–25 μm) and large decrements in capillary density.

Both aging and hypertension in this model were also found to compromise maximal myocardial perfusion and

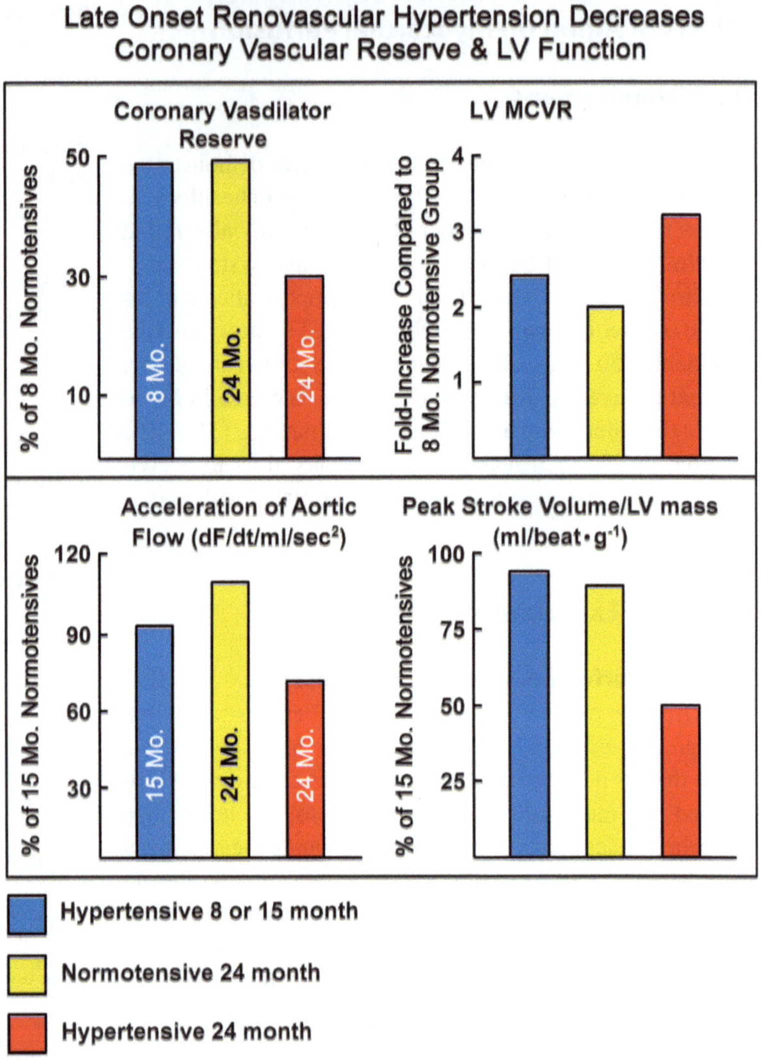

Fig. 7.4 Aging and hypertension each cause impairments in coronary reserve and maximal myocardial perfusion (*top panel*). Coronary vasodilator reserve in 24-month-old normotensive rats is only 50% of that of 8-month-old normotensive rats. This is the same degree of impairment seen in 8-month-old rats that are hypertensive. Similar increases in minimal coronary vascular resistance (MCVR) occur in these two groups. Imposition of hypertension late in life (at 21 months of age) causes a further reduction in coronary vasodilator reserve and an increase in MCVR. The data are from Tomanek et al. Am. J. Physiol. 264:H1854, 1993 [118]. The *bottom panel* illustrates the changes in cardiac function associated with aging and hypertension. Note that peak stroke volume is little affected by aging, but is compromised in the old (24 month), but not middle-aged (15 month) hypertensive rats. The data are from Tomanek et al. Am. J. Physiol. 262:H538, 1992 [125]

coronary reserve [118]. These changes (summarized in Fig. 7.4) occurred despite the fact that systolic arterial pressure in the rats with renal hypertension was normalized midway through the 3-month experimental period and that LV/body weight ratios were similar to those of the normotensive rats. Ventricular function (stroke index, stroke volume, and dP/dt) was depressed in senescent (24 month), but not middle-aged (15 month) rats with renovascular hypertension [125]. Hypertension evoked ventricular remodeling in both senescent and middle-aged rats, as indicated by cardiomyocyte loss, hypertrophy of surviving cardiomyocytes, and myocardial fibrosis. These changes were more marked in the senescent group. Similarly, Isoyama et al. [126] found that pressure overload induced by banding the ascending aorta decreased maximal myocardial perfusion and coronary reserve in both young (7 month) and old (18 month) rats. However, a marked twofold cardiac hypertrophy occurred in the young rats, whereas hypertrophy did not occur in the old rats. Thus, the attenuation of coronary reserve in young rats can be attributed, at least for the most part, to increased heart mass. In contrast, the limited coronary reserve in the aged rats was associated with the increased arterial pressure.

Further supportive evidence that aging and hypertension contribute to vascular alterations that underlie impairments of myocardial perfusion comes from SHR [50]. Maximal myocardial perfusion in both normotensive WKY and SHR were found to decline during the aging process, but the decline was greater in SHR than in WKY. An increase in wall/lumen ratio of arterioles <50 μm in the senescent (22 month) SHR and WKY was reported; the increase was 30% greater in the SHR. These data reveal that arteriolar remodeling occurring as a component of the aging process and in response to hypertension is a structural change that contributes to impaired maximal myocardial perfusion. The age effect occurs in SHR and WKY between 1 and 2 years since vasodilator reserve in SHR is attenuated during developing and peak cardiac hypertrophy at 7 months of age, but improves after the hypertrophy is stabilized at 12 months [127].

In conclusion, age-related changes, such as a reduced coronary vasodilator reserve, in the coronary vasculature are similar, to those of hypertension. Moreover, hypertension exacerbates aging changes and is less tolerated in the aged.

Effects of Age on Ischemia and Myocardial Infarction

Ischemia/Reperfusion

Both prevalence and mortality of ischemic heart disease is increased in the elderly as cardiomyocytes undergo several cellular and molecular changes (reviewed in [128]). Myocardial tolerance to ischemia and hypoxia is reduced in humans older than 60 years, as documented in atrial pectinate trabeculae from patients harvested during surgery [129]. Recovery of developed force in these muscle specimens, compared to patients ≤59 years in age, was only 75% in the 60–69 year group and 53% in the 70–89 year group. The incidence of death for patients undergoing surgery (n = 13,625) increased dramatically after the age of 70 years [130]. In the 60–69 age group, mortality was 1.9% and rose to 5.0% and 8.3% in the next 2 decades. The effects of a graded reduction in myocardial perfusion pressure, resulting in ischemia, were compared in isolated hearts from adult and senescent rats [131]. In hearts from senescent rats, developed pressure recovered more slowly, even though coronary flow was restored. These data suggest that the ischemic threshold was not altered in the senescent rats, but that rats were more vulnerable to myocardial stunning.

The effect of aging on ischemic tolerance was investigated in isolated hearts from mice aged 2 to 28 months subjected to ischemia/reperfusion [132]. Postischemic flow recovery declined during postnatal maturation (first 8 months of postnatal life). After that point, the greatest decline in postischemic flow recovery occurred between 12 months and 24–28 months and was preceded by an increase in LDH efflux, a marker on oncosis, at 12 months. On the other hand, developed pressure during recovery was already lower in 12- than in 8-month-old mice and did not decrease further with aging. A decrease in ischemic tolerance in rat hearts was also found to occur by 50 months of age and was exacerbated by 100 months, based on evidence of irreversible cardiomyocyte damage and a lower recovery of function [133]. Taken together, the data signify that recovery of flow is not necessarily impaired by aging. Rather, most of the ischemia-related structural and functional defects appear to be the result of cardiomyocyte maladaptations to the stress of ischemia. One such change is DNA fragmentation and higher levels of Bcl-2 and Bax proteins at baseline in senescent compared to young adult rats [134].

Other maladaptations may include a defective sensing mechanism for ischemia in the aged heart, as suggested by diminished heat shock protein 70 mRNA induction [135]and ischemia-induced increases in intracellular Na^+ [133] and NO [136]. The latter may be of particular significance for several reasons. First both basal and stimulated release of NO is reduced in senescent rats [137]. Second, exercise-induced increases in eNOS in the senescent rat heart improved postischemic recovery [138]. Third, NO plays a key role in ischemic preconditioning [139]. Fourth, an age-related decrease in NO production is associated with an increase in cardiomyocyte apoptosis [136]. An enhanced sensitivity to ischemia was found as early as middle age (50 weeks) in rats [140]. Hearts of middle-aged rats subjected to global ischemia followed by reperfusion had greater decreases in left ventricular systolic pressure, ATP and LV peak positive dP/dt, and peak negative dP/dt compared to the hearts of the young rats. In senescent (24 months) compared to adult (6 months) rats, ischemia/reperfusion caused greater injury, as evidenced by an increased release of creatine kinase, total protein, and lactate dehydrogenase (LDH).

The reduced capacity of cardiomyocytes to tolerate and adapt to ischemia during senescence is associated with impaired mitochondrial function, a topic reviewed by Pepe [141]. In aged rat hearts, mitochondrial inner membrane permeability to solutes causes swelling of the organelle, a proton leak and reduced efficacy of the respiratory chain, and oxidative phosphorylation uncoupling. Mitochondrial Ca^{2+} is elevated and, along with increased dehydrogenase activation, contributes to mitochondrial inefficiency. Age also has been shown to play a role in the remodeling of coronary arteries of patients with acute coronary syndrome [142]. A comparison of patients aged <60 vs. those 60 years and older revealed that age and remodeling index were inversely correlated and that low-density lipoproteins or triglycerides may be associated with attenuated remodeling in the aged patients.

In conclusion, myocardial tolerance to ischemia and hypoxia declines during the aging process. This reduced tolerance is linked to both structural and functional defects in cardiomyocytes, including mitochondrial and contractile impairments, as well as a decline in flow recovery following an ischemic event.

Ischemic Preconditioning

Data from Humans

Ischemic preconditioning, defined as brief ischemic episodes to protect the heart from future myocardial ischemia episodes, is discussed in Chap. 10. Most of the evidence from clinical and experimental studies indicates that preconditioning does not result in cardioprotection in the heart of the old individuals (reviewed in [128, 143–145]). Data from five studies comparing cardioprotection in young and aged patients revealed that only one of the five studies was able to show a protective effect of ischemic preconditioning in the elderly (reviewed in [128]).

The observation that prodromal angina may be protective by serving as a preconditioning event in older individuals was reported in several studies [146–149]. However, the findings from other studies are not in agreement. Evidence that this protection is lost in the elderly was based on data from 990 patients who underwent coronary angiography shortly before the onset of acute myocardial infarction [148]. It was concluded that prodromal angina was associated with cardioprotective effects (i.e., lower peak creatine kinase levels and lower in-hospital mortality rates) in patients <70, but not in those over the age of 70 years. Similarly, evaluation of 505 patients who experienced angina prior to acute MI revealed that those aged <65 years had a lower incidence of in-hospital deaths, congestive heart failure, or shock [146]. However, patients aged ≥65 years were less likely to benefit from prodromal angina. In contrast, a study on 557 elderly patients found that a high level of physical activity in those patients with preinfarction angina was strongly associated with a reduction in hospital mortality [150].

Data from Experimental Animals

Similarly, most data from experimental animals indicate that age limits or precludes the effects of ischemic preconditioning. Preconditioning was not cardioprotective in senescent rats that were calorie restricted [151]. Although preconditioning reduced infarct size in 12-month-old rats, this effect did not occur in 18–20-month-old rats [152]. Moreover, preconditioning had no effect on myocardial necrosis or contractile function in senescent (22 month) rats [153]. Reduced levels of connexin 43 (Cx43) may contribute to the loss of ischemic preconditioning in the aged heart [154], as evidenced by the finding that the reduction in infarct size is prevented by genetically reducing this protein in mice. In aged mice, Cx43 was decreased and was associated with the loss of cardioprotection provided by preconditioning.

Factors Influencing the Reduction in Cardioprotection

The age-dependent reduction in cardioprotection from ischemic preconditioning has been attributed to factors such as cardiac hypertrophy [155], diastolic dysfunction [156], and impaired angiogenesis [157]. More specifically, an age-related decline in catecholamine release [158] due to factors such as diminished catecholamine synthesis has been shown to occur in hearts of aged rats during ischemic preconditioning [159]. In this regard, exercise training may restore ischemic preconditioning-induced cardioprotection by increasing norepinephrine release. Age-related alterations in several proteins, key to the cardioprotective process, have been shown in the myocardium, e.g., bradykinin receptor, interleukin 6, heat shock protein, NOS, sodium–hydrogen exchanger, some mitogen-activated protein kinases, extracellular signal-regulated kinase, and p38 (reviewed in [128, 160]). A lack of appropriate genomic responses in the senescent myocardium to preconditioning may also limit or preclude cardioprotection, as indicated by a lack of expression in 31 of 32 genes concerning transcriptional regulation, growth regulation, cytokines, remodeling, and cell adhesion in 20–24-month-old rats [161]. Impaired activation of K_{ATP} channels in patients aged ≥65 years has been reported to cause the loss of preconditioning [162]. The conclusion is supported by data revealing the effectiveness of a K_{ATP} channel agonist (nicorandil) in mimicking the ischemic preconditioning effects.

Mitochondria play a major role in the links between ischemia damage, protection, and aging; see recent review by Wojtovich et al. [163]. The aged heart experiences large increases in ROS production and decreases in mitochondrial antioxidant defenses, which may limit ischemic preconditioning. Mitochondrial K_{ATP} channel is one critical component for ischemic preconditioning and has been shown to decline with aging in the rat heart [164]. Protein kinase C (PKC) mediates mitochondrial K_{ATP} and has been shown to contribute to ischemic preconditioning in young (12 weeks), but not middle-aged (50 weeks) rats, partly due to a failure to translocate PKC isoforms [165]. The finding that dysregulation of mitochondrial (1) Ox-Phos, (2) Ca^{2+} handling, and (3) ROS generation occur both in aging and ischemic-reperfusion injury suggests that molecular mechanisms underlying these phenomena are likely the same [163].

Conclusion Regarding Ischemic Preconditioning

Data from both humans and experimental animals support the conclusion that ischemic preconditioning is either not protective in the aged heart or that the protection is limited. Discrepancies in data from humans may be largely due to age groups studied. If the study considers subjects ≥70 years of age, the findings support the conclusion stated above, whereas if 60 years of age is the cutoff point, then some protection may be indicated. The age-associated reduction in cardioprotection is not surprising considering changes in gene expression, mitochondrial function, and impaired angiogenesis.

Myocardial Infarction

It is well known that elderly patients have an increased rate of mortality following a myocardial infarction. Age is the most significant factor influencing mortality 30 days after infarction [166], and the increased mortality rate occurs despite opening of coronary arteries by thrombolysis [167]. Data from 2,312 patients with acute MI indicate that those over the age of 79 years have mortality rates of 44 and 77% 28 days and 1 year, respectively, after an acute myocardial infarction [168] (Fig. 7.5). Hospital mortality for patients with first myocardial infarction is 1.9% for those 40 years or younger, but increases to 31.9% among those over the age of 80 years [169]. Findings in another study of 3,256 patients hospitalized for acute myocardial infarction indicate a jump in in-hospital mortality rates from 4.6% in the 55–64 age group to 12.3% in the 65–74 age group and 17.8% in those ≥75 years [170]. Moreover, cardiac rupture is more than fourfold greater in patients over the age of 70 compared to those aged ≤60. The susceptibility to myocardial ischemia/reperfusion injury has also been shown to be greater in the aged [171]. Senescent mice (22–24 months) had larger areas of infarcted myocardium and a greater extent of contraction band necrosis than the young adult (6–8 months) mice. Moreover, mortality was higher after ischemia and reperfusion in the senescent mice, as was DNA fragmentation.

Impairment of Growth Factors

Work by Edelberg et al. [172] has defined a platelet-derived growth factor-AB (PDGF-AB)-mediated communication between coronary microvascular ECs and cardiomyocytes, which revealed cardiomyocyte-inducted PDGF-B expression in ECs. Formation of the PDGF-AB heterodimer results in EC expression of VEGF and VEGFR-2. PDGF levels decrease during aging [173] and EC dysregulation of the PDGF communication pathway is linked to impaired angiogenesis in the senescent heart [174]. ECs from senescent mouse hearts did not express PDGF-B when cocultured with cardiomyocytes. In vivo experiments demonstrated that intramyocardial delivery of PDGF-AB promoted angiogenesis and minimized the extent of myocardial infarction in the hearts of senescent mice.

Collateral Circulation

Collateral circulations are known to increase myocardial salvage during ischemia and infarction [175–177], and therefore play a key role in recovery. The hypothesis that aging limits collateral flow to infarct-related artery in elderly patients with acute myocardial infarction was tested in 1,934 patients [178]. Advanced age was an independent predictive factor for limited collateral circulation to the infarct-related artery. The prevalence of collaterals in patients aged <50 years was 48%, but only 34% in those aged >70 years. Another study evaluated coronary collateral development in 102 patients within 12 h after the first acute myocardial infarction [179]. The prevalence of well-developed collateral circulation in patients ≤64 years was significantly higher (69%) compared to patients ≥65 years (39%). These studies suggest that the development of coronary collaterals is impaired during aging. Whether a rarefaction of collaterals occurs during the aging process is not evident from these studies involving myocardial ischemia. However, age-related collateral rarefaction in mice hindlimbs is suggested by the finding that a greater drop in perfusion occurred in 16-month-old mice compared to those aged 3 months immediately after femoral artery ligation [180]. Moreover, arteriolar density declined significantly between 24 and 31 months of age. Impairment of collateral vessel development with age in this model has also been documented in middle-aged (4–5 years) compared to young (6–8 months) rabbits [157]. Forty days after femoral artery resection, hindlimb perfusion and the number of angiographically visible vessels were lower in the older group of rabbits.

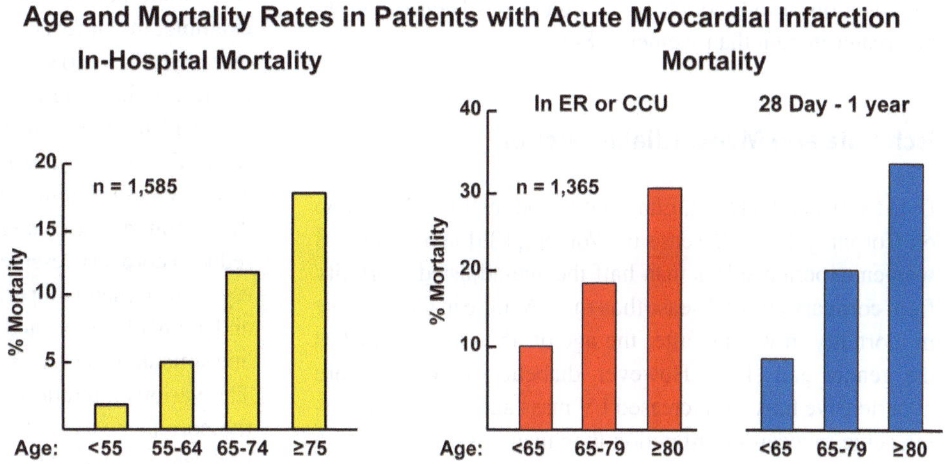

Fig. 7.5 Mortality rates increase with age in patients with acute myocardial infarctions. The data on in-hospital mortality are from Weaver et al. J. Am. Coll. Cardiol. 18:657, 1991 [170]. The data regarding mortality in the ER or CCU and 28 and 1 year follow-up are from Yang et al. Acta Cardiol. 42:59, 1987 [168]

-

Advanced age is a risk factor for survival from myocardial infarction and is associated with larger infarct size. Limitations in the size of the vascular bed in general and impairments in the development of the coronary collateral vessels in particular are contributing factors to the poor postinfarction outcomes in the elderly.

Influence of Gender on Aging of Coronary Vessels

Aging Processes in Myocardium and Coronary Vessels

It has long been recognized that males and females differ with regard to some cardiovascular parameters and susceptibility to disease (reviewed in [181]). For example, independent of age and menopause, myocardial remodeling is more favorable in females, whereas they are more likely to present with diastolic dysfunction. A morphometric study on hearts of individuals aged 17–95 years demonstrated that aging in women was associated with the preservation of the number of cardiomyocytes and ventricular mass [182]. In contrast, data from men indicated a substantial loss of cardiomyocytes with hypertrophy of the surviving cardiomyocytes during aging. A large retrospective analysis of patients in their mid-sixties with chronic stable angina compared men and women [183]. Women had a lower incidence of angina than men when their ejection fractions were above 55%, but a much higher incidence than men when ejection fractions were <45%. Moreover, an end systolic volume >43 ml/m^2 also was associated with a greater risk of heart failure in women than in men. The investigators concluded that a greater adverse remodeling in women contributed to the increased incidence of heart failure. The incidence of coronary artery calcification in individuals 65 and older has been shown to be greater in men than women [184].

Ischemia and Myocardial Infarction

Data from an NIH Heart, Lung and Blood Institute Workshop on Coronary Heart Disease in Women [185] show that US women experience less than half the age-adjusted mortality from coronary artery disease than men. A surge in the increase in mortality in women after the age of 45 years diminishes the gender gap [186]. However, diabetic women who are hypertensive have an increased LV mass and fare worse during acute myocardial infarction than men [187]. Similarly, a study regarding calcification of coronary arteries concluded that women with both diabetes and hypertension experience an increase in LV mass and fare worse during acute myocardial infarction than men [187]. Some of the differences in conclusions regarding gender and myocardial infarctions are most likely due to unadjusted mortality rates. For example, much of the greater early mortality after myocardial infarction in women can be explained by the older age in women who experience the infarctions [188]. Control for age and other factors indicate that the survival rates are higher for women than men.

The reduced tolerance to myocardial ischemia in the aged has also been confirmed in a study in mice exposed to 20 min of ischemia and 60 min of reperfusion [132]. Consistent with that study is the finding in rats that by 12 months of age the recovery of myocardial contractility (e.g., developed pressure) after ischemia/reperfusion was impaired. By 18 months, flow recovery was attenuated and decreased further in the 24–28-month age group. The data were similar for males and females with the exception that LDH efflux was greater in females. These findings indicate that age-related changes in myocardial ischemic tolerance develop before senescence.

-

In conclusion, there is evidence that males and females do not experience identical changes in the coronary vasculature during aging. The lower risk of coronary artery disease in women is lost after menopause and women then have less favorable outcomes after myocardial infarction than men if they have diabetes and hypertension.

Summary

Aging of the coronary vasculature is characterized by both structural and functional changes that are dependent on the specific coronary vessel type (i.e., large and small arteries, arterioles, and capillaries). For example, the fibrosis, due to increases in collagen and extracellular matrix in large arteries, is generally lacking in arterioles; in the latter, length density decreases and wall thickness increases. Endothelial dysfunction, reduced eNOS, impaired dilation, and augmented responses to calcium are also characteristic of aging in the coronary vasculature. These changes underlie a reduced coronary reserve. Ischemic tolerance and recovery from ischemia/reperfusion are impaired with aging and are likely associated with both limited angiogenesis and structural and functional changes in cardiomyocytes. The various alterations occurring during aging render the coronary vasculature and the heart less adaptable to diseases, such as hypertension.

References

1. Tomanek RJ, Karlsson UL. Myocardial ultrastructure of young and senescent rats. J Ultrastruct Res. 1973;42:201–20.
2. Brandes RP, Fleming I, Busse R. Endothelial aging. Cardiovasc Res. 2005;66:286–94.
3. Cosentino F, Osto E. Aging and endothelial dysfunction. Clin Hemorheol Microcirc. 2007;37:143–7.
4. Lee HY, Oh BH. Aging and arterial stiffness. Circ J. 2010;74: 2257–62.
5. Lakatta EG, Wang M, Najjar SS. Arterial aging and subclinical arterial disease are fundamentally intertwined at macroscopic and molecular levels. Med Clin North Am. 2009;93:583–604, table of contents.
6. Karavidas A, Lazaros G, Tsiachris D, Pyrgakis V. Aging and the cardiovascular system. Hellenic J Cardiol. 2010;51:421–7.
7. Edelberg JM, Reed MJ. Aging and angiogenesis. Front Biosci. 2003;8:s1199–209.
8. Hoenig MR, Bianchi C, Rosenzweig A, Sellke FW. Decreased vascular repair and neovascularization with ageing: mechanisms and clinical relevance with an emphasis on hypoxia-inducible factor-1. Curr Mol Med. 2008;8:754–67.
9. Marin J, Rodriguez-Martinez MA. Age-related changes in vascular responses. Exp Gerontol. 1999;34:503–12.
10. Marin J. Age-related changes in vascular responses: a review. Mech Ageing Dev. 1995;79:71–114.
11. Benetos A, Waeber B, Izzo J, Mitchell G, Resnick L, Asmar R, et al. Influence of age, risk factors, and cardiovascular and renal disease on arterial stiffness: clinical applications. Am J Hypertens. 2002;15:1101–8.
12. Wolinsky H. Long-term effects of hypertension on the rat aortic wall and their relation to concurrent aging changes. Morphological and chemical studies. Circ Res. 1972;30:301–9.
13. McEniery CM, Wilkinson IB, Avolio AP. Age, hypertension and arterial function. Clin Exp Pharmacol Physiol. 2007;34:665–71.
14. O'Rourke MF, Safar ME, Dzau V. The Cardiovascular Continuum extended: aging effects on the aorta and microvasculature. Vasc Med. 2010;15:461–8.
15. Minamino T, Miyauchi H, Yoshida T, Tateno K, Komuro I. The role of vascular cell senescence in atherosclerosis: antisenescence as a novel therapeutic strategy for vascular aging. Curr Vasc Pharmacol. 2004;2:141–8.
16. Erusalimsky JD, Kurz DJ. Cellular senescence in vivo: its relevance in ageing and cardiovascular disease. Exp Gerontol. 2005;40:634–42.
17. Campisi J, d'Adda di Fagagna F. Cellular senescence: when bad things happen to good cells. Nat Rev Mol Cell Biol. 2007;8:729–40.
18. Ogrunc M, di Fagagna F. Never-ageing cellular senescence. Eur J Cancer. 2011;47:1616–22.
19. Ogami M, Ikura Y, Ohsawa M, Matsuo T, Kayo S, Yoshimi N, et al. Telomere shortening in human coronary artery diseases. Arterioscler Thromb Vasc Biol. 2004;24:546–50.
20. Thorin E, Thorin-Trescases N. Vascular endothelial ageing, heartbeat after heartbeat. Cardiovasc Res. 2009;84:24–32.
21. Vanhoutte PM. Endothelial dysfunction: the first step toward coronary arteriosclerosis. Circ J. 2009;73:595–601.
22. Ungvari Z, Kaley G, de Cabo R, Sonntag WE, Csiszar A. Mechanisms of vascular aging: new perspectives. J Gerontol A Biol Sci Med Sci. 2010;65:1028–41.
23. Donato AJ, Eskurza I, Silver AE, Levy AS, Pierce GL, Gates PE, et al. Direct evidence of endothelial oxidative stress with aging in humans: relation to impaired endothelium-dependent dilation and upregulation of nuclear factor-kappaB. Circ Res. 2007;100:1659–66.
24. Cosentino F, Luscher TF. Maintenance of vascular integrity: role of nitric oxide and other bradykinin mediators. Eur Heart J. 1995;16(Suppl K):4–12.
25. Csiszar A, Ungvari Z, Edwards JG, Kaminski P, Wolin MS, Koller A, et al. Aging-induced phenotypic changes and oxidative stress impair coronary arteriolar function. Circ Res. 2002;90:1159–66.
26. Yildiz O. Vascular smooth muscle and endothelial functions in aging. Ann N Y Acad Sci. 2007;1100:353–60.
27. Sun M, Dawood F, Wen WH, Chen M, Dixon I, Kirshenbaum LA, et al. Excessive tumor necrosis factor activation after infarction contributes to susceptibility of myocardial rupture and left ventricular dysfunction. Circulation. 2004;110:3221–8.
28. Yang YM, Huang A, Kaley G, Sun D. eNOS uncoupling and endothelial dysfunction in aged vessels. Am J Physiol Heart Circ Physiol. 2009;297:H1829–36.
29. Collins C, Tzima E. Hemodynamic forces in endothelial dysfunction and vascular aging. Exp Gerontol. 2011;46:185–8.
30. Nichols WW, O'Rourke MF, Avolio AP, Yaginuma T, Murgo JP, Pepine CJ, et al. Effects of age on ventricular-vascular coupling. Am J Cardiol. 1985;55:1179–84.
31. Merillon JP, Motte G, Masquet C, Azancot I, Guiomard A, Gourgon R. Relationship between physical properties of the arterial system and left ventricular performance in the course of aging and arterial hypertension. Eur Heart J. 1982;3(Suppl A):95–102.
32. Virmani R, Avolio AP, Mergner WJ, Robinowitz M, Herderick EE, Cornhill JF, et al. Effect of aging on aortic morphology in populations with high and low prevalence of hypertension and atherosclerosis. Comparison between occidental and Chinese communities. Am J Pathol. 1991;139:1119–29.
33. Franklin SS, Gustin WT, Wong ND, Larson MG, Weber MA, Kannel WB, et al. Hemodynamic patterns of age-related changes in blood pressure. The Framingham Heart Study. Circulation. 1997;96:308–15.
34. Lakatta EG, Levy D. Arterial and cardiac aging: major shareholders in cardiovascular disease enterprises: part I: aging arteries: a "set up" for vascular disease. Circulation. 2003;107:139–46.
35. Toda T, Tsuda N, Nishimori I, Leszczynski DE, Kummerow FA. Morphometrical analysis of the aging process in human arteries and aorta. Acta Anat (Basel). 1980;106:35–44.
36. Wang M, Zhang J, Jiang LQ, Spinetti G, Pintus G, Monticone R, et al. Proinflammatory profile within the grossly normal aged human aortic wall. Hypertension. 2007;50:219–27.
37. Kojimahara M, Sekiya K, Ooneda G. Age-induced changes of cerebral arteries in rats. An electron microscope study. Virchows Arch A Pathol Pathol Anat. 1973;361:11–8.
38. Waller BF, Morgan R. The very elderly heart. Cardiovasc Clin. 1988;18:361–410.
39. Muller-Delp JM, Gurovich AN, Christou DD, Leeuwenburgh C. Redox balance in the aging microcirculation: new friends, new foes, and new clinical directions. Microcirculation. 2012;19: 19–28.
40. Safciuc F, Constantin A, Manea A, Nicolae M, Popov D, Raicu M, et al. Advanced glycation end products, oxidative stress and metalloproteinases are altered in the cerebral microvasculature during aging. Curr Neurovasc Res. 2007;4:228–34.
41. Riddle DR, Sonntag WE, Lichtenwalner RJ. Microvascular plasticity in aging. Ageing Res Rev. 2003;2:149–68.
42. Hutchins PM, Lynch CD, Cooney PT, Curseen KA. The microcirculation in experimental hypertension and aging. Cardiovasc Res. 1996;32:772–80.
43. Urbieta Caceres VH, Syed FA, Lin J, Zhu XY, Jordan KL, Bell CC, et al. Age-dependent renal cortical microvascular loss in female mice. Am J Physiol Endocrinol Metab. 2012;302(8):E979–86.
44. Chang E, Yang J, Nagavarapu U, Herron GS. Aging and survival of cutaneous microvasculature. J Invest Dermatol. 2002;118:752–8.
45. Tomanek RJ, Aydelotte MR, Torry RJ. Remodeling of coronary vessels during aging in purebred beagles. Circ Res. 1991; 69:1068–74.
46. Valenta J, Vitek K, Cihak R, Konvickova S, Sochor M, Horny L. Age related constitutive laws and stress distribution in human

main coronary arteries with reference to residual strain. Biomed Mater Eng. 2002;12:121–34.
47. Scott AD, Keegan J, Mohiaddin RH, Firmin DN. Noninvasive detection of coronary artery wall thickening with age in healthy subjects using high resolution MRI with beat-to-beat respiratory motion correction. J Magn Reson Imaging. 2011;34:824–30.
48. Wilens SL, Plair CM, Henderson D. Size of the major epicardial coronary arteries at necropsy. Relation to age, heart weight, and myocardial infarction. JAMA. 1966;198:1325–9.
49. Tracy RE, Eigenbrodt ML. Coronary artery circumferential stress: departure from Laplace expectations with aging. Scientific World J. 2009;9:946–60.
50. Vitullo JC, Penn MS, Rakusan K, Wicker P. Effects of hypertension and aging on coronary arteriolar density. Hypertension. 1993;21:406–14.
51. Rakusan K, Nagai J. Morphometry of arterioles and capillaries in hearts of senescent mice. Cardiovasc Res. 1994;28:969–72.
52. Joris I, Majno G. Cellular breakdown within the arterial wall. An ultrastructural study of the coronary artery in young and aging rats. Virchows Arch A Pathol Anat Histol. 1974;364:111–27.
53. Uno H, Poff B. Coronary arterial ectasia, a predominant type of coronary sclerosis in aged captive rhesus monkeys (*Macaca mulatta*). Am J Pathol. 1983;111:315–22.
54. Patek PR, De Mignard VA, Bernick S. Changes in structure of coronary arteries: susceptibility to arteriosclerosis in old rats. Arch Pathol. 1968;85:388–96.
55. Cavallotti C, Nuti F, Bruzzone P, Mancone M. Age-related changes in dopamine D2 receptors in rat heart and coronary vessels. Clin Exp Pharmacol Physiol. 2002;29:412–8.
56. Poelaert JI, Mungroop HE, Koolen JJ, Van den Berg PC. Hemodynamic effects of dopexamine in patients following coronary artery bypass surgery. J Cardiothorac Anesth. 1989;3:441–3.
57. Bruzzone P, Cavallotti C, Mancone M, Tranquilli Leali FM. Age-related changes in catecholaminergic nerve fibers of rat heart and coronary vessels. Gerontology. 2003;49:80–5.
58. Amenta F, Mione MC. Age-related changes in the noradrenergic innervation of the coronary arteries in old rats: a fluorescent histochemical study. J Auton Nerv Syst. 1988;22:247–51.
59. Biernacka A, Frangogiannis NG. Aging and cardiac fibrosis. Aging Dis. 2011;2:158–73.
60. Schwartzkopff B, Motz W, Frenzel H, Vogt M, Knauer S, Strauer BE. Structural and functional alterations of the intramyocardial coronary arterioles in patients with arterial hypertension. Circulation. 1993;88:993–1003.
61. Frohlich ED. Fibrosis and ischemia: the real risks in hypertensive heart disease. Am J Hypertens. 2001;14:194S–9.
62. Schwartzkopff B, Brehm M, Mundhenke M, Strauer BE. Repair of coronary arterioles after treatment with perindopril in hypertensive heart disease. Hypertension. 2000;36:220–5.
63. Ito N, Isoyama S, Takahashi T, Takishima T. Coronary dilator reserve and morphological changes after relief of pressure-overload in rats. J Mol Cell Cardiol. 1993;25:3–14.
64. Jalil JE, Janicki JS, Pick R, Weber KT. Coronary vascular remodeling and myocardial fibrosis in the rat with renovascular hypertension. Response to captopril. Am J Hypertens. 1991;4:51–5.
65. Varagic J, Frohlich ED, Diez J, Susic D, Ahn J, Gonzalez A, et al. Myocardial fibrosis, impaired coronary hemodynamics, and biventricular dysfunction in salt-loaded SHR. Am J Physiol Heart Circ Physiol. 2006;290:H1503–9.
66. Csiszar A, Ungvari Z, Koller A, Edwards JG, Kaley G. Proinflammatory phenotype of coronary arteries promotes endothelial apoptosis in aging. Physiol Genomics. 2004;17:21–30.
67. Lee MY, Wang Y, Vanhoutte PM. Senescence of cultured porcine coronary arterial endothelial cells is associated with accelerated oxidative stress and activation of NFkB. J Vasc Res. 2010;47: 287–98.
68. Hinschen AK, Rose'Meyer RB, Headrick JP. Age-related changes in adenosine-mediated relaxation of coronary and aortic smooth muscle. Am J Physiol Heart Circ Physiol. 2001;280:H2380–9.
69. Jenner TL, Rose'Meyer RB. Adenosine A(3) receptor mediated coronary vasodilation in the rat heart: changes that occur with maturation. Mech Ageing Dev. 2006;127:264–73.
70. Kristo G, Yoshimura Y, Keith BJ, Mentzer Jr RM, Lasley RD. Aged rat myocardium exhibits normal adenosine receptor-mediated bradycardia and coronary vasodilation but increased adenosine agonist-mediated cardioprotection. J Gerontol A Biol Sci Med Sci. 2005;60:1399–404.
71. Lorbar M, Fenton RA, Duffy AJ, Graybill CA, Dobson Jr JG. Effect of aging on myocardial adenosine production, adenosine uptake and adenosine kinase activity in rats. J Mol Cell Cardiol. 1999;31:401–12.
72. Fenton RA, Dobson Jr JG. Reduced adenosine release from the aged mammalian heart. J Cell Physiol. 2012;227(11):3709–14.
73. Toda N, Miyazaki M. Senescent beagle coronary arteries in response to catecholamines and adrenergic nerve stimulation. J Gerontol. 1987;42:210–8.
74. Saetrum Opgaard O, Ytterberg HT, Saxena PR, Edvinsson L. Influence of ageing on vasomotor responses of human epicardial coronary arteries. Pharmacol Toxicol. 2000;86:183–91.
75. Murohara T, Yasue H, Ohgushi M, Sakaino N, Jougasaki M. Age related attenuation of the endothelium dependent relaxation to noradrenaline in isolated pig coronary arteries. Cardiovasc Res. 1991;25:1002–9.
76. Egashira K, Inou T, Hirooka Y, Kai H, Sugimachi M, Suzuki S, et al. Effects of age on endothelium-dependent vasodilation of resistance coronary artery by acetylcholine in humans. Circulation. 1993;88:77–81.
77. Machii H, Saitoh S, Kaneshiro T, Takeishi Y. Aging impairs myocardium-induced dilation in coronary arterioles: role of hydrogen peroxide and angiotensin. Mech Ageing Dev. 2010;131:710–7.
78. Zeiher AM, Drexler H, Saurbier B, Just H. Endothelium-mediated coronary blood flow modulation in humans. Effects of age, atherosclerosis, hypercholesterolemia, and hypertension. J Clin Invest. 1993;92:652–62.
79. Yasue H, Matsuyama K, Okumura K, Morikami Y, Ogawa H. Responses of angiographically normal human coronary arteries to intracoronary injection of acetylcholine by age and segment. Possible role of early coronary atherosclerosis. Circulation. 1990;81:482–90.
80. Kang LS, Reyes RA, Muller-Delp JM. Aging impairs flow-induced dilation in coronary arterioles: role of NO and H(2)O(2). Am J Physiol Heart Circ Physiol. 2009;297:H1087–95.
81. Kang LS, Chen B, Reyes RA, Leblanc AJ, Teng B, Mustafa SJ, et al. Aging and estrogen alter endothelial reactivity to reactive oxygen species in coronary arterioles. Am J Physiol Heart Circ Physiol. 2011;300:H2105–15.
82. Adler A, Messina E, Sherman B, Wang Z, Huang H, Linke A, et al. NAD(P)H oxidase-generated superoxide anion accounts for reduced control of myocardial O_2 consumption by NO in old Fischer 344 rats. Am J Physiol Heart Circ Physiol. 2003;285:H1015–22.
83. Liu Y, Zhao H, Li H, Kalyanaraman B, Nicolosi AC, Gutterman DD. Mitochondrial sources of H_2O_2 generation play a key role in flow-mediated dilation in human coronary resistance arteries. Circ Res. 2003;93:573–80.
84. Widlansky ME, Gutterman DD. Regulation of endothelial function by mitochondrial reactive oxygen species. Antioxid Redox Signal. 2011;15:1517–30.
85. LeBlanc AJ, Shipley RD, Kang LS, Muller-Delp JM. Age impairs Flk-1 signaling and NO-mediated vasodilation in coronary arterioles. Am J Physiol Heart Circ Physiol. 2008;295:H2280–8.
86. Mieno S, Boodhwani M, Clements RT, Ramlawi B, Sodha NR, Li J, et al. Aging is associated with an impaired coronary microvascular

response to vascular endothelial growth factor in patients. J Thorac Cardiovasc Surg. 2006;132:1348–55.
87. Cook BH, Granger HJ, Taylor AE. Metabolism of coronary arteries and arterioles: a histochemical study. Microvasc Res. 1977;14: 145–59.
88. Amenta D, Lucreziotti R, Ramacci MT, Ricci A, Amenta F. Metabolism of coronary vasculature in senescent rats–a histochemical study. Arch Gerontol Geriatr. 1987;6:123–32.
89. Nyborg NC. Ageing is associated with increased 5-HT2-receptor affinity and decreased receptor reserve in rat isolated coronary arteries. Br J Pharmacol. 1991;102:282–6.
90. Nyborg NC, Mikkelsen EO. Serotonin response increases with age in rat coronary resistance arteries. Cardiovasc Res. 1988;22:131–7.
91. Tschudi MR, Luscher TF. Age and hypertension differently affect coronary contractions to endothelin-1, serotonin, and angiotensins. Circulation. 1995;91:2415–22.
92. Simonsen AH, Sheykhzade M, Berg Nyborg NC. Age- and endothelium-dependent changes in coronary artery reactivity to serotonin and calcium. Vascul Pharmacol. 2004;41:43–9.
93. Korzick DH, Muller-Delp JM, Dougherty P, Heaps CL, Bowles DK, Krick KK. Exaggerated coronary vasoreactivity to endothelin-1 in aged rats: role of protein kinase C. Cardiovasc Res. 2005;66:384–92.
94. Goodwin AT, Amrani M, Marchbank AJ, Gray CC, Jayakumar J, Yacoub MH. Coronary vasoconstriction to endothelin-1 increases with age before and after ischaemia and reperfusion. Cardiovasc Res. 1999;41:554–62.
95. Donoso MV, Fournier A, Peschke H, Faundez H, Domenech R, Huidobro-Toro JP. Aging differentially modifies arterial sensitivity to endothelin-1 and 5-hydroxytryptamine: studies in dog coronary arteries and rat arterial mesenteric bed. Peptides. 1994;15:1489–95.
96. Shipley RD, Muller-Delp JM. Aging decreases vasoconstrictor responses of coronary resistance arterioles through endothelium-dependent mechanisms. Cardiovasc Res. 2005;66:374–83.
97. Marijic J, Li Q, Song M, Nishimaru K, Stefani E, Toro L. Decreased expression of voltage- and Ca(2+)-activated K(+) channels in coronary smooth muscle during aging. Circ Res. 2001;88:210–6.
98. Nishimaru K, Eghbali M, Lu R, Marijic J, Stefani E, Toro L. Functional and molecular evidence of MaxiK channel beta1 subunit decrease with coronary artery ageing in the rat. J Physiol. 2004;559:849–62.
99. Albarwani S, Al-Siyabi S, Baomar H, Hassan MO. Exercise training attenuates ageing-induced BKCa channel downregulation in rat coronary arteries. Exp Physiol. 2010;95:746–55.
100. Toro L, Marijic J, Nishimaru K, Tanaka Y, Song M, Stefani E. Aging, ion channel expression, and vascular function. Vascul Pharmacol. 2002;38:73–80.
101. Rakusan K, Poupa O. Capillaries and muscle fibres in the heart of old rats. Gerontologia. 1964;69:107–12.
102. Tomanek RJ. Effects of age and exercise on the extent of the myocardial capillary bed. Anat Rec. 1970;167:55–62.
103. Tomanek RJ, Hovanec JM. The effects of long-term pressure-overload and aging on the myocardium. J Mol Cell Cardiol. 1981;13:471–88.
104. Vandewoude MF, Buyssens N. Effect of ageing and malnutrition on rat myocardium. II. The microvasculature. Virchows Arch A Pathol Anat Histopathol. 1992;421:189–92.
105. Khan AS, Lynch CD, Sane DC, Willingham MC, Sonntag WE. Growth hormone increases regional coronary blood flow and capillary density in aged rats. J Gerontol A Biol Sci Med Sci. 2001;56:B364–71.
106. Besse S, Boucher F, Linguet G, Riou L, De Leiris J, Riou B, et al. Intramyocardial protein therapy with vascular endothelial growth factor (VEGF-165) induces functional angiogenesis in rat senescent myocardium. J Physiol Pharmacol. 2010;61:651–61.
107. Tomanek RJ, Aydelotte R, Burrwea CA. Late onset renal hypertension in old rats alters myocardial microvessels. Am J Physiol. 259:H1681–H1687, 1990;(3Pt2):H1062–73.
108. Rakusan K, Korecky B. The effect of growth and aging on functional capillary supply of the rat heart. Growth. 1982;46:275–81.
109. Tomanek RJ, Connell PM, Butters CA, Torry RJ. Compensated coronary microvascular growth in senescent rats with thyroxine-induced cardiac hypertrophy. Am J Physiol. 1995;268:H419–25.
110. Ahluwalia A, Narula J, Jones MK, Deng X, Tarnawski AS. Impaired angiogenesis in aging myocardial microvascular endothelial cells is associated with reduced importin alpha and decreased nuclear transport of HIF1 alpha: mechanistic implications. J Physiol Pharmacol. 2010;61:133–9.
111. Ahluwalia A, Tarnawski AS. Activation of the metabolic sensor-AMP activated protein kinase reverses impairment of angiogenesis in aging myocardial microvascular endothelial cells. Implications for the aging heart. J Physiol Pharmacol. 2011;62:583–7.
112. Garfinkel S, Hu X, Prudovsky IA, McMahon GA, Kapnik EM, McDowell SD, et al. FGF-1-dependent proliferative and migratory responses are impaired in senescent human umbilical vein endothelial cells and correlate with the inability to signal tyrosine phosphorylation of fibroblast growth factor receptor-1 substrates. J Cell Biol. 1996;134:783–91.
113. Augustin-Voss HG, Voss AK, Pauli BU. Senescence of aortic endothelial cells in culture: effects of basic fibroblast growth factor expression on cell phenotype, migration, and proliferation. J Cell Physiol. 1993;157:279–88.
114. Uren NG, Camici PG, Melin JA, Bol A, de Bruyne B, Radvan J, et al. Effect of aging on myocardial perfusion reserve. J Nucl Med. 1995;36:2032–6.
115. Ishida S, Hamasaki S, Kamekou M, Yoshitama T, Nakano F, Yoshikawa A, et al. Advancing age is associated with diminished vascular remodeling and impaired vasodilation in resistance coronary arteries. Coron Artery Dis. 2003;14:443–9.
116. Weisfeldt ML, Wright JR, Shreiner DP, Lakatta E, Shock NW. Coronary flow and oxygen extraction in the perfused heart of senescent male rats. J Appl Physiol. 1971;30:44–9.
117. Hachamovitch R, Wicker P, Capasso JM, Anversa P. Alterations of coronary blood flow and reserve with aging in Fischer 344 rats. Am J Physiol. 1989;256:H66–73.
118. Tomanek RJ, Aydelotte MR, Anderson KE, Torry RJ. Coronary blood flow in senescent rats with late-onset hypertension. Am J Physiol. 1993;264:H1854–60.
119. Isoyama S, Sato F, Takishima T. Effect of age on coronary circulation after imposition of pressure-overload in rats. Hypertension. 1991;17:369–77.
120. Susic D, Nunez E, Hosoya K, Frohlich ED. Coronary hemodynamics in aging spontaneously hypertensive and normotensive Wistar-Kyoto rats. J Hypertens. 1998;16:231–7.
121. Gao Z, Wilson TE, Drew RC, Ettinger J, Monahan KD. Altered coronary vascular control during cold stress in healthy older adults. Am J Physiol Heart Circ Physiol. 2012;302:H312–8.
122. Muller MD, Gao Z, Mast JL, Blaha CA, Drew RC, Leuenberger UA, et al. Aging attenuates the coronary blood flow response to cold air breathing and isometric handgrip in healthy humans. Am J Physiol Heart Circ Physiol. 2012;302(8):H1737–46.
123. Amrani M, Chester AH, Jayakumar J, Yacoub MH. Aging reduces postischemic recovery of coronary endothelial function. J Thorac Cardiovasc Surg. 1996;111:238–45.
124. Anversa P, Li P, Sonnenblick EH, Olivetti G. Effects of aging on quantitative structural properties of coronary vasculature and microvasculature in rats. Am J Physiol. 1994;267(3Pt2): H1062–73.
125. Tomanek RJ, Aydelotte MR. Late onset renal hypertension in old rats alters left ventricular structure and function. Am J Physiol. 1992;262:H531–8.

126. Isoyama S, Ito N, Komatsu M, Nitta Y, Abe K, Aoki M, et al. Responses to hemodynamic stress in the aged heart. Jpn Heart J. 1994;35:403–18.
127. Peters KG, Wangler RD, Tomanek RJ, Marcus ML. Effects of long-term cardiac hypertrophy on coronary vasodilator reserve in SHR rats. Am J Cardiol. 1984;54:1342–8.
128. Boengler K, Schulz R, Heusch G. Loss of cardioprotection with ageing. Cardiovasc Res. 2009;83:247–61.
129. Mariani J, Ou R, Bailey M, Rowland M, Nagley P, Rosenfeldt F, et al. Tolerance to ischemia and hypoxia is reduced in aged human myocardium. J Thorac Cardiovasc Surg. 2000;120:660–7.
130. Weintraub WS, Craver JM, Cohen CL, Jones EL, Guyton RA. Influence of age on results of coronary artery surgery. Circulation. 1991;84(III226).
131. Abete P, Cioppa A, Calabrese C, Pascucci I, Cacciatore F, Napoli C, et al. Ischemic threshold and myocardial stunning in the aging heart. Exp Gerontol. 1999;34:875–84.
132. Willems L, Zatta A, Holmgren K, Ashton KJ, Headrick JP. Age-related changes in ischemic tolerance in male and female mouse hearts. J Mol Cell Cardiol. 2005;38:245–56.
133. Tani M, Suganuma Y, Hasegawa H, Shinmura K, Ebihara Y, Hayashi Y, et al. Decrease in ischemic tolerance with aging in isolated perfused Fischer 344 rat hearts: relation to increases in intracellular Na+ after ischemia. J Mol Cell Cardiol. 1997;29:3081–9.
134. Liu L, Azhar G, Gao W, Zhang X, Wei JY. Bcl-2 and Bax expression in adult rat hearts after coronary occlusion: age-associated differences. Am J Physiol. 1998;275:R315–22.
135. Nitta Y, Abe K, Aoki M, Ohno I, Isoyama S. Diminished heat shock protein 70 mRNA induction in aged rat hearts after ischemia. Am J Physiol. 1994;267:H1795–803.
136. Tevzadze N, Gujabidze N, Giorgadze S, Rukhadze R. The age related changes of nitric oxide and apoptosis in experiment. Georgian Med News. 2009;169:87–90.
137. Amrani M, Goodwin AT, Gray CC, Yacoub MH. Ageing is associated with reduced basal and stimulated release of nitric oxide by the coronary endothelium. Acta Physiol Scand. 1996;157:79–84.
138. Le Page C, Noirez P, Courty J, Riou B, Swynghedauw B, Besse S. Exercise training improves functional post-ischemic recovery in senescent heart. Exp Gerontol. 2009;44:177–82.
139. Bolli R. Cardioprotective function of inducible nitric oxide synthase and role of nitric oxide in myocardial ischemia and preconditioning: an overview of a decade of research. J Mol Cell Cardiol. 2001;33:1897–918.
140. Tani M, Suganuma Y, Hasegawa H, Shinmura K, Hayashi Y, Guo X, et al. Changes in ischemic tolerance and effects of ischemic preconditioning in middle-aged rat hearts. Circulation. 1997; 95:2559–66.
141. Pepe S. Mitochondrial function in ischaemia and reperfusion of the ageing heart. Clin Exp Pharmacol Physiol. 2000;27:745–50.
142. Song D, Kang W, Woelki H, Li M, Guo X. Biomarkers, age, and coronary artery remodeling in patients with acute coronary syndrome. Am J Geriatr Cardiol. 2008;17:71–7.
143. Abete P, Testa G, Cacciatore F, Della-Morte D, Galizia G, Langellotto A, et al. Ischemic preconditioning in the younger and aged heart. Aging Dis. 2011;2:138–48.
144. Abete P, Calabrese C, Ferrara N, Cioppa A, Pisanelli P, Cacciatore F, et al. Exercise training restores ischemic preconditioning in the aging heart. J Am Coll Cardiol. 2000;36:643–50.
145. Juhaszova M, Rabuel C, Zorov DB, Lakatta EG, Sollott SJ. Protection in the aged heart: preventing the heart-break of old age? Cardiovasc Res. 2005;66:233–44.
146. Abete P, Ferrara N, Cacciatore F, Madrid A, Bianco S, Calabrese C, et al. Angina-induced protection against myocardial infarction in adult and elderly patients: a loss of preconditioning mechanism in the aging heart? J Am Coll Cardiol. 1997;30:947–54.
147. Kloner RA, Przyklenk K, Shook T, Cannon CP. Protection conferred by preinfarct angina is manifest in the aged heart: evidence from the TIMI 4 trial. J Thromb Thrombolysis. 1998;6:89–92.
148. Ishihara M, Sato H, Tateishi H, Kawagoe T, Shimatani Y, Ueda K, et al. Beneficial effect of prodromal angina pectoris is lost in elderly patients with acute myocardial infarction. Am Heart J. 2000;139:881–8.
149. Jimenez-Navarro M, Gomez-Doblas JJ, Alonso-Briales J, Hernandez Garcia JM, Gomez G, Alcantara AG, et al. Does angina the week before protect against first myocardial infarction in elderly patients? Am J Cardiol. 2001;87:11–5.
150. Abete P, Ferrara N, Cacciatore F, Sagnelli E, Manzi M, Carnovale V, et al. High level of physical activity preserves the cardioprotective effect of preinfarction angina in elderly patients. J Am Coll Cardiol. 2001;38:1357–65.
151. Abete P, Testa G, Ferrara N, De Santis D, Capaccio P, Viati L, et al. Cardioprotective effect of ischemic preconditioning is preserved in food-restricted senescent rats. Am J Physiol Heart Circ Physiol. 2002;282:H1978–87.
152. Schulman D, Latchman DS, Yellon DM. Effect of aging on the ability of preconditioning to protect rat hearts from ischemia-reperfusion injury. Am J Physiol Heart Circ Physiol. 2001;281: H1630–6.
153. Fenton RA, Dickson EW, Meyer TE, Dobson Jr JG. Aging reduces the cardioprotective effect of ischemic preconditioning in the rat heart. J Mol Cell Cardiol. 2000;32:1371–5.
154. Boengler K, Konietzka I, Buechert A, Heinen Y, Garcia-Dorado D, Heusch G, et al. Loss of ischemic preconditioning's cardioprotection in aged mouse hearts is associated with reduced gap junctional and mitochondrial levels of connexin 43. Am J Physiol Heart Circ Physiol. 2007;292:H1764–9.
155. Gerstenblith G, Frederiksen J, Yin FC, Fortuin NJ, Lakatta EG, Weisfeldt ML. Echocardiographic assessment of a normal adult aging population. Circulation. 1977;56:273–8.
156. Tresch DD, McGough MF. Heart failure with normal systolic function: a common disorder in older people. J Am Geriatr Soc. 1995;43:1035–42.
157. Rivard A, Fabre JE, Silver M, Chen D, Murohara T, Kearney M, et al. Age-dependent impairment of angiogenesis. Circulation. 1999;99:111–20.
158. Dawson Jr R, Meldrum MJ. Norepinephrine content in cardiovascular tissues from the aged Fischer 344 rat. Gerontology. 1992;38:185–91.
159. Abete P, Ferrara N, Cioppa A, Ferrara P, Bianco S, Calabrese C, et al. Preconditioning does not prevent postischemic dysfunction in aging heart. J Am Coll Cardiol. 1996;27:1777–86.
160. Taylor RP, Starnes JW. Age, cell signalling and cardioprotection. Acta Physiol Scand. 2003;178:107–16.
161. Liu L, Zhu J, Glass PS, Brink PR, Rampil IJ, Rebecchi MJ. Age-associated changes in cardiac gene expression after preconditioning. Anesthesiology. 2009;111:1052–64.
162. Lee TM, Su SF, Chou TF, Lee YT, Tsai CH. Loss of preconditioning by attenuated activation of myocardial ATP-sensitive potassium channels in elderly patients undergoing coronary angioplasty. Circulation. 2002;105:334–40.
163. Wojtovich AP, Nadtochiy SM, Brookes PS, Nehrke K. Ischemic preconditioning: the role of mitochondria and aging. Exp Gerontol. 2012;47:1–7.
164. Krylova IB, Kachaeva EV, Rodionova OM, Negoda AE, Evdokimova NR, Balina MI, et al. The cardioprotective effect of uridine and uridine-5′-monophosphate: the role of the mitochondrial ATP-dependent potassium channel. Exp Gerontol. 2006;41:697–703.
165. Tani M, Honma Y, Hasegawa H, Tamaki K. Direct activation of mitochondrial K(ATP) channels mimics preconditioning but

protein kinase C activation is less effective in middle-aged rat hearts. Cardiovasc Res. 2001;49:56–68.

166. Lee KL, Woodlief LH, Topol EJ, Weaver WD, Betriu A, Col J, et al. Predictors of 30-day mortality in the era of reperfusion for acute myocardial infarction. Results from an international trial of 41,021 patients. GUSTO-I Investigators. Circulation. 1995; 91:1659–68.
167. Lesnefsky EJ, Lundergan CF, Hodgson JM, Nair R, Reiner JS, Greenhouse SW, et al. Increased left ventricular dysfunction in elderly patients despite successful thrombolysis: the GUSTO-I angiographic experience. J Am Coll Cardiol. 1996;28:331–7.
168. Yang XS, Willems JL, Pardaens J, De Geest H. Acute myocardial infarction in the very elderly. A comparison with younger age groups. Acta Cardiol. 1987;42:59–68.
169. Maggioni AP, Maseri A, Fresco C, Franzosi MG, Mauri F, Santoro E, et al. Age-related increase in mortality among patients with first myocardial infarctions treated with thrombolysis. The Investigators of the Gruppo Italiano per lo Studio della Sopravvivenza nell'Infarto Miocardico (GISSI-2). N Engl J Med. 1993;329: 1442–8.
170. Weaver WD, Litwin PE, Martin JS, Kudenchuk PJ, Maynard C, Eisenberg MS, et al. Effect of age on use of thrombolytic therapy and mortality in acute myocardial infarction. The MITI Project Group. J Am Coll Cardiol. 1991;18:657–62.
171. Azhar G, Gao W, Liu L, Wei JY. Ischemia-reperfusion in the adult mouse heart influence of age. Exp Gerontol. 1999;34:699–714.
172. Edelberg JM, Aird WC, Wu W, Rayburn H, Mamuya WS, Mercola M, et al. PDGF mediates cardiac microvascular communication. J Clin Invest. 1998;102:837–43.
173. Sarzani R, Arnaldi G, Takasaki I, Brecher P, Chobanian AV. Effects of hypertension and aging on platelet-derived growth factor and platelet-derived growth factor receptor expression in rat aorta and heart. Hypertension. 1991;18:III93–9.
174. Edelberg JM, Lee SH, Kaur M, Tang L, Feirt NM, McCabe S, et al. Platelet-derived growth factor-AB limits the extent of myocardial infarction in a rat model: feasibility of restoring impaired angiogenic capacity in the aging heart. Circulation. 2002;105: 608–13.
175. Pedelty L, Gorelick PB. Management of hypertension and cerebrovascular disease in the elderly. Am J Med. 2008;121:S23–31.
176. Eliason JL, Wainess RM, Proctor MC, Dimick JB, Cowan Jr JA, Upchurch Jr GR, et al. A national and single institutional experience in the contemporary treatment of acute lower extremity ischemia. Ann Surg. 2003;238:382–9, discussion 9–90.
177. Ohta T, Hosaka M, Ishibashi H, Sugimoto I, Mihara E, Hida K, et al. Limb salvage and survival rates among elderly patients with advanced limb ischemia. Surgery today. 1998;28:156–61.
178. Kurotobi T, Sato H, Kinjo K, Nakatani D, Mizuno H, Shimizu M, et al. Reduced collateral circulation to the infarct-related artery in elderly patients with acute myocardial infarction. J Am Coll Cardiol. 2004;44:28–34.
179. Nakae I, Fujita M, Miwa K, Hasegawa K, Kihara Y, Nohara R, et al. Age-dependent impairment of coronary collateral development in humans. Heart Vessels. 2000;15:176–80.
180. Faber JE, Zhang H, Lassance-Soares RM, Prabhakar P, Najafi AH, Burnett MS, et al. Aging causes collateral rarefaction and increased severity of ischemic injury in multiple tissues. Arterioscler Thromb Vasc Biol. 2011;31:1748–56.
181. Piro M, Della Bona R, Abbate A, Biasucci LM, Crea F. Sex-related differences in myocardial remodeling. J Am Coll Cardiol. 2010;55:1057–65.
182. Olivetti G, Giordano G, Corradi D, Melissari M, Lagrasta C, Gambert SR, et al. Gender differences and aging: effects on the human heart. J Am Coll Cardiol. 1995;26:1068–79.
183. Ky B, Kirwan BA, de Brouwer S, Lubsen J, Poole-Wilson P, Otterstad JE, et al. Gender differences in cardiac remodeling and clinical outcomes in chronic stable angina pectoris (from the ACTION Trial). Am J Cardiol. 2010;105:943–7.
184. Kim BJ, Lee SH, Kim CK, Ryu WS, Kwon HM, Choi SY, et al. Advanced coronary artery calcification and cerebral small vessel diseases in the healthy elderly. Circ J. 2011;75:451–6.
185. Eaker ED, Packard B, Wenger NK, Clarkson TB, Tyroler HA. Coronary artery disease in women. Am J Cardiol. 1988;61: 641–4.
186. Lerner DJ, Kannel WB. Patterns of coronary heart disease morbidity and mortality in the sexes: a 26-year follow-up of the Framingham population. Am Heart J. 1986;111:383–90.
187. Motro M, Shemesh J. Prevalence of coronary calcification in relation to age, gender and risk factor profile in the insight population. Br J Clin Pract Suppl. 1997;88:1–5.
188. Vaccarino V, Krumholz HM, Berkman LF, Horwitz RI. Sex differences in mortality after myocardial infarction. Is there evidence for an increased risk for women? Circulation. 1995;91: 1861–71.

8 Adaptations to Exercise Training

Abbreviations

EC Endothelial cell
ET Exercise training
LV Left ventricle
MI Myocardial infarction
NO Nitric oxide
RV Right ventricle
VEGF Vascular endothelial growth factor

Introduction

Repeated bouts of exercise are widely recognized as a factor that reduces the risk of ischemic heart disease [1–5]. Exercise training (ET) cardiovascular benefits include improved cardiac function and O_2 utilization and greater cardiac efficiency associated with a reduced resting heart rate. In patients with coronary heart disease, a 3-month program of exercise conditioning significantly reduced the exercise angina threshold, suggesting an increased myocardial O_2 supply [6]. Meta-analysis of 51 studies involving 8,440 patients who participated in exercise-based cardiac rehabilitation programs revealed a 31% reduction in cardiovascular mortality [7]. Cardiac responses to increased O_2 demands depend on both adequate myocardial perfusion and transcapillary exchange at the cellular level [8]. Accordingly, improved O_2 delivery to myocardial cells resulting from exercise training could result from biochemical/physiological and/or structural adaptations, which could occur at various levels of the coronary hierarchy. Such adaptations can include several levels of control, e.g. endothelial, neurohumoral, metabolic, and myogenic, as well as at several levels of the coronary hierarchy, i.e. conduit arteries, arterioles, and the capillary bed. This chapter reviews the adaptations that occur in healthy as well as diseased hearts.

One of the problems in drawing generalized conclusions from studies on exercise training-induced adaptations is that the data are based on studies that have employed various species, age groups, methodological approaches, and different types of ET programs (i.e., different training intensities, types, and durations). In reviewing the data from these studies, attention must be paid to these variables. A priority, in this regard, is an exercise training program of sufficient duration and intensity to produce a "training effect," such as documented by development of resting bradycardia, increased exercise tolerance, increased VO_2 max, and improved cardiac function. Another consideration is the sensitivity of the measurements used to document various adaptations. This chapter focuses on the coronary vasculature. A review of activity and inactivity on other vascular beds is provided by Thijssen et al. [9].

Coronary Responses During Acute Exercise

A comprehensive review of this topic was published by Duncker and Bache [10] and Duncker et al. [11]. This section is intended as a brief review of the responses during an exercise bout that may underlie adaptations to exercise training (ET). Aerobic exercise, when severe, may increase coronary blood flow by as much as fivefold to meet the increase in oxygen demand, which is determined by contractility, heart rate, muscle shortening, and wall tension. Augmented blood flow during exercise is the primary contributor to O_2 delivery in humans and swine because any increase in O_2 extraction is negligible. In contrast, dogs are able to increase O_2 extraction from 79 ± 2 to $93 \pm 1\%$ [12]. Moreover, an increase in hemoglobin during exercise in some species, e.g. a 40% increase in dogs [13], provides additional O_2. This is especially noteworthy because dogs have been used extensively in studies on exercise.

Vascular Resistance

The increase in coronary blood flow, as occurs during exercise, is facilitated by dilation of resistance vessels and an increase

R.J. Tomanek, *Coronary Vasculature: Development, Structure-Function, and Adaptations*,
DOI 10.1007/978-1-4614-4887-7_8, © Springer Science+Business Media New York 2013

in mean arterial pressure. The increase in pressure at the coronary ostia, i.e., intravascular distending pressure, is compromised by extravascular compression in transmural arteries and arterioles. This phenomenon, discussed in Chap. 4, is known as the "vascular waterfall" [14]. It limits blood flow to the endocardial side of the myocardium during systole. In the healthy heart, vasodilator reserve is not compromised during exercise because the drop in coronary vascular resistance is sufficient to elevate blood flow to levels needed to maintain adequate O_2 delivery [10, 11]. Recent data signify that ATP and its breakdown products ADP and AMP contribute to the feedback control that matches coronary flow to O_2 consumption, both at rest and during exercise [15]. This conclusion is based on the finding that purinergic receptor blockade, in combination with NOS inhibition, decreases O_2 delivery and consumption.

Neural and Humoral Factors

Coronary blood flow during exercise is increased by sympathetic β-adrenergic-mediated arteriolar vasodilation (reviewed by [16]). Vasoconstriction of medium and large coronary arteries, mediated by α-adrenoceptor, helps to maintain blood flow to the vulnerable subepicardium when heart rate and myocardial contractility are elevated during high O_2 demand. In large coronary arteries, NO is activated in response to elevated shear stress acting on endothelial cells (ECs). Despite the accumulation of a wealth of data on exercise-induced hyperemia in the heart, our understanding of the underlying mechanisms is incomplete due to some species differences [17]. For example, in dogs, K_{ATP} channel activation, adenosine, and nitric oxide (NO) contribute to exercise hyperemia in a nonlinear redundant fashion, whereas in swine, exercise hyperemia involves K_{Ca} channel opening mediated, in part, by β-adrenergic activation. Evidence for a role of K_{ATP} channels, NO, and adenosine in human exercise hyperemia is inconclusive. During continuous treadmill exercise in swine, endothelin production decreases and appears to contribute to metabolic coronary vasodilation [18].

Mechanical Factors

Aerobic exercise increases mechanical factors that affect coronary ECs, vascular smooth muscle (VSM), and the extracellular matrix (ECM). As discussed in Chaps. 1 and 11, increased blood flow is accompanied by enhanced shear stress, stretch, and compression of cells due to elevated pressure. These variables are not equally effective in all coronary vessels. Exercise-induced vasodilation in the small arteries and arterioles increases their diameters and thereby stretches cells of the vascular wall. Thus, activation of stretch receptors triggers signals which promote vascular growth. When these forces become chronic, they promote cell growth via the release of growth factors, and consequently angiogenesis, arteriogenesis, and vascular remodeling. One should keep in mind that the position of a particular vessel in the hierarchy of the coronary vasculature, as well as its location in the heart (i.e., epicardial, transmural, or subendocardial), determines in part, the vascular responses to these mechanical forces. Shear stress during exercise is evident in the larger coronary arteries, whereas stretch due to vasodilation is a characteristic of arterioles.

Species Differences

A recent review of coronary resistance vessel tone in response to exercise notes that in humans, K_{ATP} channels, NO, and adenosine do not appear to be critical for exercise hyperemia, whereas in dogs, they do contribute in a nonlinear, redundant fashion [11]. In swine, β-adrenergic activation and exercise-induced blunting of endothelin-mediated vasoconstriction mediate vasodilation.

Maximal Myocardial Perfusion

Maximal myocardial perfusion, a measure of blood flow capacity, has been evaluated by several different approaches (see review by [19]). One common method is the pharmacological induction of maximal coronary vasodilation. Perfusion under this condition must be adjusted for pressure to obtain a valid measure of "conductance." Another approach is to measure hyperemic blood flow, i.e. the increase in flow after the release of temporary occlusion of a coronary artery. Finally, blood flow during "maximal" exercise has been used. However, the latter two approaches are only indirect estimates of coronary flow capacity. Most studies on rats trained either by running or swimming on 5 days/week over a 6–18-week period, have documented an increased maximal myocardial perfusion. In these studies, vasodilation was achieved by administration of adenosine or dipyridamole [20–22], increased cardiac work [23, 24], or hypoxia [25]. Exercise training (ET) in dogs also was found to increase maximal myocardial perfusion, as determined by adenosine-induced vasodilation [26, 27], reactive hyperemia [28], or elevating heart rate [29]. Similarly, increased maximal myocardial perfusion after training was reported to occur in pigs [30, 31].

In contrast, unchanged maximal myocardial perfusion was reported in some studies on trained dogs [32–38], rats [39], and pigs [40]. In many of these studies, maximal vasodilation may not have been reached, which indicates that maximal perfusion was not achieved. Of the 12 studies that documented a higher coronary blood flow capacity, 7 [20–22, 26, 27, 30, 41] provided good evidence that maximal vasodilation was attained. Thus, one explanation for the negative results is failure to achieve maximal vasodilation. Another explanation for the contradictory results is the presence or absence of cardiac hypertrophy. For example, the exercise-trained pigs in the study by Breisch et al. [40] had larger ventricles than the controls, but similar minimal coronary resistances; this finding indicates that the growth of resistance vessels actually paralleled the increase in cardiac mass.

In conclusion, there are sufficient data that indicate improvement in maximal myocardial perfusion in exercise-trained animals. The specific adaptations that may underlie this improvement are discussed in the following sections of this chapter.

Artery and Arteriole Adaptations

General Concepts

Data from Experimental Animals

The microvasculature plays a prominent role in the regulation of coronary flow. During baseline conditions, as revealed in cats, 55% of coronary vascular resistance is distal to arterioles 100 μm in diameter [42]. During maximal vasodilation, resistance falls by 79%, with nearly the entire drop occurring in arteries and arterioles [43]. Therefore, the formation of new arterioles and/or the remodeling of arteries and arterioles to increase their diameters is structural adaptation that provides a mechanism for increased maximal perfusion and coronary flow reserve. Adaptations that enhance collateralization are critical for perfusion of specific myocardial regions that have limited flow reserve.

The well-documented finding that ET increases the volume of coronary arteries was first demonstrated by Tepperman et al. [44, 45], who utilized coronary corrosion casts to estimate the volume of the coronary arteries. These authors reported that rats exposed to an exercise wheel or trained by swimming had larger coronary trees than their sedentary controls. Subsequently, Stevenson [46] repeated the swim-training experiments and found that even 60-min swim bouts, twice per week, increased the size of the coronary arterial tree. Coronary casts in rats exposed to a running wheel for 16 weeks were significantly heavier than those of their cage-restricted controls [47]. A study on monkeys trained by running 3 times/week over a 42-month period documented nearly a twofold increase in the diameters of major coronary arteries [48]. ET did not affect total serum cholesterol, but increased high-density lipoprotein and lowered low-density lipoprotein and triglyceride. The trained monkeys had lower resting heart rates, indicative of a "training effect" and a lower incidence of coronary atherosclerosis.

Data from Humans

Studies on humans are consistent with those on experimental animals. For example, the unusually large coronary arteries of the famed long distance runner Clarence DeMar noted more than 50 years ago are consistent with subsequent studies that repeatedly demonstrated proximal coronary arteries to be larger in endurance athletes than in nonathletes [49–51]. Moreover, these vessels in the endurance athletes dilate much more in response to adenosine or dipyridamole than those of non-trained individuals [49–51]. Similarly, a comparison of ultradistance runners and sedentary men revealed that the proximal segments of the runners dilated much more in response to nitroglycerin than those of the sedentary group [52]. The dilating capacity of the runners was positively correlated with aerobic capacity and negatively with resting heart rate.

Flow as a Stimulus

The findings of these studies are not surprising in that increased flow in other vascular beds, e.g. carotids, has been shown to activate remodeling, resulting in an increased vessel diameter [53]. Moreover, it is well established that exercise stress evokes a reactive dilation of large coronary arteries, demonstrated in dogs [54], and that the dilation is flow dependent [55]. Such a repeated acute response may be a sufficient stimulus for the remodeling process, leading to a structural increase in the diameters of these large vessels. Increased compliance of large noncoronary arteries has been shown to occur in exercise-trained men [56].

In conclusion, the data from human and experimental animals indicate that ET evokes both structural (remodeling to increase vessel diameters and arteriogenesis) and functional (greater vasodilatory response) adaptations in coronary arteries. The responses of various components of the arterial/arteriolar tree to ET are discussed in subsequent sections of this chapter.

Exercise Training Affects Both Vessel Formation and Remodeling

A review of this topic [57] stressed that both angiogenesis and remodeling of the coronary vasculature are characteristic adaptations to ET. A training period lasting 6–12 weeks has been shown to affect several structural changes in coronary vessels. As mentioned above, remodeling to increase diameter, especially in major arteries, is one structural adaption to ET, which has been reported in trained rats [58] and dogs [39, 59]. A second adaptation is an increase in arteriolar numerical or length density, as documented in ET mice [60] and pigs [40, 61–63]. The last cited study explored the growth of various sized arterioles by quantifying endothelial and smooth muscle cell DNA labeling, and arteriolar numerical densities, diameters, and cross-sectional areas after 1, 3, 8, and 16 weeks of training. Arteriolar EC DNA labeling increased about 20-fold during the first week of training, then declined after 8 weeks. Arteriolar smooth muscle cell labeling followed a similar course and showed a sixfold increase by the third week. Arteriolar numerical density increased significantly by 16 weeks in arterioles with diameters 31–40 μm, but not those larger than 40 μm, whereas arteriolar cross-sectional area increased in all diameter ranges. Thus, remodeling to increase diameter was the common response in all arterioles, while the smallest arterioles increased in number. These morphological changes were accompanied by increases in maximal coronary perfusion, already evident after 3 weeks of training.

White et al. [61] trained young mini pigs on a treadmill 5 days/week for 10 weeks. A moderate ET program caused a 16.5% increase in LV/BW ratio, whereas an intense ET program evoked a 35.2% increase. Exercise time to exhaustion increased about twofold in both groups, and similar decreases in serum lactates also occurred. Arteriolar length density increased 56% and 40% in the moderate ET and intense ET groups, respectively. These data indicate that ET can evoke substantial arteriolar growth in young, growing pigs that exceeds the magnitude of cardiac hypertrophy.

Effects of Exercise Training on Vasodilation of Arteries and Arterioles

An important adaptation by the coronary arterial system is an improved vasodilation that may provide the capacity for a greater myocardial perfusion in response to increased O_2 demand. The responses of arteries and arterioles of different diameters to vasoactive substances vary. Therefore, the diameters of arteries and arterioles need to be considered in evaluating the effects of ET on the coronary arterial tree.

The vasodilatory response to norepinephrine in preconstricted, isolated canine coronary arteries was examined in a preparation in which α_1- and β-receptors were blocked so that the responses involving the norepinephrine α_2-receptor could be determined [64]. No differences were noted between exercise-trained and control dogs in the responses to norepinephrine in the isolated arteries. However, an in vivo study documented a greater dose-dependent vasodilation in trained than in non-trained dogs [65]. In contrast to the previous study, these dogs were trained only for 7–10 days, which may suggest that this adaptation was an early response to training, or that the vascular responses differ in vivo and in vitro. Oltman, et. al. [66], who isolated coronary arteries from ET pigs, found that their responses to several endothelium-dependent vasodilators (serotonin, substance P, bradykinin, and clonidine, an alpha 2 agonist) were not different than those of their sedentary counterparts. In contrast, the coronary rings from the ET group were more sensitive to adenosine and less sensitive to nitroprusside [67]. These effects were noted in arteries with either intact or denuded endothelium. Endothelium-dependent vasodilation was then shown to be unaffected by ET in female swine as documented by vasodilator responses of vascular rings to bradykinin, substance P, clonidine, serotonin, and the Ca^{2+} ionophose A-23187 [67]. Microvascular exchange capacity as a function of permeability was shown to be regulated by ET [68]. Exposure to adenosine in ET swine resulted in enhanced permeability in arterioles of both males and females, but enhancement of venular permeability occurred only in females. This permeability response was NO pathway dependent since it did not occur when NOS was blocked.

ET Enhances Dilatory Responses of Large Arteries

Several studies have documented that reactive dilation of large coronary arteries from ET dogs is greater than that in their sedentary controls. Four weeks of ET in dogs enhanced the vasodilatory response to adenosine as well as to β_2-adrenergic agonists and enhanced flow in the left circumflex coronary artery [41]. These responses occurred in the absence of any myocardial metabolic changes. Studies in Hintze's lab used a brief chronic ET program, i.e., 7 days, which they showed increases the release of L-arginine-derived nitrite from both large coronary arteries and microvessels [69]. They documented an enhanced acetylcholine-induced dilation that was NO dependent since the dilation was eliminated by nitro-L-arginine [70]. ET was also found to increase coronary blood flow during activation of the Bezold-Jarisch reflex, i.e., activation of vagal pathways, which was blunted by nitro-L-arginine [71]. This dilatory effect, however, was probably related to the increase in microvessel NO. A study in pigs demonstrated that after only 7 days of ET, endothelium-dependent dilation was enhanced in coronary arteries, but not arterioles [72]. This improved dilatory response was not mediated by changes in SOD-1 or endothelial nitric oxide synthase (eNOS) expression. A subsequent study [73] found that large coronary arteries in ET dogs demonstrated an enhanced vasodilation in response to acetylcholine, associated with improved elastic properties.

ET as a Regulator of NO in Arterioles and Arteries

In their review paper, Zanesco and Antunes [74] suggested that increases in endothelial-derived NOS and antioxidant enzyme expression are the main contributors to improved endothelium-dependent vasodilatory responses in trained individuals or animals. This suggestion fits with the idea that ET improves endothelial function in patients with coronary artery disease (CAD) by enhancing NO production and reducing superoxide anion [75]. The role of NO in VSMC relaxation is well established. Its diffusion into VSMC stimulates cGMP, thereby evoking Ca^{2+} extrusion from the cell and consequently relaxation. An increase in bioavailability of NO is a consequence of increased antioxidant enzyme expression in ET animals [76, 77]. These studies indicate the importance of NO as a vasodilator that may be enhanced by ET. There are two caveats, however, that need to be pointed out. First, much of the evidence on NO effects in ET organisms is based on arteries other than coronaries. Second, there still exist conflicting data on the responses of coronary arteries to endothelium-dependent vasodilators. ET did not affect the contractile responses of large coronary arteries to K^+, acetylcholine, or endothelin, but it increased their responsiveness to adenosine [78]. Since resistance arterioles <150 μm in diameter were not affected by ET, it appears that the effects are selective, occurring only upstream of the major resistance vessels.

In contrast to the failure of ET to affect vasodilation of large coronary arteries (pigs) in response to bradykinin [66], the vasodilator responses to this agent were enhanced in arterioles in ET pigs [79]. Since this enhancement was prevented when NOS was blocked, it was suggested that the underlying mechanism of the ET effect may be an increase in NOS synthase or NOS activation. That ET increases eNOS protein expression in pig coronary arteries and arterioles was documented, but the increase occurred downstream of coronary conduit arteries [80]. ET has been documented to upregulate EC NOS in arterioles [81]. Since nitric oxide half-life depends partly on SOD-1 management of O_2 load, the hypothesis that ET increases SOD-1 was tested [76]. ET in pigs enhanced SOD-1 protein and mRNA, as well as SOD-1 enzymatic activity in coronary arterioles. These data, then, support the idea that enhanced SOD-1 levels contribute to arteriolar dilation. Moreover, ET in dogs has been shown to improve the vasodilatory response of coronary arteries to bradykinin [82]. This effect was NOS dependent, since its inhibition attenuated the vasodilation. The authors concluded that ET augments the sensitivity of coronary arteries to the endothelium-dependent effects of bradykinin, which may reflect an increased role of NO and endothelium-derived hyperpolarizing factor (EDHF).

ET Reduces Constrictor Responses of Arteries

Several studies provided evidence that coronary arteries of ET animals show a blunted response to vasoconstrictive agents. Constrictor responses to phenylephrine in the LAD and circumflex arteries were blunted in exercise-trained dogs [83]. Moreover, isolated proximal aortic rings from trained dogs showed the same blunted response when exposed to either epinephrine or phenylephrine [64]. Similarly, exercise training reduced the contractile responses to endothelin-1 in male pigs [84]. However, this training effect did not occur in females even though other training effects (endurance time and citrate synthase activity) were similar in males and females. An earlier study also demonstrated that ET did not alter the responsiveness of conduit coronary arteries of female pigs to endothelin [78].

Role of Calcium

The role of Ca^{2+} unloading in vascular smooth muscle cells (VSMC), a phenomenon in which sarcoplasmic reticular Ca^{2+} is slowly released through ryanodine receptors and extruded through the cell and is not subsequently sequestered, has been studied as a possible mechanism underlying the diminished responses of coronary arteries to vasoconstrictors. In this regard, Stehno-Bittel et al. [85, 86] were the first to demonstrate that exercise training caused a decline in the caffeine-releasable Ca^{2+} from the sarcoplasmic reticulum in coronary artery smooth muscle cells. The authors concluded that the blunted responses of coronary arteries to vasoconstrictors after ET are due to (1) lower SR Ca^{2+} release, and (2) an elevated buffering of the Ca^{2+} influx. However, ET was found to increase, rather than decrease, in the Ca^{2+} influx that occurs in response to endothelin [87, 88]. Despite this increased influx, intracellular Ca^{2+} and contractile responses were decreased. In female swine, ET has been documented to increase L-type calcium current density in smooth muscle cells from conduit and small coronary arteries, as well as arterioles, and to increase voltage-gated Ca^{2+} channels [89]. This effect did not result in changes in voltage-dependent activation or inactivation. These changes were later shown to be sex dependent since they did not occur in male ET swine [90]. Wamhoff et al. [91] demonstrated that ET enhanced nuclear Ca^{2+} regulation and mediated coronary VSMC phenotype and the calcium responses to endothelin-1. An important role for ET in diabetic dyslipidemia is suggested by a study that found the impaired intracellular Ca^{2+} extrusion of porcine coronary smooth muscle was corrected by a 20-week program of treadmill running [92]. A previous study from that laboratory revealed that ET in this model of diabetic dyslipidemia prevented the increased coupling of Ca^{2+} release to K_{Ca} channel activation [93]. A summary of ET-induced changes in coronary VSMCs is provided in Fig. 8.1.

Potassium Channels

K^+ sarcolemmal channels are important determinants of intracellular calcium by their effects on membrane potential since they affect membrane hyperpolarization. In large coronary arteries, contractions were evoked by blocking K_{Ca} and K_v channels; the magnitude of these contractions was greater in ET swine than in their sedentary controls [89]. Thus, another

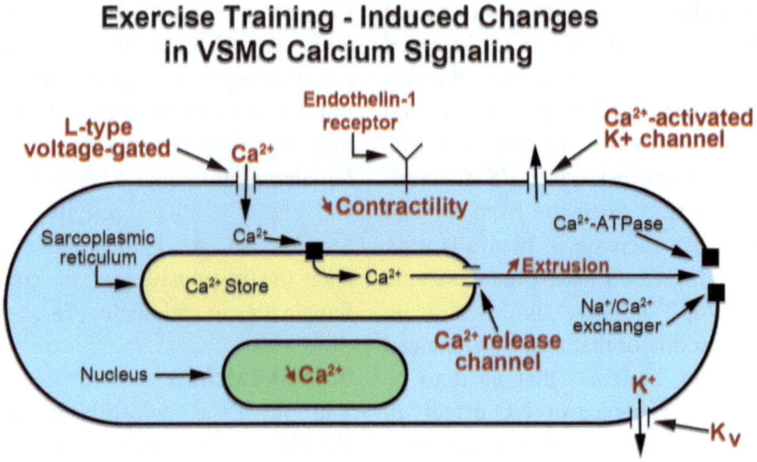

Fig. 8.1 Effects of exercise training (ET) on calcium signaling in coronary VSMC that result in attenuated vasoconstriction. These effects include increased subsarcolemmal Ca^{2+} cycling, decreased responses to endothelin-1 and nuclear Ca^{2+}, and increased Ca^{2+} release from the sarcoplasmic reticulum and its extrusion from the cell. Although Ca^{2+} entry into the cell is increased by ET, K^+ extrusion via its Ca^{2+}-activated channel is increased. This summary is based on: Wamhoff et al. [91], Bowles et al. [87], and Bowles and Wamhoff [182]. For details, see text

In conclusion, ET induces changes in VSMCs of large (conduit) coronary arteries that decrease the sensitivity of these vessels to α-adrenergic agonists and endothelin-1. These adaptations appear to be related to sarcoplasmic Ca^{2+} unloading. ET enhancement of vasodilation in these vessels is species dependent. Both humans and experimental animals show endothelium-dependent vasodilatory responses for ET that is related to enhanced NO production and antioxidant enzyme expression. The fact that discordant results have been published regarding ET effects on coronary artery vasoreactivity is due to a variety of factors: species employed, in vitro vs. in vivo conditions, specific agonist employed, and male and female differences. Figure 8.2 summarizes the effects of ET on coronary arterial constriction and dilation.

benefit of ET is an increase in the contribution of these channels to basal tone. Aging is associated with downregulation of large-conductance voltage- and calcium-activated K^+ channels. Low-intensity ET in senescent rats was shown to attenuate this decline, a finding that suggests it may restore the age-related decline in coronary artery vasodilation [94].

Collateral Growth and Adaptations in Humans

As discussed in Chaps. 4, 5, and 10, collateral coronary arterial growth is the most significant adaptive process that can compensate for arterial obstruction and therefore is of great clinical significance. The importance of inter-arterial collaterals is well supported by various data that indicate that patients who have extensive collaterals and coronary obstruction have prolonged survival. More than 50 years ago, postmortem angiography documented collaterals, with greater diameters in individuals with coronary artery narrowing [95].

Most of the observations and data from humans with ischemic heart disease have not produced a clear consensus regarding the role of exercise in producing collateral growth, as indicated by a recent review [96]. This is not surprising because the methods of assessment available for use in human subjects are limited. Cohen's review [97] details the findings on humans and the various methods employed. In many studies, the patients with obstructive CAD participated only in very mild exercise programs. Not surprisingly, angiographic evaluation, the criteria for accessing the abundance of collaterals, did not provide conclusive evidence that ET affected collateral development [6, 98, 99] because angiography does not effectively demonstrate transmural vessels, nor can it identify microvessels, i.e., those smaller than 100 μm. Moreover, an investigation on patients with stenotic CAD found no conclusive evidence that intensive ET and low fat diet for 1 year enhanced collateral growth [100].

However, there is strong evidence that ET in the ischemic environment enhances coronary collateral flow. As summarized by Sasayama [101], patients with stable effort angina who trained on a treadmill and received heparin treatment experienced an increase in coronary collateral circulation. More recent studies have also indicated that collateral flow is enhanced in patients with CAD. These studies have utilized coronary flow index, a measure of collateral function. Senti et al. [102] used this approach in patients undergoing percutaneous transmural coronary angioplasty and reported that

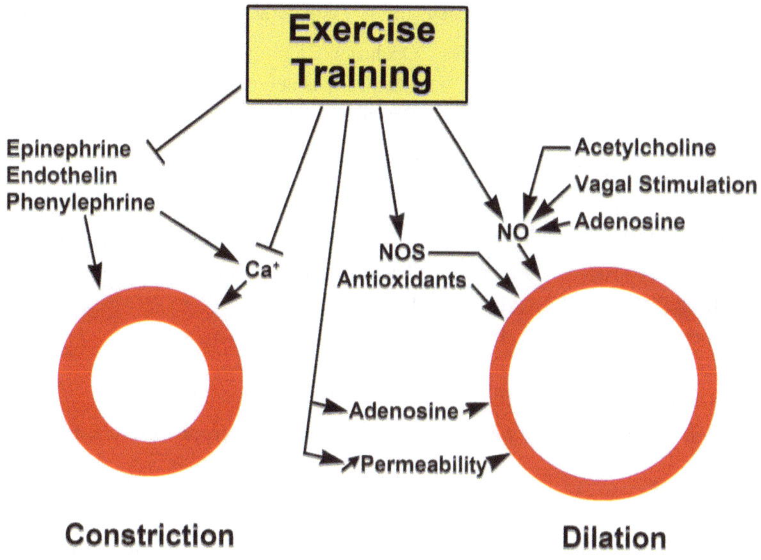

Fig. 8.2 Exercise training facilitates adaptations in coronary arteries. These include decreased responses to vasoconstrictors and enhanced responses to vasodilators. NO plays a key role in these adaptations

long-term physical activity during leisure time and the severity of the stenosis were determinants of the degree of coronary collateral flow. Consistent with these data, collateral flow, based on the collateral flow index, was found to be greater in patients with CAD who completed a 3-month ET program than in a sedentary group [103].

At best, the human studies are inconclusive for several reasons. First, improvements in maximal oxygen consumption may be the consequence of determinants other than collateral flow improvements (e.g., biochemical adaptations). Second, many of the studies did not use standardized training programs and did not provide evidence of "training effects." Third, subject variability with regard to the degree of arterial blockage, ventricular mass, and pharmacological agents prescribed reduce the probability of acceptable standard deviations. Finally, as previously stated, much of the data are based on indirect assessment of collateral growth, which is a limitation. Thus, animal studies are much more likely to provide reliable data.

Collateral Growth and Adaptations in Experimental Animals

Collateral Growth

Most of the data regarding collateral growth in response to ET is based on canine or porcine studies. This topic has been recently reviewed by Heaps and Parker [96]. The classical study of Eckstein [104] demonstrated for the first time that exercise training in hearts with coronary artery narrowing induced collateral growth. He trained 44 dogs on a treadmill 5 days per week for 6–8 weeks and found that circumflex retrograde flow was higher in the trained group, a finding that reflected an increase in the collateral vascular bed. That exercise training in the absence of myocardial ischemia does not stimulate collateral growth has been documented by many laboratories in dogs [38, 105, 106], swine [107], and rats [108]. Postmortem angiograms in trained and sedentary dogs also did not reveal differences in collaterals [109]. These findings are not surprising since exercise in healthy subjects is unlikely to cause ischemia and therefore does not provide the primary stimulus for collateral growth.

As noted in Table 8.1, many studies have concurred with Eckstein's work that ET in animals with coronary occlusion enhances collateral development and/or coronary flow in dogs [38, 110–112], pigs [113, 114], and rats [108]. However, two studies on dogs [115, 116] did not find significant effects of training on collateral development. Although an increase in epicardial collaterals was noted in trained dogs by Neill and Oxendine [111], they could not document an increase in perfusion. The lack of agreement from the dog studies is not surprising because of differences in the types of measurements utilized and the time of ET onset after occlusion. The failure to find a training effect on collateral formation [115] was likely due to the dependence entirely on angiograms of epicardial vessels; therefore data on intramural collaterals were not included. Moreover, no quantitative data were provided. However, even when similar approaches were utilized to measure collateral flow, i.e., radioactive microspheres [112, 116], the conclusions were not always consistent.

The dog is probably not the appropriate model for studies addressing factors that influence the development of coronary collateral vessels. First, the dog has an extensive col-

Table 8.1 Exercise training-induced coronary collateral growth in experimental animals with coronary occlusion

References	Species	Occlusion/ET program	Findings
Eckstein [104]	Dogs	LCx, various degrees occlusion/6–8 weeks	↑ Retrograde flow proportioned to degree of constriction
Heaton et al. [110]	Dogs	Gradual LAD/6 weeks	39% ↑ in retrograde flow during exercise
Neill and Oxendine [111]	Dogs	Gradual LCx/5 and 8 weeks	↑ epi collaterals; no effect on flow
Cohen et al. [112]	Dogs	LCx—75–85% stenosis/10–12 weeks	2× ↑ in flow to ischemic region
Bloor et al. [113]	Pigs	Gradual—LCx/5 months	2× ↑ in flow to border region; ET pigs had smaller infarcts
Roth et al. [114]	Pigs	Gradual LCx/5 weeks, severe or moderate	58, 35, 29% ↑ in epi, mid, and endo flows—severe ET
Koerner et al. [108]	Rats	Acute/12–24 weeks ligation	16% ↑in flow to border zone
Kaplinsky et al. [115]	Dogs	Ligation LAD	Angiograms (qualitative);no effect
Schaper [116]	Dogs	Gradual LCx and RCA/14 weeks	No effect—subepi and subendo flows (Langendorff)
Scheel et al. [38]	Dogs	Gradual LCx/6 weeks	2× ↑ in collateral conductance
Lu et al. [118]	Pigs	Intermittent occlusion/8 weeks	1.8× ↑ in ischemic region flow

LCx left circumflex artery; *LAD* left anterior descending artery; *ET* exercise training

lateral vasculature and already undergoes development of large collaterals when coronary artery occlusion occurs. Second, the dog is normally a very active animal (compared to pigs). Third, the collateral vasculature in the pig is more similar to humans than that of dogs. Its innate collateral circulation is very limited and it lacks the large epicardial collaterals characteristic of dogs [117]. Thus, the porcine studies from Bloor's laboratory [113, 114] provide a comparison with the numerous canine studies. Gradual coronary occlusion of the circumflex artery was induced in pigs and then one group of the animals was subjected to a 5-month program of exercise training. Compared to the non-trained control group, the ET pigs had smaller infarcts and a greater increase in collateral flow in or near the ischemic zone. The endomyocardial/epimyocardial blood flows in the tissue region served by the occluded left circumflex coronary artery were not altered. Most importantly, the time to exhaustion during a stress test in the ET group was double that of the non-trained pigs.

The role of intermittent myocardial ischemia combined with ET was explored in miniature swine [118]. One group was subjected to daily 2-min coronary artery occlusions during an 8-week period, while a second group underwent the same procedure and was also exposed to a program of treadmill exercise. The authors concluded that ET promoted collateral formation, as evidenced by higher blood flow to the collateral-dependent region associated with increases in vascular endothelial growth factor (VEGF) and VEGFR-2 expression. Although intermittent occlusions in the non-trained pigs also caused improvements in blood flow, those in the ET group were greater.

> Based on the various studies cited here and in Table 8.1, there is fairly good evidence that ET can induce collateral development in ischemic, but not in nonischemic, hearts. Thus, ischemia is a requisite for ET to facilitate collateralization in the coronary vasculature. Differences in the coronary arterial hierarchy and the extent and types of native collaterals in different animal species (defined in Chap. 4) may underlie some of the discordant findings.

Changes in Collateral-Dependent Vessel Function

Impairment of Collateral-Dependent Arteries

Many laboratories have documented impaired vasomotor responses in collateral-dependent arteries of dogs [119–122] and swine [72, 123–126]. These are downstream vessels that receive flow from collaterals. Compared to arteries and arterioles from non-collateral-dependent regions of the myocardium, they show an impaired vasorelaxation in response to adenosine and an enhanced α-adrenergic-induced vasoconstriction [119]. Similarly, constriction to vasopressin was elevated, while relaxation to acetylcholine or ADP was impaired in microvessels [121]. In a porcine model, altered vasoactive responses in microvessels from collateral-dependent myocardial regions have also been documented [121]. Relaxation to the endothelium-independent agent sodium nitroprusside was enhanced, while relaxation evoked by endothelium-dependent agents bradykinin and ADP was impaired. These data demonstrate that changes in the vascular responses to vasoactive substances in collateral-dependent vessels are specific. They suggest that blood flow to the collateral-dependent myocardium may be impaired when O_2 demand is increased.

ET Improves Impaired Relaxation of Collateral-Dependent Coronary Arteries

The finding that ET enhances the sensitivity of porcine arteries to adenosine [67] brought to focus the hypothesis that the impaired responses of collateral-dependent arteries to adenosine may be improved by ET [127]. Ameroid occluders were placed on the left circumflex artery of female swine, and 8 weeks later, an ET program of treadmill running that occurred over a 16-week period was initiated. ET prevented the impaired relaxation to two cAMP-dependent vasodilators, adenosine, and isoproterenol. The likely mechanism underlying a reversal of the impaired relaxation in response to adenosine was suggested to be a greater reduction in intracellular Ca^{2+} concentration, which these investigators found to parallel the decline in developed tension of the isolated arterial rings. ET has a positive effect on several parameters in collateral-dependent arterioles in pigs. It restores coronary arteriolar dilation in response to NOS activation and at the same time increases H_2O_2 production [126]. Moreover, ET causes an increase in endothelial NOS in arterioles [125]. $VEGF_{165}$-induced vasodilation of collateral-dependent arterioles is enhanced by ET and is dependent on NO synthase and tyrosine kinase activity [123]. The $VEGF_{165}$-mediated vasodilation in these arterioles is dependent on neuropilin-1, as demonstrated by the finding that inhibition of $VEGF_{165}$-neuropilin interaction prevents the enhanced vasodilation in the arterioles of the ET pigs [124].

Griffin et al. [128] documented improved endothelium-mediated relaxation in collateral-dependent arterioles from exercised pigs. Their study demonstrated that vasorelaxation was improved in response to bradykinin and that the improvement contributed to the enhanced expression of EC NOS mRNA. Coronary artery (~1 mm lumen diameter) segments from collateral-dependent and -independent arteries were studied in order to test hypotheses regarding larger components of the arterial hierarchy [129]. A 14-week ET program increased EC Ca^{2+}, eNOS protein, and the distribution of eNOS-to-caveolin-1 ratio at the plasma membrane in ECs of both collateral-dependent and -independent arteries. The possibility that collateral growth associated with ET may involve recruitment of bone marrow cells may be consistent with data that showed a nearly fourfold increase in these cells after a single bout of intense exercise [130]. Cultured/circulating angiogenic cells were enhanced 2.5-fold. Of particular clinical relevance is the finding that patients with CAD and cardiovascular risk factors experienced a 2.9-fold increase in circulating putative endothelial progenitor cells (EPCs) [131]. This enhancement was associated with improved vascular function and increased NO synthesis. Patients with chronic heart failure who completed a 6-month training program that corrected endothelial dysfunction experienced a 77% increase in the migration of circulating angiogenic cells [132]. Prior to training a single bout of exercise elevated circulating angiogenic cells; but after training, this acute change did not occur. The authors suggested that the repetitive bouts of exercise lead to a progressive endothelial repair.

Paradoxically, collateral-dependent arteries in ET pigs also enhance contractile responses of collateral-dependent coronary arteries [133]. This adaptation was attributed to a greater PKC-mediated Ca^{2+} sensitization. Contractile responses to endothelin-1 were enhanced in these arteries in ET pigs.

In conclusion, collateral-dependent arteries/arterioles are characterized by vasomotor impairment that may limit perfusion. ET in humans and experimental animals has been shown to improve impaired relaxation of these vessels primarily via eNOS. In humans, endothelial repair may occur by ET-induced recruitment of putative EPCs.

Capillary Formation and Remodeling

Assessment of capillary neoformation has most often been based on capillary counts expressed per area of tissue, i.e., numerical density. This approach requires that acceptable tissue cross sections are obtained. A more sensitive measurement is length density, which defines the total capillary length in a given volume of tissue. EC proliferation in capillary profiles based on DNA technology has also been used. However, this parameter requires that the time point of assessment corresponds to the phase of ET when proliferation is occurring.

Quantification of the myocardial capillary bed also requires that all capillaries are readily identified either by labeling or evaluated in thin plastic-embedded sections. To determine if capillary growth has occurred when quantifying numerical or length densities, one needs to know whether cardiomyocyte growth occurred. If so, no change in capillary density would actually indicate capillary growth proportional to the growth of the myocardium. Moreover, in comparing capillary data from trained experimental animals, it is important to consider species, sex, and age as determinates of the outcome observed.

The necessity of a very rich capillary supply to the myocardium in organisms with a high O_2 demand is consistent with the importance of short intercapillary distances for O_2 diffusion. This supposition is supported by data that have documented a higher myocardial capillary density in wild compared to domestic animals, e.g., wild vs. laboratory rat [134] and hare vs. domestic rabbit [135]. Early studies on the

Table 8.2 Effects of exercise training on myocardial capillarization: studies on rats

References	Exercise program	Sex–age	Cardiac hypertrophy	Findings
Leon and Bloor [148]	10 weeks—swim daily or 2×/week	M-young	Yes-daily	C/F ratio ↑—most
		M-young	No-2×/week	in daily group
Bloor and Leon [143]	10 weeks—swim daily or 2×/week	M-1 month	Yes	C/F ratio ↑
		M-3 months	Yes	C/F ratio ↑
		M-12 months	Yes	C/F ratio—no change
Tomanek [142]	12 weeks—treadmill	M-3 months	No	C/F ratio and CD ↑
		M-7 months	No	C/F ↑
		M-22 months	No	C/F ↑
Frenzel et al. [153]	9 weeks—swim	F-young	Yes	CD ↓, cap diam ↑
Jacobs et al. [237]	3 or 6 weeks	M-young	No	CD ↑
		M-adult	No	CD ↑
Anversa et al. [146]	7 weeks—treadmill	M-young	Yes RV	CD ↑
Anversa et al. [145]	7 weeks—treadmill strenuous exercise	M-young	Yes RV	CD ↓
Anversa et al. [147]	7 weeks—treadmill strenuous exercise	M-young	Yes LV	CD↓
Mattfeldt et al. [157]	18 weeks—treadmill	F-young	Yes	CD, Vol. dens. no change C/F ratio ↑
Mandache et al. [139]	4 weeks and 3 months—swim	F-young	Yes	↑ EC mitoses
Suzuki [238]	6 weeks—treadmill	M-yes	No	C/F ratio no change
Unge et al. [140]	3 weeks—swim	M-young	Yes	↑ EC mitoses
		M-adult	No	↑ EC mitoses
		M-old	Yes	No□ in mitoses
Carlsson et al. [150]	2 weeks—swim	F-young	No	↑ EC mitoses
Kayar [158]	6 weeks—treadmill	M-young	Yes	CD ↓
Bell and Rasmussen [239]	6–11 weeks	M-10 weeks	?	C/F ratio ↑
		M-15 weeks	?	C/F ratio ↑
Tittle et al. [149]	16 weeks	M and F	Yes	CD ↑
White et al. [62]	5 months—treadmill swim	M-adult	Yes	CD ↑
		F-adult	Yes	CD ↑
Ljungqvist and Unge [141]	4 weeks—swim	F-young	Yes	↑ EC mitoses
Tornling [166]	3 weeks—swim	M-young	Yes	CF ↑
		M-adult		CF ↑
Tharpe and Wagner [160]	8 weeks—treadmill 3–5 days/week	Young	Yes	CD ↓
Belabbas et al. [178]	10 weeks—treadmill	Young	Yes	CD ↑
Rakusan et al. [151]	6 weeks—swimming	F-young	Yes	Total capillary length ↑
Rakusan et al. [152]	5–6 weeks—swimming	F-young	Yes	# Capillaries/arteriole ↑ CD—no □
Marcus and Tipton [175]	12 weeks—treadmill	M-young	Yes	CD—no□
McElroy et al. [188]	5 weeks—swimming	M-young	No	C/F ratio ↑

M male; *F* female; *C/F* capillary/fiber (cardiomyocyte); *CD* capillary density; *EC* endothelial cell

effects of ET on myocardial capillary density in guinea pigs reported both increases [136, 137] and decreases in this parameter [138].

Studies in Rodents

Since that time, many studies have exercise-trained rats by running on a treadmill or by swimming (Table 8.2). The majority of these studies have documented increases in capillary density and/or capillary density/cardiomyocyte fiber ratio, or proliferation as indicated by EC mitoses in the trained animals. In some studies, but not in others, cardiac hypertrophy occurred in response to the training protocol. In the studies listed in Table 8.3, capillary growth is documented in every study but one where cardiac hypertrophy was absent and in most studies where hypertrophy was present. That ET stimulated capillary EC mitoses was documented in all studies that evaluated this index of growth [139–141]. The role of age as a determinant of capillary growth is indicated by several studies beginning with the work of Tomanek [142] and Bloor and Leon [143] who showed that capillary growth was restricted in older exercise-trained rats. The limiting effect of age on capillary proliferation in response to ET was also demonstrated by Unge et al. [140], who reported endothelial cell (EC) mitoses in young and

Table 8.3 Effects of exercise training on myocardial capillarization: studies on dogs and pigs

References	Exercise program	Sex–age	Cardiac hypertrophy	Findings
Thörner [162]		12–24 months	Yes	CD ↑
Wyatt and Mitchell [59]	Dogs—12 weeks treadmill	M and F—adult	?	CD no change
Laughlin and Tomanek [27]	Dogs—18 weeks treadmill	M and F—adult	No	CD no change
				C/F ratio no change
White et al. [61]	Pigs—10 weeks treadmill	?—Young	Yes	CD ↑
	moderate treadmill intense		Yes	CD ↓
Breisch et al. [40]	Pigs—12 weeks treadmill	M and F	Yes	CD ↓
White et al. [63]	Pigs treadmill	3 weeks	No	CD ↑, EC mitoses ↑
		8 weeks	Yes	CD—no change

Abbreviations are the same as in Table 8.2

adult, but not old rats. Studies that did not find exercise-induced increases in capillarity density all reported increased heart mass, which indicates that capillary growth paralleled the growth of cardiomyocytes. Studies in mice also showed that ET consisting of running [144] or swimming [60] over a 3- or 4-week period increased capillary density.

Variables Influencing ET Results

The type of ET program, its intensity, and its frequency are important determinants of capillary growth. Studies by Anversa et al. [145–147] demonstrated that moderate exercise training was associated with a 16% increase in capillary density while strenuous exercise affected a 14% decrease in this parameter. At the same time, frequency of training plays a role in the response of the capillary bed. For example, daily swim-training affected a greater capillary proliferation than semiweekly sessions even though the former, but not the latter, caused cardiac hypertrophy [148]. Although more studies included male than female rats, those that included both sexes documented capillary growth in both [62, 149]. Most studies that included only female rats also provided evidence that ET induces capillary growth as documented by increases in EC mitoses [139, 141, 150], total capillary length [151], and number of capillaries per arteriole [152]. In contrast, Frenzel [153] reported no change in capillary/cardiomyocyte ratio and a drop in capillary density. However, ET evoked an increase in capillary diameter in response to a high degree (72%) of cardiac hypertrophy.

ET in Mothers Affects Capillarization in Offspring

The effect of ET during pregnancy on myocardial capillarization of the offspring was determined in a series of studies by Parizkova [154–156]. Male offspring of ET mothers had higher capillary/cardiomyocyte ratios and shorter diffusion distances than offspring from non-ET mothers. ET in the offspring of ET mothers caused a further increase in capillary density. Male and female offspring did not differ with regard to these parameters. Thus, the in utero environment is effected by the mother's physical activity and in this case promoted the growth of myocardial capillaries of the fetuses.

Deconditioning Decreases Capillary Density

To maintain the increase in capillary density derived from a 10-week ET program, some level and frequency of ET must be employed. Rats trained by swimming for 60 min/5 days per week had significant increases in capillary density, and the number of capillaries/cardiomyocyte, and were able to maintain these gains only if they swam at least 30 min, twice per week.

Summary: ET-induced Capillary Growth in Rodents

In sum, a lack of or inadequate growth of the capillary bed in exercised rats is the exception rather than the rule, and when this finding was reported, it always involved hypertrophied hearts [153, 157–160]. Based on studies that quantified EC proliferation, the evidence indicates that ET triggers this response. When cardiac hypertrophy is also evoked by ET, the EC proliferative response may or may not be adequate to fully compensate for the increased cardiac mass. Whereas males and females appear to respond similarly to ET with regard to capillarization, age is a determinant of myocardial capillary growth in response to ET as documented in studies on guinea pigs [137] and rats [140, 142, 143]. The intensity or duration is also a determinant of ET-induced capillary growth as already recognized more than 7 decades ago [137]. In that study, mild ET was ineffective for angiogenesis. However, if exercise is too strenuous, angiogenesis is also lacking or inadequate in the right [145] and left [161] ventricle.

Studies on Dogs and Swine (Table 8.3)

Although Thorner [162] reported a greater capillary density in his two trained dogs, subsequent studies by Wyatt [59] and Laughlin and Tomanek [27] were unable to confirm this finding. Since myocardial capillary diffusion capacity is increased in ET dogs [26, 27], this increase is related to determinants of capillary blood flow and/or the relationship between capillary area available for exchange and capillary perfusion rather than capillary density. Studies on swine from Bloor's lab indicated that exercise training in farm pigs with cardiac hypertrophy resulted in a decreased capillary density [40], while in Yucatan pigs, capillary density was increased by moderate training and decreased in severe training [61]. In mini-pigs, exercise training of just 3 weeks resulted in increased EC mitoses and capillary density [62]. This occurred prior to significant cardiac hypertrophy. With establishment of cardiac hypertrophy at 8 weeks, capillary density was normalized. However, capillary diameter showed a gradual increase between 3 and 16 weeks of training.

Taken together, these studies indicate that ET induces capillary growth in swine. However, whether this growth fully compensates for the presence of cardiac hypertrophy depends on the magnitude of the growth. In contrast, ET in dogs has not been shown to enhance capillary density.

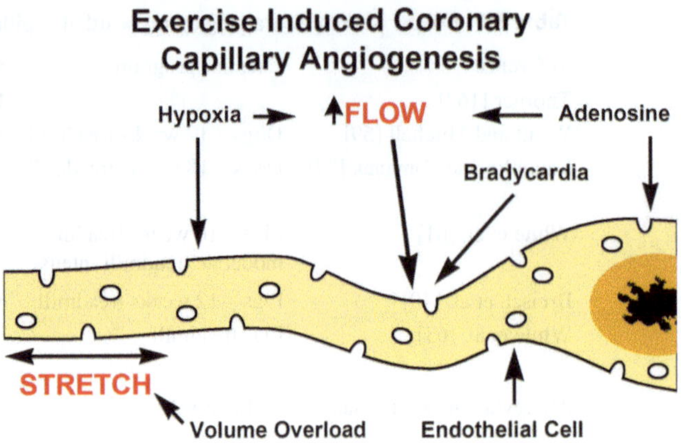

Fig. 8.3 Coronary capillary angiogenesis is a response to endurance exercise training as indicated by most studies. Increased flow due to hypoxia or adenosine provides a mechanical stimulus. Hypoxia and adenosine, independent of flow, may also provide a primary stimulus by the activation of growth factors, although this is less likely. The volume overload, due to increased venous return, causes stretch of ECs which is known to trigger angiogenic growth factors. Finally, training-induced resting bradycardia also increases venous return, which stretches ECs and cardiomyocytes, thus providing a mechanical stimulus for growth factor upregulation

ET-Induced Mechanisms of Capillary Growth

For a discussion of ET-induced vascular growth in skeletal muscle and heart, see Prior et al. [163].

Enhanced Blood Flow

Based on these data, one can conclude that the capillary bed proliferates in response to chronic exercise in rats and pigs, but not dogs. Possible explanations for the failure of ET to evoke capillary angiogenesis in dogs are that (1) they have an unusually well-developed collateral circulation, (2) their capillary bed adapts by increasing its diffusion capacity, and (3) enhanced O_2 extraction occurs in dogs during high workloads. As discussed in Chaps. 1 and 9, metabolic (hypoxia) and mechanical factors serve as stimuli for vascular growth. As reviewed by Tomanek [164] and Hudlicka et al. [165], enhanced blood flow is a key stimulus for capillary growth, as occurs in response to ET, hypoxia, and elevated thyroid hormone levels. Increases in coronary blood flow via chronic administration of the vasodilator drug, dipyridamole, increases capillary growth in the rat heart [166–168]. Two daily injections over a 5-week period were reported to increase capillary/cardiomyocyte ratio by 24% [166]. In rats with cardiac hypertrophy due to renal hypertension, chronic dipyridamole administration increased endomyocardial capillary length density by 33% [168]. These studies documenting capillary growth in response to increased blood flow support the argument that growth that occurs in response to ET is mediated by increased blood flow.

Prolonged Diastolic Filling and Stretch

Another important consideration is the lower resting heart rate that characterizes aerobic ET. Lowering heart rate by chronic pacing at 60% of normal resting heart rates caused a substantial increase in capillary density [169]. Pharmacologically lowered heart rate also has been shown to stimulate myocardial capillary growth after myocardial infarction in young rats [170]. While total flow through capillaries is not increased during bradycardia, the prolongation of diastole increases two forces on the capillary wall (1) the period of dilation is prolonged and (2) stretch is increased due to prolonged diastolic filling. Myocardial ECs exposed to cyclic stretch have enhanced VEGFR-2 (flk-1) and Tie-1 and Tie-2 protein levels consistent with their increased proliferation [171]. VEGF and its receptors are required for an adequate capillary density, as evidenced in VEGF deficient mice that have a 60% reduction in capillary density [172]. These mice have a severe (81%) decrease in endurance running capacity.

Conclusions Regarding ET Effects on Capillary Growth
Mechanisms underlying ET-induced capillary growth are summarized in Fig. 8.3. ET provides stimuli, such as those accompanying increased blood flow, that increase EC proliferation as well as (in some cases) capillary remodeling to increase luminal diameter. These stimuli include shear stress and stretch. Limiting or modifying factors include age, intensity and duration of ET, and species.

Neovascularization and Blood Flow in Pressure-Overloaded, Ischemic and Postinfarcted Hearts

Pressure Overload

Capillary Growth

More than 3 decades ago Ljungqvist et al. [173] showed that whereas ET by swimming in normotensive rats causes neoformation of myocardial capillaries, this response does not occur in rats with aortic constriction. The magnitude of the resulting hypertrophy is a factor that limits compensatory growth, as evidenced in the aortic constriction model of pressure overload [174]. A 40% LV hypertrophy did not cause a reduction in capillary density, whereas an 80% LV hypertrophy did. Thus, a compensatory capillary growth occurred in the former, but not the latter. An 8-week exercise program (voluntary running in an exercise wheel) failed to increase capillary density in these rats. Similarly, rats with renal hypertension trained by running [175] or swimming [151, 152] did not experience capillary neovascularization. In spontaneously hypertensive rats (SHR), capillary density was increased by ET in young (6 week old) rats [176], but not in 7-month-old rats [177]. These two studies from the same laboratory indicate differential responses that are dependent on the age of the animal and/or the stage of hypertension. In both studies, training effects, indicated by an increased O_2 consumption, were documented and the magnitude of hypertrophy was not significantly enhanced in the trained SHR in either age group. Some evidence for ET-induced capillarization has been reported by two more recent studies. In one, hypertension was induced in 6-week-old rats by chronic infusion of angiotensin II, which caused left ventricular mass to increase by 34% [178]. A 10-week ET program of treadmill running did not enhance the magnitude of hypertrophy, but tended to increase “vessel density” (these were mainly capillaries). That the stage of hypertension may be a determinant of capillary growth in response to ET is suggested by another study that found capillary density and capillary/myocyte ratio in the right ventricle of young rats with stable hypertension to increase with a 4-week program [179]. In contrast, ET rats with progressive hypertension and the development of heart failure did not experience capillary growth as indicated by these indices.

ET Protection Against Ischemia/Reperfusion

To test the hypothesis that the effects of ischemia/reperfusion are attenuated in an exercise-trained animal, mice were housed for 4 weeks in cages with exercise wheels and then subjected to 45 min of coronary artery occlusion followed by 24 h of reperfusion [180]. Compared to mice with no access to an exercise wheel, the ET group had smaller infarcts, and increases in the expression of cardioprotective molecules CuZnSOD and AMP-activated protein kinase. The cardioprotective effects of ET were mediated by alterations in eNOS phosphorylation (an increase in serine 1177 and a decrease in threonine 495), leading to an increase in NO generation and storage of NO metabolites (nitrites and nitrosothiols). The increase in nitrite represents a reversal of the characteristic reduction of nitrite during ischemia reperfusion. The study also revealed that β_3 adrenergic blockade prevented the increase in eNOS and resulted in a loss of cardioprotection.

Myocardial Perfusion

A more critical question is whether ET can improve maximal coronary perfusion and coronary reserve. Studies in Scheuer's laboratory [21, 181] addressed the effects of ET on myocardial blood flow in female rats with hypertension induced by the 1 kidney, 1 clip procedure. The rats trained by a swim protocol over 10–12-week period had higher maximal blood flows during maximal vasodilation with adenosine, despite an increased magnitude of cardiac hypertrophy, than the non-trained hypertensive controls. Another group of investigators used young female Sprague–Dawley rats in which they induced renal hypertension by banding one renal artery and leaving the other untouched [22, 151, 152]. ET, also consisting of moderate swimming, improved maximal coronary resistance in normotensive rats, but not in the hypertensives [22]. Although ET attenuated left ventricular hypertrophy, coronary vasodilator reserve was not altered. Moreover, the higher wall/lumen ratio of coronary arterioles in the hypertensive rats was not affected by ET [152].

Postinfarcted and/or Ischemic Hearts: Studies in Experimental Animals

Postischemic Recovery

ET has been shown to provide a cardioprotective effect for postischemic recovery (reviewed by [182]). This cardioprotection is likely related, in part, to vascular adaptations that occur during ET. One example of such a training effect is a decreased response of microvessels in ET animals to endothelin and the thromboxane A2 analog, U44619 following ischemia [183]. This finding is consistent with data that reveal a lower Ca^{2+} response in coronary smooth muscle cells from ET swine compared to their sedentary controls [184]. Since acute exercise induces heat shock protein (HSP) 70, male and female rats were subjected to a bout of exercise on a treadmill and their hearts removed and evaluated after global ischemia and reperfusion [185]. In males, the exercise-induced increase in HSP 70 was double that of the increase in females, whereas in ovariectomized females, the increase in HSP 70 was similar to that of males. Postischemic left ventricular function was improved in the exercised males, but not in the females with intact ovaries. These findings suggest that estrogen may have negative effects on the heart, which are related to the coronary circulation and are consistent with data that indicate premenopausal women have higher postinfarction mortality rates than men [186]. Most importantly, moderate ET in senescent (24 months) rats was shown to enhance both coronary flow and active tension during reperfusion following a 45-min period of low coronary flow [187]. The data also revealed that ET in the senescent rats decreased LV protein carbonylation, a modification induced by ROS, and increased myocardial HSP 70 and eNOS content.

Myocardial Infarction

Infarct size 48 h after coronary occlusion was studied in previously trained and non-trained rats [188]. Myocardial infarct size was 31% smaller in the trained group, a finding that was considered to be due, at least in part, to the fact that ET enhanced the capillary/cardiomyocyte ratio. The effect of ET on neovascularization after infarction was studied by Przyklenk and Groom [189, 190]. They subjected rats with myocardial infarction to 4 weeks of voluntary exercise in activity cages and found that capillary density and capillary/fiber ratio was normalized in the hypertrophic border (transition) zone if the rats ran 5–10 km during the 4-week period. When rats with myocardial infarctions were trained on a treadmill over a 20-week period, their coronary flow rates and ventricular function were better preserved during and after transient myocardial ischemia than their sedentary counterparts [191]. Moreover, infarct size was smaller. ET has been shown to preserve the heart against ischemia reperfusion injury [192]. A 12-week program of resistance training (using a squat apparatus) in rats was found to increase coronary flow and decrease infarct size following 40 min of ischemia and 80 min of reperfusion.

Leosco et al. [193] induced myocardial infarction in rats that subsequently showed signs of heart failure at the onset of a 10-week program of treadmill running. Data from these experiments documented improvements in LV contractility in response to β-adrenergic stimulation, maximal myocardial perfusion, coronary reserve, capillary density, and arteriolar length density at the conclusion of the ET program. One possible underlying mechanism for the vascular growth was the finding that ET increased VEGF, Akt activation, and Akt-induced eNOS phosphorylation. A role for eNOS in the improvement in ventricular function and attenuation of fibrosis and apoptosis in ET postinfarcted mice has also been reported [194]. A mechanism underlying the more favorable remodeling was not identified. Since NO is important for vascular tone and function, it is possible that the failure of ET in eNOS$^{+/-}$ and eNOS$^{-/-}$ mice to prevent apoptosis and fibrosis may be related to a decline in vascular function. Increases in VEGF and VEGF receptors Flt- and Flk-1 induced by ET have been documented to improve angiogenesis and attenuate infarct size in mice [195]. VEGF and its receptors were upregulated by exercise in mice with infarction, but not in mice that were not infarcted. This finding indicates that this ET effect requires the context of ischemia.

Postinfarcted and/or Ischemic Hearts: Studies in Humans

ET in Patients with Coronary Disease

ET is commonly prescribed for patients with CAD and has been studied to determine its effects on myocardial oxygenation. Detry and Bruce [196] studied the effects of 3 months ET on the relationship between ST segment depression to the product of heart rate and systolic blood pressure in patients with CAD and did not find a significant ET effect. Subsequently, Ehsani and colleagues [197] noted that the studies employing mild, intermittent, or brief ET programs [99, 198] also did not consistently find an improvement in myocardial ischemia, and suggested that a prolonged program of ET of increasing intensity duration and frequency would improve indicators of myocardial ischemia. To test this hypothesis, they [197] recruited 10 patients, who participated in intense endurance ET lasting 12 months. Initially (3 months) ET consisted of a patient's exercise intensity requiring a 50–70% VO_2 max for 30 min, then increasing to 70–80% of a patient's VO_2 max and lasting 50–60 min with additional, shorter intervals of exercise requiring a 80–90% VO_2 max. A summary of key data is illustrated in Fig. 8.4. VO_2 max increased in every patient (mean = 35%), as did the time to exhaustion (mean = 34%). ET increased the level of heart rate required to reach the threshold for ischemic ST-segment displacement. Finally, the double product ($HR \times SBP \times 10^{-3}$) threshold for ischemic ST-segment depression required to induce 0.1 mV of segment depression increased. This important study documents that a long-term ET program of sufficient intensity in patients with antecedent myocardial ischemia attributable to CAD elicits responses indicative of attenuated myocardial ischemia. These include (1) elevation of the double-product threshold for ischemic ST-segment depression, (2) decrease of ST-segment depression at same double product, and (3) a reduced or unchanged maximal ST-segment depression despite large increases in the maximum double product.

Coronary Function

Chronic heart failure, as often occurs following large myocardial infarctions, is characterized by impaired endothelium-dependent dilation of resistance vessels [199, 200]. On the other hand, exercise has been shown to restore endothelial function in chronic heart failure patients in both peripheral [201] and coronary vessels [202]. ET in patients

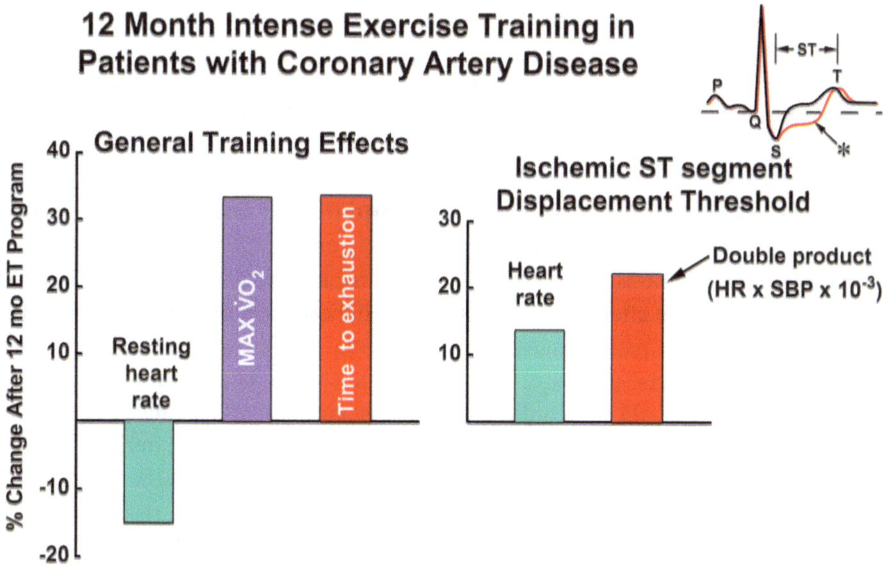

Fig. 8.4 Data summary from an exercise training program study in patients with ischemic ST-segment depression (shown at the *top right* corner of this figure). Data are from Ehasani et al. [197] who utilized a an exercise program involving jogging or bicycle ergometer that required VO_2 max of 50–70% initially and then 80–90%, which is considered intense for this group of ten patients, nine of which had previously experienced a single myocardial infarction. The program resulted in a reduction in resting heart rate, an increase in max VO_2, and a reduction in ST-segment displacement. The double product threshold for an ischemic ST-segment response was defined as the product of systolic blood pressure and heart rate at which ischemic ST-segment displacement first appeared

with recent myocardial infarction was found to improve endothelial function as measured by flow-mediated dilation and von Willebrand factor levels in the brachial artery [203]. These effects did not persist when training was discontinued. Whether endothelial function was affected in the coronary vasculature was not addressed. Some of the benefits of exercise, however, may be due to training effects other than improved coronary vessel function, e.g., a higher exercise capacity and maximal oxygen uptake can be a consequence of adaptations in cardiac and skeletal muscle and neurohumoral control. Nevertheless, ET in patients with CAD or after myocardial infarction has been documented to improve coronary circulation. Postinfarction patients who trained 3×/week for 12 weeks had 20% and 28% improvements in coronary vasodilator reserve in the infarcted and remote myocardial regions, respectively [204]. Additionally, maximal perfusion in the myocardial remote region was increased by 33% in the ET group [205]. Early onset (9 ± 3 days) of ET after acute MI in 50 patients over a 6-month period was shown to reduce stress-induced ischemia and to improve LV wall motion and thickness [206].

Coronary Structure

The relationship between the size of the coronary vasculature and myocardial infarction has also been studied. When coronary arteries were injected with ink in 216 necropsy cases, several findings of interest were noted [207]. First, coronary artery cross-sectional areas increased with age. Second, the group with myocardial infarction had smaller coronary artery cross-sectional areas than the noninfarcted group. Finally, those individuals in the infarct group identified as physically active (including those doing heavy work) had coronary artery cross-sectional areas that were 75% greater than in those individuals whose lifestyle was labeled as inactive. The observation that the size of coronary arteries increases with age was also observed in another study [208]. The subjects for that study were Masi men who led very active lives, but had a high fat diet. At autopsy, coronary artery intimal thickening was found to be similar to American men, but these vessels were enlarged and thus appeared to compensate for the atherosclerosis.

Is ET in patients with CAD as effective as percutaneous coronary angioplasty? This question was addressed in 101 male patients aged 70 and older [209]. In the group that trained for 12 months, only 6 of 51 patients reported ischemic events, compared to 21 of 50 in PCI group. While both groups demonstrated symptom-free exercise tolerance, the ET patients had a higher exercise capacity and maximal oxygen uptake. These findings suggest that ET has some advantages over PCI in event-free survival and exercise capacity.

ET Increases Bone Marrow-Derived Cells

Enhancement of bone marrow-derived cells (BMDCs) as a therapeutic aid for patients with ischemic heart disease has received considerable attention during the last decade. These cells have been found to improve endothelial function, enhance angiogenesis, and promote vascular repair. Healthy young male volunteers were trained according to one of three protocols [210]. When the subjects ran for 30 min 4–5 times per week, their circulating BMDCs increased about 2.5-fold. The maximum elevation in these cells was noted 10–30 min after intensive running. Another study on healthy subjects documented a nearly fourfold increase in BMDCs and a 2.5-fold increase in cultured angiogenic cells after a single bout of exhaustive exercise [130]. Studies on patients have also provided data demonstrating the beneficial effects of exercise on angiogenic cells. Patients with CAD and cardiovascular risk factors were subjected to a 12-week program consisting of running [131]. BMDCs were enhanced 2.9-fold by ET and correlated with the increase in NO_x (the degradation products of the NO pathway). Encouraging results were also obtained in patients with chronic heart failure [132]. Circulating angiogenic cells from these patients were impaired as documented by migration assays. However, following a single exercise bout, migration of these cells was normalized. The 6-month ET program increased the number of BMDCs.

Conclusions Regarding ET in Overloaded and Ischemic Hearts

Data regarding ET as a stimulus for myocardial capillary neoformation in the pressure overloaded heart require careful scrutiny, since there are a number of variables to be considered. Both age and the stage of hypertension are limiting factors. Similarly, the role of ET in improving coronary blood flow is not clearly established in the hypertensive heart. In contrast, the ET appears to be effective in decreasing infarct size, increasing maximal perfusion and coronary reserve, restoring EC function, and increasing the number of BMDCs in the circulation.

Exercise Training Effects on Coronary Artery Disease

Prevention and Treatment in Humans

ET has been shown to be beneficial for the prevention and treatment of CAD and is advocated by the NIH [211] and the American Heart Association [212]. As noted in an AHA Scientific Statement [213], the importance of physical activity in reducing the incidence of CAD has been consistently documented and a reduction of atherosclerotic risk factors has also been established. However, the specific mechanisms underlying the preventative and restorative effects of ET on the coronary vasculature are not fully understood. Therefore, most of the evidence regarding the effects of ET on atherosclerosis is based on overall functional improvement, a reduction in angina and a higher exercise tolerance.

ET and Risk of Coronary Artery Disease

A study on over 28,000 women explored the relationship of physical activity, as indicated by kcal expenditure/week and the reduction in cardiovascular events [214]. After obtaining the initial laboratory data, the women were reevaluated 11 years later. The data revealed that lowering of inflammatory/hemostatic biomarkers (high-sensitivity C-reactive protein, fibrinogen, and soluble intracellular molecule-1) was the greatest contributor to the inverse relationship between physical activity and the risk of cardiovascular disease, followed by blood pressure and lipids. Although study limitations included dependence on self-estimates of activity levels by participants and a lack of data on training effects, the large number of women enrolled provides for some valuable insights. Of special significance are data from a meta-analysis of 26 studies that included 500,000 individuals who were followed up for 4–25 years [215]. The focus of the analysis was the relationship between physical activity and primary prevention of coronary heart disease. This meta-analysis indicated that a high level of physical activity was associated with a 27% lower risk of coronary heart disease and that even a moderate level of physical activity was found to be associated with a 17% decline in risk. Further evidence that aerobic fitness is associated with a reduced incidence of atherosclerosis comes from an evaluation of middle-aged men [216]. That study found that the individuals with the greatest aerobic fitness had less advanced atherosclerosis.

Specific Cardiovascular Benefits

A recent review has considered the effects of ET on the causal factors of atherosclerosis, i.e., lipoproteins, inflammation, and thrombosis, and concluded that ET is effective in reducing triglycerides, apolipoprotein B (the primary apolipoprotein of low density lipoproteins), and coronary artery calcium [217]. Programs in heart disease rehabilitation have also documented a reduction in total cholesterol and triglycerides, inflammation and homocysteine levels, and improvements in exercise capacity in ET patients [218]. Evidence that high intensity interval ET reduces systemic inflammation in patients after percutaneous coronary intervention was obtained from 40 patients who trained for 6 months [219]. The findings indicated that (1) ET reduced inflammatory markers interleukin-6 and -8 and C-reactive protein and (2) these reductions correlated significantly with attenuation in luminal reduction at 6 months. Although not established in these studies, these improvements in inflammatory markers may contribute to or reflect improved coronary circulation. There is substantial evidence that ET reduces vascular wall inflammation (reviewed in [220]). C-reactive protein, produced in response to inflammatory cytokines, primarily IL-6, has been shown by many investigators to be reduced by ET (for review, see [220]). A study of particular importance in this regard is that of Walther et al. [221]. A comparison of percutaneous intervention with stent and ET in 101 patients with stable CAD revealed that ET reduced C-reactive protein by 41%, whereas the percutaneous intervention failed to affect any change. The improvement in the ET group was independent of statin therapy and weight loss. Sedentary individuals are at high risk of acute coronary syndromes, such as coronary plaque rupture, whereas those who sustain ET are at lower risk because of reduced platelet reactivity and better fibrinolytic systems which limit plaque formation [222].

One important benefit of ET was found to be a lower need for further revascularization after both stent and percutaneous transluminal coronary angioplasty, as determined in 118 patients [223]. The study also reported that the ET was associated with improved perfusion of the territory distal to the stenosis and a lower rate of new epicardial coronary stenoses.

Endothelial Dysfunction

ET has numerous favorable effects on the endothelium that contribute, in large part, to the prevention or attenuation of atherosclerosis. These effects, both in humans and experimental animals, have been recently reviewed [224]. Disturbances in endothelial dysfunction, common in patients with CAD (e.g., atherosclerosis), is characterized by a reduced availability of NO associated with vasoconstriction (reviewed in [220]). Work by Hambrecht and colleagues [201] has documented improved endothelial function in patients with CAD who exercise regularly and found that this improvement was due to increases in eNOS phosphorylation. Impairment of NO production in combination with excessive oxidative stress contributes to endothelial dysfunction and consequently myocardial ischemia [225]. The increase in myocardial perfusion in patients with CAD after a program of ET is largely attributable to improved endothelial dysfunction. A hospital-based ET program improved endothelium-dependent vasodilation (response to acetylcholine) fourfold [226]. Ribeiro et al. [220] suggested that exercise induces both an increase in NO production and a decrease in NO degradation associated with increased SOD. Endothelial dysfunction was improved in 39 patients with CAD who participated in a 4-week ET program [227], based on the finding that blood flow velocity in the internal mammary artery in response to acetylcholine increased 93% after ET. Moreover, the improvement correlated with serum concentrations of erythropoietin and VEGF. ET has also been shown, by numerous studies, to downregulate EC proinflammatory activities in humans and laboratory animals [228].

Data from Experimental Animals

There is considerable evidence, from both in vitro and in vivo studies, that hemodynamic stimuli are the major players in adaptations that occur in the vascular wall in response to ET [224]. Since ET can attenuate EC dysfunction, the hypothesis that ET would improve endothelial function of porcine coronary arterioles exposed to a high-fat, high-cholesterol diet was tested [229]. ET enhanced eNOS protein and endothelium-dependent dilation in the coronary arterioles of the pigs fed a high fat diet. The study was based on an early stage of coronary disease. ET near the time of stenting has been shown to prevent stent-induced microvascular dysfunction and to attenuate native atheroma [230]. Hypercholesterolemic swine were characterized by impaired coronary vasodilation in response to adenosine or bradykinin and lower microvascular density. In contrast, the swine that completed a 4-week training program prior to angiography had normal coronary vasodilatory responses to these endothelium-dependent and -independent agents, respectively, and demonstrated a preserved microvascular density. Moreover, native atheroma was reduced by the exercise regimen and the training effects were independent of plasma cholesterol. The study provides a key insight into the preservation of endothelial dysfunction by ET prior to stenting.

Dyslipidemia

The role of ET in prevention of dyslipidemia associated with coronary artery smooth muscle impairment was addressed in Sturek's laboratory [92, 93, 231]. Their experiments showed that ET prevents the increased coupling of Ca^{2+} release to K_{Ca} channel activation in swine with dyslipidemia [93] and restores Ca^{2+} extrusion [92]. They demonstrated that ET specifically prevents diabetic dyslipidemia-induced decreases in Ca^{2+} efflux via the plasma membrane, increases Ca^{+}-ATPase activity and protein expression, and decreases voltage-gated Ca^{2+} channel current density [231]. These effects of ET on Ca^{2+} are consistent with the finding that ET reduces coronary artery maximal responses to endothelin-1 [232]. A recent review of exercise protection against CAD in metabolic syndrome and diabetes concludes that ET either prevents or reverses Ca^{2+} signaling abnormalities [233]. Accordingly, ET modulates the coronary artery VSMC phenotype.

Studies in ET apolipoprotein E mice have documented a reduction in the neointimal growth and severity of atherosclerosis [234–236]. The data from these studies, based on systemic arteries, indicate that ET decreased intimal/media ratio and luminal stenosis [234] and suppressed the atherosclerosis by its antioxidant effects via NO [235]. More recently, ET was found to decrease macrophage concentration and MMP-9 and to increase metalloproteinases in atherosclerotic plaques [236]. These authors considered these changes as responsible for the reduction in plaque severity noted in this study.

Conclusions: ET and Coronary Artery Disease

The benefits of ET on cardiovascular health have long been recognized. More recent data have begun to provide some insights into mechanisms that contribute to the prevention and reversal of CAD. One important finding in both humans and experimental animals is that ET attenuates endothelial dysfunction. Studies have documented that ET corrects Ca^{2+} abnormalities in coronary VSM of swine with dyslipidemia and decreases maximal contractile response to endothelin in coronary atherosclerotic arteries (Fig. 8.1). ET, when properly administered, has both preventative and attenuating effects on parameters of coronary disease.

References

1. Paffenbarger Jr RS, Hyde RT, Wing AL, Hsieh CC. Physical activity, all-cause mortality, and longevity of college alumni. N Engl J Med. 1986;314:605–13.
2. Leon S, Connett J, Jacobs DR, Rauramaa R. Leisure-time physical activity levels and risk of coronary heart disease and death. JAMA. 1987;258:2388–95.
3. Powell KE, Thompson PD, Caspersen CJ, Kendrick JS. Physical activity and the incidence of coronary heart disease. Annu Rev Public Health. 1987;8:253–87.
4. Kavanagh T. Exercise in the primary prevention of coronary artery disease. Can J Cardiol. 2001;17:155–61.
5. Laughlin MH, Bowles DK, Duncker DJ. The coronary circulation in exercise training. Am J Physiol Heart Circ Physiol. 2012; 302:H10–23.
6. Sim DN, Neill WA. Investigation of the physiological basis for increased exercise threshold for angina pectoris after physical conditioning. J Clin Invest. 1974;54:763–70.
7. Jolliffe JA, Rees K, Taylor RS, Thompson D, Oldridge N, Ebrahim S. Exercise-based rehabilitation for coronary heart disease. Cochrane Database Syst Rev 2001;CD001800
8. Renkin EM. Capillary blood flow and transcapillary exchange. Physiologist. 1966;9:361–6.
9. Thijssen DH, Maiorana AJ, O'Driscoll G, Cable NT, Hopman MT, Green DJ. Impact of inactivity and exercise on the vasculature in humans. Eur J Appl Physiol. 2010;108:845–75.
10. Duncker DJ, Bache RJ. Regulation of coronary blood flow during exercise. Physiol Rev. 2008;88:1009–86.
11. Duncker D, Bache R, Merkus D. Regulation of coronary resistance vessel tone in response to exercise. J Mol Cell Cardiol. 2012;52:P802–13.
12. von Restorff W, Holtz J, Bassenge E. Exercise induced augmentation of myocardial oxygen extraction in spite of normal coronary dilatory capacity in dogs. Pflugers Arch. 1977;372:181–5.
13. Vatner SF, Higgins CB, Millard RW, Franklin D. Role of the spleen in the peripheral vascular response to severe exercise in untethered dogs. Cardiovasc Res. 1974;8:276–82.
14. Downey JM, Kirk ES. Inhibition of coronary blood flow by a vascular waterfall mechanism. Circ Res. 1975;36:753–60.
15. Gorman MW, Rooke GA, Savage MV, Jayasekara MP, Jacobson KA, Feigl EO. Adenine nucleotide control of coronary blood flow during exercise. Am J Physiol Heart Circ Physiol. 2010;299: H1981–9.
16. Tune JD, Gorman MW, Feigl EO. Matching coronary blood flow to myocardial oxygen consumption. J Appl Physiol. 2004;97: 404–15.
17. Duncker DJ, Merkus D. Exercise hyperaemia in the heart: the search for the dilator mechanism. J Physiol. 2007;583:847–54.
18. deBeer VJ, Bender SB, Taverne YJ, Gao F, Dunker DJ, Laughlin MH, Merkus D. Exercise limits the production of endothelin in the coronary vasculature. Am J Physiol. 2011;300:H1950–9.
19. Laughlin MH, McAllister RM. Exercise training-induced coronary vascular adaptation. J Appl Physiol. 1992;73:2209–25.
20. Baur TS, Brodowicz GR, Lamb DR. Indomethacin suppresses the coronary flow response to hypoxia in exercise trained and sedentary rats. Cardiovasc Res. 1990;24:733–6.
21. Buttrick PM, Levite HA, Schaible TF, Ciambrone G, Scheuer J. Early increases in coronary vascular reserve in exercised rats are independent of cardiac hypertrophy. J Appl Physiol. 1985;59: 1861–5.
22. Wicker P, Abdul-Samad M, Rakusan K, Tarazi RC, Healy B. Effects of chronic exercise on the coronary circulation in conscious rats with renovascular hypertension. Hypertension. 1987;10:74–81.
23. Schaible TF, Scheuer J. Effects of physical training by running or swimming on ventricular performance of rat hearts. J Appl Physiol. 1979;46:854–60.
24. Penpargkul S, Scheuer J. The effect of physical training upon the mechanical and metabolic performance of the rat heart. J Clin Invest. 1970;49:1859–68.
25. Spear KL, Koerner JE, Terjung RL. Coronary blood flow in physically trained rats. Cardiovasc Res. 1978;12:135–43.
26. Laughlin MH. Effects of exercise training on coronary transport capacity. J Appl Physiol. 1985;58:468–76.
27. Laughlin MH, Tomanek RJ. Myocardial capillarity and maximal capillary diffusion capacity in exercise-trained dogs. J Appl Physiol. 1987;63:1481–6.
28. Laughlin MH, Diana JN, Tipton CM. Effects of exercise training on coronary reactive hyperemia and blood flow in the dog. J Appl Physiol. 1978;45:604–10.
29. Liang IY, Stone HL. Effect of exercise conditioning on coronary resistance. J Appl Physiol. 1982;53:631–6.
30. Laughlin MH, Overholser KA, Bhatte MJ. Exercise training increases coronary transport reserve in miniature swine. J Appl Physiol. 1989;67:1140–9.
31. Overholser KA, Laughlin MH, Bhatte MJ. Exercise training-induced increase in coronary transport capacity. Med Sci Sports Exerc. 1994;26:1239–44.
32. Bove AA, Hultgren PB, Ritzer TF, Carey RA. Myocardial blood flow and hemodynamic responses to exercise training in dogs. J Appl Physiol. 1979;46:571–8.
33. Stone HL. Coronary flow, myocardial oxygen consumption, and exercise training in dogs. J Appl Physiol. 1980;49:759–68.
34. Barnard RJ, Duncan HW, Baldwin KM, Grimditch G, Buckberg GD. Effects of intensive exercise training on myocardial performance and coronary blood flow. J Appl Physiol. 1980;49:444–9.
35. Carey RA, Santamore WP, Michele JJ, Bove AA. Effects of endurance training on coronary resistance in dogs. Med Sci Sports Exerc. 1983;15:355–9.
36. Liang IY, Hamra M, Stone HL. Maximum coronary blood flow and minimum coronary resistance in exercise-trained dogs. J Appl Physiol. 1984;56:641–7.
37. Cohen MV. Coronary vascular reserve in the greyhound with left ventricular hypertrophy. Cardiovasc Res. 1986;20:182–94.
38. Scheel KW, Ingram LA, Wilson JL. Effects of exercise on the coronary and collateral vasculature of beagles with and without coronary occlusion. Circ Res. 1981;48:523–30.

39. Yipintsoi T, Rosenkrantz J, Codini MA, Scheuer J. Myocardial blood flow responses to acute hypoxia and volume loading in physically trained rats. Cardiovasc Res. 1980;14:50–7.
40. Breisch EA, White FC, Nimmo LE, McKirnan MD, Bloor CM. Exercise-induced cardiac hypertrophy: a correlation of blood flow and microvasculature. J Appl Physiol. 1986;60:1259–67.
41. DiCarlo SE, Blair RW, Bishop VS, Stone HL. Daily exercise enhances coronary resistance vessel sensitivity to pharmacological activation. J Appl Physiol. 1989;66:421–8.
42. Chilian WM, Eastham CL, Marcus ML. Microvascular distribution of coronary vascular resistance in beating left ventricle. Am J Physiol. 1986;251:H779–88.
43. Chilian WM, Layne SM, Klausner EC, Eastham CL, Marcus ML. Redistribution of coronary microvascular resistance produced by dipyridamole. Am J Physiol. 1989;256:H383–90.
44. Tepperman J, Pearlman D. Effects of exercise and anemia on coronary arteries of small animals as revealed by the corrosion-cast technique. Circ Res. 1961;9:576–84.
45. Tepperman J, Pearlman D. Effects of exercise and anemia on coronary arteries of small animals as revealed by the corrosion-cast technique. Circ Res. 1961;9:576–84.
46. Stevenson JA, Box BM, Feleki V, Beaton JR. Bouts of exercise and food intake in the rat. J Appl Physiol. 1966;21:118–22.
47. Ho KW, Roy RR, Taylor JF, Heusner WW, Van Huss WD. Differential effects of running and weight-lifting on the rat coronary arterial tree. Med Sci Sports Exerc. 1983;15:472–7.
48. Kramsch DM, Aspen AJ, Abramowitz BM, Kreimendahl T, Hood Jr WB. Reduction of coronary atherosclerosis by moderate conditioning exercise in monkeys on an atherogenic diet. N Engl J Med. 1981;305:1483–9.
49. Pelliccia A, Spataro A, Granata M, Biffi A, Caselli G, Alabiso A. Coronary arteries in physiological hypertrophy: echocardiographic evidence of increased proximal size in elite athletes. Int J Sports Med. 1990;11:120–6.
50. Kozakova M, Galetta F, Gregorini L, Bigalli G, Franzoni F, Giusti C, et al. Coronary vasodilator capacity and epicardial vessel remodeling in physiological and hypertensive hypertrophy. Hypertension. 2000;36:343–9.
51. Hildick-Smith DJ, Johnson PJ, Wisbey CR, Winter EM, Shapiro LM. Coronary flow reserve is supranormal in endurance athletes: an adenosine transthoracic echocardiographic study. Heart. 2000;84:383–9.
52. Haskell WL, Sims C, Myll J, Bortz WM, St Goar FG, Alderman EL. Coronary artery size and dilating capacity in ultradistance runners. Circulation. 1993;87:1076–82.
53. Tronc F, Wassef M, Esposito B, Henrion D, Glagov S, Tedgui A. Role of NO in flow-induced remodeling of the rabbit common carotid artery. Arterioscler Thromb Vasc Biol. 1996;16:1256–62.
54. Hintze TH, Vatner SF. Reactive dilation of large coronary arteries in conscious dogs. Circ Res. 1984;54:50–7.
55. Holtz J, Forstermann U, Pohl U, Giesler M, Bassenge E. Flow-dependent, endothelium-mediated dilation of epicardial coronary arteries in conscious dogs: effects of cyclooxygenase inhibition. J Cardiovasc Pharmacol. 1984;6:1161–9.
56. Tanaka H, Dinenno FA, Monahan KD, Clevenger CM, DeSouza CA, Seals DR. Aging, habitual exercise, and dynamic arterial compliance. Circulation. 2000;102:1270–5.
57. Brown M. Exercise and coronary vascular remodeling in the healthy heart. Exp Physiol. 2003;88(5):645–58.
58. Haslam RW, Cobb RB. Frequency of intensive, prolonged exercise as a determinant of relative coronary circumference index. Int J Sports Med. 1982;3:118–21.
59. Wyatt HL, Mitchell J. Influences of physical conditioning and deconditioning on coronary vasculature of dogs. J Appl Physiol. 1978;45:619–25.
60. Gigante B, Tarsitano M, Cimini V, De Falco S, Persico MG. Placenta growth factor is not required for exercise-induced angiogenesis. Angiogenesis. 2004;7:277–84.
61. White FC, McKirnan MD, Breisch EA, Guth BD, Liu YM, Bloor CM. Adaptation of the left ventricle to exercise-induced hypertrophy. J Appl Physiol. 1987;62:1097–110.
62. White FC, Witzel G, Breisch EA, Bloor CM, Nimmo LE. Regional capillary and myocyte distribution in normal and exercise trained male and female rat hearts. Am J Cardiovasc Pathol. 1988;2: 247–53.
63. White FC, Bloor CM, McKirnan MD, Carroll SM. Exercise training in swine promotes growth of arteriolar bed and capillary angiogenesis in heart. J Appl Physiol. 1998;85:1160–8.
64. Rogers PJ, Miller TD, Bauer BA, Brum JM, Bove AA, Vanhoutte PM. Exercise training and responsiveness of isolated coronary arteries. J Appl Physiol. 1991;71:2346–51.
65. Wang DH, Prewitt RL. Alterations of mature arterioles associated with chronically reduced blood flow. Am J Physiol. 1993;264: H40–4.
66. Oltman CL, Parker JL, Laughlin MH. Endothelium-dependent vasodilation of proximal coronary arteries from exercise-trained pigs. J Appl Physiol. 1995;79:33–40.
67. Oltman CL, Parker JL, Adams HR, Laughlin MH. Effects of exercise training on vasomotor reactivity of porcine coronary arteries. Am J Physiol. 1992;263:H372–82.
68. Huxley VH, Wang JJ, Sarelius IH. Adaptation of coronary microvascular exchange in arterioles and venules to exercise training and a role for sex in determining permeability responses. Am J Physiol Heart Circ Physiol. 2007;293:H1196–205.
69. Sessa WC, Pritchard K, Seyedi N, Wang J, Hintze TH. Chronic exercise in dogs increases coronary vascular nitric oxide production and endothelial cell nitric oxide synthase gene expression. Circ Res. 1994;74:349–53.
70. Wang J, Wolin MS, Hintze TH. Chronic exercise enhances endothelium-mediated dilation of epicardial coronary artery in conscious dogs. Circ Res. 1993;73:829–38.
71. Zhao G, Zhang X, Xu X, Ochoa M, Hintze TH. Short-term exercise training enhances reflex cholinergic nitric oxide-dependent coronary vasodilation in conscious dogs. Circ Res. 1997;80:868–76.
72. Laughlin MH, Rubin LJ, Rush JW, Price EM, Schrage WG, Woodman CR. Short-term training enhances endothelium-dependent dilation of coronary arteries, not arterioles. J Appl Physiol. 2003;94:234–44.
73. Stewart JM, Xu X, Ochoa M, Hintze TH. Exercise reduces epicardial coronary artery wall stiffness: roles of cGMP and cAMP. Med Sci Sports Exerc. 1998;30:220–8.
74. Zanesco A, Antunes E. Effects of exercise training on the cardiovascular system: pharmacological approaches. Pharmacol Ther. 2007;114:307–17.
75. Erbs S, Linke A, Hambrecht R. Effects of exercise training on mortality in patients with coronary heart disease. Coron Artery Dis. 2006;17:219–25.
76. Rush JW, Laughlin MH, Woodman CR, Price EM. SOD-1 expression in pig coronary arterioles is increased by exercise training. Am J Physiol Heart Circ Physiol. 2000;279:H2068–76.
77. Fukai T, Siegfried MR, Ushio-Fukai M, Cheng Y, Kojda G, Harrison DG. Regulation of the vascular extracellular superoxide dismutase by nitric oxide and exercise training. J Clin Invest. 2000;105:1631–9.
78. Parker JL, Oltman CL, Muller JM, Myers PR, Adams HR, Laughlin MH. Effects of exercise training on regulation of tone in coronary arteries and arterioles. Med Sci Sports Exerc. 1994;26:1252–61.
79. Muller JM, Myers PR, Laughlin MH. Vasodilator responses of coronary resistance arteries of exercise-trained pigs. Circulation. 1994;89:2308–14.

80. Laughlin MH, Pollock JS, Amann JF, Hollis ML, Woodman CR, Price EM. Training induces nonuniform increases in eNOS content along the coronary arterial tree. J Appl Physiol. 2001; 90:501–10.
81. Woodman CR, Muller JM, Laughlin MH, Price EM. Induction of nitric oxide synthase mRNA in coronary resistance arteries isolated from exercise-trained pigs. Am J Physiol. 1997;273: H2575–9.
82. Mombouli JV, Nakashima M, Hamra M, Vanhoutte PM. Endothelium-dependent relaxation and hyperpolarization evoked by bradykinin in canine coronary arteries: enhancement by exercise-training. Br J Pharmacol. 1996;117:413–8.
83. Bove AA, Dewey JD. Proximal coronary vasomotor reactivity after exercise training in dogs. Circulation. 1985;71:620–5.
84. Jones AW, Rubin LJ, Magliola L. Endothelin-1 sensitivity of porcine coronary arteries is reduced by exercise training and is gender dependent. J Appl Physiol. 1999;87:1172–7.
85. Stehno-Bittel L, Laughlin MH, Sturek M. Exercise training alters Ca release from coronary smooth muscle sarcoplasmic reticulum. Am J Physiol. 1990;259:H643–7.
86. Stehno-Bittel L, Laughlin MH, Sturek M. Exercise training depletes sarcoplasmic reticulum calcium in coronary smooth muscle. J Appl Physiol. 1991;71:1764–73.
87. Bowles DK, Laughlin MH, Sturek M. Exercise training alters the Ca^{2+} and contractile responses of coronary arteries to endothelin. J Appl Physiol. 1995;78:1079–87.
88. Heaps CL, Bowles DK, Sturek M, Laughlin MH, Parker JL. Enhanced L-type Ca^{2+} channel current density in coronary smooth muscle of exercise-trained pigs is compensated to limit myoplasmic free Ca^{2+} accumulation. J Physiol. 2000;528:435–45.
89. Bowles DK, Hu Q, Laughlin MH, Sturek M. Exercise training increases L-type calcium current density in coronary smooth muscle. Am J Physiol. 1998;275:H2159–69.
90. Bowles L, Kopelman P. Leptin: of mice and men? J Clin Pathol. 2001;54:1–3.
91. Wamhoff BR, Bowles DK, Dietz NJ, Hu Q, Sturek M. Exercise training attenuates coronary smooth muscle phenotypic modulation and nuclear Ca2+ signaling. Am J Physiol Heart Circ Physiol. 2002;283:H2397–410.
92. Witczak CA, Sturek M. Exercise prevents diabetes-induced impairment in superficial buffer barrier in porcine coronary smooth muscle. J Appl Physiol. 2004;96:1069–79.
93. Mokelke EA, Hu Q, Song M, Toro L, Reddy HK, Sturek M. Altered functional coupling of coronary K^+ channels in diabetic dyslipidemic pigs is prevented by exercise. J Appl Physiol. 2003;95:1179–93.
94. Albarwani S, Al-Siyabi S, Baomar H, Hassan MO. Exercise training attenuates ageing-induced BKCa channel downregulation in rat coronary arteries. Exp Physiol. 2010;95:746–55.
95. Fulton WF. Chronic generalized myocardial ischaemia with advanced coronary artery disease. Br Heart J. 1956;18:341–54.
96. Heaps CL, Parker JL. Effects of exercise training on coronary collateralization and control of collateral resistance. J Appl Physiol. 2011;111:587–98.
97. Cohen MV. Coronary and collateral blood flows during exercise and myocardial vascular adaptations to training. Exerc Sport Sci Rev. 1983;11:55–98.
98. Ferguson RJ, Petitclerc R, Choquette G, Chaniotis L, Gauthier P, Huot R, et al. Effect of physical training on treadmill exercise capacity, collateral circulation and progression of coronary disease. Am J Cardiol. 1974;34:764–9.
99. Nolewajka AJ, Kostuk WJ, Rechnitzer PA, Cunningham DA. Exercise and human collateralization: an angiographic and scintigraphic assessment. Circulation. 1979;60:114–21.
100. Niebauer J, Hambrecht R, Marburger C, Hauer K, Velich T, von Hodenberg E, et al. Impact of intensive physical exercise and low-fat diet on collateral vessel formation in stable angina pectoris and angiographically confirmed coronary artery disease. Am J Cardiol. 1995;76:771–5.
101. Sasayama S. Effect of coronary collateral circulation on myocardial ischemia and ventricular dysfunction. Cardiovasc Drugs Ther. 1994;8 Suppl 2:327–34.
102. Senti S, Fleisch M, Billinger M, Meier B, Seiler C. Long-term physical exercise and quantitatively assessed human coronary collateral circulation. J Am Coll Cardiol. 1998;32:49–56.
103. Zbinden R, Zbinden S, Meier P, Hutter D, Billinger M, Wahl A, et al. Coronary collateral flow in response to endurance exercise training. Eur J Cardiovasc Prev Rehabil. 2007;14:250–7.
104. Eckstein RW. Effect of exercise and coronary artery narrowing on coronary collateral circulation. Circ Res. 1957;5:230–5.
105. Burt JJ, Jackson R. The effects of physical exercise on the coronary collateral circulation of dogs. J Sports Med Phys Fitness. 1965;4:203.
106. Cohen MV, Yipintsoi T, Malhotra A, Penpargkul S, Scheuer J. Effect of exercise on collateral development in dogs with normal coronary arteries. J Appl Physiol. 1978;45:797–805.
107. Sanders M, White FC, Peterson TM, Bloor CM. Effects of endurance exercise on coronary collateral blood flow in miniature swine. Am J Physiol. 1978;234:H614–9.
108. Koerner JE, Terjung RL. Effect of physical training on coronary collateral circulation of the rat. J Appl Physiol. 1982;52:376–87.
109. Amann L, Meesmann W, Schulz FW, Schley G, Wilde A, Tuttemann J. Studies on the formation of collaterals in the healthy heart following physical training. Verh Dtsch Ges Kreislaufforsch. 1971;37:151–4.
110. Heaton WH, Marr KC, Capurro NL, Goldstein RE, Epstein SE. Beneficial effect of physical training on blood flow to myocardium perfused by chronic collaterals in the exercising dog. Circulation. 1978;57:575–81.
111. Neill WA, Oxendine JM. Exercise can promote coronary collateral development without improving perfusion of ischemic myocardium. Circulation. 1979;60:1513–9.
112. Cohen MV, Yipintsoi T, Scheuer J. Coronary collateral stimulation by exercise in dogs with stenotic coronary arteries. J Appl Physiol. 1982;52:664–71.
113. Bloor CM, White FC, Sanders TM. Effects of exercise on collateral development in myocardial ischemia in pigs. J Appl Physiol. 1984;56:656–65.
114. Roth DM, White FC, Nichols ML, Dobbs SL, Longhurst JC, Bloor CM. Effect of long-term exercise on regional myocardial function and coronary collateral development after gradual coronary artery occlusion in pigs. Circulation. 1990;82:1778–89.
115. Kaplinsky E, Hood Jr WB, McCarthy B, McCombs HL, Lown B. Effects of physical training in dogs with coronary artery ligation. Circulation. 1968;37:556–65.
116. Schaper W. Influence of physical exercise on coronary collateral blood flow in chronic experimental two-vessel occlusion. Circulation. 1982;65:905–12.
117. Unger EF. Experimental evaluation of coronary collateral development. Cardiovasc Res. 2001;49:497–506.
118. Lu X, Wu T, Huang P, Lin S, Qiu F, Meng X, et al. Effect and mechanism of intermittent myocardial ischemia induced by exercise on coronary collateral formation. Am J Phys Med Rehabil. 2008;87:803–14.
119. Rapps JA, Sturek M, Jones AW, Parker JL. Altered reactivity of coronary arteries located distal to a chronic coronary occlusion. Am J Physiol. 1997;273:H1879–87.
120. Peters KG, Marcus ML, Harrison DG. Vasopressin and the mature coronary collateral circulation. Circulation. 1989;79:1324–31.
121. Sellke FW, Quillen JE, Brooks LA, Harrison DG. Endothelial modulation of the coronary vasculature in vessels perfused via mature collaterals. Circulation. 1990;81:1938–47.
122. Sellke FW, Kagaya Y, Johnson RG, Shafique T, Schoen FJ, Grossman W, et al. Endothelial modulation of porcine coronary

microcirculation perfused via immature collaterals. Am J Physiol. 1992;262:H1669–75.
123. Fogarty JA, Muller-Delp JM, Delp MD, Mattox ML, Laughlin MH, Parker JL. Exercise training enhances vasodilation responses to vascular endothelial growth factor in porcine coronary arterioles exposed to chronic coronary occlusion. Circulation. 2004;109:664–70.
124. Fogarty JA, Delp MD, Muller-Delp JM, Laine GA, Parker JL, Heaps CL. Neuropilin-1 is essential for enhanced VEGF(165)-mediated vasodilatation in collateral-dependent coronary arterioles of exercise-trained pigs. J Vasc Res. 2009;46:152–61.
125. Heaps CL, Mattox ML, Kelly KA, Meininger CJ, Parker JL. Exercise training increases basal tone in arterioles distal to chronic coronary occlusion. Am J Physiol Heart Circ Physiol. 2006;290:H1128–35.
126. Thengchaisri N, Shipley R, Ren Y, Parker J, Kuo L. Exercise training restores coronary arteriolar dilation to NOS activation distal to coronary artery occlusion: role of hydrogen peroxide. Arterioscler Thromb Vasc Biol. 2007;27:791–8.
127. Heaps CL, Sturek M, Rapps JA, Laughlin MH, Parker JL. Exercise training restores adenosine-induced relaxation in coronary arteries distal to chronic occlusion. Am J Physiol Heart Circ Physiol. 2000;278:H1984–92.
128. Griffin KL, Woodman CR, Price EM, Laughlin MH, Parker JL. Endothelium-mediated relaxation of porcine collateral-dependent arterioles is improved by exercise training. Circulation. 2001;104:1393–8.
129. Zhou M, Widmer RJ, Xie W, Jimmy Widmer A, Miller MW, Schroeder F, et al. Effects of exercise training on cellular mechanisms of endothelial nitric oxide synthase regulation in coronary arteries after chronic occlusion. Am J Physiol Heart Circ Physiol. 2010;298:H1857–69.
130. Rehman J, Li J, Parvathaneni L, Karlsson G, Panchal VR, Temm CJ, et al. Exercise acutely increases circulating endothelial progenitor cells and monocyte-/macrophage-derived angiogenic cells. J Am Coll Cardiol. 2004;43:2314–8.
131. Steiner S, Niessner A, Ziegler S, Richter B, Seidinger D, Pleiner J, et al. Endurance training increases the number of endothelial progenitor cells in patients with cardiovascular risk and coronary artery disease. Atherosclerosis. 2005;181:305–10.
132. Van Craenenbroeck EM, Hoymans VY, Beckers PJ, Possemiers NM, Wuyts K, Paelinck BP, et al. Exercise training improves function of circulating angiogenic cells in patients with chronic heart failure. Basic Res Cardiol. 2010;105:665–76.
133. Robles JC, Sturek M, Parker JL, Heaps CL. Ca2+ sensitization and PKC contribute to exercise training-enhanced contractility in porcine collateral-dependent coronary arteries. Am J Physiol Heart Circ Physiol. 2011;300:H1201–9.
134. Wachtlova M, Rakusan K, Roth Z, Poupa O. The terminal vascular bed of the myocardium in the wild rat (Rattus norvegicus) and the laboratory rat (*Rattus norvegicus* lab.). Physiol Bohemoslov. 1967;16:548–54.
135. Wachtlova M, Rakusan K, Poupa O. The coronary terminal vascular bed in the heart of the hare (*Lepus europeus*) and the rabbit (*Oryctolagus domesticus*). Physiol Bohemoslov. 1965;14:328–31.
136. Hakkila J. Studies on the myocardial capillary concentration in cardiac hypertrophy due to training. An experimental study with guinea pigs. Ann Med Exp Biol Fenn. 1955;33:10.
137. Petren T, Sjostrand T, Sylven B. Der Einfluss des Trainings auf die Haufigkeit de Kapillaren in Herz-und Skellettmuskatur. Arbeitsphysiologie. 1936;9:376–86.
138. Frank A. Experimentelle herz hypertrophie. Ges Exp Med. 1950;115:312–49.
139. Mandache E, Unge G, Ljungqvist A. Myocardial blood capillary reaction in various forms of cardiac hypertrophy. An electron microscopical investigation in the rat. Virchows Arch B Cell Pathol. 1972;11:97–110.
140. Unge G, Carlsson S, Ljungqvist A, Tornling G, Adolfsson J. The proliferative activity of myocardial capillary wall cells in variously aged swimming-exercised rats. Acta Pathol Microbiol Scand A. 1979;87:15–7.
141. Ljungqvist A, Unge G. Capillary proliferative activity in myocardium and skeletal muscle of exercised rats. J Appl Physiol. 1977;43:306–7.
142. Tomanek RJ. Effects of age and exercise on the extent of the myocardial capillary bed. Anat Rec. 1970;167:55–62.
143. Bloor CM, Leon AS. Interaction of age and exercise on the heart and its blood supply. Lab Invest. 1970;22:160–5.
144. Tagarakis CV, Bloch W, Hartmann G, Hollmann W, Addicks K. Testosterone-propionate impairs the response of the cardiac capillary bed to exercise. Med Sci Sports Exerc. 2000;32:946–53.
145. Anversa P, Beghi C, Levicky V, McDonald SL, Kikkawa Y. Morphometry of right ventricular hypertrophy induced by strenuous exercise in rat. Am J Physiol. 1982;243:H856–61.
146. Anversa P, Levicky V, Beghi C, McDonald SL, Kikkawa Y. Morphometry of exercise-induced right ventricular hypertrophy in the rat. Circ Res. 1983;52:57–64.
147. Anversa P, Beghi C, Levicky V, McDonald SL, Kikkawa Y, Olivetti G. Effects of strenuous exercise on the quantitative morphology of left ventricular myocardium in the rat. J Mol Cell Cardiol. 1985;17:587–95.
148. Leon AS, Bloor CM. Effects of exercise and its cessation on the heart and its blood supply. J Appl Physiol. 1968;24:485–90.
149. Tittle K, Knacke K, Brauer B, Otto H. Der Einfluss Korperlicker Belastengen Uterschiedlicker dauer und Intersitof auf die kapillarisierung der herzund skelettmuskulatur bei albino ratten. Hannover: XVI International World Congress for Sports Medicine; 1966. p. 181–8.
150. Carlsson S, Ljungqvist A, Tornling G, Unge G. The myocardial capillary vasculature in repeated physical exercise. An experimental investigation in the rat. Acta Pathol Microbiol Scand A. 1978;86:117–9.
151. Rakusan K, Wicker P, Abdul-Samad M, Healy B, Turek Z. Failure of swimming exercise to improve capillarization in cardiac hypertrophy of renal hypertensive rats. Circ Res. 1987;61:641–7.
152. Rakusan K, Wicker P. Morphometry of the small arteries and arterioles in the rat heart: effects of chronic hypertension and exercise. Cardiovasc Res. 1990;24:278–84.
153. Frenzel H, Schwartzkopff B, Holtermann W, Schnurch HG, Novi A, Hort W. Regression of cardiac hypertrophy: morphometric and biochemical studies in rat heart after swimming training. J Mol Cell Cardiol. 1988;20:737–51.
154. Parizkova J. Impact of daily work-load during pregnancy on the microstructure of the rat heart in male offspring. Eur J Appl Physiol Occup Physiol. 1975;34:323–6.
155. Parizkova J. The impact of daily work load during pregnancy and/or postnatal life on the heart microstructure of rat male offspring. Basic Res Cardiol. 1978;73:433–41.
156. Parizkova J. Cardiac microstructure in female and male offspring of exercised rat mothers. Acta Anat (Basel). 1979;104:382–7.
157. Mattfeldt T, Kramer KL, Zeitz R, Mall G. Stereology of myocardial hypertrophy induced by physical exercise. Virchows Arch A Pathol Anat Histopathol. 1986;409:473–84.
158. Kayar SR, Conley KE, Claassen H, Hoppeler H. Capillarity and mitochondrial distribution in rat myocardium following exercise training. J Exp Biol. 1986;120:189–99.
159. Kayar SR, Banchero N. Volume overload hypertrophy elicited by cold and its effects on myocardial capillarity. Respir Physiol. 1985;59:1–14.
160. Tharp GD, Wagner CT. Chronic exercise and cardiac vascularization. Eur J Appl Physiol Occup Physiol. 1982;48:97–104.
161. Anversa P, Beghi C, Kikkawa Y, Olivetti G. Myocardial response to infarction in the rat. Morphometric measurement of infarct size and myocyte cellular hypertrophy. Am J Pathol. 1985;118:484–92.

162. Thorner W. Training Versuch an Huden. III Histologische Beobachtungen an Herz und Skelettmuske. Arbeitsphysiologie. 1935;8:359–70.
163. Prior BM, Yang HT, Terjung RL. What makes vessels grow with exercise training? J Appl Physiol. 2004;97:1119–28.
164. Tomanek RJ, Torry RJ. Growth of the coronary vasculature in hypertrophy: mechanisms and model dependence. Cell Mol Biol Res. 1994;40:129–36.
165. Hudlicka O, Brown MD, Walter H, Weiss JB, Bate A. Factors involved in capillary growth in the heart. Mol Cell Biochem. 1995;147:57–68.
166. Tornling G. Capillary neoformation in the heart and skeletal muscle during dipyridamole–treatment and exercise. Acta Pathol Microbiol Immunol Scand Suppl. 1982;278:1–63.
167. Mall G, Schikora I, Mattfeldt T, Bodle R. Dipyridamole-induced neoformation of capillaries in the rat heart. Quantitative stereological study on papillary muscles. Lab Invest. 1987;57:86–93.
168. Torry RJ, O'Brien DM, Connell PM, Tomanek RJ. Dipyridamole-induced capillary growth in normal and hypertrophic hearts. Am J Physiol. 1992;262:H980–6.
169. Wright AJ, Hudlicka O. Capillary growth and changes in heart performance induced by chronic bradycardial pacing in the rabbit. Circ Res. 1981;49:469–78.
170. Lei L, Zhou R, Zheng W, Christensen LP, Weiss RM, Tomanek RJ. Bradycardia induces angiogenesis, increases coronary reserve, and preserves function of the postinfarcted heart. Circulation. 2004;110:796–802.
171. Zheng W, Christensen LP, Tomanek RJ. Stretch induces upregulation of key tyrosine kinase receptors in microvascular endothelial cells. Am J Physiol Heart Circ Physiol. 2004;287:H2739–45.
172. Olfert IM, Howlett RA, Tang K, Dalton ND, Gu Y, Peterson KL, et al. Muscle-specific VEGF deficiency greatly reduces exercise endurance in mice. J Physiol. 2009;587:1755–67.
173. Ljungqvist A, Unge G, Carlsson S. The myocardial capillary vasculature in exercising animals with increased cardiac pressure load. Acta Pathol Microbiol Scand A. 1976;84:244–6.
174. van Deel ED, de Boer M, Kuster DW, Boontje NM, Holemans P, Sipido KR, et al. Exercise training does not improve cardiac function in compensated or decompensated left ventricular hypertrophy induced by aortic stenosis. J Mol Cell Cardiol. 2011; 50:1017–25.
175. Marcus KD, Tipton CM. Exercise training and its effects with renal hypertensive rats. J Appl Physiol. 1985;59:1410–5.
176. Crisman RP, Rittman B, Tomanek RJ. Exercise-induced myocardial capillary growth in the spontaneously hypertensive rat. Microvasc Res. 1985;30:185–94.
177. Tomanek RJ, Gisolfi CV, Bauer CA, Palmer PJ. Coronary vasodilator reserve, capillarity, and mitochondria in trained hypertensive rats. J Appl Physiol. 1988;64:1179–85.
178. Belabbas H, Zalvidea S, Casellas D, Moles JP, Galbes O, Mercier J, et al. Contrasting effect of exercise and angiotensin II hypertension on in vivo and in vitro cardiac angiogenesis in rats. Am J Physiol Regul Integr Comp Physiol. 2008;295:R1512–8.
179. Handoko ML, de Man FS, Happe CM, Schalij I, Musters RJ, Westerhof N, et al. Opposite effects of training in rats with stable and progressive pulmonary hypertension. Circulation. 2009;120:42–9.
180. Calvert JW, Condit ME, Aragon JP, Nicholson CK, Moody BF, Hood RL, et al. Exercise protects against myocardial ischemia-reperfusion injury via stimulation of beta(3)-adrenergic receptors and increased nitric oxide signaling: role of nitrite and nitrosothiols. Circ Res. 2011;108:1448–58.
181. Schaible TF, Ciambrone GJ, Capasso JM, Scheuer J. Cardiac conditioning ameliorates cardiac dysfunction associated with renal hypertension in rats. J Clin Invest. 1984;73:1086–94.
182. Bowles DK, Wamhoff BR. Coronary smooth muscle adaptation to exercise: does it play a role in cardioprotection? Acta Physiol Scand. 2003;178:117–21.
183. Symons JD, Rendig SV, Stebbins CL, Longhurst JC. Microvascular and myocardial contractile responses to ischemia: influence of exercise training. J Appl Physiol. 2000;88:433–42.
184. Underwood FB, Laughlin MH, Sturek M. Altered control of calcium in coronary smooth muscle cells by exercise training. Med Sci Sports Exerc. 1994;26:1230–8.
185. Paroo Z, Haist JV, Karmazyn M, Noble EG. Exercise improves postischemic cardiac function in males but not females: consequences of a novel sex-specific heat shock protein 70 response. Circ Res. 2002;90:911–7.
186. Vaccarino V, Parsons L, Every NR, Barron HV, Krumholz HM. Sex-based differences in early mortality after myocardial infarction. National registry of myocardial infarction 2 participants. N Engl J Med. 1999;341:217–25.
187. Le Page C, Noirez P, Courty J, Riou B, Swynghedauw B, Besse S. Exercise training improves functional post-ischemic recovery in senescent heart. Exp Gerontol. 2009;44:177–82.
188. McElroy CL, Gissen SA, Fishbein MC. Exercise-induced reduction in myocardial infarct size after coronary artery occlusion in the rat. Circulation. 1978;57:958–62.
189. Przyklenk K, Groom AC. Can exercise promote revascularization in the transition zone of infarcted rat hearts? Can J Physiol Pharmacol. 1984;62:630–3.
190. Przyklenk K, Groom AC. Effects of exercise frequency, intensity, and duration on revascularization in the transition zone of infarcted rat hearts. Can J Physiol Pharmacol. 1985;63:273–8.
191. Brown DA, Jew KN, Sparagna GC, Musch TI, Moore RL. Exercise training preserves coronary flow and reduces infarct size after ischemia-reperfusion in rat heart. J Appl Physiol. 2003;95: 2510–8.
192. Soufi FG, Saber MM, Ghiassie R, Alipour M. Role of 12-week resistance training in preserving the heart against ischemia-reperfusion-induced injury. Cardiol J. 2011;18:140–5.
193. Leosco D, Rengo G, Iaccarino G, Golino L, Marchese M, Fortunato F, et al. Exercise promotes angiogenesis and improves beta-adrenergic receptor signalling in the post-ischaemic failing rat heart. Cardiovasc Res. 2008;78:385–94.
194. de Waard MC, van Haperen R, Soullie T, Tempel D, de Crom R, Duncker DJ. Beneficial effects of exercise training after myocardial infarction require full eNOS expression. J Mol Cell Cardiol. 2010;48:1041–9.
195. Wu G, Rana JS, Wykrzykowska J, Du Z, Ke Q, Kang P, et al. Exercise-induced expression of VEGF and salvation of myocardium in the early stage of myocardial infarction. Am J Physiol Heart Circ Physiol. 2009;296:H389–95.
196. Detry JM, Bruce RA. Effects of physical training on exertional S-T-segment depression in coronary heart disease. Circulation. 1971;44:390–6.
197. Ehsani AA, Heath GW, Hagberg JM, Sobel BE, Holloszy JO. Effects of 12 months of intense exercise training on ischemic ST-segment depression in patients with coronary artery disease. Circulation. 1981;64:1116–24.
198. Hellerstein HK. Exercise therapy in coronary disease. Bull N Y Acad Med. 1968;44:1028–47.
199. Landmesser U, Drexler H. The clinical significance of endothelial dysfunction. Curr Opin Cardiol. 2005;20:547–51.
200. Carville C, Adnot S, Sediame S, Benacerraf S, Castaigne A, Calvo F, et al. Relation between impairment in nitric oxide pathway and clinical status in patients with congestive heart failure. J Cardiovasc Pharmacol. 1998;32:562–70.
201. Hambrecht R, Wolf A, Gielen S, Linke A, Hofer J, Erbs S, et al. Effect of exercise on coronary endothelial function in patients with coronary artery disease. N Engl J Med. 2000;342:454–60.
202. Hambrecht R, Hilbrich L, Erbs S, Gielen S, Fiehn E, Schoene N, et al. Correction of endothelial dysfunction in chronic heart failure: additional effects of exercise training and oral L-arginine supplementation. J Am Coll Cardiol. 2000;35:706–13.

203. Vona M, Codeluppi GM, Iannino T, Ferrari E, Bogousslavsky J, von Segesser LK. Effects of different types of exercise training followed by detraining on endothelium-dependent dilation in patients with recent myocardial infarction. Circulation. 2009;119:1601–8.
204. Lee BC, Chen SY, Hsu HC, Su MY, Wu YW, Chien KL, et al. Effect of cardiac rehabilitation on myocardial perfusion reserve in postinfarction patients. Am J Cardiol. 2008;101:1395–402.
205. Lee BC, Hsu HC, Tseng WY, Su MY, Chen SY, Wu YW, et al. Effect of cardiac rehabilitation on angiogenic cytokines in postinfarction patients. Heart. 2009;95:1012–8.
206. Giallauria F, Acampa W, Ricci F, Vitelli A, Maresca L, Mancini M, Grieco A et al. Effects of exercise training started within 2 weeks after acute myocardial infarction on myocardial perfusion and left ventricular function: a gated SPECT imaging study. Eur J Cardiovas Prev Rehab. 2011, in press.
207. Rose G, Prineas RJ, Mitchell JR. Myocardial infarction and the intrinsic calibre of coronary arteries. Br Heart J. 1967;29:548–52.
208. Mann GV, Spoerry A, Gray M, Jarashow D. Atherosclerosis in the Masai. Am J Epidemiol. 1972;95:26–37.
209. Hambrecht R, Walther C, Mobius-Winkler S, Gielen S, Linke A, Conradi K, et al. Percutaneous coronary angioplasty compared with exercise training in patients with stable coronary artery disease: a randomized trial. Circulation. 2004;109:1371–8.
210. Laufs U, Urhausen A, Werner N, Scharhag J, Heitz A, Kissner G, et al. Running exercise of different duration and intensity: effect on endothelial progenitor cells in healthy subjects. Eur J Cardiovasc Prev Rehabil. 2005;12:407–14.
211. Health NIo. Physical activity and cardiovascular health. NIH Consens Statement. 19995;13(3):1–33.
212. Fletcher GF, Balady G, Blair SN, Blumenthal J, Caspersen C, Chaitman B, et al. Statement on exercise: benefits and recommendations for physical activity programs for all Americans. A statement for health professionals by the Committee on Exercise and Cardiac Rehabilitation of the Council on Clinical Cardiology, American Heart Association. Circulation. 1996;94:857–62.
213. Thompson PD, Buchner D, Pina IL, Balady GJ, Williams MA, Marcus BH, et al. Exercise and physical activity in the prevention and treatment of atherosclerotic cardiovascular disease. A statement from the Council on Clinical Cardiology (Subcommittee on Exercise, Rehabilitation, and Prevention) and the Council on Nutrition, Physical Activity, and Metabolism (Subcommittee on Physical Activity). Circulation. 2003;107:3109–16.
214. Mora S, Cook N, Buring JE, Ridker PM, Lee IM. Physical activity and reduced risk of cardiovascular events: potential mediating mechanisms. Circulation. 2007;116:2110–8.
215. Sofi F, Capalbo A, Cesari F, Abbate R, Gensini GF. Physical activity during leisure time and primary prevention of coronary heart disease: an updated meta-analysis of cohort studies. Eur J Cardiovasc Prev Rehabil. 2008;15:247–57.
216. Sung J, Cho SJ, Choe YH, Choi YH, Hong KP. Prevalence of coronary atherosclerosis in asymptomatic middle-age men with high aerobic fitness. Am J Cardiol. 2012;109(6):839–43.
217. Ahmed HM, Blaha MJ, Nasir K, Rivera JJ, Blumenthal RS. Effects of physical activity on cardiovascular disease. Am J Cardiol. 2012;109(2):288–95.
218. Lavie CJ, Milani RV. Cardiac rehabilitation and exercise training in secondary coronary heart disease prevention. Prog Cardiovasc Dis. 2011;53:397–403.
219. Munk PS, Breland UM, Aukrust P, Ueland T, Kvaloy JT, Larsen AL. High intensity interval training reduces systemic inflammation in post-PCI patients. Eur J Cardiovas Prev Rehabit. 2011;18:850–7.
220. Ribeiro F, Alves AJ, Duarte JA, Oliveira J. Is exercise training an effective therapy targeting endothelial dysfunction and vascular wall inflammation? Int J Cardiol. 2010;141:214–21.
221. Walther C, Mobius-Winkler S, Linke A, Bruegel M, Thiery J, Schuler G, et al. Regular exercise training compared with percutaneous intervention leads to a reduction of inflammatory markers and cardiovascular events in patients with coronary artery disease. Eur J Cardiovasc Prev Rehabil. 2008;15:107–12.
222. Kumar A, Kar S, Fay WP. Thrombosis, physical activity, and acute coronary syndromes. J Appl Physiol. 2011;111:599–605.
223. Belardinelli R, Paolini I, Cianci G, Piva R, Georgiou D, Purcaro A. Exercise training intervention after coronary angioplasty: the ETICA trial. J Am Coll Cardiol. 2001;37:1891–900.
224. Newcomer SC, Thijssen DH, Green DJ. Effects of exercise on endothelium and endothelium/smooth muscle cross talk: role of exercise-induced hemodynamics. J Appl Physiol. 2011;111: 311–20.
225. Linke A, Erbs S, Hambrecht R. Exercise and the coronary circulation-alterations and adaptations in coronary artery disease. Prog Cardiovasc Dis. 2006;48:270–84.
226. Gielen S, Erbs S, Linke A, Mobius-Winkler S, Schuler G, Hambrecht R. Home-based versus hospital-based exercise programs in patients with coronary artery disease: effects on coronary vasomotion. Am Heart J. 2003;145:E3.
227. Beck EB, Erbs S, MÖbiuis-Winkler S, Adams V, Woitek FJ, Walther T, Hambrecht P, Mohr FW, Stumvoll M, BlÜher M, Schuler G, Linke A. Exercise restores the endothelial response to vascular growth factors in patients with stable coronary artery disease. Eur J Prev Cardiol. 2011;19:412–8.
228. Smith JK. Exercise and cardiovascular disease. Cardiovasc Hematol Disord Drug Targets. 2010;10:269–72.
229. Henderson KK, Turk JR, Rush JW, Laughlin MH. Endothelial function in coronary arterioles from pigs with early-stage coronary disease induced by high-fat, high-cholesterol diet: effect of exercise. J Appl Physiol. 2004;97:1159–68.
230. Long X, Bratz IN, Alloosh M, Edwards JM, Sturek M. Short-term exercise training prevents micro- and macrovascular disease following coronary stenting. J Appl Physiol. 2010;108: 1766–74.
231. Witczak CA, Wamhoff BR, Sturek M. Exercise training prevents Ca^{2+} dysregulation in coronary smooth muscle from diabetic dyslipidemic yucatan swine. J Appl Physiol. 2006;101:752–62.
232. Bunker AK, Laughlin MH. Influence of exercise and perivascular adipose tissue on coronary artery vasomotor function in a familial hypercholesterolemic porcine atherosclerosis model. J Appl Physiol. 2010;108:490–7.
233. Sturek M. Ca2+ regulatory mechanisms of exercise protection against coronary artery disease in metabolic syndrome and diabetes. J Appl Physiol. 2011;111:573–86.
234. Pynn M, Schafer K, Konstantinides S, Halle M. Exercise training reduces neointimal growth and stabilizes vascular lesions developing after injury in apolipoprotein e-deficient mice. Circulation. 2004;109:386–92.
235. Okabe TA, Shimada K, Hattori M, Murayama T, Yokode M, Kita T, et al. Swimming reduces the severity of atherosclerosis in apolipoprotein E deficient mice by antioxidant effects. Cardiovasc Res. 2007;74:537–45.
236. Kadoglou NP, Kostomitsopoulos N, Kapelouzou A, Moustardas P, Katsimpoulas M, Giagini A, et al. Effects of exercise training on the severity and composition of atherosclerotic plaque in apoE-deficient mice. J Vasc Res. 2011;48:347–56.
237. Jacobs TB, Bell RD, McClements JD. Exercise, age and the development of the myocardial vasculature. Growth. 1984;48:148–57.
238. Suzuki J. Microvascular angioadaptation after endurance training with L-arginine supplementation in rat heart and hindleg muscles. Exp Physiol. 2005;90:763–71.
239. Bell RD, Rasmussen RL. Exercise and the myocardial capillary-fiber ratio during growth. Growth. 1974;38:237–44.

Hypoxia

9

Abbreviations

EC	Endothelial cell
ECM	Extracellular matrix
EPO	Erythropoietin
HIF	Hypoxia inducible factor
NO	Nitric oxide
PHDs	Propyl hydroxylase proteins
VEGF	Vascular endothelial growth factor
VSMC	Vascular smooth muscle cell

Introduction

The overall goal of this chapter is to explore the effects of acute and chronic hypoxia on the coronary vasculature and coronary blood flow. Chapter 1 included a section regarding the general effects of hypoxia on the vasculature. Other chapters address the effects of hypoxia as they pertain to exercise (Chap. 8) and ischemia and infarction (Chap. 10).

Hypoxia and Ischemia

Hypoxia is defined as a condition in which O_2 levels lower than required for tissue and cell metabolic requirements. Hypoxia indicates a decreased availability of O_2, whereas anoxia indicates an absence of O_2. The types of hypoxia include (1) systemic—low PO_2 in arterial blood, (2) anemic—decreased concentration of functional hemoglobin or a reduction in erythrocytes, (3) ischemic—a tissue hypoxia due to inadequate blood supply to tissues, and (4) oxygen affinity—a reduction in O_2 release from hemoglobin.

Although hypoxia is a major determinant of tissue responses to ischemia, the latter is more complex because it is influenced by other important factors, e.g., inadequate removal of metabolic products and the influence of flow, shear stress, and pressure. Ischemia results in an accumulation of metabolites, and consequently a drop in cellular pH and the development of hyperosmolarity. In contrast, hypoxia, in the absence of ischemia, washes out the products of glycolysis and thereby retards the development of acidosis.

It is important to recognize that oxygen sensing relates to a host of processes in addition to neovascularization; these include pH homeostasis, erythropoiesis, metabolism growth and development. Air entering the upper respiratory tract contains about 21% O_2, whereas most tissues experience much reduced levels of O_2, usually about 6% or 40 mm Hg PO_2 [1]. Hypoxia can act as a friend or foe, depending on its severity, the molecules that are activated, and the tissue or organ involved.

Continuous and Intermittent Hypoxia

Hypoxia can be continuous, e.g., residence at a high altitude, or intermittent, e.g., as occurs during sleep apnea or swimming. In this chapter, the term "intermittent hypoxia" is also used to refer to studies utilizing periods of hypoxia interspersed with periods of normoxia. The acute phase of hypoxia involves transient responses mediated by posttranslational modification of proteins, whereas the chronic phase is characterized by altered gene transcription and protein synthesis. Details of these types and phases of hypoxia are provided in reviews on oxygen homeostasis [2, 3].

Hypoxia-Inducible Factor and Gene Activation

Discovery of HIF-1

Cellular sensing of hypoxia involving the transcription factor, hypoxia-inducible factor (HIF-1), composed of HIF-1α and HIF-1β subunits, was first documented by Wang and Semenza [4] to occur in all mammalian cell types. The long-recognized importance of hypoxia in the production of erythrocytes led to the discovery of a protein complex (HIF-1) which

R.J. Tomanek, *Coronary Vasculature: Development, Structure-Function, and Adaptations*,
DOI 10.1007/978-1-4614-4887-7_9, © Springer Science+Business Media New York 2013

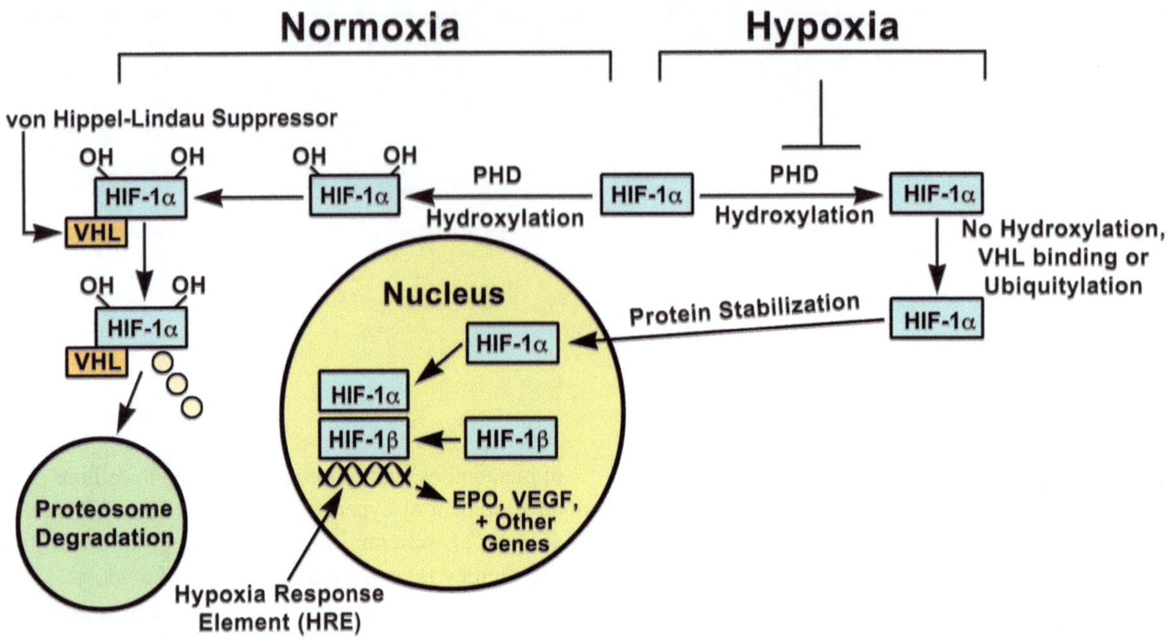

Fig. 9.1 Hypoxia causes protein stabilization of HIF-1α, its translocation to the nucleus, dimerization with HIF-1β, and finally the activation of hypoxia response elements of genes such as erythropoietin (EPO) and VEGF. Hypoxia inhibits the hydroxylation of HIF-1α by inhibiting oxygen-sensing prolyl hydroxylase domain proteins (PHDs), thereby preventing binding of the von-Hippel-Lindau (VHL) tumor suppressor protein (which regulates polyubiquitination). The latter is required for HIF-1α degradation in proteosomes. See text for further details

binds to the 3′ enhancer of the erythropoietin (EPO) region only during hypoxia [5–8]. HIF-1 was found to increase EPO mRNA transcription and production (reviewed in [9]). Moreover, this response was shown to occur in most cell types [10].

Cellular Responses to Hypoxia

As noted in Chap. 1, cellular responses to hypoxia involve many steps and transcription factors. A general summary of these steps, provided in Fig. 9.1, illustrates that in the context of normoxia HIF-1α is degraded via a pathway that involves HIF-1α polyubiquitination. This process is initiated by hydroxylation of HIFα subunits on key protein residues via members of the oxygen-sensing propyl hydroxylase domain proteins (PHDs) family. This then facilitates interaction with von-Hippel-Lindau (pVHL) tumor suppressor protein, which regulates the polyubiquitination steps. In the context of hypoxia, HIF-1α is stabilized due to the inhibition of hydroxylase activity, inactivation of the PHDs, and neutralization of pVHL. Thus, HIF-1α is resistant to ubiquitination and degradation does not occur [11, 12]. This leaves the protein free for translocation to the nucleus, where it dimerizes with HIF-1β (also known as ARNT) and associates with transcription coactivators and mediates responses at the cellular, tissue, and systems levels (reviewed in [13, 14]). This HIF-1-driven adaptation establishes a shift toward glycolytic metabolism to maximize ATP production and minimize increases in ROS.

Hypoxia-Inducible Factor in the Heart

Systemic hypoxia produces organ-specific regulation of HIF-1 expression [15]. Cardiac adaptations to hypoxia, many of which are mediated by HIF-1α, are influenced by both the magnitude and duration of hypoxia. Ning and colleagues [16] used a short-cycle hypoxia protocol in isolated rabbit hearts to test the hypothesis that relatively mild short-cycle hypoxia, which does not disrupt the energy state or cause significant cardiac dysfunction, can induce HIF-α activation. Their work revealed that a 10-s hypoxia/110-s reoxygenation cycle induced an eightfold increase in HIF-1α, whereas severe hypoxia (60 s hypoxia/60 s reoxygenation) induced a smaller, fourfold increase in HIF-1α. Moreover, although the mild short, but not the severe, hypoxic cycle increased vascular endothelial growth factor (VEGF) protein significantly, it was defined as subthreshold because it did not stimulate coronary vasodilation or enhance lactate production. These data support the concept that hypoxia can, but does not necessarily produce favorable adaptations in the heart and that its effect may, therefore, be either physiological or pathological. The idea that HIF-1α may induce coronary collateral growth, a topic covered in Chap. 10, is supported by data from patients with at least 70% narrowing of one or more coronary arteries [17]. Patients in this group who exhibited demonstrable coronary artery collaterals had significantly higher monocyte and lymphocyte HIF-1α levels than patients without demonstrable collaterals. These data are consistent with the concept that HIF-1α induction plays a key role in coronary neovascularization.

Hypoxia and Neovascularization: General Concepts

Hypoxia serves as a trigger for vascularization during (1) prenatal and postnatal growth and (2) remodeling necessary for optimal coronary flow and reserve during pathological states, e.g., ischemic heart disease, cardiomyopathy, and cardiac hypertrophy. A role for HIF-1-regulated hypoxia in vasculogenesis, angiogenesis, and arteriogenesis is well established (reviewed in [18, 19]). HIF-1 triggers angiogenesis locally in response to inadequate oxygen by activating multiple growth factors. Not surprisingly, this process is of great clinical interest with regard to both promoting and preventing neovascularization. HIF-1α is essential for embryonic survival, since its deletion causes degeneration of the developing vascular plexus and fetal death [20]. Cellular responses to the activated growth factors are temporally and spatially regulated and their activation by HIF-1α influences not only vasculogenesis and angiogenesis but also arteriogenesis. Hypoxia has been shown to stimulate a variety of steps leading to vascularization (reviewed by [21]); these include increased permeability, endothelial sprouting, EC proliferation and migration, pericyte and smooth muscle recruitment, and degradation of the ECM. HIF also plays a role in hypoxia-induced pulmonary arterial remodeling that is unique for these vessels (reviewed in [19]).

HIFs: The Link between Hypoxia and Vascular Growth Factors

HIF-1 Activates Multiple Genes

The key role of HIF-1 in the activation of angiogenic growth factors is evident from the fact that HIF-1 transcription induced by hypoxia results in upregulation of VEGF, stromal-derived factor-1 (SDF-1), angiogpoietin-2, placental growth factor (PIGF), platelet-derived growth factor B (PDGF-B), and stem cell factor (reviewed in [14, 18]). Gene activation of VEGF, SDF-1, and angiopoietin-2 and stem cell factor occurs by direct binding of HIF-1.

To test the hypothesis that HIF-1 mediates cell autonomous activation of ECs, these cells were infected with a constitutively active form of HIF-1 under normoxia [22]. This experiment certified that HIF-1 increased the expression of 245 genes to the same level as hypoxia. Kelly et al. [23] found that ECs infected with HIF-1 migrated across basement membranes similar to ECs cultured under hypoxia, and demonstrated that a constitutively active form of HIF-1α is sufficient for the induction of angiogenesis in nonhypoxic tissue. In the mouse ischemic limb model, a partial HIF-1α deficiency was associated with marked declines in VEGF, PIGF, Angiopoietin-1 and -2, stromal-derived factor-1 (SDF-1), and stem cell factor [24]. These declines were associated with impaired recovery from ischemia, but the impairment was restored by administration of a constitutively active form of HIF-1α, which resulted from an increase in the number of circulating angiogenic cells. Hypoxia enhances VEGF expression not only in cardiomyocytes and ECs but also in pericytes [25, 26]. In pericytes, the levels of VEGF mRNA increase as O_2 tension decreases and pericyte proliferation increases in response to the application of exogenous VEGF [27].

HIF-2α Plays a Role in Vascular Development

Vascular development requires this HIF as demonstrated in HIF-2α$^{-/-}$ mouse embryos [28]. These mice develop severe vascular defects and die before E12.5, and endothelium-specific expression of HIF-2α restores normal vascular development and function. An important finding from this study was that Tie-2 expression was reduced in the HIF-2α $^{-/-}$ mutants, but restored by HIF-2α cDNA expression in ECs. Thus, both HIF-1α and HIF-2α mediate transcriptional responses to hypoxia. Despite high levels of sequence conservation between these HIF genes, the proteins they encode appear to have unique transcriptional targets [29]. HIF-2α knockout mice die at midgestation [28] and are characterized by bradycardia and reduced noradrenaline [30]; they also develop cardiac hypertrophy, retinopathy, and are characterized by increased oxidative stress [31]. Moreover, HIF-2α has shown to be the physiological regulator of erythropoietin production [32] and couples erythropoiesis with iron homeostasis [33]. Haploinsufficiency of HIF-2α results in dysregulation of the autonomic responses associated with enhanced oxidative stress [34], a finding that implicates this HIF in antioxidant function. Therefore, prolonged HIF-2α accumulation may facilitate adaptation to chronic hypoxia [29].

VEGF and VEGFR-1 Signaling Are Upregulated By Hypoxia

The importance of VEGFR-1 signaling in the angiogenic response to hypoxia has been delineated in ECs [35]. This reported assay-based work revealed an upregulation of VEGFR-1, but not VEGFR-2, during EC exposure to hypoxia. Further support for a role of VEGFR-1 in angiogenesis comes from experiments that used Flt-1 (VEGFR-1) intraceptors (endoplasmic retention signal-coupled VEGF receptors) in corneal epithelial cells and showed that this led to suppression of hypoxia-induced VEGF secretion [36]. The link between VEGF and hypoxia in coronary vessels was provided by Marti and Risau [37], who exposed adult mice to 6% oxygen for 6 h and demonstrated that both VEGF and VEGFR-1 mRNA were upregulated in the heart. In contrast, VEGFR-2 mRNA levels were unchanged. Evidence that PIGF is effective in enhancing EC migration [38] also supports a role for VEGFR-1 in angiogenesis. Moreover, a 12-h exposure of neonatal cardiomyocytes to hypoxia enhances their PlGF mRNA nearly fourfold [39]. Hypoxia has also been shown to resolve thrombi, which have a PO_2 that is only 10% of that found in venous blood [40]. Among 13 HIF-1 regulated angiogenic factors, VEGF and VEGFR-1 expressions were upregulated twofold when the HIF-1α stabilizer, prolyl hydroxylase, was inhibited. Thus, increased HIF-1α levels enhance thrombus resolution and vein recanalization, at least in part, by increasing VEGF and VEGFR-1 expression.

In summary, it is well established that hypoxia upregulates VEGF by increasing both its transcriptional activity and stability [37, 41–43]. The data also suggest that VEGF/VEGFR-1 signaling and HIF-1α activity participate in an autocrine loop. Further support for this notion comes from experiments in which neuroblastoma cells were exposed to hypoxia. This environment sustains ERK (MAPK) activation [44], and is necessary for EC survival and migration [45]. Notably, treatment of the cultures with anti-VEGF and anti-VEGFR-1 antibodies reduced ERK 1/2 activation and the cell survival molecule bcl-2. Thus, VEGFR-1 is the key receptor for angiogenic and survival phenomena triggered by HIF-1α. Finally, HIF-2α is important for normal organ development and survival and may facilitate adaptations to chronic hypoxia.

Hypoxia and Vessel Sprouting

A description of the formation of vascular branches by sprouting is described in Chap. 1. A vascular sprout consists of ECs in a stalk with tip cells with filopodia in the leading front of the branch sensing a hypoxic microenvironment to which they migrate [46]. As already noted in this chapter, the degradation of HIFs under normal oxygen concentrations involves hydroxylation of HIFs by prolyl hydroxylases (PHDs). These proteins are oxygen sensors that are downregulated in the tip cells present in hypoxic tissue regions, thus allowing stabilization of HIF-1α, which facilitates sprouting. There is evidence that loss of HIF-1α, which attenuates VEGF and VEGFR-2 expression in ECs, disrupts hypoxia-induced angiogenesis in tumor cells [47]. Incidentally, HIF-2α levels are not enhanced in the absence of HIF-1α, and HIF-2α is not able to rescue the vascular defects that occur in embryos that lack HIF-1α (reviewed in [48]). These findings suggest that HIF-2α plays a role in sprout stabilization, a notion supported by the finding that HIF-1α deficiency in ECs causes an increase in vessel permeability [49].

In the adult mouse heart, administration of fibroblast growth factor (FGF-2), $VEGF_{164}$, or platelet-derived growth factor-BB (PDGF-BB) in the context of hypoxia was found to enhance vascular sprouting significantly more than hypoxia alone [50]. Surprisingly, PDGF-BB enhanced sprouting in the hypoxic environment more than the other two growth factors.

Effects of Hypoxia on Vascular Cells

Endothelial Cells

The severity of hypoxia is a determinant of EC responses. For example, severe hypoxia (near anaerobic conditions) will stimulate apoptosis. Such a response occurs in vitro when hypoxia results in stabilization of p53, which in turn inhibits HIF-1α/CBP interaction [51, 52]. Hypoxia-associated EC apoptosis occurs when expression of the bcl-2 proto-oncogene, an inhibitor of apoptosis, is suppressed [53]. Although these data are meaningful in that they identify some of the mechanisms evoking apoptosis, it must be noted that they were derived in vitro under extreme hypoxia and, for this reason, do not necessarily reflect changes that occur during more physiological conditions. In contrast, moderate hypoxia has been repeatedly shown to promote angiogenesis by activating molecules that play key roles in EC survival, proliferation, and migration (reviewed in [54]). Hypoxia upregulates many genes that affect the scaffolding of the extracellular matrix (ECM) during angiogenesis [55]. These ECM components include collagens, fibronectin, heparin sulfate proteoglycans, enzymes, and growth factors. Release of the latter by proteinases, such as matrix metalloproteinases, is an important ECM event that facilitates angiogenesis by enabling the extension of tip cells at the leading edge of the vascular sprout.

Vascular Smooth Muscle Cells

Hypoxia has been shown to enhance the proliferation of pulmonary VSMCs in response to FGF-2, PDGF, and epidermal growth factor [18, 56]. These experiments revealed that although HIF-1α contributes to EC proliferation, it is not crucial for its occurrence. Pulmonary VSMC proliferation during hypoxia-induced remodeling has been shown to increase in the presence of transforming growth factor-β (TGF-β1), which induces COX-2 via the p38MAPK pathway [57]. In contrast, BMP-4 (bone morphogenic protein) inhibited

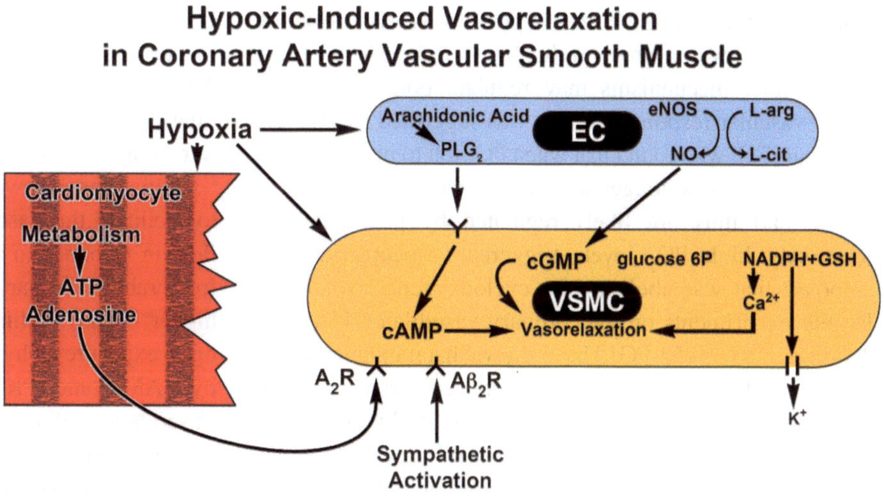

Fig. 9.2 Hypoxia activates several signaling pathways in three cell types in the heart: the endothelial cell (EC), the vascular smooth muscle (VSMC), and the cardiomyocyte. The activation occurs via adenosine from cardiomyocytes, prostacyclin (PLG_2) and NO from ECs, and potassium channels in VSMCs. VSMC vasorelaxation occurs via reductions in Ca^{2+}, opening of K^+ channels, and increases in cGMP and cAMP. Sympathetic activation of $A\beta_2R$ on ECs also occurs during hypoxia

the hypoxic induction of COX-2 by a MAPK-independent pathway. The finding that human pulmonary VSMCs proliferate in a moderately low PO_2 environment, independent of IL-1 [58], is consistent with pulmonary hypertension that characterizes organisms subjected to high altitude. In contrast, arteries of the systemic circulation vasodilate in response to HIF-1α.

Macrophages

When tissues become hypoxic, they release attractants such as monocyte chemotactic protein-1 (MCP-1). ECs and VSMCs secrete macrophage colony stimulating factor (MCSF), which may enhance macrophage survival and proliferation [59]. Macrophages not only function in phagocytosis, but secrete a wide range of growth factors, cytokines and enzymes; thus, their role in angiogenesis, arteriogenesis, and tissue remodeling is not surprising.

Mechanisms of Hypoxic Induction of Coronary Artery Dilation and Coronary Flow

Contributing Signaling Pathways

Hypoxia is a well-documented vasodilator of coronary arteries and has been shown to trigger several signaling pathways in ECs, VSMCs, and cardiomyocytes (reviewed by [60]). However, the relaxation of coronary VSMCs does not require activation of all of these pathways. Moreover, the endothelium does not play a compulsory role, as evidenced by data that certify hypoxia-induced coronary artery relaxation in the absence of an endothelium [61–63]. Nevertheless, the endothelium releases two important vasodilators, NO and prostacyclin, during hypoxia [64–66]. The subsequent sections address the role of several vasodilators that have been shown to play a role in hypoxia-induced coronary artery vasodilation and coronary flow. A summary of hypoxia-induced signaling involved in VSMC relaxation is provided in Fig. 9.2.

Prostaglandins

Several studies have investigated the role of prostaglandins as mediators of coronary artery vasodilation during hypoxia. Experiments on isolated rabbit hearts revealed that blocking prostacyclin with indomethacin did not prevent anoxia-induced increases in coronary blood flow [67], whereas it did prevent the increase in flow attributed to hypoxia [68]. An important consideration in this regard is the timing of prostanoid production, as indicated by the finding that in isolated hearts, indomethacin suppressed the increase in coronary blood flow only during the early phase of hypoxia [69].

In studies of isolated bovine [70, 71] and porcine [72] coronary arteries, the precise coronary response was found to be a function of the extent of PO_2 reduction. Collectively, these studies support the conclusion that coronary arteries relax during hypoxic exposure, associated with an increase in prostacyclin, but constrict when hypoxia is severe. For example, in bovine coronary artery strips during hypoxia (5% O_2), sustained vasorelaxation occurred, whereas anoxia evoked only a brief vasorelaxation followed by constriction [71]. The arterial relaxation was associated with enhanced prostacyclin synthesis and its inhibition, with indomethacin, decreased the hypoxia-induced relaxation. Moreover, the relationship between the magnitude of hypoxia, coronary artery reactivity, and prostacyclin was demonstrated in experiments indicating that a decrease in PO_2 from 580 mmHg to 47 mmHg led to increases in prostacyclin and the magnitude of vasorelaxation. Yet, a PO_2 reduction to 9 mmHg inhibited prostacyclin synthesis and induced arterial constriction. The decrease in coronary vascular resistance in isolated rabbit hearts during hypoxia was also found to depend on elevated prostacyclin levels [65]. The idea that two distinct mechanisms may regulate porcine coronary artery vascular responses to PO_2 was suggested by Rubanyi and Paul [72], who found that when PO_2 fell to near zero, vasorelaxation was no longer sensitive to cyclooxygenase inhibition, and thus not likely regulated by prostaglandins. Relatively high PO_2 levels triggered vasoconstriction, a response that was abolished by cyclooxygenase inhibitors. Recent experiments on the coronary vasodilator 15-deoxy-Δ-prostaglandin (15d-PGJ_2) have shown that it inhibits soluble epoxide hydrolase during hypoxia-induced coronary vasodilation [73]. The vessels of soluble epoxide hydrolase-null mice are basally dilated compared to wild-type controls and fail to dilate in response to 15d-PGJ_2 and during hypoxia.

Adenosine

A role for adenosine in hypoxia-mediated coronary vasodilation is indicated by experiments in which adenosine A_2 receptor blockade attenuated vasodilation in porcine arteries [74]. Since adenosine production in the artery was not enhanced by hypoxia, the investigators concluded that hypoxia only enhances the sensitivity of the A_2 receptor. However, these experiments were inconclusive because they utilized isolated arteries and they were not able to address adenosine production by cardiomyocytes. Notably, Kamekura et al. [75] had previously documented an increase in adenosine production in isolated rat hearts following the opening of K_{ATP} channels. It is well established that adenosine release is elevated exponentially as the severity of hypoxia increases [76], a fact that supports the role of this nucleotide in triggering coronary vasodilation.

K^+ Channels

As recently reviewed [77], the main role of K^+ channels in coronary vasodilation is to determine resting membrane potential and to mediate vasodilator signals. Ca^{2+} influx and consequently arterial tone change as K^+ channel activity is altered. Hypoxic induction of coronary vasodilation in perfused hearts is inhibited by the K_{ATP} channel blocker glibenclamide and facilitated by the K_{ATP} channel opener cromakalin [78, 79]. Smani et al. [80] suggested that any circumstance, like protracted hypoxia, that reduces intracellular ATP levels will lead to opening of K_{ATP} channels; this in turn causes hyperpolarization of the cell membrane, closure of voltage-dependent Ca^{2+} channels, and consequently vasorelaxation. In isolated rat hearts, K_{ATP} channel-dependent flow is suppressed by glibenclamide during hypoxia [75]. Moreover, low O_2 tension decreased basal cytosolic and transmembrane Ca^{2+}, indicating that the established voltage-gated Ca^{2+} channels in coronary VSMCs are controlled by O_2 tension [80]. A review of the role of potassium channels in coronary vasodilation also concludes that K_{ATP} channels do not play a role in resting coronary blood flow [77].

Activation of inward rectifier K^+ channels has been shown to facilitate the vasodilation and increased coronary blood flow in response to acute hypoxia in rabbits [81, 82]. Cells from rabbit coronary arterioles (<100 μm in diameter) had higher inward rectifier K^+ current than arterioles >100 μm upon exposure to hypoxia and these currents were mediated by cAMP and PKA-dependent signaling cascades [81]. Vasodilation of coronary arteries was abolished when K^+ channels were blocked, whereas Ca^{2+} blockade of either small or large channels was without effect [62]. These effects were independent of an intact endothelium. When glycolysis was blocked by replacing glucose with deoxyglucose, coronary arteries reached a near-maximum dilation; the effect was reversed by glibenclamide [79]. This finding suggests that a reduction in the pentose phosphate pathway (PPP) affects K^+ channels and thereby facilitates coronary artery vasodilation. In contrast, a study on human atrial appendage arterioles (70–180 μm in diameter) reported that glibenclamide was without effect on hypoxia-induced vasodilation [83].

Nitric Oxide

The role of NO in hypoxia-induced coronary vasodilation has been well established in several animal models, including guinea pigs [84, 85], dogs [86–88], and rats [83]. The dependence of hypoxia-induced coronary vasodilation on NO has been shown to range from partial in guinea pigs [85] to complete in rats [83]. Park et al. [84] studied the role of NO in relation to other vasodilators and discovered that NO is most important for the early phase of hypoxia-induced vasodilation, whereas adenosine contributes to the late phase. The production of NO in the coronary vasculature differs in ECs from microvascular and epicardial vessels [89]. Although hypoxia increased NO and eNOS levels in the cells from both types of vessels, the increases were less in microvascular ECs. A major difference noted between the two vessel types was the change in total mRNA in response to hypoxia, i.e., the level increased more than twofold in the epicardial endothelium, but stayed at control levels in the microvascular ECs. The authors concluded that the O_2-sensitive response mechanisms that modulate NO production may differ in the EC's lining resistance vs. those lining large arteries.

Cardiac mitochondria adapt to high altitude by increasing their NOS activity and expression by >75% and mitochondrial cytochrome complex I activity by 34% [90]. Since mitochondrial NOS constitutes a substantial (about 50%) source of NO in cardiomyocytes, elevated NO levels in high altitude dwellers may serve to maintain sufficient O_2 supply by enhancing myocardial perfusion. The right ventricle (RV) has a somewhat unique ability to adapt to decreased PO_2 because it extracts only about 50% of O_2 from the circulation during basal conditions, compared to the 75% extracted by the left ventricle (LV) [91]. During exercise, however, RV vasodilation does not occur until pO_2 falls to about 20 mm Hg. Thus, the RV has an extraction reserve. A study on isolated perfused hearts found that NO was a major factor in coronary vasodilation during normoxia, but not during hypoxia [75]. The vasodilation that occurred immediately after hypoxia was associated with K_{ATP} channel opening and subsequent enhanced adenosine production. However, the role of NO in vascular responses is not fully resolved because of differences in the experimental protocols, species, magnitude of hypoxia, and vascular beds studied.

Reactive Oxygen Species

Vascular cells produce reactive oxygen species (ROS), via NAD(P)H oxidases (reviewed in [92]). Superoxide and hydrogen peroxide are particularly important for signaling molecules in cardiovascular cells, and contribute to vascular tone and remodeling. Coronary artery VSMCs exposed to acute (5–10 min) hypoxia undergo decreased ROS production, which may reflect a lower oxygen substrate available for ROS production [93]. Consistent with these data is the observation that high arterial O_2 tension increases vascular tone by generating reactive O_2 species in the vessel's wall [94], and the finding that reactive O_2 species reduce NO availability [95, 96]. A study on patients with stable angina reported that the constrictor responses observed during hyperoxia could be abolished by administering the antioxidant Vitamin C [97]. Moreover, Vitamin C administration, which reduces free radicals, has been found to restore NO in ECs [98, 99]. Wolin and colleagues [100] found that changes in O_2 levels affect the production of superoxide and superoxide anion-derived hydrogen peroxide and a cGMP-mediated relaxation response. Work from that laboratory in calves also established that (1) NADH oxidoreductase is a major source of superoxide anion [101] and (2) NADH-derived superoxide contributes to relaxation during posthypoxic reoxygenation, but not during hypoxia [102]. The data indicated that changes in PO_2 regulate vascular superoxide anion by two processes: first, during hypoxia superoxide anion levels are suppressed due to a decrease in PO_2; second, during reoxygenation the superoxide anion is transiently produced, apparently by a flavoprotein containing NADH oxidoreductase. A review of the studies from Wolin's lab [103] indicates that glucose 6P activity of the PPP promotes oxidation of cytosolic NADH and lowering the Ca^{2+} concentration, resulting in coronary artery relaxation.

Oxidation of NADPH and Glutathione

The role of PPP inhibition in coronary artery vasodilation was investigated in a series of studies [63, 104, 105]. Endothelium-denuded bovine coronary arteries were found to relax during hypoxia in the absence of EC-derived mediators or changes in superoxide or peroxidase [102, 105]. Subsequently, a role for PPP was established, based on the finding that its inhibition results in the oxidation of NADPH and glutathione that appears to activate coordination of redox-controlled mechanisms of relaxation [104]. The data suggested that the relaxation is mediated via a decrease in intracellular Ca^{2+}. Hypoxia was shown to decrease glucose-6-phosphate, but not ATPase and it was concluded that hypoxia promotes a systolic NADPH oxidation by reducing the availability of substrate for NADPH production via the glucose-6-phosphate dehydrogenase reaction of PPP. Pyruvate increased glucose-6-phosphate and NADPH, and also attenuated the hypoxia-induced relaxation. In sum, these studies reveal a novel mechanism of bovine coronary artery relaxation that is independent of mitochondrial energy metabolism and changes in ROS generation.

Role of O_2 and CO_2 Synergism in Coronary Blood Flow

Coronary vascular resistance was originally shown to correlate with venous oxygen and carbon dioxide gas tensions [106, 107]; subsequently, Broten et al. [108] demonstrated that it is the combined tensions that determine coronary blood flow during cardiac pacing. In closed-chest dogs, the left main coronary artery was perfused at a constant pressure, while coronary arterial gas tensions were controlled at a constant myocardial O_2 consumption. The data revealed a hyperbolic relation between venous O_2 and CO_2 tension and coronary blood flow during constant myocardial metabolism, and that coronary venous O_2 and CO_2 tensions interact synergistically in producing steady-state changes in coronary blood flow.

> Hypoxia is a powerful stimulus for coronary vasodilation, especially when arterial tension falls below 40 mmHg. The mediators of increased coronary flow during hypoxia involve several signaling pathways. A decrease in arterial PO_2 increases NO and PGI_2 in the endothelium, whereas enhanced cardiomyocyte contractility and the consequential decrease in PO_2 increases adenosine. Activation of sympathetic nerves and release of norepinephrine activates β-adrenergic receptors of VSMCs. These events lead to vasorelaxation as intracellular Ca^{2+} is reduced, cAMP and cGMP are increased, and K^+ channels are activated, as summarized in Fig. 9.2.

Hypoxia During Prenatal and Perinatal Coronary Development

Tissue expansion is a characteristic of growth and requires enhanced O_2 availability. This is obvious during the rapid myocardial growth that occurs during the prenatal–perinatal period, as described in Chaps. 2 and 3. As cells proliferate and hypertrophy, passive diffusion of O_2 and nutrients from the heart chamber lumen are no longer adequate. The resulting relative intermittent hypoxia is a signal for a cascade of events that facilitate vascularization of the tissue regions experiencing inadequate levels of O_2 (Fig. 9.3). However, it is evident that chronic hypoxia during pregnancy has many deleterious effects on the embryo or fetus, e.g., suppression of cardiac function, increased apoptosis, and premature exit of cardiomyocytes from the cell cycle [109]. This apparent paradox is explained by considering the levels of hypoxia and their duration, since as noted earlier, severe hypoxia is lethal, whereas moderate hypoxia facilitates vascular growth.

The term "normal" hypoxia, indicating lower oxygen tension in the fetus compared to the adult, has been used to indicate the physiological nature of the hypoxia [110]. As discussed in reviews [111, 112], the immature heart is relatively resistant to hypoxia as documented in many species. The survival time for animals during the early postnatal period exposed to anoxic environments is inversely related to age. Similarly, the cardiac sensitivity to ischemia is also less in the immature heart, i.e., postischemic recovery of developed force is highest in the newborn and declines during the first week of postnatal life [113].

Embryonic Coronary Development

Experimentally Induced Hypoxia In Vitro

To determine the influence of hypoxia on the formation of coronary vascular tubes by epicardial-derived cells (vasculogenesis), we explanted embryonic day 6 quail ventricular apexes onto collagen gels and cultured them under hypoxic or normoxic conditions [114, 115]. In this model, angioblasts delaminate from the epicardium and form vascular tubes in the collagen gel. In these cultured heart explants, aggregate tube length was >2-fold higher in 5% or 10% O_2 than in those cultured at 20% O_2 [115]. In contrast, explants cultured in a hyperoxic environment (95% O_2) had a markedly reduced tubulogenesis (Fig. 9.4). The hypoxia-induced tubulogenesis was VEGF-A dependent since addition of neutralizing antibodies to this growth factor resulted in aggregate tube length similar to the explants cultured under normoxic conditions (Fig. 9.5). Since we noted that the mRNAs of three VEGF splice variants 122, 166, and 190 were increased by hypoxia, we tested the effects of these specific splice variants on tubulogenesis and found that $VEGF_{165}$ enhanced tubulogenesis in a dose-dependent manner, whereas $VEGF_{121}$ had no effect. These data indicate that $VEGF_{165}$ is the most important VEGF-A splice variant for tubulogenesis in this model. Although tubulogenesis was enhanced by either hypoxia (5 or 10% O_2) or $VEGF_{165}$, the diameters of tubes in cultures containing exogenous VEGF were more than 2 times larger than those from hypoxic or normoxic environments (Fig. 9.5). Notably, exposure to both hypoxia and $VEGF_{165}$ resulted in formation of tubes larger than those formed in the context of normoxia, but smaller than those formed in cultures containing

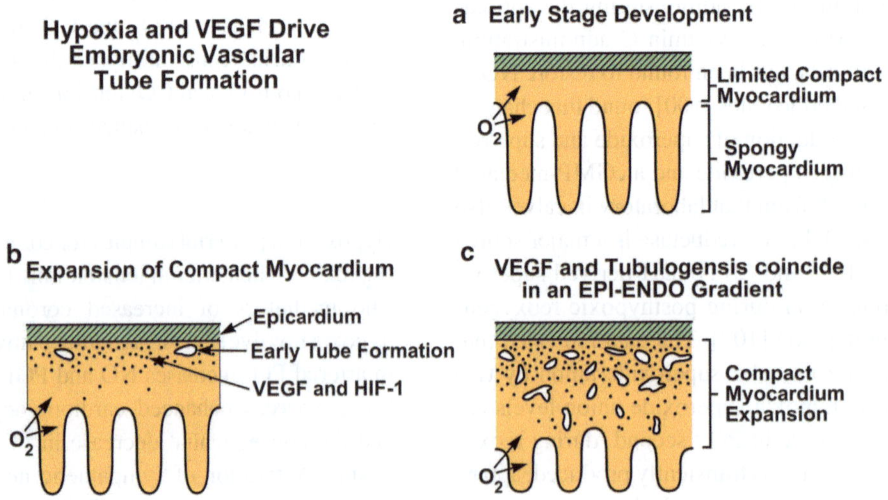

Fig. 9.3 Hypoxia activates VEGF in the developing heart. During the early stage of embryonic heart development (**a**) the compact portion of the ventricle is only a few cells thick and therefore O_2 diffusion from the lumen is sufficient. As the compact myocardium increases in thickness (**b**) the cells nearest the epicardium become hypoxic and release HIF-1, which triggers upregulation of VEGF and stimulates the formation of vascular tubes. Further growth (expansion) of the compact myocardium (**c**) causes formation of a hypoxia gradient toward the endocardium, which stimulates HIF-1 and VEGF, and consequently additional tubulogenesis

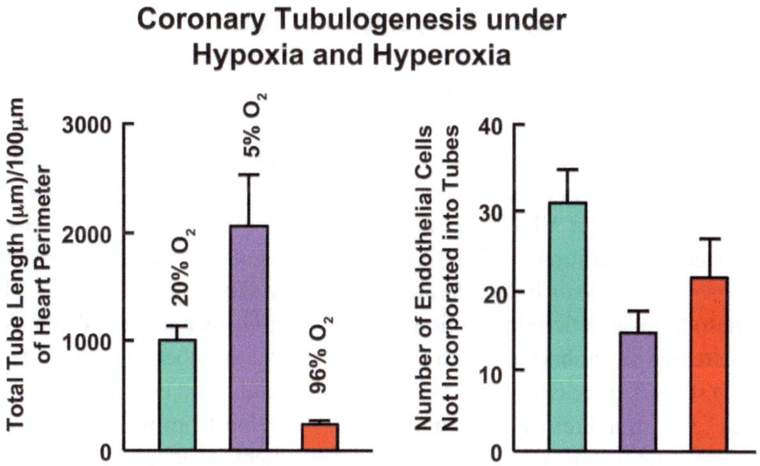

Fig. 9.4 Hypoxia stimulates and hyperoxia inhibits tubulogenesis in explanted quail embryonic hearts. Total tube length is twofold greater in a hypoxic environment, whereas hyperoxia inhibits tubulogenesis by 77%. The number of ECs not incorporated into tubes is reduced by hypoxia, a finding consistent with their incorporation into vascular tubes and the greater aggregate tube length in the hypoxic group. Data are from Yue and Tomanek 1999 [116].

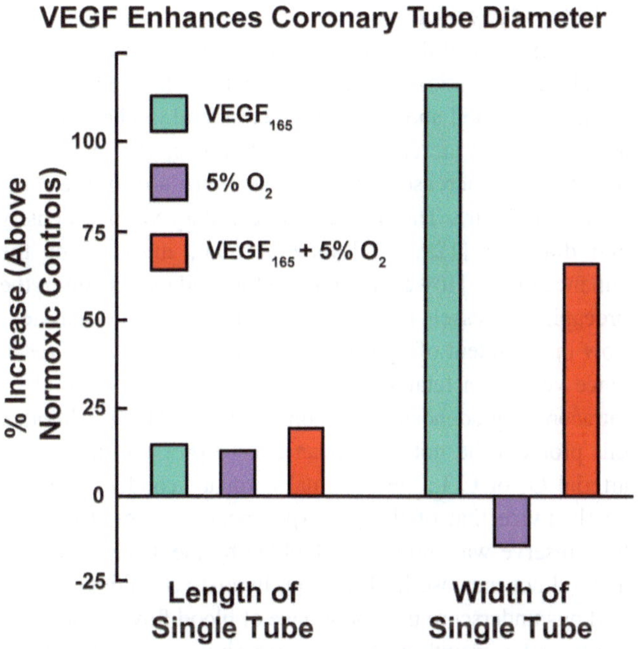

Fig. 9.5 Hypoxia and VEGF have similar effects on the lengths of individual tubes but contrasting effects on their diameters. $VEGF_{165}$ and 5% O_2 lengthen individual vascular tubes by about 13–15% compared to that in normoxic controls. However, $VEGF_{165}$ more than doubles tube width, whereas 5% O_2 causes a slight reduction in tube width. A combination of $VEGF_{165}$ and hypoxia is associated with tube widths that are intermediate to those produced by treatment with $VEGF_{165}$ and hypoxia treatments. Data are from Yue and Tomanek 2001 [115]

exogenous $VEGF_{165}$. These data indicate that although hypoxia enhances tubulogenesis by upregulating VEGF, the influence of at least one VEGF splice variant exerts unique characteristics.

As noted in Chap. 2, VEGFs A, B, and C, and VEGFR-1 play a role in coronary tubulogenesis [117]. VEGF-B, VEGF-A, and PlGF are all ligands for VEGFR-1. Because hypoxia upregulates VEGFR-1, but not VEGFR-2 in coronary ECs [37], the increase in this receptor facilitates the binding of both VEGFs A and B. The hypoxic effect on VEGF-B is both organ specific [37] and cell-type specific [118]. In addition to VEGF family members, other growth factors (e.g., FGFs and angiopoietin) contribute to the coronary vascularization process in the embryo [119, 120]. Thus, hypoxia-induced myocardial tubulogenesis involves multiple ligands and signaling pathways.

Tissue Hypoxia Characterizes Developing Embryos (In Vivo Studies)

Activation of HIF signaling in the developing heart is an important consideration since the rapidly expanding tissue mass becomes relatively hypoxic. When Lee et al. [121] used the nitroimidazole hypoxic marker, pimonidazole, to locate areas of hypoxia in embryonic mice, they discovered hypoxic regions that coincided with VEGF and HIF-1α expression and that these regions were sites of EC proliferation and vessel formation. Another contribution of this study was the finding that hypoxia induced both HIF-1α and VEGF in cell cultures of F9 embryonic teratocarcinoma stem cells. Nanka et al. [122] also found hypoxic areas in the myocardium of quail embryos developing under normoxic conditions and noted that these regions were characterized by elevated VEGF and HIF-1 expression. Moreover, when the embryos were exposed to hypoxia, HIF-1 and VEGF were overexpressed. However, prolonged exposure to hypoxia (16% ambient O_2) during the embryonic period was lethal by E9, and usually associated with failure of one coronary artery stem to form [123]. Similar results from another lab in embryonic chick hearts were obtained when the embryos were exposed to hypoxia [124]. These investigators also discovered that hypoxia, hyperoxia, and overactive HIF-1 resulted in similar types and frequencies of coronary anomalies. Their study underscores that a precise window of O_2 level is required for the formation and development of coronary arteries.

Hypoxic Induction of Embryonic Stem Cells

Hypoxia has been found to accelerate the expression of VEGFR-2 (FLK-1), a marker of hemangioblasts in embryonic stem cell cultures [125]. The same experiments revealed that a documented hypoxic regulation of the number of hemangioblasts is dependent on HIF-1, since its deficiency resulted in fewer VEGFR-2^+ cells under both hypoxic and normoxic conditions. Moreover, hypoxia regulates other mesodermal events by accelerating Brachyury expression, a mesoderm-specific transcription factor. When O_2 levels are decreased in embryonic stem cell cultures, the number of $CD31^+$ ECs increases [126]. Moreover, when embryoid bodies (3-D structures of embryonic tissues) develop from the embryonic stem cells, a hypoxic environment enhances angiogenic sprouts, and an increase in VEGFR-1 and VEGFR-2 occurs in cells derived from the embryoid bodies. These data suggest that embryonic hypoxia may enhance progenitor cell numbers, which in turn accelerate angiogenesis. This conclusion is consistent with the evidence that both VEGF receptors function in embryonic vascular development as demonstrated by embryonic lethality and defects in hematopoietic and angiogenic lineages in VEGFR-$2^{-/-}$ mice [127] and a disorganized vasculature in VEGFR-$1^{-/-}$ mice [128]. However, as noted previously, hypoxia upregulates VEGFR-1, but not VEGFR-2 [35].

Fetal Coronary Development and Responses

Vessel Formation and Growth

During fetal life, the coronary circulation is intact and provides nutrition to the compact region of the ventricles (external to the trabecular spongy myocardium). To test the hypothesis that coronary vessels and flow adapt to decreases in O_2 and hematocrit, a number of studies have produced anemia in sheep at late gestational stages by daily isovolemic hemorrhage; this results in marked declines in hematocrit and O_2, e.g., from 36% to 19% and from 8% to 2%, respectively [129]. In this model of chronic fetal hypoxemia, cardiac output is increased, vascular resistance is decreased, and capillary hydrostatic pressure is increased [130]. The loss of blood causes (1) a reduction in blood O_2 carrying capacity and (2) a compensatory increase in cardiac work necessary to maintain O_2 delivery to tissues. These two effects cause a marked reduction in the myocardial O_2 supply/demand ratio. Maximal coronary conductance was increased threefold after 7 days of anemia and increased further in response to adenosine [131]; these findings indicate that coronary vasodilator reserve (the difference between maximal and resting flow) was maintained during anemia, despite a very large increase in resting flow. This increase in vascular capacity suggests that vascular growth can compensate for the defects in the coronary circulation. Hearts of anemic fetuses had greater capillary densities and diameters compared to nonanemic controls [129]. Coronary blood flow increased progressively during the 7-day period, and, most importantly, coronary reserve was preserved. HIF-1α protein was elevated after 7 days of anemia, whereas VEGF, VEGFR-1, and LDH (which catalyzes the last step of glycolysis) were elevated by the third day. These data support the earlier findings by Martin et al. [132] that had revealed a relationship between VEGF, HIF-1α, and vascularization in chronically anemic sheep. Moreover, the data are consistent with a study that documented an increase in maximal coronary perfusion in late gestational sheep that were hypoxemic for 5–8 days [133]. That study also verified a preservation of coronary vasodilator reserve despite the doubling of resting (baseline) flow in the hypoxemic lambs.

Hypoxia and Blood Flow Induce Coronary Growth in Fetal Myocardium

Vascularization of the fetal myocardium is a response to both metabolic (hypoxia) and mechanical (shear stress and stretch) stimuli. As noted above, hypoxemia in fetal lambs is associated with large increases in maximal myocardial perfusion, indicating an increase in the cross-sectional area of the coronary vasculature. The increases in capillary volume density and diameter [129, 132] may account, in part, for the enhanced flow. However, a remodeling and expansion of the precapillary vessels is the major contributor. To determine if flow independent of hypoxia stimulates the growth of resistance vessels in fetal sheep, flow was increased twofold by intracoronary adenosine infusion for 4 days [134]. Although this protocol did not alter mean arterial pressure, heart rate, arterial O_2 or CO_2, the maximal coronary conductance was nearly twice that of the pre-experimental values. Coronary flow reserve was more than doubled by the 4-day treatment and did not increase further under hypoxic conditions. These findings underscore the importance of blood flow in modulating vascular growth in the fetus, which is consistent with its role in adults [135]. Hypoxia may nevertheless exert a role independent of the increases in blood flow because ECs sense low O_2 levels and upregulate genes that are associated with angiogenesis [136, 137]. The independent role of hypoxia is supported by the previously cited in vitro studies on explanted embryonic hearts [114, 115] and by the evidence that a constitutively active form of HIF-1 induces tube formation [22].

Vasoactive Responses

Reller et al. [138] established nitric oxide as a determinant of coronary flow both at rest and during hypoxia in fetal lambs. This group demonstrated that the enhanced flow in response to hypoxia was prevented by blocking NOS, despite the fact that L-NNA, a NOS competitor, caused an increase in arterial pressure. Moreover, their data revealed that acute hypoxemia increased coronary blood flow to a level greater than that induced by adenosine. Inhibition of NOS reduced coronary flow to values similar to those attributed to adenosine alone. Consistent with these findings, a role for eNOS, an O_2-sensitive synthase [139] that is activated during chronic hypoxia, was documented in a study in which fetal guinea pigs were housed in a 10.5% O_2 environment for 14 days [140]. In coronary arteries, this exposure led to increases in both mRNA and protein eNOS expressions in coronary arteries, but in the myocardium, both were decreased, indicating that the response to hypoxia was tissue specific. The importance of the enhanced production of NO due to eNOS upregulation is that it contributes to acetylcholine-induced coronary vasodilation, as documented in fetal guinea pig hearts [141]. These findings confirm the observation of Thornburg and Reller [142] that the large production of NO in the fetal heart contributes to the high coronary flows during acute hypoxemia.

Chronic hypoxia in fetal sheep (as a consequence of exposure to high altitude) has also been shown to reduce the vasoconstrictive responses to a thromboxane mimetic [143]. The mechanism underlying attenuated constriction was found to be a NO-independent sensitivity. Enhanced coronary perfusion has been established as a compensatory adaptation to arterial hypoxemia in fetal lambs [144]. When arterial O_2 was reduced by 50%, blood flow increased twofold to sixfold, and myocardial consumption of O_2, glucose, and lactate was maintained at normal, aerobic levels. These findings are consistent with (1) an increase in blood flow in fetal lambs when O_2 levels decline [145] and (2) a 31% decrease in Ca^{2+} channel density in coronary arteries of fetal lambs whose mothers resided at an altitude of 3,820 m for 110 days [146]. Arterial intracellular levels of Ca^{2+} in these lambs were reduced, as was contraction in response to KCl.

> These data support the conclusion that NOS plays a key role in dilating coronary vessels and increasing blood flow during hypoxia in prenatal and perinatal hearts. The upregulation of eNOS and production of NO contribute to acetylcholine-induced coronary vasodilation. Another adaptation of the fetal coronary vasculature to hypoxia is a decline in calcium sensitivity, which is independent of NO.

High Altitude Hypoxia

General Characteristics

The partial pressure of oxygen is reduced by approximately 7 mmHg for every km increase in altitude (each km increase affects a 2.5% drop in ambient O_2). Residing at a high altitude, i.e., 2,700–5,500 m above sea level, or a hypobaric exposure simulating such altitudes, causes a number of predictable biological changes (reviewed in [147]). These include (1) a drop in arterial PO_2, which induces polycythemia; (2) an increase in myocardial myoglobin content; and (3) anaerobic glycolysis and glucose utilization. Constriction of pulmonary arteries causes a pressure overload in the right ventricle and results in hypertrophy of that chamber. Other cellular responses are similar to those observed in non-altitude hypoxemia.

The low O_2 partial pressure (pO_2) encountered by individuals native to low altitudes when they are exposed to high altitude requires adaptations that are aimed at normalizing cellular oxygenation. Chronic exposure to high altitude leads to systemic hypoxia rather than being limited to one organ or tissue region, as is the case in most other forms of injury-associated hypoxia. Systemic hypoxia results in (1) elevated hematocrit and hemoglobin, due to increased erythropoietin (EPO), (2) reduced heart rate, and (3) pulmonary hypertension. TNF-α is elevated in the right ventricle (RV) during hypoxia and is a mediator of the pulmonary hypertension as evidenced by the failure of TNF-$\alpha^{-/-}$ mice to develop increased systolic RV pressure [148]. The specific changes occurring in the RV and LV during adaptation to high altitude depend on the duration of exposure, whether the exposure is intermittent or constant and the magnitude of the simulated altitude.

Effects of High Altitude on Coronary Flow

Calves born and raised at an altitude of 3,500 m were studied under both hypoxemia and normoxia [149]. Despite RV/body weight ratios that were 77% higher in these calves than in their sea-level controls, maximal coronary vasodilation in all transmural RV layers (epimyocardium, midmyocardium, and endomyocardium) was similar to the controls. These data indicate that the cross-sectional area of the coronary vasculature increased in the calves that sojourned at the high altitude, and facilitated a maximal perfusion proportional to the increase in RV mass. However, the hypoxic environment required a higher (twofold) resting (baseline) blood flow compared to that in the calves raised at sea level and, consequently, caused a decrease in coronary flow reserve.

High Altitude and Gene Expression

In adult rats, intermittent hypoxia has been shown to modulate gene expression differently in the RV and LV [150]. Although hypertrophy developed in the RV, but not LV, both ventricles exhibited upregulation of heme-oxygenase-1 (HO-1), a microsomal enzyme that catalyzes the first (rate-limiting) reaction in heme metabolism. However, LDH-A, which like HO-1 contains a HIF-1 binding site [151], was upregulated only in the RV. VEGF-A mRNA levels were significantly elevated after 3 days of intermittent hypoxia in both ventricles, whereas a significant increase in VEGFR-2 (Flk-1) levels occurred only in the RV. In contrast, TGF-β1 was elevated by day 1 in the RV and by day 3 in the LV. These data suggest that intermittent hypoxia upregulates some of the genes that are important for angiogenesis independently of ventricular hypertrophy. The role of TGF-β1, which is upregulated by hypoxia in both ventricles, is most likely to induce fibrosis, which has been shown to be present in both ventricles in chronically hypoxic rats [152].

Changes in regulatory proteins in response to intermittent hypoxia (25 exposures of 8 h/day, 5 days/week) in adult rats were addressed by Strniskova et al. [153]. The simulated altitude of 7,000 m, which resulted in a 15% decrease in body weight and also a marked increase in RV/body weight ratio, caused tissue hypoxia in the RV, as indicated by an enhanced level of carbonic anhydrase. Other changes limited to the hypertrophic RV were increases in the levels of proteins associated with cell signaling (JNK) and angiogenesis. The observed increase in RV MMP levels is consistent with ECM turnover, which facilitates angiogenesis. Whereas extracellular regulated kinase (ERK) was enhanced in both ventricles, an increase in phosphorylated Akt (which facilitates cell survival, migration, and tube formation) was documented in the LV, but not RV.

In sum, intermittent hypoxia induces tissue hypoxia in the pressure-overloaded RV that evokes changes in protein expression that cause hypertrophy, remodeling, and angiogenesis. The LV also undergoes some of the changes that occur in the RV, e.g., upregulation of TGF-β1 and VEGF-A mRNAs, but not those associated with cardiac hypertrophy.

Influence of Altitude-Induced Hypoxia on the Heart and Its Capillaries

Degree and Organ Specificity of Hypoxia

As noted earlier in this chapter, some level of hypoxia, such as that which occurs when the compact myocardium expands, is required for vascularization of the embryonic heart. In this circumstance, the hypoxia is local rather than systemic. Since altitude hypoxia or O_2 restrictions by placental limitations cause a number of changes in the organism, the effects on the coronary system and the heart are more complex. Hypoxemia in chick embryos disrupts hemodynamics and growth and leads to dilated cardiomyopathy and a decline in cardiac contractility [154]. The latter condition is associated with increases in the levels of VEGF-A splice variants 166 and 190. Mouse fetuses made hypoxic by reducing the inspired air of the mothers experienced a decrease in cardiomyocyte proliferation resulting in a quantity of myocardial tissue that was only 50% of that in nonhypoxic controls [155]. This vulnerability to a 24-h exposure to hypoxia was most evident at midgestation, as evidenced by 89% and 51% mortality at E13.5 and E17.5, respectively, but only 5% mortality at E11.5. These effects were likely due to the epicardial detachment that occurred early during hypoxemia, which negated the source of progenitor cells required for coronary vessel formation.

As noted earlier, the timing and magnitude of the hypoxia are determinants of the effects on the heart. For example, mouse fetus survival is markedly reduced when maternal inspired air is reduced from 8% to 7% O_2 [155], a seemingly subtle difference, but is consistent with studies demonstrating the importance of the magnitude and timing of hypoxia with respect to cardiac hypoplasia and reduced ventricular mass [154, 155], as well as biventricular hypertrophy [156].

Prenatal Life

To test the hypothesis that the offspring of animals acclimatized to high altitude also undergo coronary capillary adaptations, Becker and colleagues [157] studied canine neonates born at a simulated altitude of 20,000 ft. Both mother and pups had elevated hemoglobin values. Morphometry of heart sections (the LV and RV were not separated) revealed that capillary/tissue areas of the pups born at high altitude were 38% larger than those of their counterparts born at sea level. In another study [158], pregnant ewes were exposed to an altitude of 3,820 m between days 30 and 139 of gestation and then the coronary capillary beds of the ovine fetuses were evaluated. Notably, the ventricles of these fetuses were not enlarged and capillary parameters were not altered. The discrepancies between the findings from these studies in dogs and sheep can potentially be accounted for by the fact that the former were neonates, whereas the latter were fetuses.

Early Postnatal Life

A number of subsequent studies have documented that capillary growth in the RV is increased when animals are either born and raised, or transferred to a simulated high altitude. This adaptation is usually limited to the RV which undergoes enhanced growth in response to pulmonary hypertension. That capillary proliferation is enhanced in the RV in rats born and raised at simulated high altitude has been repeatedly documented [159–162]. In some cases, the extent of capillary growth has even exceeded the growth of the RV myocardium as indicated by an enhanced capillary density despite a substantial increase in RV mass [159, 160, 163]. RV mass has been found to increase by as much as twofold or threefold in rats born and raised at a high altitude [160, 163]. This RV enlargement is due to both increases in cross-sectional areas of cardiomyocytes [159, 160, 163] and the number of cardiomyocytes [162]. The rats that were born and raised for 3 months in a low pressure chamber had a greater number of cardiomyocytes and a higher capillary density than their controls [162], findings that demonstrate both cardiomyocyte and capillary EC proliferation in response to hypoxia.

Young and Adult Animals

Several studies have explored the coronary adaptations that occur in young or adult animals chronically exposed to high altitude. Capillary growth in the RV, like that reported in neonate, is indicated by the data from rats [164–167] and guinea pigs [168]. Capillary growth was found to parallel the growth of the RV in young rats exposed to a 3,500-m simulated altitude as evidenced by capillary densities that were similar to [165] or exceeded [164] those in the controls. Kayar and Banchero [169] compared cardiac and myocardial capillary growth in guinea pigs exposed to hypobaric hypoxia at 5 weeks of age to that of their normobaric controls. RV cardiomyocyte cross-sectional area increased more in the hypobaric group than in controls, but the capillary/cardiomyocyte ratio also increased in fairly close proportion to cardiomyocyte growth. These data indicate that in most of the guinea pigs, capillary growth fully compensated for the hypoxia-induced increase in RV mass. However, when the RV hypertrophy was extreme, a favorable diffusion distance was not maintained, indicating that capillary compensatory growth is limited. In adult rats exposed to simulated high altitude, capillary density decreased and therefore did not keep pace with the more than twofold increase in RV weight [166].

Studies on intermittent hypoxia have reported increases in capillary density and the absence of ventricular hypertrophy [167, 170]. Young rats exposed to intermittent (6 h/day, for 28 or 42 days) high altitude (5,000 m) were shown to have a better flow recovery following 30 min of ischemia and increased capillary densities in both ventricles [167]. Adult rats subjected to intermittent hypoxia (4 h/day, 5 days/week for 22 days) also had higher capillary densities, which persisted during the 40-day period following the treatment protocol [170].

Hypoxia and Capillary Growth in the Left Ventricle

RV hypertrophy in response to altitude-induced hypoxia is mainly a consequence of pulmonary hypertension; in contrast, the LV is not exposed to notable pressure overload during hypoxic exposure. Most studies that have addressed adaptations to chronic hypoxia in the LV have reported increased capillary density [171–175]. Rats maintained for 10 or 30 days in a chamber with 9% O_2 experienced capillary density increases of 14 and 37%, respectively [172]. Moreover, mitochondrial/myofibril ratio and mitochondrial surface density of cardiomyocytes were enhanced by exposure to hypoxia, indicating a structural adaptation enhances O_2 delivery in mitochondria. Exposure of rats to a simulated altitude of 6,100 m for 6 weeks evoked a 20% increase in LV cardiomyocyte diameter, but capillary density was similar to that in the nonhypoxic controls, indicating that capillary growth was proportional to the magnitude of the hypertrophy [173]. Young mice exposed to a 10% O_2 over a 3-week period demonstrated a marked (about 40%) increase in capillary density in the LV which did not undergo hypertrophy [175]. Similarly, LV capillary density increased in newborn rabbits exposed to hypoxia for a period of 3 weeks despite the fact that LV mass was not increased [174]. Another study addressed the role of altitude hypoxia on LV capillary growth in guinea pigs born at high altitude and in those exposed postnatally to simulated high altitude [176]. Neither of the two groups differed with respect to capillary density or capillary/cardiomyocyte ratio; however, the presence of LV hypertrophy indicates that capillary growth was proportional to the increase in myocardial mass. Taken together, these data support the role of hypoxia as a stimulus of capillary growth in the hypertrophic LV, and also indicate that most robust response occurs in the young.

There is no consensus regarding the development of LV hypertrophy in response to hypobaria; LV hypertrophy was not found in some studies [160, 174, 177, 178], but was evident in others [164, 173, 176]. The hypothesis that VEGF upregulation is a requisite for the angiogenic response to chronic hypoxia was tested by Birot et al. [179], who found some increase in $VEGF_{188}$ mRNA in the hypertrophied RV and evidence of angiogenesis. In the LV, $VEGF_{188}$ mRNA was not enhanced and angiogenesis could not be documented. However, VEGF protein was unchanged in either ventricle of hypoxia-exposed rats. Three week old rabbits exposed to hypoxia for 8 weeks demonstrated an increase in capillary density, HIF-1α, HIF-2α, VEGFR-2, but not VEGF protein in the non-hypertrophied LV [174]. Thus, increases in VEGFR-2 may have sufficed for the induction of angiogenesis.

Relationship Between Hypoxia and Pre-existing Cardiac Hypertrophy

We raised the issue of the relationship between cardiac hypertrophy and the hypoxic induction of capillary growth [173]. Rats with LV hypertrophy resulting from spontaneous hypertension (SHR) or aortic constriction were exposed to simulated high altitude for 6 weeks. Systolic blood pressure was decreased in all three groups exposed to chronic hypoxia (Fig. 9.6); the largest decrease (34%) occurred in the SHR group. Heart rate declined by 30% in the normotensive rats and by 22% in the SHR group, whereas no change occurred in the aortic constricted rats. Figure 9.6 also indicates both the increase in cardiomyocyte diameter due to pressure

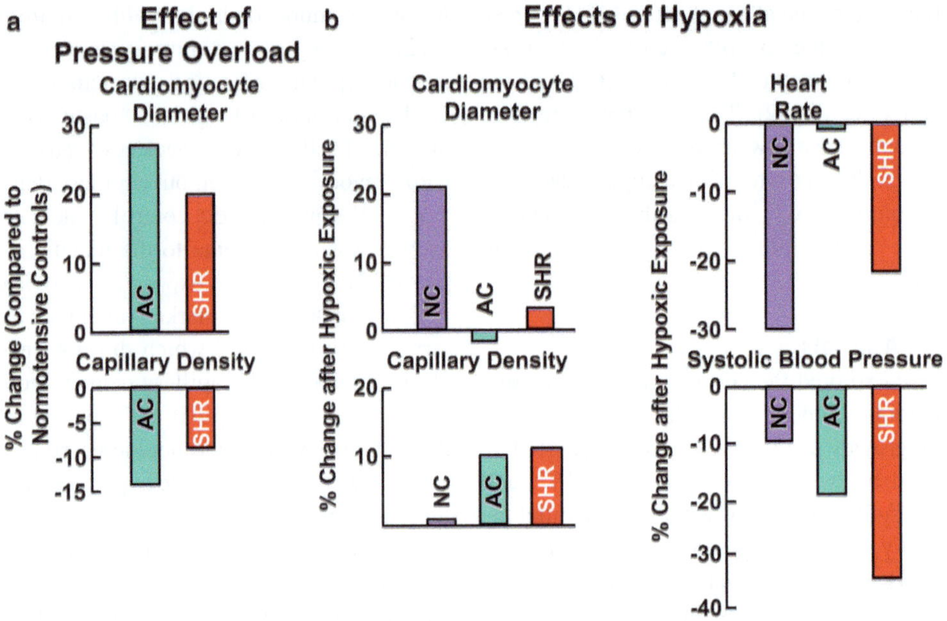

Fig. 9.6 Hypoxia enhances capillary growth in pressure-overloaded rat hearts. (**a**) A chronic increase in systolic pressure due to aortic constriction (AC) or spontaneous hypertension (SHR) increases cardiomyocyte diameter and decreases capillary density. (**b**) When hypertensive rats are exposed to chronic hypoxia, cardiomyocyte diameter is not increased further, whereas normotensive controls (NC) experience a 20% increase in cardiomyocyte diameter. Hypoxia causes a small but significant increase in capillary density in the two hypertensive groups. In the normotensive controls hypoxia does not alter capillary density, despite the increase in cardiomyocyte diameter; this finding indicates that capillary growth is proportional to cardiomyocyte hypertrophy when hypoxia is the factor inducing cardiac hypertrophy. Data are from Lund and Tomanek 1980 [173]

oveload and the associated decrease in capillary density. However, hypoxic exposure for 6 weeks enhanced cardiomyocyte diameters only in the normotensive controls, resulting in similar mean diameters in all three groups. Hypobaric hypoxia stimulated capillary growth sufficiently to normalize capillary density in SHR and significantly increase capillary density in rats with aortic constriction (Fig. 9.6). In the normotensive group, capillary density was unchanged despite a 23% increase in cardiomyocyte diameter, indicating that capillary growth fully compensated for the myocardial hypertrophy. These data indicate that hypoxia promotes capillary growth in the LV both (1) during the development of cardiac hypertrophy and (2) afterward.

Ultrastructural analysis of the hearts from the 3 groups of rats exposed to chronic hypoxia and described above revealed a number of cardiomyocyte adaptations. Longitudinal splitting of cardiomyocytes permitted capillaries to become incorporated between the newly formed cell branches (Fig. 9.7). The splits emanated from intercalated discs, which frequently extended longitudinally; double intercalated discs were also encountered in the hearts from the hypoxic groups. Vesicles in and beneath the sarcolemma were more numerous, and lateral infolding of the sarcolemma also was encountered. Like Friedman and colleagues [172], we found that the number of cardiomyocyte mitochondria was increased by hypoxia. These data indicate that hypoxia can promote adaptations that decrease the O_2 diffusion distance by stimulating proliferation of capillaries and their indentation into cardiomyocyte grooves and by increased cardiomyocyte branching. The greater number of mitochondria results in a larger surface area of these organelles for respiration, which may benefit aerobic metabolism.

Interpretation of Data Regarding Hypoxic Effects on the Hypertrophied Heart

Chronic exposure to hypobaric hypoxia evokes RV hypertrophy and pulmonary hypertension and is associated with capillary growth. The increase in myocardial mass, together with hypoxia, stimulates capillary proliferation. Because compensatory growth of capillaries in the LV that had been enlarged by pressure overload occurred during chronic exposure to hypoxia, the data implicate decreased O_2 in capillary growth in this model of hypertrophy. Two changes that occurred in the LV with hypoxic exposure may have contributed to the adaptations that occurred. First, a decrease in systolic pressure reduced both the afterload on the LV and the heart rate. Second, the reduction in heart rate increased end diastolic filling, thereby increased both ventricular and stroke volume. As previously documented, chronic bradycardia is associated with enhanced coronary capillary growth [180–182]. Moreover, data from newborn rabbits exposed to hypoxia for 3 weeks revealed an increase in capillary density despite an absence of LV hypertrophy [174].

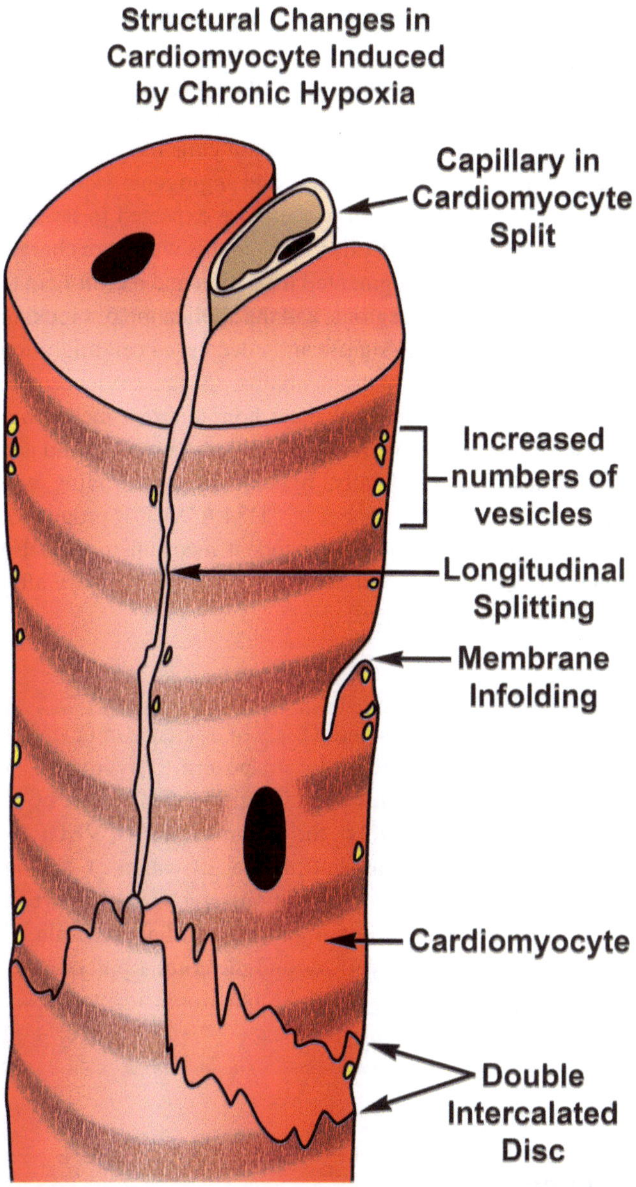

Fig. 9.7 Hypoxia evokes structural adaptations in cardiomyocytes. Exposure of hypertensive rats to hypoxia (see also Fig. 9.6) causes alterations in myocyte morphology that reduce the diffusion distance from capillaries. These include (1) longitudinal splitting of cardiomyocytes, which allows capillaries to be positioned in the resulting clefts, (2) membrane infolding, which decreases the distance between the center of the cardiomyocyte and the extracellular compartment, and (3) an increase in the number of sarcolemmal vesicles and the presence of double intercalated discs

Cardioprotective Effect of Hypoxic Exposure

Preservation of Cardiac Structure and Function

A role for ischemic preconditioning in limiting myocardial cell injury due to subsequent ischemia is well established [183–186]. This topic is addressed in Chap. 10. Exposure to hypoxia has also been shown to protect the heart during subsequent exposure to hypoxia or ischemia (reviewed in [111]). Ostadal and Kolar [187] reviewed data from humans and experimental animals and concluded that high altitude hypoxia enhances cardiac tolerance to the deleterious consequences of acute oxygen deprivation. Evidence for the protective effects of sustained or intermittent hypoxia was provided 4 decades ago [188, 189]. However, these investigators observed that the benefits were age dependent and that hypoxia may be harmful if extreme or persistent. They pointed out that intermittent hypoxia is initially associated with oxidative stress and increased adrenergic stimulation, events that are currently considered to be linked with the development of the ischemia-resistant cardiac phenotype.

Interest in hypoxic exposure as a protective modality against ischemic injury was heightened by evidence that it is as effective as ischemic preconditioning [190], and many subsequent studies have provided evidence that it improves myocardial tolerance to ischemia [190–197]. This topic is detailed in Chap. 10.

Mechanisms Facilitating Cardioprotective Effects of Hypoxic Exposure

Several mechanisms have been proposed to explain the improved cardiac function during hypoxia in hearts exposed to either continuous or intermittent hypoxia [111]. These include the heart's enhanced anaerobic capacity and glycogen reserves, better recovery from ischemia, and its decreased production of free radicals. However, these favorable changes do not necessarily mean that favorable adaptations of the coronary vasculature underlie the improved cardiac function. Rather than using continuous or intermittent exposure to hypoxia for cardioprotection, one study subjected rats to a single hypoxic exposure for 4 h followed by 24 h of normoxia and then coronary artery ligation [198]. In the preconditioned group, capillary and arteriolar densities were elevated by the second day after coronary artery ligation. Moreover, the hypoxic exposures also decreased the levels of EC apoptosis and attenuated the decline in contractile functional reserve as demonstrated by max dP/dt during dobutamine stress. This single exposure to hypoxia prior to coronary artery ligation increased the expression of VEGFR-1 (flt-1) and Tie-1 fivefold [199].

Cardiac protection against myocardial ischemia induced by intermittent hypoxia requires HIF-1α, as documented in HIF-1$\alpha^{+/-}$ mice [200]. In these mice, exposure to hypoxia failed to trigger a rise in EPO. A decrease in O_2 and an increase in mitochondrial ROS levels led to the enhancement of HIF-1-dependent transcription genes encoding several proteins that decrease mitochondrial ROS [201]. Therefore, HIF-1-dependent regulation of mitochondrial metabolism also appears to play a role in protecting the heart from injury.

A Role for NO

More relevant for cardioprotection is activation of NO and angiogenic growth factors. In recent years, HIF-1 has been recognized as a factor that mediates cardioprotection, especially by its induction of iNOS, heme oxygenase, and EPO [202]. Intermittent hypoxia has been shown to increase HIF-1 levels, which targets the iNOS gene, stimulates coronary flow at reperfusion, and reduces infarct size [203]. That study established the interaction of HIF-1 with iNOS as a consequence of hypoxic exposures. A role for NO in cardioprotection by exposure to hypoxia is well established. Both iNOS mRNA and protein expression increase after intermittent hypoxia and this results in an elevation of NO [194]. The importance of enhancing NO prior to reperfusion was highlighted by a study that found that improved tolerance to ischemia following intermittent hypoxia is abolished when NOS is inhibited by L-NAME [192]. Notably, in mice with myocardial infarctions, inducible nitric oxide synthase expression (NOS2) was increased in the preconditioned mouse hearts, and the reduction in infarct size was abolished when NOS2 was blocked.

K_{ATP} Channel Activation

Baker and colleagues [204] found that chronic exposure to hypoxia in neonatal rabbits is associated with enhanced K_{ATP} activity in the heart. They subsequently provided evidence that chronic hypoxia increased myocardial NO and decreased the action potentials in Purkinje fibers [205]. Their data showed that the effects on the sarcolemmal K_{ATP} channel that result in hyperpolarization were abolished by glibenclamide and by NO inhibitors. Activation of the K_{ATP} channel by hypoxia in this model is associated with an increased tolerance to ischemia and was suggested to be the consequence of increased lactate production [204]. This suggests that the increase in NO provides tolerance to ischemia via K_{ATP} channel activation, a conclusion supported by the findings that NO activates K_{ATP} channels in normoxic, as well as hypoxic hearts through a cyclic GMP-dependent mechanism [205].

Other Mechanisms

Additional mechanisms have been proposed to contribute to the favorable effects of hypoxic exposure. VEGF and erythropoietin levels increase within 3 h of hypoxic exposure [206], a finding that fits with data linking myocardial protection from ischemic injury in mice to the evidence that chronic hypoxia increases both capillary and arteriolar density and maximal myocardial perfusion [175]. A more efficient O_2 delivery is also indicated by an increased capillary density and decreased diffusion distance after a 22-day program of intermittent hypoxia [170].

Hypoxic Preconditioning of Angiogenic Cells

The utilization of progenitor cells for cell-based therapy is a topic receiving much attention and is discussed in Chap. 12. Hypoxic preconditioning of progenitor cells has been shown to upregulate many antiapoptotic and angiogenic factors (for references, see [207]), and is therefore expected to be very useful for this purpose. Cells treated in this way were characterized by markedly augmented migration and recruitment to ischemic myocardial regions, and the application of blocking antibodies for CXCR4 significantly decreased cell migration [208]. Consistent with these findings is the evidence that hypoxic preconditioning enhances bone-marrow mesenchymal stem cell migration, homing to injured myocardium and angiogenesis [209]. Finally, hypoxic preconditioning was shown to increase the number of $CD34^+/CXCR4^+$ progenitor cells, via an erythropoietin-dependent mechanism that also enhances cell homing and decreases myocardial injury after ischemia reperfusion [196].

In conclusion, a substantial body of evidence indicates that sustained or intermittent exposure to hypoxia is cardioprotective. This protection is facilitated by mechanisms that involve the activities of NO, VEGF, and erythropoietin, as well as the activation of K_{ATP} channels. The resulting adaptation, which is protective in the context of hypoxia and myocardial ischemia, affects both cardiomyocytes and the coronary vessels, with the latter undergoing both functional adaptations and growth.

References

1. Simon MC, Keith B. The role of oxygen availability in embryonic development and stem cell function. Nat Rev Mol Cell Biol. 2008;9:285–96.
2. Semenza GL. Does loss of CD151 expression promote the metastasis of hypoxic colon cancer cells? Clin Cancer Res. 2008;14:7969–70.
3. Semenza GL. Oxygen homeostasis. Wiley Interdiscip Rev Syst Biol Med. 2010;2:336–61.
4. Wang GL, Semenza GL. General involvement of hypoxia-inducible factor 1 in transcriptional response to hypoxia. Proc Natl Acad Sci USA. 1993;90:4304–8.
5. Semenza GL, Nejfelt MK, Chi SM, Antonarakis SE. Hypoxia-inducible nuclear factors bind to an enhancer element located 3′ to the human erythropoietin gene. Proc Natl Acad Sci USA. 1991;88:5680–4.
6. Beck I, Ramirez S, Weinmann R, Caro J. Enhancer element at the 3′-flanking region controls transcriptional response to hypoxia in the human erythropoietin gene. J Biol Chem. 1991;266:15563–6.
7. Pugh CW, Tan CC, Jones RW, Ratcliffe PJ. Functional analysis of an oxygen-regulated transcriptional enhancer lying 3′ to the mouse erythropoietin gene. Proc Natl Acad Sci USA. 1991;88:10553–7.

8. Semenza GL, Wang GL. A nuclear factor induced by hypoxia via de novo protein synthesis binds to the human erythropoietin gene enhancer at a site required for transcriptional activation. Mol Cell Biol. 1992;12:5447–54.
9. Semenza GL, Shimoda LA, Prabhakar NR. Regulation of gene expression by HIF-1. Novartis Found Symp. 2006;272:2–8. discussion –14, 33–6.
10. Maxwell PH, Pugh CW, Ratcliffe PJ. Inducible operation of the erythropoietin 3′ enhancer in multiple cell lines: evidence for a widespread oxygen-sensing mechanism. Proc Natl Acad Sci USA. 1993;90:2423–7.
11. Salceda S, Caro J. Hypoxia-inducible factor 1alpha (HIF-1alpha) protein is rapidly degraded by the ubiquitin-proteasome system under normoxic conditions. Its stabilization by hypoxia depends on redox-induced changes. J Biol Chem. 1997;272:22642–7.
12. Maxwell PH, Wiesener MS, Chang GW, Clifford SC, Vaux EC, Cockman ME, et al. The tumour suppressor protein VHL targets hypoxia-inducible factors for oxygen-dependent proteolysis. Nature. 1999;399:271–5.
13. Semenza GL. Regulation of oxygen homeostasis by hypoxia-inducible factor 1. Physiology. 2009;24:97–106.
14. Semenza GL. Vascular responses to hypoxia and ischemia. Arterioscler Thromb Vasc Biol. 2010;30:648–52.
15. Stroka DM, Burkhardt T, Desbaillets I, Wenger RH, Neil DA, Bauer C, et al. HIF-1 is expressed in normoxic tissue and displays an organ-specific regulation under systemic hypoxia. FASEB J. 2001;15:2445–53.
16. Ning XH, Chen SH, Buroker NE, Xu CS, Li FR, Li SP, et al. Short-cycle hypoxia in the intact heart: hypoxia-inducible factor 1alpha signaling and the relationship to injury threshold. Am J Physiol Heart Circ Physiol. 2007;292:H333–41.
17. Chen SM, Li YG, Zhang HX, Zhang GH, Long JR, Tan CJ, et al. Hypoxia-inducible factor-1alpha induces the coronary collaterals for coronary artery disease. Coron Artery Dis. 2008;19:173–9.
18. Rey S, Semenza GL. Hypoxia-inducible factor-1-dependent mechanisms of vascularization and vascular remodelling. Cardiovasc Res. 2010;86:236–42.
19. Hanze J, Weissmann N, Grimminger F, Seeger W, Rose F. Cellular and molecular mechanisms of hypoxia-inducible factor driven vascular remodeling. Thromb Haemost. 2007;97:774–87.
20. Iyer NV, Kotch LE, Agani F, Leung SW, Laughner E, Wenger RH, et al. Cellular and developmental control of O_2 homeostasis by hypoxia-inducible factor 1 alpha. Genes Dev. 1998;12:149–62.
21. Pugh CW, Ratcliffe PJ. Regulation of angiogenesis by hypoxia: role of the HIF system. Nat Med. 2003;9:677–84.
22. Manalo DJ, Rowan A, Lavoie T, Natarajan L, Kelly BD, Ye SQ, et al. Transcriptional regulation of vascular endothelial cell responses to hypoxia by HIF-1. Blood. 2005;105:659–69.
23. Kelly BD, Hackett SF, Hirota K, Oshima Y, Cai Z, Berg-Dixon S, et al. Cell type-specific regulation of angiogenic growth factor gene expression and induction of angiogenesis in nonischemic tissue by a constitutively active form of hypoxia-inducible factor 1. Circ Res. 2003;93:1074–81.
24. Bosch-Marce M, Okuyama H, Wesley JB, Sarkar K, Kimura H, Liu YV, et al. Effects of aging and hypoxia-inducible factor-1 activity on angiogenic cell mobilization and recovery of perfusion after limb ischemia. Circ Res. 2007;101:1310–8.
25. Nomura M, Yamagishi S, Harada S, Hayashi Y, Yamashima T, Yamashita J, et al. Possible participation of autocrine and paracrine vascular endothelial growth factors in hypoxia-induced proliferation of endothelial cells and pericytes. J Biol Chem. 1995;270:28316–24.
26. Yamagishi S, Yonekura H, Yamamoto Y, Fujimori H, Sakurai S, Tanaka N, et al. Vascular endothelial growth factor acts as a pericyte mitogen under hypoxic conditions. Lab Invest. 1999;79:501–9.
27. Ando K, Nakajima Y, Yamagishi T, Yamamoto S, Nakamura H. Development of proximal coronary arteries in quail embryonic heart: multiple capillaries penetrating the aortic sinus fuse to form main coronary trunk. Circ Res. 2004;94:346–52.
28. Duan LJ, Zhang-Benoit Y, Fong GH. Endothelium-intrinsic requirement for Hif-2alpha during vascular development. Circulation. 2005;111:2227–32.
29. Patel SA, Simon MC. Biology of hypoxia-inducible factor-2alpha in development and disease. Cell Death Differ. 2008;15:628–34.
30. Tian H, Hammer RE, Matsumoto AM, Russell DW, McKnight SL. The hypoxia-responsive transcription factor EPAS1 is essential for catecholamine homeostasis and protection against heart failure during embryonic development. Genes Dev. 1998;12: 3320–4.
31. Scortegagna M, Ding K, Oktay Y, Gaur A, Thurmond F, Yan LJ, et al. Multiple organ pathology, metabolic abnormalities and impaired homeostasis of reactive oxygen species in Epas1−/− mice. Nat Genet. 2003;35:331–40.
32. Gruber M, Hu CJ, Johnson RS, Brown EJ, Keith B, Simon MC. Acute postnatal ablation of Hif-2alpha results in anemia. Proc Natl Acad Sci USA. 2007;104:2301–6.
33. Rolfs A, Kvietikova I, Gassmann M, Wenger RH. Oxygen-regulated transferrin expression is mediated by hypoxia-inducible factor-1. J Biol Chem. 1997;272:20055–62.
34. Peng YJ, Nanduri J, Khan SA, Yuan G, Wang N, Kinsman B, et al. Hypoxia-inducible factor 2alpha (HIF-2alpha) heterozygous-null mice exhibit exaggerated carotid body sensitivity to hypoxia, breathing instability, and hypertension. Proc Natl Acad Sci USA. 2011;108:3065–70.
35. Gerber HP, Condorelli F, Park J, Ferrara N. Differential transcriptional regulation of the two vascular endothelial growth factor receptor genes. Flt-1, but not Flk-1/KDR, is up-regulated by hypoxia. J Biol Chem. 1997;272:23659–67.
36. Singh N, Amin S, Richter E, Rashid S, Scoglietti V, Jani PD, et al. Flt-1 intraceptors inhibit hypoxia-induced VEGF expression in vitro and corneal neovascularization in vivo. Invest Ophthalmol Vis Sci. 2005;46:1647–52.
37. Marti HH, Risau W. Systemic hypoxia changes the organ-specific distribution of vascular endothelial growth factor and its receptors. Proc Natl Acad Sci USA. 1998;95:15809–14.
38. Li B, Sharpe EE, Maupin AB, Teleron AA, Pyle AL, Carmeliet P, et al. VEGF and PlGF promote adult vasculogenesis by enhancing EPC recruitment and vessel formation at the site of tumor neovascularization. FASEB J. 2006;20:1495–7.
39. Torry RJ, Tomanek RJ, Zheng W, Miller SJ, Labarrere CA, Torry DS. Hypoxia increases placenta growth factor expression in human myocardium and cultured neonatal rat cardiomyocytes. J Heart Lung Transplant. 2009;28:183–90.
40. Evans CE, Humphries J, Mattock K, Waltham M, Wadoodi A, Saha P, et al. Hypoxia and upregulation of hypoxia-inducible factor 1{alpha} stimulate venous thrombus recanalization. Arterioscler Thromb Vasc Biol. 2010;30:2443–51.
41. Brogi E, Wu T, Namiki A, Isner JM. Indirect angiogenic cytokines upregulate VEGF and bFGF gene expression in vascular smooth muscle cells, whereas hypoxia upregulates VEGF expression only. Circulation. 1994;90:649–52.
42. Ladoux A, Frelin C. Hypoxia is a strong inducer of vascular endothelial growth factor mRNA expression in the heart. Biochem Biophys Res Commun. 1993;195:1005–10.
43. Ikeda E, Achen MG, Breier G, Risau W. Hypoxia-induced transcriptional activation and increased mRNA stability of vascular endothelial growth factor in C6 glioma cells. J Biol Chem. 1995;270:19761–6.
44. Das B, Yeger H, Tsuchida R, Torkin R, Gee MF, Thorner PS, et al. A hypoxia-driven vascular endothelial growth factor/Flt1 autocrine loop interacts with hypoxia-inducible factor-1alpha

through mitogen-activated protein kinase/extracellular signal-regulated kinase 1/2 pathway in neuroblastoma. Cancer Res. 2005;65:7267–75.
45. Mavria G, Vercoulen Y, Yeo M, Paterson H, Karasarides M, Marais R, et al. ERK-MAPK signaling opposes Rho-kinase to promote endothelial cell survival and sprouting during angiogenesis. Cancer Cell. 2006;9:33–44.
46. Gerhardt H, Golding M, Fruttiger M, Ruhrberg C, Lundkvist A, Abramsson A, et al. VEGF guides angiogenic sprouting utilizing endothelial tip cell filopodia. J Cell Biol. 2003;161:1163–77.
47. Tang N, Wang L, Esko J, Giordano FJ, Huang Y, Gerber HP, et al. Loss of HIF-1alpha in endothelial cells disrupts a hypoxia-driven VEGF autocrine loop necessary for tumorigenesis. Cancer Cell. 2004;6:485–95.
48. Coulon C, Georgiadou M, Roncal C, De Bock K, Langenberg T, Carmeliet P. From vessel sprouting to normalization: role of the prolyl hydroxylase domain protein/hypoxia-inducible factor oxygen-sensing machinery. Arterioscler Thromb Vasc Biol. 2010;30:2331–6.
49. Skuli N, Liu L, Runge A, Wang T, Yuan L, Patel S, et al. Endothelial deletion of hypoxia-inducible factor-2alpha (HIF-2alpha) alters vascular function and tumor angiogenesis. Blood. 2009;114:469–77.
50. Kiefer FN, Munk VC, Humar R, Dieterle T, Landmann L, Battegay EJ. A versatile in vitro assay for investigating angiogenesis of the heart. Exp Cell Res. 2004;300:272–82.
51. Stempien-Otero A, Karsan A, Cornejo CJ, Xiang H, Eunson T, Morrison RS, et al. Mechanisms of hypoxia-induced endothelial cell death. Role of p53 in apoptosis. J Biol Chem. 1999;274:8039–45.
52. An WG, Kanekal M, Simon MC, Maltepe E, Blagosklonny MV, Neckers LM. Stabilization of wild-type p53 by hypoxia-inducible factor 1alpha. Nature. 1998;392:405–8.
53. Matsushita H, Morishita R, Nata T, Aoki M, Nakagami H, Taniyama Y, et al. Hypoxia-induced endothelial apoptosis through nuclear factor-kappaB (NF-kappaB)-mediated bcl-2 suppression: in vivo evidence of the importance of NF-kappaB in endothelial cell regulation. Circ Res. 2000;86:974–81.
54. Fong GH. Mechanisms of adaptive angiogenesis to tissue hypoxia. Angiogenesis. 2008;11:121–40.
55. Germain S, Monnot C, Muller L, Eichmann A. Hypoxia-driven angiogenesis: role of tip cells and extracellular matrix scaffolding. Curr Opin Hematol. 2010;17:245–51.
56. Schultz K, Fanburg BL, Beasley D. Hypoxia and hypoxia-inducible factor-1alpha promote growth factor-induced proliferation of human vascular smooth muscle cells. Am J Physiol Heart Circ Physiol. 2006;290:H2528–34.
57. Sheares KK, Jeffery TK, Long L, Yang X, Morrell NW. Differential effects of TGF-beta1 and BMP-4 on the hypoxic induction of cyclooxygenase-2 in human pulmonary artery smooth muscle cells. Am J Physiol Lung Cell Mol Physiol. 2004;287:L919–27.
58. Cooper AL, Beasley D. Hypoxia stimulates proliferation and interleukin-1alpha production in human vascular smooth muscle cells. Am J Physiol. 1999;277:H1326–37.
59. Clinton SK, Underwood R, Hayes L, Sherman ML, Kufe DW, Libby P. Macrophage colony-stimulating factor gene expression in vascular cells and in experimental and human atherosclerosis. Am J Pathol. 1992;140:301–16.
60. Larsen BT, Gutterman DD. Hypoxia, coronary dilation, and the pentose phosphate pathway. Am J Physiol Heart Circ Physiol. 2006;290:H2169–71.
61. Close LA, Bowman PS, Paul RJ. Reoxygenation-induced relaxation of coronary arteries. A novel endothelium-dependent mechanism. Circ Res. 1994;74:870–81.
62. Lee YH, Kim JT, Kang BS. Mechanisms of relaxation of coronary artery by hypoxia. Yonsei Med J. 1998;39:252–60.
63. Gupte SA, Wolin MS. Hypoxia promotes relaxation of bovine coronary arteries through lowering cytosolic NADPH. Am J Physiol Heart Circ Physiol. 2006;290:H2228–38.
64. Busse R, Forstermann U, Matsuda H, Pohl U. The role of prostaglandins in the endothelium-mediated vasodilatory response to hypoxia. Pflugers Arch. 1984;401:77–83.
65. Nakhostine N, Lamontagne D. Contribution of prostaglandins in hypoxia-induced vasodilation in isolated rabbit hearts. Relation to adenosine and KATP channels. Pflugers Arch. 1994;428:526–32.
66. Nakhostine N, Laurent CE, Nadeau R, Cardinal R, Lamontagne D. Hypoxia-induced release of prostaglandins: mechanisms and sources of production in coronary resistance vessels of the isolated rabbit heart. Can J Physiol Pharmacol. 1995;73:1742–9.
67. Block AJ, Feinberg H, Herbaczynska-Cedro K, Vane JR. Anoxia-induced release of prostaglandins in rabbit isolated hearts. Circ Res. 1975;36:34–5.
68. Wennmalm A. Prostacyclin-dependent coronary vasodilation in rabbit and guinea pig hearts. Acta Physiol Scand. 1979;106:47–52.
69. Okada T. Hypoxia-induced change in prostanoids production and coronary flow in isolated rat heart. J Mol Cell Cardiol. 1991;23: 939–48.
70. Kalsner S. The effect of hypoxia on prostaglandin output and on tone in isolated coronary arteries. Can J Physiol Pharmacol. 1977;55:882–7.
71. Roberts AM, Messina EJ, Kaley G. Prostacyclin (PGI2) mediates hypoxic relaxation of bovine coronary arterial strips. Prostaglandins. 1981;21:555–69.
72. Rubanyi G, Paul RJ. Two distinct effects of oxygen on vascular tone in isolated porcine coronary arteries. Circ Res. 1985;56:1–10.
73. Charles RL, Burgoyne JR, Mayr M, Weldon SM, Hubner N, Dong H, et al. Redox regulation of soluble epoxide hydrolase by 15-deoxy-delta-prostaglandin J2 controls coronary hypoxic vasodilation. Circ Res. 2011;108:324–34.
74. Frobert O, Haink G, Simonsen U, Gravholt CH, Levin M, Deussen A. Adenosine concentration in the porcine coronary artery wall and A2A receptor involvement in hypoxia-induced vasodilatation. J Physiol. 2006;570:375–84.
75. Kamekura I, Okumura K, Matsui H, Murase K, Mokuno S, Toki Y, et al. Mechanisms of hypoxic coronary vasodilatation in isolated perfused rat hearts. J Cardiovasc Pharmacol. 1999;33: 836–42.
76. Tune JD. Control of coronary blood flow during hypoxemia. Adv Exp Med Biol. 2007;618:25–39.
77. Dick GM, Tune JD. Role of potassium channels in coronary vasodilation. Exp Biol Med. 2010;235:10–22.
78. Daut J, Maier-Rudolph W, von Beckerath N, Mehrke G, Gunther K, Goedel-Meinen L. Hypoxic dilation of coronary arteries is mediated by ATP-sensitive potassium channels. Science. 1990;247:1341–4.
79. von Beckerath N, Cyrys S, Dischner A, Daut J. Hypoxic vasodilatation in isolated, perfused guinea-pig heart: an analysis of the underlying mechanisms. J Physiol. 1991;442:297–319.
80. Smani T, Hernandez A, Urena J, Castellano AG, Franco-Obregon A, Ordonez A, et al. Reduction of Ca($^{2+}$) channel activity by hypoxia in human and porcine coronary myocytes. Circ Res. 2002;53:97–104.
81. Park WS, Han J, Kim N, Ko JH, Kim SJ, Earm YE. Activation of inward rectifier K+ channels by hypoxia in rabbit coronary arterial smooth muscle cells. Am J Physiol Heart Circ Physiol. 2005;289:H2461–7.
82. Park WS, Son YK, Kim N, Ko JH, Kang SH, Warda M, et al. Acute hypoxia induces vasodilation and increases coronary blood flow by activating inward rectifier K(+) channels. Pflugers Arch. 2007;454:1023–30.
83. Lynch FM, Austin C, Heagerty AM, Izzard AS. Adenosine- and hypoxia-induced dilation of human coronary resistance arteries:

evidence against the involvement of K(ATP) channels. Br J Pharmacol. 2006;147:455–8.
84. Park KH, Rubin LE, Gross SS, Levi R. Nitric oxide is a mediator of hypoxic coronary vasodilatation. Relation to adenosine and cyclooxygenase-derived metabolites. Circ Res. 1992;71:992–1001.
85. Brown IP, Thompson CI, Belloni FL. Role of nitric oxide in hypoxic coronary vasodilatation in isolated perfused guinea pig heart. Am J Physiol. 1993;264:H821–9.
86. Huckstorf C, Zanzinger J, Fink B, Bassenge E. Reduced nitric oxide formation causes coronary vasoconstriction and impaired dilator responses to endogenous agonists and hypoxia in dogs. Naunyn Schmiedebergs Arch Pharmacol. 1994;349:367–73.
87. Audibert G, Saunier CG, Siat J, Hartemann D, Lambert J. Effect of the inhibitor of nitric oxide synthase, NG-nitro-L-arginine methyl ester, on cerebral and myocardial blood flows during hypoxia in the awake dog. Anesth Anal. 1995;81:945–51.
88. Martinez RR, Setty S, Zong P, Tune JD, Downey HF. Nitric oxide contributes to right coronary vasodilation during systemic hypoxia. Am J Physiol Heart Circ Physiol. 2005;288:H1139–46.
89. Justice JM, Tanner MA, Myers PR. Endothelial cell regulation of nitric oxide production during hypoxia in coronary microvessels and epicardial arteries. J Cell Physiol. 2000;182:359–65.
90. Zaobornyj T, Valdez LB, Iglesias DE, Gasco M, Gonzales GF, Boveris A. Mitochondrial nitric oxide metabolism during rat heart adaptation to high altitude: effect of sildenafil, L-NAME, and L-arginine treatments. Am J Physiol Heart Circ Physiol. 2009; 296:H1741–7.
91. Zong P, Tune JD, Downey HF. Mechanisms of oxygen demand/supply balance in the right ventricle. Exp Biol Med. 2005;230:507–19.
92. Griendling KK, Sorescu D, Lassegue B, Ushio-Fukai M. Modulation of protein kinase activity and gene expression by reactive oxygen species and their role in vascular physiology and pathophysiology. Arterioscler Thromb Vasc Biol. 2000;20: 2175–83.
93. Wu W, Platoshyn O, Firth AL, Yuan JX. Hypoxia divergently regulates production of reactive oxygen species in human pulmonary and coronary artery smooth muscle cells. Am J Physiol Lung Cell Mol Physiol. 2007;293:L952–9.
94. Lee PJ, Choi AM. Pathways of cell signaling in hyperoxia. Free Radic Biol Med. 2003;35:341–50.
95. Rubanyi GM, Vanhoutte PM. Superoxide anions and hyperoxia inactivate endothelium-derived relaxing factor. Am J Physiol. 1986;250:H822–7.
96. Ting HH, Timimi FK, Boles KS, Creager SJ, Ganz P, Creager MA. Vitamin C improves endothelium-dependent vasodilation in patients with non-insulin-dependent diabetes mellitus. J Clin Invest. 1996;97:22–8.
97. McNulty PH, Robertson BJ, Tulli MA, Hess J, Harach LA, Scott S, et al. Effect of hyperoxia and vitamin C on coronary blood flow in patients with ischemic heart disease. J Appl Physiol. 2007;102: 2040–5.
98. Levine GN, Frei B, Koulouris SN, Gerhard MD, Keaney Jr JF, Vita JA. Ascorbic acid reverses endothelial vasomotor dysfunction in patients with coronary artery disease. Circulation. 1996;93: 1107–13.
99. Taddei S, Virdis A, Ghiadoni L, Magagna A, Salvetti A. Vitamin C improves endothelium-dependent vasodilation by restoring nitric oxide activity in essential hypertension. Circulation. 1998;97: 2222–9.
100. Wolin MS, Burke-Wolin TM, Mohazzab HK. Roles for NAD(P)H oxidases and reactive oxygen species in vascular oxygen sensing mechanisms. Respir Physiol. 1999;115:229–38.
101. Mohazzab KM, Kaminski PM, Wolin MS. NADH oxidoreductase is a major source of superoxide anion in bovine coronary artery endothelium. Am J Physiol. 1994;266:H2568–72.
102. Mohazzab HK, Kaminski PM, Fayngersh RP, Wolin MS. Oxygen-elicited responses in calf coronary arteries: role of H_2O_2 production via NADH-derived superoxide. Am J Physiol. 1996;270:H1044–53.
103. Wolin MS. Reactive oxygen species and the control of vascular function. Am J Physiol Heart Circ Physiol. 2009;296:H539–49.
104. Gupte SA, Arshad M, Viola S, Kaminski PM, Ungvari Z, Rabbani G, et al. Pentose phosphate pathway coordinates multiple redox-controlled relaxing mechanisms in bovine coronary arteries. Am J Physiol Heart Circ Physiol. 2003;285:H2316–26.
105. Mohazzab HK, Agarwal R, Wolin MS. Influence of glutathione peroxidase on coronary artery responses to alterations in PO_2 and H_2O_2. Am J Physiol. 1999;276:H235–41.
106. Case RB, Greenberg H. The response of canine coronary vascular resistance to local alterations in coronary arterial P CO_2. Circ Res. 1976;39:558–66.
107. Case RB, Felix A, Wachter M, Kyriakidis G, Castellana F. Relative effect of CO_2 on canine coronary vascular resistance. Circ Res. 1978;42:410–8.
108. Broten TP, Romson JL, Fullerton DA, Van Winkle DM, Feigl EO. Synergistic action of myocardial oxygen and carbon dioxide in controlling coronary blood flow. Circ Res. 1991;68:531–42.
109. Zhang L. Prenatal hypoxia and cardiac programming. J Soc Gynecol Investig. 2005;12:2–13.
110. Patterson AJ, Zhang L. Hypoxia and fetal heart development. Curr Mol Med. 2010;10:653–66.
111. Ostadal B, Ostadalova I, Dhalla NS. Development of cardiac sensitivity to oxygen deficiency: comparative and ontogenetic aspects. Physiol Rev. 1999;79:635–59.
112. Ostadal B, Ostadalova I, Kolar F, Charvatova Z, Netuka I. Ontogenetic development of cardiac tolerance to oxygen deprivation—possible mechanisms. Physiol Res. 2009;58 Suppl 2:S1–12.
113. Ostadalova I, Ostadal B, Kolar F, Parratt JR, Wilson S. Tolerance to ischaemia and ischaemic preconditioning in neonatal rat heart. J Mol Cell Cardiol. 1998;30:857–65.
114. Yue X, Tomanek RJ. Stimulation of coronary vasculogenesis/angiogenesis by hypoxia in cultured embryonic hearts. Dev Dyn. 1999;216:28–36.
115. Yue X, Tomanek RJ. Effects of VEGF(165) and VEGF(121) on vasculogenesis and angiogenesis in cultured embryonic quail hearts. Am J Physiol Heart Circ Physiol. 2001;280:H2240–7.
116. Tomanek RJ, Ratajska A, Kitten GT, Yue X, Sandra A. Vascular endothelial growth factor expression coincides with coronary vasculogenesis and angiogenesis. Dev Dyn. 1999;215:54–61.
117. Tomanek RJ, Holifield JS, Reiter RS, Sandra A, Lin JJ. Role of VEGF family members and receptors in coronary vessel formation. Dev Dyn. 2002;225:233–40.
118. Enholm B, Paavonen K, Ristimaki A, Kumar V, Gunji Y, Klefstrom J, et al. Comparison of VEGF, VEGF-B, VEGF-C and Ang-1 mRNA regulation by serum, growth factors, oncoproteins and hypoxia. Oncogene. 1997;14:2475–83.
119. Tomanek RJ, Zheng W, Peters KG, Lin P, Holifield JS, Suvarna PR. Multiple growth factors regulate coronary embryonic vasculogenesis. Dev Dyn. 2001;221:265–73.
120. Tomanek RJ, Christensen LP, Simons M, Murakami M, Zheng W, Schatteman GC. Embryonic coronary vasculogenesis and angiogenesis are regulated by interactions between multiple FGFs and VEGF and are influenced by mesenchymal stem cells. Dev Dyn. 2010;239:3182–91.
121. Lee YM, Jeong CH, Koo SY, Son MJ, Song HS, Bae SK, et al. Determination of hypoxic region by hypoxia marker in developing mouse embryos in vivo: a possible signal for vessel development. Dev Dyn. 2001;220:175–86.
122. Nanka O, Valasek P, Dvorakova M, Grim M. Experimental hypoxia and embryonic angiogenesis. Dev Dyn. 2006;235:723–33.

123. Nanka O, Krizova P, Fikrle M, Tuma M, Blaha M, Grim M, et al. Abnormal myocardial and coronary vasculature development in experimental hypoxia. Anat Rec (Hoboken). 2008;291:1187–99.
124. Wikenheiser J, Wolfram JA, Gargesha M, Yang K, Karunamuni G, Wilson DL, et al. Altered hypoxia-inducible factor-1 alpha expression levels correlate with coronary vessel anomalies. Dev Dyn. 2009;238:2688–700.
125. Ramirez-Bergeron DL, Runge A, Dahl KD, Fehling HJ, Keller G, Simon MC. Hypoxia affects mesoderm and enhances hemangioblast specification during early development. Development. 2004;131:4623–34.
126. Han Y, Kuang SZ, Gomer A, Ramirez-Bergeron DL. Hypoxia influences the vascular expansion and differentiation of embryonic stem cell cultures through the temporal expression of vascular endothelial growth factor receptors in an ARNT-dependent manner. Stem Cells. 2010;28:799–809.
127. Shalaby F, Rossant J, Yamaguchi TP, Gertsenstein M, Wu XF, Breitman ML, et al. Failure of blood-island formation and vasculogenesis in Flk-1-deficient mice. Nature. 1995;376:62–6.
128. Fong GH, Rossant J, Gertsenstein M, Breitman ML. Role of the Flt-1 receptor tyrosine kinase in regulating the assembly of vascular endothelium. Nature. 1995;376:66–70.
129. Mascio CE, Olison AK, Ralphe JC, Tomanek RJ, Scholz TD, Segar JL. Myocardial vascular and metabolic adaptations in chronically anemic fetal sheep. Am J Physiol Regul Integr Comp Physiol. 2005;289:R1736–45.
130. Davis LE, Hohimer AR. Hemodynamics and organ blood flow in fetal sheep subjected to chronic anemia. Am J Physiol. 1991;261:R1542–8.
131. Davis LE, Hohimer AR, Morton MJ. Myocardial blood flow and coronary reserve in chronically anemic fetal lambs. Am J Physiol. 1999;277:R306–13.
132. Martin C, Yu AY, Jiang BH, Davis L, Kimberly D, Hohimer AR, et al. Cardiac hypertrophy in chronically anemic fetal sheep: increased vascularization is associated with increased myocardial expression of vascular endothelial growth factor and hypoxia-inducible factor 1. Am J Obstet Gynecol. 1998;178:527–34.
133. Reller MD, Morton MJ, Giraud GD, Wu DE, Thornburg KL. Maximal myocardial blood flow is enhanced by chronic hypoxemia in late gestation fetal sheep. Am J Physiol. 1992;263: H1327–9.
134. Wothe D, Hohimer A, Morton M, Thornburg K, Giraud G, Davis L. Increased coronary blood flow signals growth of coronary resistance vessels in near-term ovine fetuses. Am J Physiol Regul Integr Comp Physiol. 2002;282:R295–302.
135. Torry RJ, O'Brien DM, Connell PM, Tomanek RJ. Dipyridamole-induced capillary growth in normal and hypertrophic hearts. Am J Physiol. 1992;262:H980–6.
136. Kourembanas S, Morita T, Liu Y, Christou H. Mechanisms by which oxygen regulates gene expression and cell-cell interaction in the vasculature. Kidney Int. 1997;51:438–43.
137. Pohl U. Endothelial cells as part of a vascular oxygen-sensing system: hypoxia-induced release of autacoids. Experientia. 1990;46:1175–9.
138. Reller MD, Burson MA, Lohr JL, Morton MJ, Thornburg KL. Nitric oxide is an important determinant of coronary flow at rest and during hypoxemic stress in fetal lambs. Am J Physiol. 1995;269:H2074–81.
139. Xue C, Rengasamy A, Le Cras TD, Koberna PA, Dailey GC, Johns RA. Distribution of NOS in normoxic vs. hypoxic rat lung: upregulation of NOS by chronic hypoxia. Am J Physiol. 1994;267:L667–78.
140. Dong Y, Thompson LP. Differential expression of endothelial nitric oxide synthase in coronary and cardiac tissue in hypoxic fetal guinea pig hearts. J Soc Gynecol Investig. 2006;13:483–90.
141. Thompson LP, Aguan K, Pinkas G, Weiner CP. Chronic hypoxia increases the NO contribution of acetylcholine vasodilation of the fetal guinea pig heart. Am J Physiol Regul Integr Comp Physiol. 2000;279:R1813–20.
142. Thornburg KL, Reller MD. Coronary flow regulation in the fetal sheep. Am J Physiol. 1999;277:R1249–60.
143. Garcia FC, Stiffel VM, Gilbert RD. Effects of long-term high-altitude hypoxia on isolated fetal ovine coronary arteries. J Soc Gynecol Investig. 2000;7:211–7.
144. Fisher DJ, Heymann MA, Rudolph AM. Regional myocardial blood flow and oxygen delivery in fetal, newborn, and adult sheep. Am J Physiol. 1982;243:H729–31.
145. Peeters LL, Sheldon RE, Jones Jr MD, Makowski EL, Meschia G. Blood flow to fetal organs as a function of arterial oxygen content. Am J Obstet Gynecol. 1979;135:637–46.
146. Kono S, Stiffel VM, Gilbert RD. Effects of long-term, high-altitude hypoxia on tension and intracellular calcium responses in coronary arteries of fetal and adult sheep. J Soc Gynecol Invest. 2006;13:11–8.
147. Sarkar S, Banerjee PK, Selvamurthy W. High altitude hypoxia: an intricate interplay of oxygen responsive macroevents and micromolecules. Mol Cell Biochem. 2003;253:287–305.
148. Smith RM, McCarthy J, Sack MN. TNF alpha is required for hypoxia-mediated right ventricular hypertrophy. Mol Cell Biochem. 2001;219:139–43.
149. Manohar M. Transmural coronary vasodilator reserve, and flow distribution during tachycardia in conscious young swine with right ventricular hypertrophy. Cardiovasc Res. 1985;19:104–12.
150. Deindl E, Kolar F, Neubauer E, Vogel S, Schaper W, Ostadal B. Effect of intermittent high altitude hypoxia on gene expression in rat heart and lung. Physiol Res. 2003;52:147–57.
151. Levy AP, Levy NS, Wegner S, Goldberg MA. Transcriptional regulation of the rat vascular endothelial growth factor gene by hypoxia. J Biol Chem. 1995;270:13333–40.
152. Ostadal B, Mirejovska E, Hurych J, Pelouch V, Prochazka J. Effect of intermittent high altitude hypoxia on the synthesis of collagenous and non-collagenous proteins of the right and left ventricular myocardium. Cardiovasc Res. 1978;12:303–8.
153. Strniskova M, Ravingerova T, Neckar J, Kolar F, Pastorekova S, Barancik M. Changes in the expression and/or activation of regulatory proteins in rat hearts adapted to chronic hypoxia. Gen Physiol Biophys. 2006;25:25–41.
154. Tintu AN, Noble FA, Rouwet EV. Hypoxia disturbs fetal hemodynamics and growth. Endothelium. 2007;14:353–60.
155. Ream M, Ray AM, Chandra R, Chikaraishi DM. Early fetal hypoxia leads to growth restriction and myocardial thinning. Am J Physiol Regul Integr Comp Physiol. 2008;295:R583–95.
156. Villamor E, Kessels CG, Ruijtenbeek K, van Suylen RJ, Belik J, de Mey JG, et al. Chronic in ovo hypoxia decreases pulmonary arterial contractile reactivity and induces biventricular cardiac enlargement in the chicken embryo. Am J Physiol Regul Integr Comp Physiol. 2004;287:R642–51.
157. Becker EL, Cooper RG, Hataway GD. Capillary vascularization in puppies born at a simulated altitude of 20,000 feet. J Appl Physiol. 1955;8:166–8.
158. Lewis AM, Mathieu-Costello O, McMillan PJ, Gilbert RD. Effects of long-term, high-altitude hypoxia on the capillarity of the ovine fetal heart. Am J Physiol. 1999;277:H756–62.
159. Grandtner M, Turek Z, Kreuzer F. Cardiac hypertrophy in the first generation of rats native to simulated high altitude. Muscle fiber diameter and diffusion distance in the right and left ventricle. Pflugers Arch. 1974;350:241–8.
160. Smith P, Clark DR. Myocardial capillary density and muscle fibre size in rats born and raised at simulated high altitude. Br J Exp Pathol. 1979;60:225–30.

161. Moravec J, Cluzeaud F, Rakusan K, Turek Z. Capillary supply and utilization of intracellular oxygen in the left ventricular myocardium from rats adapted to high altitude. Adv Exp Med Biol. 1983;159:243–52.
162. Moravec M, Turek Z, Moravec J. Persistence of neoangiogenesis and cardiomyocyte divisions in right ventricular myocardium of rats born and raised in hypoxic conditions. Basic Res Cardiol. 2002;97:153–60.
163. Pietschmann M, Bartels H. Cellular hyperplasia and hypertrophy, capillary proliferation and myoglobin concentration in the heart of newborn and adult rats at high altitude. Respir Physiol. 1985;59:347–60.
164. Turek Z, Grandtner M, Kreuzer F. Cardiac hypertrophy, capillary and muscle fiber density, muscle fiber diameter, capillary radius and diffusion distance in the myocardium of growing rats adapted to a simulated altitude of 3500 m. Pflugers Arch. 1972;335:19–28.
165. Turek Z, Hoofd L, Ringnalda B, Rakusan K. Myocardial capillarity of rats exposed to simulated high altitude. Adv Exp Med Biol. 1985;7:120–7.
166. Clark DR, Smith P. Capillary density and muscle fibre size in the hearts of rats subjected to stimulated high altitude. Cardiovasc Res. 1978;12:578–84.
167. Zhong N, Zhang Y, Zhu HF, Wang JC, Fang QZ, Zhou ZN. Myocardial capillary angiogenesis and coronary flow in ischemia tolerance rat by adaptation to intermittent high altitude hypoxia. Acta Pharmacol Sin. 2002;23:305–10.
168. Kayar SP, Banchero N. Distribution of capillaries and diffusion distances in guinea pig myocardium. Pflugers Arch. 1983; 396:350–2.
169. Kayar SR, Banchero N. Myocardial capillarity in acclimation to hypoxia. Pflugers Arch. 1985;404:319–25.
170. Panisello P, Torrella JR, Pages T, Viscor G. Capillary supply and fiber morphometry in rat myocardium after intermittent exposure to hypobaric hypoxia. High Alt Med Biol. 2007;8:322–30.
171. Miller Jr AT, Hale DM. Increased vascularity of brain, heart, and skeletal muscle of polycythemic rats. Am J Physiol. 1970;219:702–4.
172. Friedman I, Moravec J, Reichart E, Hatt PY. Subacute myocardial hypoxia in the rat. An electron microscopic study of the left ventricular myocardium. J Mol Cell Cardiol. 1973;5:125–32.
173. Lund DD, Tomanek RJ. The effects of chronic hypoxia on the myocardial cell of normotensive and hypertensive rats. Anat Rec. 1980;196:421–30.
174. Choi YH, Cowan DB, Nathan M, Poutias D, Stamm C, del Nido PJ, et al. Myocardial hypertrophy overrides the angiogenic response to hypoxia. PLoS One. 2008;3:e4042.
175. Tian F, Zhou X, Wikstrom J, Karlsson H, Sjoland H, Gan LM, et al. Protein disulfide isomerase increases in myocardial endothelial cells in mice exposed to chronic hypoxia: a stimulatory role in angiogenesis. Am J Physiol Heart Circ Physiol. 2009;297:H1078–86.
176. Rakusan K, Turek Z, Kreuzer F. Myocardial capillaries in guinea pigs native to high altitude (Junin, Peru, 4,105 m). Pflugers Arch. 1981;391:22–4.
177. Kayar SR, Banchero N. Volume overload hypertrophy elicited by cold and its effects on myocardial capillarity. Respir Physiol. 1985;59:1–14.
178. Corno AF, Milano G, Morel S, Tozzi P, Genton CY, Samaja M, et al. Hypoxia: unique myocardial morphology? J Thorac Cardiovasc Surg. 2004;127:1301–8.
179. Birot OJ, Peinnequin A, Simler N, van Cuyck-Gandre H, Hamel R, Bigard XA. Vascular endothelial growth factor expression in heart of rats exposed to hypobaric hypoxia: differential response between mRNA and protein. J Cell Physiol. 2004;200:107–15.
180. Wright AJ, Hudlicka O. Capillary growth and changes in heart performance induced by chronic bradycardial pacing in the rabbit. Circ Res. 1981;49:469–78.
181. Zheng W, Brown MD, Brock TA, Bjercke RJ, Tomanek RJ. Bradycardia-induced coronary angiogenesis is dependent on vascular endothelial growth factor. Circ Res. 1999;85:192–8.
182. Lamping KG, Zheng W, Xing D, Christensen LP, Martins J, Tomanek RJ. Bradycardia stimulates vascular growth during gradual coronary occlusion. Arterioscler Thromb Vasc Biol. 2005;25:2122–7.
183. Li GC, Vasquez JA, Gallagher KP, Lucchesi BR. Myocardial protection with preconditioning. Circulation. 1990;82:609–19.
184. Murry CE, Jennings RB, Reimer KA. Preconditioning with ischemia: a delay of lethal cell injury in ischemic myocardium. Circulation. 1986;74:1124–36.
185. Mocanu MM, Yellon DM. p53 down-regulation: a new molecular mechanism involved in ischaemic preconditioning. FEBS letters. 2003;555:302–6.
186. Yellon DM, Downey JM. Preconditioning the myocardium: from cellular physiology to clinical cardiology. Physiol Rev. 2003;83: 1113–51.
187. Ostadal B, Kolar F. Cardiac adaptation to chronic high-altitude hypoxia: beneficial and adverse effects. Respir Physiol Neurobiol. 2007;158:224–36.
188. McGrath JJ, Prochazka J, Pelouch V, Ostadal B. Physiological responses of rats to intermittent high-altitude stress: effects of age. J Appl Physiol. 1973;34:289–93.
189. Meerson FZ, Gomzakov OA, Shimkovich MV. Adaptation to high altitude hypoxia as a factor preventing development of myocardial ischemic necrosis. Am J Cardiol. 1973;31:30–4.
190. Shizukuda Y, Iwamoto T, Mallet RT, Downey HF. Hypoxic preconditioning attenuates stunning caused by repeated coronary artery occlusions in dog heart. Circ Res. 1993;27:559–64.
191. Xi L, Tekin D, Gursoy E, Salloum F, Levasseur JE, Kukreja RC. Evidence that NOS2 acts as a trigger and mediator of late preconditioning induced by acute systemic hypoxia. Am J Physiol Heart Circ Physiol. 2002;283:H5–12.
192. Beguin PC, Joyeux-Faure M, Godin-Ribuot D, Levy P, Ribuot C. Acute intermittent hypoxia improves rat myocardium tolerance to ischemia. J Appl Physiol. 2005;99:1064–9.
193. Neckar J, Szarszoi O, Herget J, Ostadal B, Kolar F. Cardioprotective effect of chronic hypoxia is blunted by concomitant hypercapnia. Physiol Res. 2003;52:171–5.
194. Ding HL, Zhu HF, Dong JW, Zhu WZ, Yang WW, Yang HT, et al. Inducible nitric oxide synthase contributes to intermittent hypoxia against ischemia/reperfusion injury. Acta Pharmacol Sin. 2005;26: 315–22.
195. Belaidi E, Beguin PC, Levy P, Ribuot C, Godin-Ribuot D. Prevention of HIF-1 activation and iNOS gene targeting by low-dose cadmium results in loss of myocardial hypoxic preconditioning in the rat. Am J Physiol Heart Circ Physiol. 2008;294:H901–8.
196. Lin JS, Chen YS, Chiang HS, Ma MC. Hypoxic preconditioning protects rat hearts against ischaemia-reperfusion injury: role of erythropoietin on progenitor cell mobilization. J Physiol. 2008;586:5757–69.
197. Berger MM, Huhn R, Oei GT, Heinen A, Winzer A, Bauer I, et al. Hypoxia induces late preconditioning in the rat heart in vivo. Anesthesiology. 2010;113:1351–60.
198. Sasaki H, Ray PS, Zhu L, Otani H, Asahara T, Maulik N. Hypoxia/reoxygenation promotes myocardial angiogenesis via an NF kappa B-dependent mechanism in a rat model of chronic myocardial infarction. J Mol Cell Cardiol. 2001;33:283–94.
199. Sasaki H, Fukuda S, Otani H, Zhu L, Yamaura G, Engelman RM, et al. Hypoxic preconditioning triggers myocardial angiogenesis: a novel approach to enhance contractile functional reserve in rat with myocardial infarction. J Mol Cell Cardiol. 2002;34:335–48.
200. Cai Z, Manalo DJ, Wei G, Rodriguez ER, Fox-Talbot K, Lu H, et al. Hearts from rodents exposed to intermittent hypoxia or

erythropoietin are protected against ischemia-reperfusion injury. Circulation. 2003;108:79–85.
201. Semenza GL. Hypoxia-inducible factor 1: regulator of mitochondrial metabolism and mediator of ischemic preconditioning. Biochim Biophys Acta. 2011;1813:1263–8.
202. Tekin D, Dursun AD, Xi L. Hypoxia inducible factor 1 (HIF-1) and cardioprotection. Acta pharmacologica Sinica. 2010;31: 1085–94.
203. Belaidi E, Beguin PC, Ribuot C, Godin-Ribuot D. Hypoxic preconditioning: role of transcription factor HIF-1alpha. Ann Cardiol Angeiol (Paris). 2006;55:70–3.
204. Baker JE, Curry BD, Olinger GN, Gross GJ. Increased tolerance of the chronically hypoxic immature heart to ischemia. Contribution of the KATP channel. Circulation. 1997;95:1278–85.
205. Baker JE, Contney SJ, Singh R, Kalyanaraman B, Gross GJ, Bosnjak ZJ. Nitric oxide activates the sarcolemmal K(ATP) channel in normoxic and chronically hypoxic hearts by a cyclic GMP-dependent mechanism. J Mol Cell Cardiol. 2001;33: 331–41.
206. Bin-Jaliah I, Ammar HI, Mikhailidis DP, Dallak MA, Al-Hashem FH, Haidara MA, et al. Cardiac adaptive responses after hypoxia in an experimental model. Angiology. 2010;61:145–56.
207. Cheng AS, Yau TM. Paracrine effects of cell transplantation: strategies to augment the efficacy of cell therapies. Semin Thorac Cardiovasc Surg. 2008;20:94–101.
208. Hung SC, Pochampally RR, Hsu SC, Sanchez C, Chen SC, Spees J, et al. Short-term exposure of multipotent stromal cells to low oxygen increases their expression of CX3CR1 and CXCR4 and their engraftment in vivo. PLoS One. 2007;2:e416.
209. Hu X, Yu SP, Fraser JL, Lu Z, Ogle ME, Wang JA, et al. Transplantation of hypoxia-preconditioned mesenchymal stem cells improves infarcted heart function via enhanced survival of implanted cells and angiogenesis. J Thorac Cardiovasc Surg. 2008;135:799–808.

Myocardial Ischemia and Infarction

10

Abbreviations

CFI	Collateral flow index
EC	Endothelial cell
FGF	Fibroblast growth factor
HIF	Hypoxia-inducible factor
IPC	Ischemic preconditioning
IPost	Ischemic postconditioning
IR	Ischemia/reperfusion
MCVR	Minimal coronary vascular resistance
MI	Myocardial infarction
ROS	Reactive oxygen species
VEGF	Vascular endothelial growth factor
VSMC	Vascular smooth muscle cell

Introduction

General Characteristics of Myocardial Ischemia

When a coronary artery is occluded, the reduction of blood flow results in (1) tissue hypoxia, (2) an accumulation of metabolic products, and (3) failure in substrate delivery. Therefore, ischemia has a greater impact on the tissue supplied by the occluded artery than does hypoxia in the absence of ischemia. The magnitude of tissue injury depends on both the degree and the duration of the ischemia. Using electron microscopy and measurements of regional myocardial perfusion, my colleagues and I correlated cardiomyocyte changes (reversible vs. irreversible) with the magnitude of the perfusion decrement [1]. Other investigators have determined that in canine hearts subjected to a <10% reduction in blood flow, cardiomyocyte death first appears after about 20 min [2, 3]. This topic is discussed in a subsequent section of this chapter. Clinically, ischemic myocardial injury is manifested by (1) cardiomyocyte death, (2) contractile dysfunction, (3) arrhythmias, and (4) microvascular dysfunction [4].

The "Stunned" and "Hibernating" Myocardium

When coronary flow is interrupted, the ischemic cardiac muscle stops contracting within seconds. The mechanism that accounts for this rapid response is still not clear, but may involve changes in calcium release [5], the development of acidosis [6], or an accumulation of inorganic phosphate [7]. The effect of this response is preservation of energy for cellular processes vital for cell survival. If the duration of ischemia is limited to a single 2-min episode, myocardial function is restored as soon as the tissue is reperfused [8]. However, when ischemia is of a greater magnitude or duration, recovery of function is delayed. For example, when flow was restored following 5 or 15 min of ischemia, myocardial contractility recovered only after 6 and 24 h, respectively [9]. Thus, the heart experiences a prolonged period of dysfunction, even once perfusion is restored; this phenomenon is termed "myocardial stunning." When a moderate level of myocardial ischemia persists, the myocardium can enter a state of "short-term hibernation" characterized by a steady level of ventricular dysfunction that initially serves to match a limited oxygen supply, reducing regional contraction, and oxygen consumption. Short-term hibernation prevents necrosis if the heart is reperfused within several hours, but invariably leads to myocyte death when extended for periods of more than 12 h [10]. Chronic dysfunction in the absence of necrosis and fibrosis can also develop following repetitive reversible ischemia [11]. Initially, moderate stenoses produce dysfunction with normal resting perfusion or chronically stunned myocardium. As stenosis severity reaches a critical level, where subendocardial flow reserve is exhausted, intrinsic adaptations lead to hibernating myocardium where resting flow, as well as resting function, is reduced. The latter adaptations reflect a downregulation in enzymes involved in myocardial energy utilization that allows the heart to remain viable at the expense of resting contractile function. Regional contractile function improves with a return to normal perfusion, but the time and extent of improvement is variable

R.J. Tomanek, *Coronary Vasculature: Development, Structure-Function, and Adaptations*,
DOI 10.1007/978-1-4614-4887-7_10, © Springer Science+Business Media New York 2013

(reviewed in [12]). In stunned myocardium and short-term hibernation, functional recovery is complete and occurs within days. Revascularization of the hibernating myocardium is more prolonged (up to 1 year) and usually results in an improvement, rather than complete normalization of function [8]. Thus, coronary stenosis in the absence of infarction can still lead to permanent ventricular dysfunction [8].

Metabolic Consequences of Myocardial Ischemia

Within 10 s of the onset of a total arrest in flow, both the microcirculation and cardiomyocytes are depleted of O_2, and this leads to cessation of oxidative phosphorylation [13, 14]. An immediate arrest of myocardial contractility serves to conserve energy in cardiomyocytes, and anaerobic glycolysis becomes a temporary source of high phosphate energy, though that ceases within 1 h (reviewed in [15]). In the complete absence of O_2, lactate produced by the anaerobic metabolism is not metabolized, but if some O_2 is available (via collaterals or because the arterial stenosis is not complete) low-level aerobic metabolism is supported; this not only provides additional ATP to the cardiomyocytes but also reduces the accumulation of glycolytic intermediates such as lactate and H^+. Nevertheless, as documented in dogs, ATP declines threefold during the first 10 min of ischemia, and lactate subsequently increases threefold [16]. Any cardiomyocyte damage incurred during the first 20 min of ischemia is usually reversible. However, when the ischemic period extended to 40 min, the damage is irreversible. Moreover, lactate levels increase >7-fold and the tissue becomes virtually depleted of ATP.

Ischemic Induction of Coronary Artery Dilation

Contribution of Several Signaling Pathways

Hypoxia is a well-documented vasodilator of coronary arteries and triggers the activities of several signaling pathways due to its effects on three cell types: endothelial cells (ECs), vascular smooth muscle cells (VSMCs), and cardiomyocytes (reviewed by [17]). However, vasodilation does not require activation of all of these pathways. For example, the signals released from ECs in the context of hypoxia (NO, prostacyclin, and adenosine) are not required, as hypoxia-induced coronary artery relaxation can occur in the absence of an endothelium [18–20]. Nevertheless, at least adenosine appears to have some role, as indicated by experiments demonstrating that blockage of the adenosine A_2 receptor attenuates vasodilation [21]. Since hypoxia did not enhance adenosine production in the artery, the investigators concluded that it instead affects the sensitivity of the A_2 receptor. However, these experiments were performed on isolated arteries and therefore did not address the possibility that adenosine might additionally be produced by cardiomyocytes.

Another important pathway regulated by O_2 levels involves reactive oxygen species (ROS). Wolin and colleagues [22] found that changes in O_2 levels affect the production of superoxide and superoxide anion-derived hydrogen, and also a cGMP-mediated relaxation response. Moreover, experiments from that laboratory established that in ovine coronary endothelia, NADH oxidoreductase is a major source of the superoxide anion [23]. They also demonstrated that in the coronary arteries of calves, NADH-derived superoxide contributes to relaxation during posthypoxic reoxygenation, but not during hypoxia [24]. The data indicated that changes in PO_2 regulate levels of the vascular superoxide anion by two different processes. First, during hypoxia, a decrease in PO_2 suppresses production of superoxide anion. However, during reoxygenation, superoxide anion is transiently overproduced, apparently by a flavoprotein-containing NADH oxidoreductase. A review of the studies from Wolin's lab [22] indicates that glucose 6P activity in the pentose phosphate pathway promotes oxidation of cytosolic NADH and a lowers Ca^{2+}, which then causes coronary arteries to relax. Finally, the group established a role for K^+ channels, demonstrating that blocking their activity abolished vasodilation, whereas blocking Ca^{2+} channels, either small or large, had no effect [19]. That study also demonstrated that the effects of K^+ are independent of an intact endothelium. Other investigators have shown that when glycolysis is blocked (by replacing glucose with deoxyglucose), coronary arteries reach a near-maximal dilation, which can be reversed by glibenclamide [25]. These findings suggest that a reduction in activity of the pentose phosphate pathway affects K^+ channels and thereby facilitates coronary artery vasodilation.

Paradoxical Constriction of the Microcirculation

Spontaneous or demand-induced ischemia in patients with coronary artery disease has been shown to induce microvascular vasoconstriction [26] [27, 28]. Application of serotonin (5-HT) to atrial arterioles isolated from patients with atherosclerosis caused relaxation in the absence of ischemia, but a potent contraction in the presence of ischemia, the latter being associated with increases in COX-2 (a prostaglandin synthesizing enzyme) at both the mRNA and protein levels [28]. The contractile response was attenuated when either COX-2 or the synthase that produces the vasoconstrictor thromboxane A_2 was inhibited, leading to the conclusion that the contractile response of coronary arterioles to 5-HT may result from thromboxane A_2 release as a secondary consequence of the enhanced COX-2 expression. In patients with stable angina, tachycardia-induced ischemia was shown to be linked to elevated coronary resistance of the microvasculature, as well as resistance of the severely stenotic arterial segment [27]. The authors suggested that enhanced extramural forces and a reduction in diastolic time do not account for the increased coronary resistance, because the administration of adenosine increased flow. To distinguish the effects of ischemia from those of coronary artery disease, Kusmic et al. [29] conducted experiments on normal, isolated mouse hearts. They reported that hypotension (a reduction in perfusion pressure from 65 mmHg to 30 mmHg) increased coronary resistance 2.2-fold, a response that was blunted by ROS; however, vasodilation occurred when either synthesis of NO or activity of the endothelin-1 ET_A receptor was inhibited. This study suggested that both the NO and endothelin-1 systems are required for the vasoconstrictive response to hypotension. Taken together, these studies support the thesis that paradoxical increases in microvascular resistance occur during reduced coronary flow. The mechanisms underlying this enhanced arteriolar contractility may include inhibition of the synthesis of NO, ET_A endothelin-1 receptors, or prostaglandins.

Conclusions: Ischemic Induction of Coronary Dilation. As noted by Duncker and Bache [30] in their review of coronary vasomotor tone during acute hypoperfusion, in the context of ischemia, coronary resistance vessels retain some vasomotor tone, a finding that indicates a defect in metabolic vasoregulation in these vessels. Thus, a failure of metabolic regulation in this portion of the coronary hierarchy during ischemia is one reason that maximal vasodilation in the resistance vasculature is not achieved. A second flow-limiting influence is the paradoxical constriction that can occur, especially in diseased vessels. Other factors, such as changes in perfusion pressure or the administration of vasodilators, might divert blood from underperfused regions (coronary steal) and exacerbate the hypoperfusion.

Vascular Alterations in the Ischemic Myocardium

Vascular Remodeling

There is now ample evidence that resistance vessels are highly plastic and able to alter their diameter through remodeling processes [31]. Specifically, coronary vessels downstream of a stenotic artery undergo biochemical and morphological changes in response to the reduction in pressure and flow [32]. Indeed, flow was documented as an important inhibitor of inward vessel remodeling, in cultured, perfused, porcine coronary arterioles [33]. Inward remodeling occurred under no-flow conditions and was inhibited by flow-dependent NO synthesis. The data from this study indicate that low-level shear stress was involved and that it does not require blood-borne cells or chemokines. Using a swine model of chronic ischemia, Hong et al. [34] demonstrated that wall thickness and proliferation were increased in arteriolar VSMCs distal to site of stenosis. Arterioles isolated from myocardial regions that had been perfused by a stenotic epicardial artery underwent inward remodeling, exhibiting exaggerated vasoconstriction in response to the application of endothelin-1 [35]. Of particular significance was the finding that even 30% coronary artery stenosis is sufficient to cause an increase in wall thickness and a reduction in the diameters of small intramyocardial arteries [34]. The fact that the lumen diameters of affected arteries correlated with the reduction in flow and the degree of fibrosis indicates that an incomplete stenosis of epicardial arteries that reduces flow but is not sufficient to cause myocardial infarction (MI) causes changes in the distal arterioles. However, clinical studies are not in agreement regarding poststenotic microvascular resistance after revascularization of a chronic stenosis. Whereas one such study reported that the increased microvascular resistance was reversed after coronary pressure was normalized via percutaneous intervention [36], others suggested that a failure to include the appropriate back pressure was responsible for an apparent increase in microvascular resistance distal to the stenosis [37]. As noted above, inward remodeling has also been shown to occur in pigs with progressive coronary occlusion, by 3–4 months of the initial stenosis [35]. In this model, the microvessels distal to a gradually occluded artery do not constrict in response to increased luminal pressure, although they exhibit increased sensitivity to endothelin-1 and normal vasodilation in response to NO and nitroprusside. Fearon and colleagues [37] found that minimal microvascular resistance at peak coronary hyperemia was not affected by increases in epicardial artery stenosis in swine when collateral flow was taken into account.

Vascular Dysfunction

Vascular Reactivity After Ischemia

Since ischemia followed by reperfusion was first reported to cause coronary endothelial dysfunction [38], such impairment has been documented in many studies, and has been shown to depend on both the component of the arterial tree that is affected and the stimulus that evokes the reactivity. Moreover, as demonstrated in dogs subjected to myocardial stunning, the degree of endothelial damage and endothelium-dependent impairment of dilation depend on the duration of the ischemia [39]. A common finding is that coronary arteries subjected to ischemia/reperfusion exhibit blunted vasodilation in response to the EC-dependent dilator acetylcholine, and enhanced constriction in response to endothelin-1 [40–43]. Although acetylcholine-induced relaxation in feline coronary arteries was not impaired after 90 min of ischemia; a 2.5-min period of reperfusion caused a 36% decrease in the response to acetylcholine, followed by a continued decline [44]. The vasodilator response to acetylcholine was preserved by applying superoxide dismutase beginning 10 min prior to reperfusion, a finding that implicates ROS in EC reperfusion injury. Significant myocardial injury occurred only after 3 h after reperfusion, indicating that impaired vasorelaxation precedes cardiomyocyte damage resulting from ischemia/reperfusion. Fernandez et al. [45] documented a reduction in coronary vasodilator reserve during partial ischemia in goats, and found that it was followed by a recovery during reperfusion. Their experiments also revealed that both vasodilation in response to acetylcholine nitroprusside and endothelin-1-mediated vasoconstriction were blunted. During reperfusion, however, both coronary vasodilator reserve and vasoreactivity recovered. The finding that endothelin-1-mediated constriction was blunted during ischemia was surprising and, according to the investigators, might be due to (1) decreases in arterial pressure and the levels of endothelial receptors or (2) increased production of NO in response to ischemia. Ischemia without reperfusion decreases the vasoreactivity of coronary arteries, as indicated in a rat model of hemorrhagic shock.

Heusch and colleagues [46] documented poststenotic adrenergic vasoconstriction and exacerbation of ischemia in dogs subjected to acute coronary occlusion of a magnitude sufficient to reduce coronary flow by 50%. Postganglionic cardiac sympathetic nerve activity was increased by 23% within 20 min of occlusion, in parallel with a 27% increase in poststenotic vascular resistance. Segmental anesthesia of cardiac sympathetic nerves prevented sympathetic activation and myocardial ischemia. These data underscore the importance of a neural response that depresses myocardial perfusion during coronary artery stenosis. This is attenuated at low perfusion pressures, since coronary pressure flow curves become nonlinear due to passive reductions in diameters, as well as the influence of extravascular pressure [47].

Nitric Oxide and Neutrophil Adhesion

Endothelial dysfunction after ischemia/reperfusion impairs NO release from ECs [44, 48], and is likely attributable to the production of O_2^- in ECs and neutrophils during reperfusion. NO interacts with O_2^- to form ONOO–, thereby limiting the amount of NO available as a source for VSMC vasorelaxation. A reduction in NO availability can last for hours or days, and leads to increased levels of adhesion molecules, thereby facilitating interactions between ECs and neutrophils, thus causing damage to ECs and cardiomyocytes [48, 49]. Adhesion between neutrophils and the endothelium is enhanced when NO is limited [50]. Moreover, coronary artery occlusion followed by reperfusion in dogs resulted in enhanced endothelin-1 constriction only when neutrophils activated with phorbol myristate were added; this finding suggests that the prolonged postinfarction angina and myocardial dysfunction after reperfusion may be due to vasospasm of the coronary arteries [40].

Ischemia and Neutrophil Activation

Neutrophil activation in combination with ischemia was shown to promote coronary vasoreactivity [51]. Specifically, ischemia attenuated the relaxation of intramyocardial, but not epicardial, arteries in response to bradykinin; the extent of EC damage correlated with impairment of artery function. Adhesion among neutrophils leads to the plugging of capillaries and provides these cells the opportunity to release vasoconstrictors [52]. However, vascular reactivity can be altered in the absence of neutrophil adherence and accumulation. Coronary artery rings from dogs subjected to ischemia (in the form of a 70% reduction in coronary artery diameter) followed by reperfusion had only a mild reduction in acetylcholine-induced relaxation, but marked reductions in ADP- and thrombin-induced vasorelaxation [53].

Cardioplegia and Endothelial Function

A review paper [54] cites the evidence that following cardioplegia-reperfusion, release of NO is impaired and COX-2 expression is induced, and that the latter is associated with enhanced contraction in the presence of serotonin [55]; this indicates that the serotonin-induced contraction observed in human microvessels is caused by both (1) release of the products of COX-2 activity and (2) impaired release of NO. When reperfusion is prolonged, contractile responses to thromboxane, serotonin, and endothelin-1 recover, whereas the impairment in endothelium-dependent relaxation is enhanced. Both the duration of cardioplegic exposure and the degree of hyperkalemia in the solution were considered determinants of the extent of impaired vasoreactivity. In this model of endothelial ischemia/reperfusion, neutrophil adherence has also been suggested to contribute to endothelial damage [56]. Sellke and Quillen [57] raised the concern that the large increase in arteriolar constriction in response to vasopressin, which is elevated during ischemia, may predispose the heart to persistent ischemia under conditions such as cardiopulmonary bypass.

Calcium and Vasoreactivity

Studies examining the role of calcium in limiting vasorelaxation of coronary arteries during ischemia/reperfusion, in which rats were treated with calcium channel blockers prior to ischemia/reperfusion, revealed that both endothelium-dependent and -independent coronary artery relaxation is enhanced in a dose-dependent manner [58]. Although the release of endothelium-derived relaxing factor (EDRF) from ECs requires an elevation in calcium [59], calcium channel antagonists do not inhibit the release of this vasodilator [60]. Moreover, the fact that smooth muscle relaxation induced by EDRF and calcium antagonists is additive [61] implies that two independent modes of action are involved. The effectiveness of adding calcium antagonists in reducing calcium overload during ischemia/reperfusion has been demonstrated [62], and cardioplegic solutions have been found to limit ischemic injury [63, 64].

Reactive Oxygen Species

Moderate amounts of ROS appear to allow "cells to adapt to environmental changes" [65]. For example, EC-derived H_2O_2 is involved in the relaxation of porcine coronary microvessels in response to bradykinin or substance P, and in both human [66] and porcine [67] coronary arteries, it triggers vasorelaxation. H_2O_2 produced by ECs in response to flow also acts as the transferrable endothelium-derived hyperpolarizing factor (EDHF), activating large conductance Ca^{2+}-activated K^+ channels on VSMCs in human arterioles [68]. H_2O_2 also plays a cardioprotective role during coronary ischemia–reperfusion by cooperating with NO to attenuate coronary ischemia/reperfusion injury, as demonstrated in an in vivo study on dogs [69]. Whereas a reduction in NOS (due to inhibition by L-NMMA) following ischemia/reperfusion attenuated the dilation of small arteries but increased vasodilation of arterioles, H_2O_2 decomposition (triggered by catalase) increased the former and decreased the latter. NADPH oxidase-derived ROS also appears to be required for endothelium-dependent coronary vasodilation [70], which is of importance for the ischemic heart.

Reactivity of Specific Coronary Artery Segments

Ischemia, per se, or ischemia/reperfusion does not necessarily affect distinct segments of the coronary arterial tree uniformly. Major hemodynamic changes that occur after chronic constriction and eventual occlusion of a coronary artery precipitate compensatory adaptations in the distal segments of the artery undergoing constriction, as shown by Li et al. [71, 72]. The responses of the segments distal to L-NAME caused a greater attenuation of substance P-induced relaxation, which the investigators suggested might be a consequence of increased NO production in these vessels. Moreover, the vasodilatory response to NO donation by SIN-1 was inhibited in proximal but not distal coronary arteries under nonischemic conditions [41]. However, the inhibition was abolished by ischemia/reperfusion, and endothelium-dependent vasodilation was attenuated in both proximal and distal coronary arteries. Quillen et al. [73] conducted experiments on conduit arteries and microvessels from dogs subjected to ischemia alone, or to ischemia followed by reperfusion. Their data revealed that endothelium-dependent relaxation in response to acetylcholine, ADP, bradykinin, A23187 (a calcium ionophore), nitroglycerin, and adenosine was not significantly altered by ischemia, regardless of whether reperfusion occurred. In contrast, in coronary arterioles (110–220 μm in diameter) this relaxation response to acetylcholine, ADP, and A23187 was inhibited by ischemia, and the effect was exacerbated when ischemia was followed by reperfusion. Thus, endothelium-dependent relaxation of coronary arterioles, but not that of conduit arteries, is impaired by ischemia and reperfusion.

Microvascular Angina

Angina-like chest pain occurring in the absence of obstructive plaques and myocardial disease is known as syndrome X. Ischemia is thought to be the cause of this pain, based on the fact that ST-segment depression is observed during episodes of angina [74], and on metabolic evidence of ischemia following pacing-induced tachycardia [75]. Moreover, a reduction in both endothelium-dependent and -independent vasodilation has been documented in patients with syndrome X [76]. Although it was not possible to verify that ischemia occurred in the patients in all of the relevant studies, Maseri et al. [77] suggested that focal ischemia in scattered regions of the myocardium is caused by dysfunction of prearteriolar vessels, which could theoretically cause a reduction or elevation in flow through the ST-segment without causing changes in wall motion. Whether all syndrome-X anginas are symptoms of ischemia is not as yet established.

Coronary vasospasm, a reversible and intense vasoconstriction that causes angina pectoris, has been reviewed by Konidala and Gutterman [78]. The mechanism underlying these vasospasms is not yet clear, but endothelial dysfunction may be a contributing (though not required) factor, in their development. Coronary vasospasms usually occur in large epicardial arteries with superimposed atherosclerosis. They can cause acute MI with normal coronary arteries, as well as contribute to thrombosis in the setting of acute plaque rupture [79]. Moreover, microvascular vasospasm also occurs in some patients, most often in postmenopausal women. Unlike vasospasm in large coronary arteries, vasospasm in the microvasculature is less responsive to calcium channel blockers [80]. They may be the consequence of arteriolar sensitivity to vasoconstrictors associated with endothelial dysfunction, as observed in a porcine model in which a large epicardial coronary artery was repeatedly denuded [81]. These animals experience microvascular spasm distal to the stenosis, with a markedly attenuated dilation in response to acetylcholine. In coronary microvessels, endothelium-dependent relaxation in response to acetylcholine is impaired during ischemia [73]. Epicardial vessels also demonstrate impaired vasodilation in response to acetylcholine, but not to the endothelium-independent nitroprusside [82].

Neovascularization in Response to Ischemia

Angiogenesis and Arteriogenesis

Coronary vessels react to chronic ischemia and infarction by two forms of arteriogenesis (1) the formation of arterioles from capillaries and (2) the remodeling of native collateral channels to form larger channels (Fig. 10.1). A limited amount of capillary neoformation may also occur in some circumstances.

Ischemic Hypoxia Triggers Growth Factors

The Role of HIF-1 as an Activator of Growth-Factor Expression

As documented in Chap. 9, hypoxia in the absence of ischemia is a powerful stimulus for angiogenesis because it activates multiple growth factors and signaling pathways. As evidenced by numerous experiments, hypoxia also activates angiogenic growth factors in the context of ischemia, this is consistent with early induction of the hypoxia-inducible factor-α (HIF-1α) during ischemia and acute MI [83]. The importance of HIF-1α as an activator of angiogenic growth factors in human ECs was demonstrated by expressing a stable form of this factor using an adenoviral vector [84]. Transduced ECs expressed higher levels of VEGF, angiopoietin-2, and angiopoietin-4, at both the mRNA and protein levels. Angiopoietin-4 expression was also increased in cardiomyocytes when treated with this vector or exposed to hypoxia. From a more physiological perspective, constitutive HIF-1α expression in mice with acute MI attenuated infarct size, accompanied by increases in capillary density as well as VEGF and iNOS levels in the peri-infarct areas [85]. Similar effects of $VEGF_{165}$ and HIF-1α on infarction were demonstrated by a study in which plasmids encoding these molecules under control of the VP16 promoter were injected

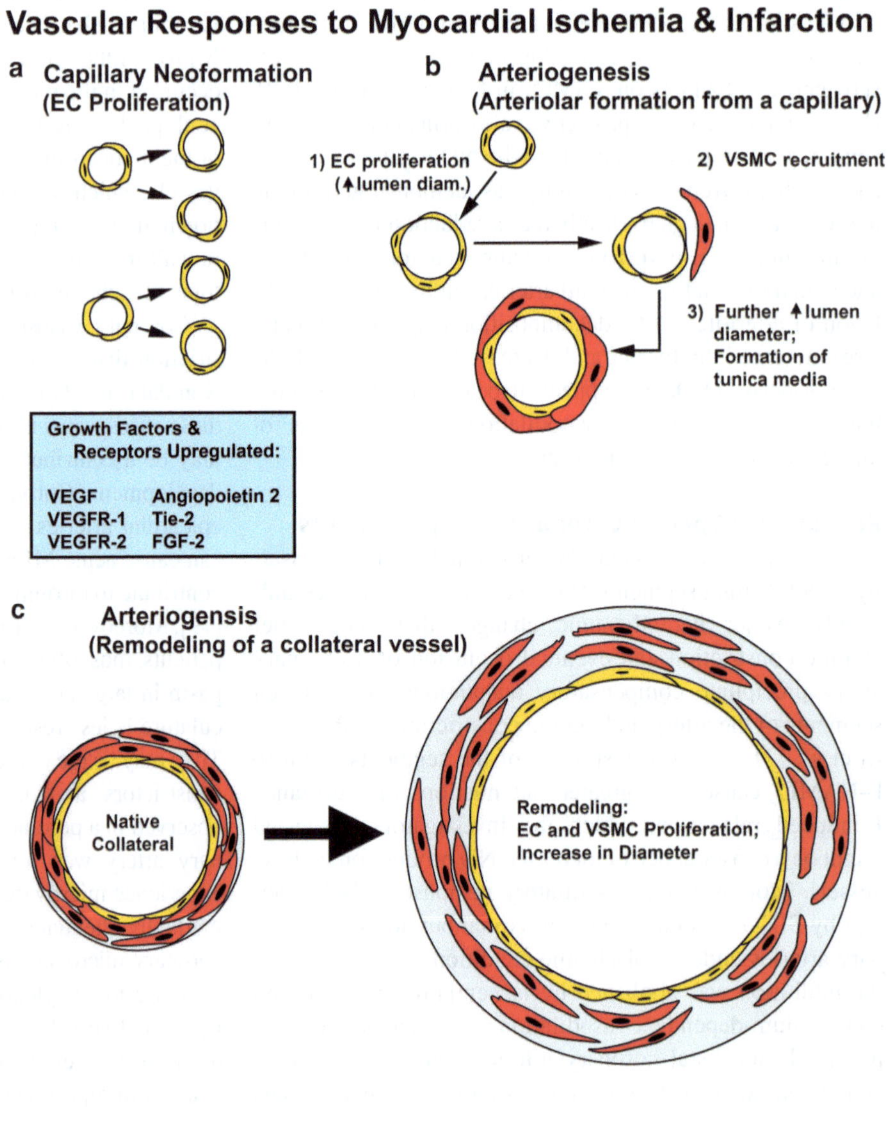

Fig. 10.1 Responses to myocardial ischemia and infarction. These include (**a**) neoformation of capillaries by EC (endothelial cell) proliferation, in response to upregulation of various growth factors and their receptors (usually a limited response); (**b**) arteriogenesis as a consequence of EC proliferation and recruitment of VSMCs encircling a capillary; and (**c**) arteriogenesis as a consequence of the proliferation of both ECs and VSMCs and their remodeling of native collateral vessels, in response to shear stress

into infarcted regions of hearts. Each of the DNA constructs reduced infarct size by a similar extent [86]. Moreover, the VEGF levels and capillary densities in those mice were higher than in untreated infarcts. Prolyl hydroxylase-2 (PHD 2) inhibits HIF-1α hydroxylation, stabilizing it and enabling it to bind HIF-1β, thereby facilitating the expression of angiogenic genes (a topic discussed in Chap. 9). The effect of increasing HIF-1α levels in this manner was studied in mice in which the genes encoding PHDs were disrupted [87]; these animals displayed highly perfusable blood vessels and "excessive" vascular growth, whereas mice in which the PHD 1- and 3-encoding genes were disrupted did not exhibit these changes.

VEGF as a Target Molecule

VEGF upregulation in response to ischemia is rapid and marked, as indicated by a fourfold increase in $VEGF_{164}$ protein 1–2 h following LAD occlusion in the dog [88]. Moreover, in rat both VEGFR-1 and VEGFR-2 are enhanced 3.5–4.0-fold within 1 h of coronary artery ligation [89]. The study in rats also revealed that VEGFR-1 was present in both large and small vessels, whereas VEGFR-2 expression was limited to small vessels. The increase in VEGF protein was found to persist for 6 weeks. TNF-α and $VEGF_{120}$ levels were increased during the first day following coronary artery ligation, and iNOS levels were increased by day 4 [90]. Moreover, two other VEGF splice variants were enhanced later, and VEGF expression was notable in the border zone of the infarct.

Coronary Collaterals

The development of collateral vessels has been reviewed by Schaper [91] and the importance of the coronary collateral circulation in humans is provided in other reviews [92–94].

Coronary Collateral Function in the Ischemic Human Heart

Contribution of Collaterals to Myocardial Perfusion

Vasodilation of coronary collaterals in response to endogenous vasoactive substances and the resulting increase in coronary flow constitute "collateral recruitment," i.e., a progressive increase in collateral flow following the establishment of a pressure gradient across the collateral artery [93]. Thus, the ability of coronary collateral to respond to vasodilators induced by ischemia is a determinant of the collateral flow. The collateral flow index (CFI) is one measure of collateral recruitment and is commonly utilized to characterize this process. In one study, CFI was recorded for 845 individuals who were undergoing a 1-min coronary balloon occlusion, and the same measurement was made 10 years later [96]. Data analysis documented that the long-term mortality in individuals with a high CFI was only 25% of that of individuals with low CFI, suggesting that functional collaterals contribute to survival. In patients undergoing angioplasty, angina pectoris occurred during balloon inflation in only 33% of patients with high levels of collateral filling, but in 100% of patients who presented with limited or undetectable collaterals [97]. A progressive increase in collateral flow has been demonstrated to result from repeated coronary artery occlusions during balloon angioplasty [98]. Collateral recruitment was also evident in a study on patients with coronary disease, in which the coronary vasodilator isosorbide dinitrate increased exercise capacity only in patients in whom a significant coronary collateral circulation was evident [99]. This is consistent with evidence that blocking serotonin increases myocardial perfusion only in patients with a good collateral circulation [100] and that collateral vessels can be more effectively dilated with nitroglycerin than can non-collateral vessels [101].

Obviously, many factors may limit the recruitment of collateral flow. Most studies evaluating collateral flow have been carried out in patients with coronary artery disease because collateral development is believed to be a response to myocardial ischemia. To test the hypothesis that functional collateral vessels exist in human hearts with angiographically normal coronary arteries, [102] measured CFI in 100 patients. During balloon occlusion, 17 patients did not exhibit signs of myocardial ischemia, and 26 did not experience angina. These data suggest that functional collaterals existed in about 25% of the patients in this group. More recently, preformed collateral vessels in 106 patients free of coronary stenoses were studied in an attempt to discover determinants of CFI [103]. In patients not using β-blockers, a low heart rate and an absence of hypertension were independent predictors of a high CFI.

Collaterals Limit Myocardial Infarction (MI) and Enhance Chances of Survival

As noted in Chap. 5, the relevance of coronary collaterals in humans was debated for many years. However, recent studies utilizing methods that have allowed more accurate measurement of collateral flow have documented a role for collaterals, in reducing infarct size, LV dysfunction, and mortality (reviewed in [92–94]). Notably, more than 3 decades ago it had been established that collaterals are one of four determinants of infarct size (the others being duration of the ischemia, size of the area at risk, and the presence or absence of ischemic preconditioning) [104]. Moreover, viability within the perfusion territory of the infarct-associated artery was linked to well-developed collaterals in patients presenting with recent myocardial infarctions [103]. Although the extent of a myocardial scar was shown to be

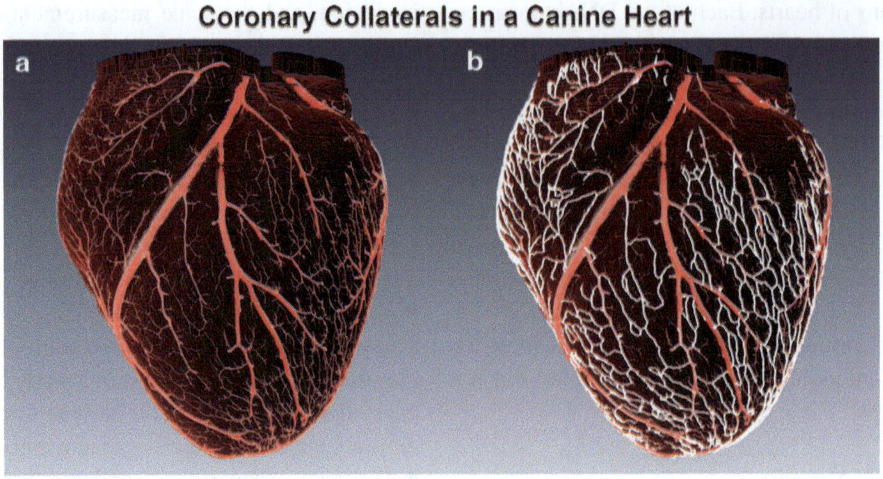

Fig. 10.2 (**a**) Reconstruction of the fluorescent intracoronary cast material showing vessels at the epicardial surface of a canine heart combined with structural outline data. (**b**) Detected collaterals (*white*) projected on top of the 3D reconstructed coronary vasculature. The vessels were filled with fluorescent cast material, the heart frozen, sliced, and imaged. The resulting stack of images containing the 3D vasculature was then skeletonized to identify the collateral connections. The images were provided by Dr. Maria Siebes, Biomedical Engineering and Physics, Academic Medical Center, University of Amsterdam

related to the severity of the coronary artery stenosis, the number of collaterals was found to be inversely related to the size of the scar [106]. Consistent with these data are findings from a study of 125 patients in whom thrombolytic therapy failed to effect reperfusion [107]. In these patients, the presence of collaterals in the early acute phase of MI was associated with a 35% reduction in infarct size. Seiler [93] noted that in 1,164 patients undergoing primary percutaneous coronary intervention, the presence of coronary collaterals significantly improved survival.

The long-term recovery of mechanical function in some patients with MIs appears to be related to the presence of collateral blood flow to the infarct region. This was demonstrated in a study where global and regional wall motion improved after MI in only those patients with a high degree of collateral filling [108]. Moreover, in a study of 450 patients with coronary artery disease, 33% demonstrated collateral flow sufficient to prevent myocardial ischemia during occlusion [109]. This study revealed that collateral flow was related to the degree of coronary artery stenosis, i.e., high collateral flows tended to occur in hearts with a marked stenosis. Ha and colleagues [110] evaluated 125 patients with total occlusion of a coronary artery branch, and compared collateral reserve between those with angina pectoris but no infarct and those who had experienced their first transmural infarction. The lack of MI (first group) was associated with well-developed collaterals. However, a subset of these patients with total coronary occlusions, but no MI, had angina during a pharmacological stress, revealing a limited collateral reserve [111]. These data led to the conclusion that while collateral growth can preserve ventricular function and prevent MI in the face of total coronary occlusion, the collateral cannot provide a normal coronary reserve.

Some Factors that Influence Collateral Development in Humans

The role of oxidative stress in the development of coronary collaterals was investigated in 176 patients with total coronary artery occlusions [112]. Data from this study revealed that the total peroxidase and oxidative stress index (the ratio of total antioxidant capacity/total peroxide) were lower in patients with poorly developed collaterals, and led to the conclusion that the oxidative stress index is independently and positively associated with the presence of a collateral circulation in patients with total coronary artery occlusion. Monocyte chemoattractant protein-1 has also been shown to be important for the development of coronary collaterals in patients with stable angina pectoris; the data revealed that it is independently related to good collateral development [113]. Another molecule related to collateralization is thymosin β4, as indicated by its higher serum levels in patients with good collaterals [114].

Coronary Collaterals in Experimental Animals

This section concerns data on coronary collaterals, derived from experimental animals with respect to the (1) recruitment of collaterals in response to myocardial ischemia, (2) development of collaterals in response to either gradually developing ischemia or brief episodes of ischemia over an extended period of time, e.g., several weeks, and (3) mechanisms that regulate collateral development. Coronary collaterals have been studied mostly in dogs and pigs, species that differ with respect to the anatomy of their collaterals. As noted in Chap. 4, the pig heart is characterized by small intramyocardial anastomoses, whereas the dog heart has large epicardial anastomoses (Fig. 10.2). Despite this difference, the development and function of collaterals in the two species are similar [115]. The growth of coronary collaterals has also been documented in rat [116, 117]. Although the mechanisms of coronary collateral growth are similar to those in other vascular beds (e.g., hindlimb, cerebral), the discussion in this chapter is limited to that in the coronary vasculature. Species vary significantly in terms of the extent of expansion of the coronary collateral circulation in response to ischemia [118]. After a major branch of the left coronary artery was ligated, innate collateral flow (as a percentage of nonischemic flow) was determined and found to be 16% in dog; 12% in cat; 6% in rat; and 0.6% in pig. In guinea pig, no area of the myocardium was found to be underperfused, a finding that indicates that collaterals in that species were able to fully compensate for the reduction in flow from one coronary artery.

Recruitment of Coronary Collaterals

Four decades ago, Cohen and colleagues [119] documented a prolonged nitroglycerin-induced vasodilation of collateral arteries that served ischemic regions in isolated dog hearts. Data from dogs [120], like those from humans [101] cited above, indicated that coronary flow increases in response to nitroglycerin, and that nitroglycerin treatment after permanent occlusion of a coronary artery reduces infarct size. There is now considerable evidence from animal experiments, consistent with that from humans, indicating that recruitment of collateral vessels occurs in response to ischemia. Many studies in dogs [121–125] and rats [116] have shown that coronary collateral flow is augmented in response to brief (typically 1 min), repetitive coronary occlusions. In dogs, the dilation of native collaterals was shown to be dependent on ischemia in the dependent bed; specifically, 30 occlusions of 10 s in duration and at 1-min intervals did not increase collateral flow, whereas a single 1-min occlusion increased flow twofold [125]. The investigators suggested that the enhanced collateral flow was a consequence of ischemia-induced accumulation of adenosine.

Collateral Development Induced By Brief, Repetitive Occlusions

As noted above, brief occlusions repeated over several days led to enhanced coronary collateral flow, suggesting that collateral recruitment had taken place. The evidence suggests that when brief occlusions are repeated for several days or weeks, or when a coronary vessel is gradually occluded, collateral vessels enlarge or proliferate. Thus, whereas acute ischemic episodes stimulate vessel dilation, chronic ischemic episodes stimulate the remodeling of native collaterals and/or the formation of new collateral channels. Schaper's monograph [126] detailed some of the earliest experiments documenting collateral growth in response to ischemia. Repetitive episodes of myocardial ischemia in dogs for over a period of up to 9 days evoked the development of coronary collaterals, and this was shown to be significant functionally since reactive hyperemia was reduced, as indicated by a lower debt repayment and an attenuation of regional myocardial dysfunction [124]. Consistent with the findings from this study, repetitive occlusions in rats over a 10-day period caused a sixfold increase in collateral flow; this was shown to be of functional significance because complete coronary occlusion failed to produce any hemodynamic irregularities or arrhythmias [116].

Collateral Development Induced By Gradual Occlusion

Application of an ameroid occluder to a coronary artery over the course of several weeks to gradually decrease vessel diameter stimulated collateral growth in dogs [126–128]. Such occlusion caused preexisting collaterals to become larger by stimulating cell division, as indicated by increases in labeling of the DNA of both ECs and VSMCs [126]. A marked increase in retrograde flow was documented in isolated dog hearts after 1 and 3 months of circumflex occlusion [127]. Moreover, a reduced antegrade resistance was noted in non-collateral LAD and right coronary vessels 1 month after occlusion, but returned to pre-occlusion values at 3 months. Gradual coronary artery constriction with an ameroid occluder in dogs initially caused regional hypokinesis and ischemia, but these disturbances diminished over time [129]. The investigators concluded that collateral development was of functional significance because it reduced ischemia and contractile abnormalities. In swine, progressive narrowing of the coronary artery resulted in a collateral flow that constituted 20% of the normal maximal coronary flow [130]. Between 4 and 8 weeks following initiation of occlusion, collateral flow increased to 60% of normal maximal flow and the presence of numerous small collateral vessels was noted in the area at risk, with some preference for the subendocardial region.

Bradycardia Facilitates the Development of Coronary Collaterals

Based on the evidence that stretch of cardiomyocytes and ECs upregulates key growth factors [131–134], we tested the hypotheses that chronic bradycardia in dogs with a gradual coronary occlusion would enhance collateral development [135]. An ameroid occluder was placed on a coronary artery of dogs with either normal heart rates (about 70–80 bpm) or bradycardia (55 bpm; caused by AV-node ablation in conjunction with implantation of a pacemaker). Adenosine-induced maximal myocardial perfusion to the collateral-dependent region of the LV was nearly twofold higher in dogs with bradycardia than in those with normal heart rates (Fig. 10.3). Collateral wall/lumen ratios were reduced, relative to those in nonbanded controls, in the

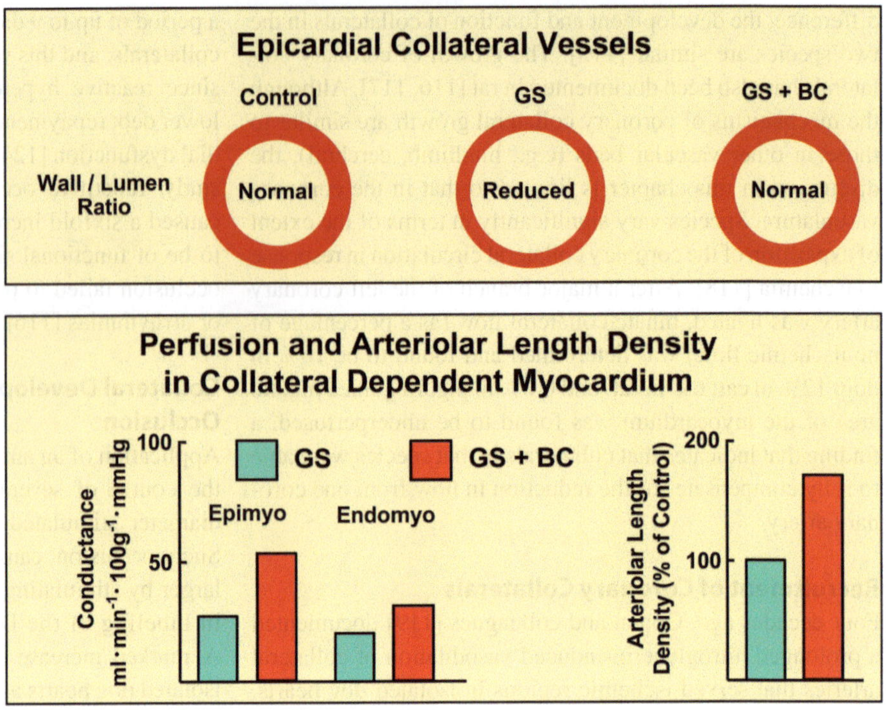

Fig. 10.3 (**a**) In dogs, gradual coronary artery occlusion (GS) using an ameroid constrictor decreases the wall/lumen ratio in coronary epicardial collateral vessels. However, in dogs with chronic bradycardia (BC) and GS, wall/lumen ratios are normal. (**b**) Chronic bradycardia (BC) in hearts undergoing gradual coronary artery occlusion improves maximal perfusion (conductance) in the collateral-dependent myocardium and enhances arteriolar length density, an indication of arteriogenesis (arteriolar growth)

banded dogs with normal heart rates, but not in the banded dogs of the bradycardia group. Finally, arteriolar length density (arteriolar length/mm^3 tissue) in the collateral-dependent region was not affected by banding in dogs with normal heart rates, but was increased by 50% in the bradycardia group. These data suggest that factors associated with bradycardia, especially the increased stretch during diastole, enhance collateral perfusion and stimulate arteriole growth.

Ischemia and Pressure Gradients as Inducers of Collateral Development

Fluid Shear Stress

Fluid shear stress (FSS), briefly reviewed in Chaps. 1, 4, and 11, and in Fig. 4.12, is well documented as a stimulus for remodeling-dependent collateral vessel growth, a theory initially advanced by Schaper and colleagues [136–139]. In this paradigm, elevated FSS activates the endothelium in a collateral vessel and sets into motion a series of events that cause proliferation of ECs and VSMCs. The elevated FSS in the collateral vessel is the consequence of decreased pressure in an occluded artery and of a resulting pressure gradient across a collateral vessel connected to an adjacent artery. The remodeling and diameter increase in the collateral artery are dependent on blood-derived monocytes that infiltrate the collateral vessel in response to monocyte chemoattractant protein (MCP-1). These events lead to the production of growth factors [140]. Incidentally, a higher serum MCP-1 level in patients is associated with good collateral development [113]. In the Schaper model, ischemia is only indirectly involved, i.e., it affects an increase in flow and FSS in the collateral channel. Most of the data in support of this paradigm come from studies in which large arteries, primarily of epicardial origin, were blocked. The remodeling required to enlarge a collateral vessel has been termed a form of arteriogenesis and, as such, differs from angiogenesis.

Ischemia, Independent of Elevated FSS

In addition to the FSS that accompanies increased blood flow, ischemia itself may play a direct role in stimulating collateral development under certain circumstances [128, 141, 142]. Although Scheel and colleagues [127, 128] concluded that the development of collaterals in dogs with gradual coronary artery occlusion was consistent with elevated pressure gradients, in some instances collateral growth occurred in the absence of such gradients. This was based on their observation that some coronary collaterals followed a tortuous course, including acute angles, factors that would limit flow. They suggested that the growth of these collaterals could be due to a gradient of hypoxia, an accumulation of metabolic end products, or some other factor. This theory was tested by Chilian et al. [141], who partially embolized the circumflex coronary perfusion territory in dogs to produce in multiple microvascular occlusions. Circumflex retrograde flow was increased after short (1–3 week)- and long (6–8 week)-term embolism. The increase in collateral flow occurred earlier, and without a pressure gradient, in the intramyocardial collaterals than in their epicardial counterparts. The authors noted that these differences are dependent on the presence of ischemia and a pressure gradient, respectively. More recently, van den Wijngaard et al. [143] used 3-dimensional reconstructions to study the development of intramural coronary collaterals in pigs in which the circumflex coronary artery had undergone gradual occlusion. They found that the collaterals developed not only in the ischemic border regions, but also distal to those regions, where FSS was unlikely to occur. The majority (62%) of the collaterals were in the subendocardial region, which is most vulnerable to ischemia. Based on these data the investigators concluded that the FSS model for collateral development needs to be modified to account for the possibility of ischemia-induced collateral formation (angiogenesis) followed by FSS-induced remodeling. This position in no way diminishes the role of FSS as the determinant in remodeling of native collaterals, but rather recognizes that some collateralization can also occur in response to metabolic stimuli.

Collateral Growth Requires Multiple Genes

Remodeling of a collateral channel into a larger vessel to facilitate greater blood flow necessitates the proliferation of ECs, both the proliferation and migration of VSMCs, and the recruitment of cells from blood and the extracellular matrix. This growth process requires an interplay of various cell types and the activation of multiple genes. Although this chapter focuses mainly on coronary collaterals, some mechanistic information from collateral development in the hindlimb ischemia model is also included.

Fibroblast Growth Factors

Since both FGF-2 and PDGF-BB participate in the development of the tunica media, it is not surprising that coadministration of these growth factors into the ischemic porcine myocardium from a slow-release polymer stimulated the formation of new collaterals that became incorporated into the vascular network [144]. Six-week treatment with these growth factors significantly improved regional blood flow. This is consistent with the fact that heparin administered during gradual coronary artery occlusion enhances collateral development [145], as it potentiates FGF-1 activity [146], releases FGF-2 from the subendothelial extracellular matrix [147], and protects FGF-1 from inactivation [148]. Notably, heparin appears to augment the collateral circulation in models of repeated ischemia, coronary occlusion, and exercise (reviewed in [149]). In dogs, chronic exogenous application of FGF-2 has been shown to enhance coronary collateral flow [150–152]. As demonstrated in an ischemic hindlimb rabbit model, FGF-2-induced VSMC migration requires the small GTP-binding protein Rap2 [153]. Rap2 appears to be similarly involved in FGFR-1-mediated effects on collateral growth, as infection with a dominant-negative FGFR-1-expressing adenovirus inhibited Rap2 upregulation and also collateral growth, and a dominant-negative Rap2 blocked arteriogenesis.

Vascular Endothelial Growth Factor

Vascular endothelial growth factor (VEGF), widely recognized as a major regulator of vasculogenesis and angiogenesis, has also been documented as a required factor for coronary collateral development, using a model of repetitive coronary artery occlusions over a 10-day period in rats [116]. Collateral flow was enhanced sixfold in this model, but the enhancement was completely prevented when an anti-VEGF antibody was administered. VEGF is not only stimulated by hypoxia, but also binds to eNOS in ECs exposed to FSS [154]. Moreover, arteriovenous fistulas stimulated by FSS can be completely prevented with pharmacological blockade of VEGF-A (reviewed in [91]). Within the hindlimb, VEGF also appears to play a role in collateral growth, as suggested by an observed upregulation of VEGFR-2 [155, 156] and VEGF-A [156] in the context of FSS. VEGF-C has likewise been implicated in the induction of coronary collateral growth, in a study on piglets that underwent a progressive stenosis of a coronary artery [157]. Intramyocardial injections of adenoviruses coding VEGF-C prevented the progression of ischemia and there was angiographic evidence of clustering of collateral vessels in the area of growth factor injection. A role for placental growth factor (PlGF), a ligand that binds only to VEGFR-1, in collateral growth is also indicated in the hindlimb ischemia model (1) PlGF gene deficiency limited the formation of collateral vessels [158] and (2) administration of PlGF enhanced collateral conductance [159].

Myocardial Infarction

A variety of cardiovascular abnormalities limit myocardial perfusion, resulting in a decline in coronary flow reserve (the difference between maximal and resting or baseline flow), which is a critical indicator of the ability of the coronary vasculature to increase myocardial perfusion in proportion to increased metabolic demand. As noted earlier in this chapter, a reduction in flow causes a number of metabolic and contractile changes in the myocardium. Timely restoration of flow may reestablish cardiomyocyte function, whereas extension of the occlusion time or additional damage during reperfusion can cause irreversible cardiomyocyte damage, i.e., infarction. These consequences of ischemia are summarized below.

Cardiomyocyte Injury: Cellular Alterations

Descriptions of cardiomyocyte injury following ischemia and/or reperfusion have commonly included the swelling of cells, denaturation of intracellular proteins, and damage and rupture of membranes. Jennings and colleagues [160] provided the first detailed account of ischemia-induced subcellular changes in cardiomyocytes. As proposed by Buja and Weerasinghe [161], cardiomyocyte injury and death can occur by apoptosis (programmed cell death Type I), autophagy (programmed cell death Type II), or oncosis (accidental or spontaneous cell death). Normally, sodium in the extracellular fluid opposes cell swelling, but in the absence of ATP the sodium-potassium pumps in the membrane become inactive and the transmembrane sodium collapses. Consequently, the ischemic cardiomyocyte swells, ending in lethal membrane rupture. Apoptosis is initiated by proteases of the caspase family, leading to destruction of the DNA within the nucleus and a slow cell death. Ischemia-induced cell death has been postulated to occur by a hybrid mode that involves both the apoptotic and oncotic pathways [162]. Even a brief interruption (5 min) of flow can cause functional abnormalities (resulting in a "stunned myocardium") that can last for a day or two (reviewed in [163]). Stunning occurs primarily at reperfusion and is associated with the formation of ROS [164]. In addition to the generation of oxygen radicals, two other mechanisms that likely contribute to the pathogenesis of myocardial stunning are an overload of calcium and attenuation of the responsiveness of contractile filaments to calcium (see review by [165]). As described below, the resulting ultrastructural changes are heterogenous, but can be seen as early as a few minutes after the onset of ischemia. For a review of the cellular responses to brief myocardial ischemia, see Kloner and Jennings [166, 167]; for a comprehensive review of the salient features of the morphology associated with myocardial infarction in humans, see Cantin and Leone [168].

Reversible Injury

The extent of permanent cellular injury is determined in part by the duration and magnitude of ischemia. When perfusion is reestablished, myocyte damage may be reversed and cellular function reestablished. Ischemic regions of the ventricle frequently contain viable cardiomyocytes next to infarcts. Some of the heterogeneity in infarction is due to mechanical compression, which limits subendocardial delivery of collateral flow, making the tissue region involved especially vulnerable. However, heterogeneity is seen even in isolated heart models of infarction, where flow is zero during ischemia. This finding indicates differing levels of vulnerability to ischemia within the ventricle arising from variations in oxygen consumption, which is greatest in the endomyocardium. Thus, the ventricle is vulnerable to ischemia for multiple reasons. Any injury to cardiomyocytes whose function is recovered is obviously reversible [15]. The temporal ultrastructural changes in cardiomyocytes subjected to ischemia have been described by numerous investigators. Ischemia lasting 15 min or less is associated with moderate glycogen depletion, cellular and mitochondrial swelling, and disruption of mitochondria [169–171]. Such changes are considered "reversible," because the cardiomyocyte will survive upon restoration of blood flow [169].

Irreversible Injury

A number of morphological and metabolic changes are characteristic of cardiomyocytes that will not regain their function following reperfusion. These include cessation of anaerobic glycolysis, a >90% decrease in ATP levels and a high H^+ concentration [15]. Cell death, i.e., irreversible injury, is also evidenced by certain ultrastructural changes. Of these, the presence of local disruptions of the sarcolemma is the clearest indicator of irreversibility, since this allows vital enzymes and contractile proteins to leak into the extracellular fluid. Associated with these disruptions are the presence of amorphous densities within swollen mitochondria, peripheral aggregation of chromatin, and the presence of prominent contraction bands within the chromatin [169].

Determinants of Irreversible Injury

Duration of Ischemic and Irreversible Injury

In dogs [169] and rabbits [171], occlusion of a coronary artery for about 45 min or longer results in some irreversible ischemic injury. The time at which irreversible injury first occurs has been difficult to predict more precisely because the exact time of cell death cannot be determined based on morphology alone. Nevertheless, it can be concluded that deprivation of blood flow for this length of time causes a significant myocardial infarction. The relationship between the degree of myocardial perfusion and the extent of myocardial infarction was studied by Rivas et al. [172], in dogs with acute coronary artery occlusion. Their data revealed that the degree of infarction varies in different transmural myocardial layers and is inversely related to blood flow. At approximately the same time, my colleagues and I [173] found, based on histological analysis of multiple tissue samples and the percent of perfusion in each sample as a percentage of flow to the normal myocardium, that the extent of myocardial necrosis 44–48 h after occlusion was closely related to the degree of perfusion 5–10 min after occlusion.

Magnitude of Ischemia and Irreversible Injury

The notion that the extent of cardiomyocyte damage correlates with the decrease in myocardial perfusion was further tested utilizing electron microscopy technology [1]. Perfusion was measured by microspheres to 99 myocardial segments before coronary artery occlusion, and also 45 min and 12 h after occlusion. Ischemia was classified into four levels, as defined

Table 10.1 Ultrastructural changes during various levels of ischemia (12 h after onset of ischemia)

Level of ischemia % of control	Mitochondria	Sarcoplasm	Myofibrils	Nuclei
Borderline (75–80%)	Rare focal disruption	Occasional mild enhancement	Normal	Normal
Mild (50–74%)	Swelling and disruption in all cells	Enhancement (swelling)	Some sarcomeres shortened	Normal
Moderate (35–49%)	Marked swelling and amorphous densities	Translucent, marked enhancement, loss of glycogen, vacuoles	Z line irregularity, contraction bands	Clumping and margination of chromatin
Severe (0–24%)	Prominent amorphous densities, vesiculation, some loss of cristae	Marked expansion, vesiculation	Disruptions, loss of Z lines, many contraction bands	As above, but all nuclei affected

Data from Tomanek et al. [1]

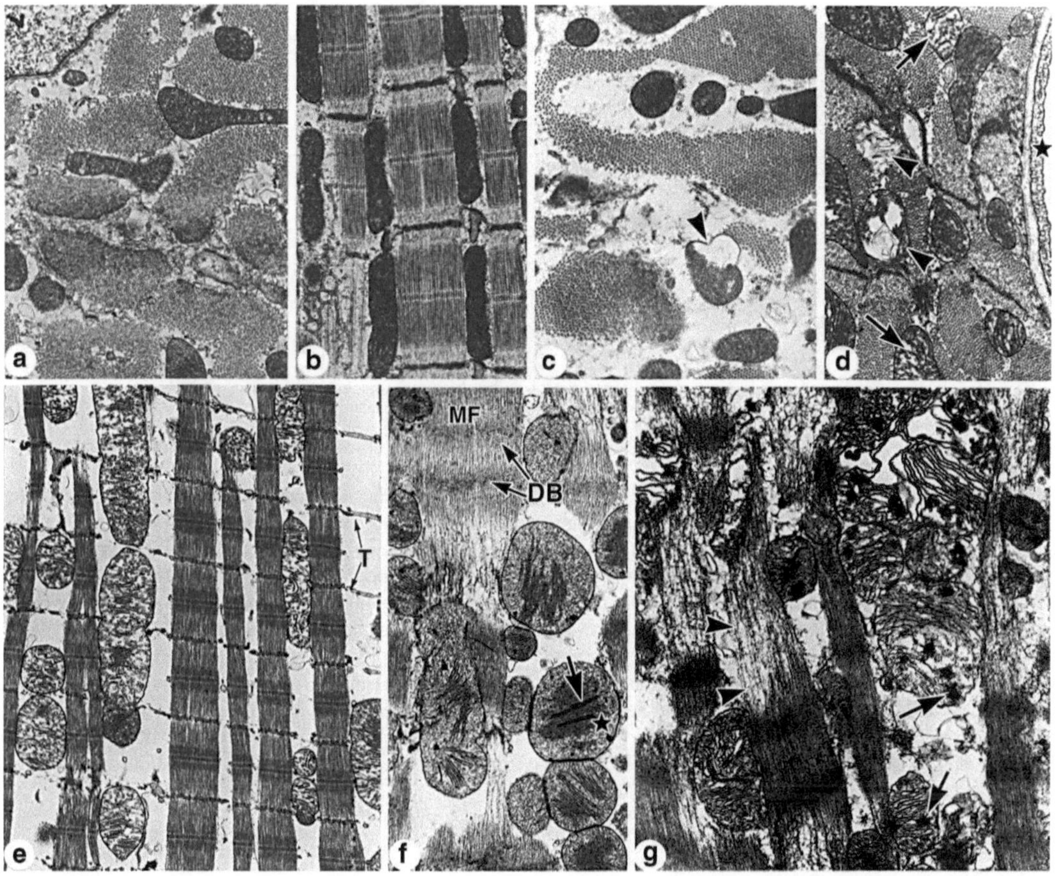

Fig. 10.4 Ultrastructural alterations in cardiomyocytes of dogs subjected to varying degrees of ischemia. (**a, b**) Cardiomyocytes from nonischemic hearts are characterized by close apposition of mitochondria and myofibrils and well-defined sarcomeres. (**c, d**) In cardiomyocytes subjected to borderline ischemia, where flow is only 75–80% of control values, some swelling occurs, causing the organelles to separate; occasionally mitochondria swell and their cristae degenerate (*arrowheads* in **c** and **d**). The star in (**d**) indicates capillary endothelium. (**e, f**) In cardiomyocytes subjected to moderate ischemia, defined by a flow of 25–49% relative to that in controls, the sarcoplasm becomes translucent and virtually all mitochondria swell. (**f**) Mitochondria alterations may include the presence of rod-like densities (*arrow*) or densities with a loss of cristae (*star* in **f**); dense bodies (DBs) in myofibrils (MF) area are signs of irreversible damage. (**g**) In cardiomyocytes subjected to severe ischemia, which occurs when perfusion falls below 25% of control values, cell death is common, as characterized by the loss of contractile proteins (*arrowheads*), the disruption and rupture of mitochondria, and dense bodies within mitochondria (*arrows*). Data from Tomanek et al. [1]

by the percentage of flow values post-occlusion compared to pre-occlusion (1) borderline (75–80%), (2) mild (50–74%), (3) moderate (25–50%), and (4) severe (0–24%). A summary of cardiomyocyte changes associated with each class of ischemia is provided in Table 10.1, and the ultrastructural alterations corresponding to various degrees of ischemia are illustrated in Fig. 10.4. The key finding of this study was that a reduction of myocardial perfusion to <50% of control for a 12-h period results in non-reversible cardiomyocyte damage, as characterized by clumping and margination of chromatin, loss of contraction bands and Z lines, disruption of myofibrils, and the presence of amorphous mitochondrial densities.

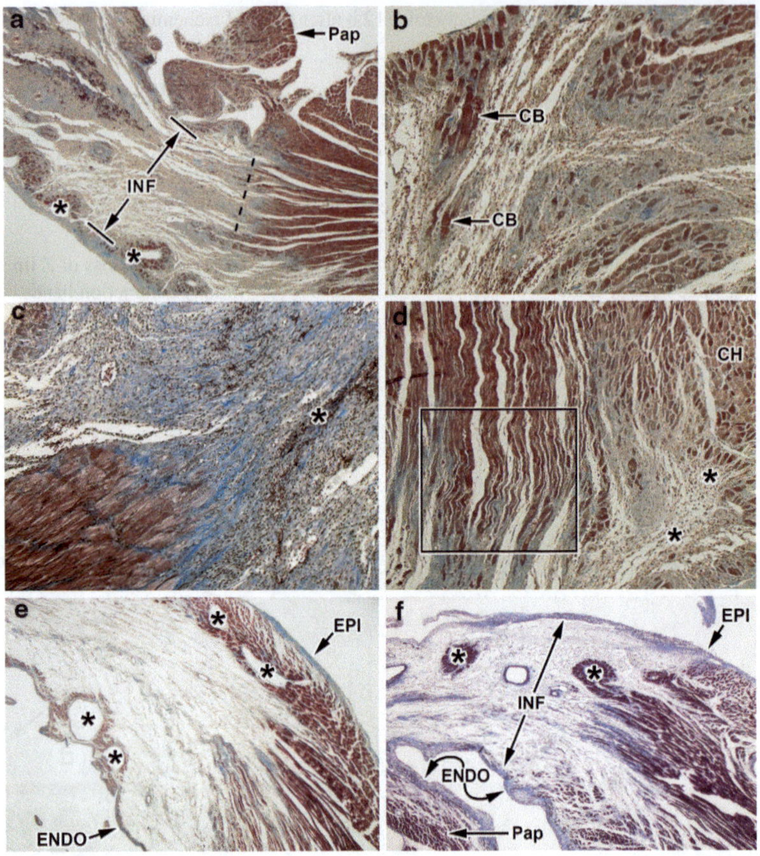

Fig. 10.5 Changes in the myocardium induced by banding the left anterior descending coronary artery in rats. Micrographs were prepared at the following postinfarction times: 1 week (**a, b**), 2 weeks (**c, d**), and 4 weeks (**e, f**). (**a**) Transmural loss of cardiomyocytes in the infarct region (INF) with surviving cells in the border zone (*right of broken line*), in the papillary muscle (Pap), along the adjacent endocardial region, and surrounding venules (*asterisks*). (**b**) Surviving cardiomyocytes with some showing contraction bands (CB), a sign of irreversible damage. The cardiomyocytes are surrounded by a fluid that contains neutrophils, which is characteristic of the inflammation occurring early following coronary stenosis. (**c, d**) 2 weeks after coronary stenosis, blood cells persist (*asterisks*) and dense collagen forms (*blue* staining regions in **c**). Cardiomyocytes adjacent to the infarct (shown within *square* in **d**) show signs of degeneration, whereas others are undergoing hypertrophy (CH). 4 weeks after coronary artery stenosis (**e, f**), the edema has resided and scars have developed. In (**e**) a band of cardiomyocytes close to or surrounding venules (*asterisks*) near the epicardium (Epi) has survived. Thus the infarct region occupies the inner 75% of the ventricular wall. In contrast, the infarct in F (INF) is transmural. Yet small clusters of cardiomyocytes surrounding venules (*asterisks*) have survived. *Pap* papillary muscle; *ENDO* endocardium. Micrographs are from hearts used in studies by Christensen et al. [175] and Zhang et al. [176]

Since our tissue samples were relatively small, the characteristics of the cardiomyocytes were more consistent than those based on large samples with less homogeneous flows. This study was the first to document that a threshold of ischemia is necessary to produce irreversible myocardial damage. Since that time, large clinical studies have confirmed that the degree of ischemia and its duration are determinants of ischemia–reperfusion injury (reviewed in [4]).

Progression of Myocardial Infarction

Because there is overlap in the perfusion territories of adjacent arteries (evidenced by end-capillary loops at the interface of the perfusion field), one might anticipate some level of partial perfusion at the periphery of an infarct. However, as demonstrated by applying a diffusible tracer in canine hearts, less than 3% of the area perfused by any artery is supplied by other branches [174]. Thus, little tissue can be salvaged by augmenting blood flow at the border zone. Reimer and Jennings [2] showed that in the moderately collateralized dog heart, infarction starts at the subendocardial region and, as the duration of ischemia increases, moves as a wave across the ischemic zone toward the epicedial surface, coincident with the transmural gradient of collateral flow. The human subendocardium has long been known to be particularly vulnerable to infarction, whereas the remaining heart layers are variably susceptible to both ischemia and infarction, as seen in infarcts with surviving cells, which are particularly common adjacent to venules. Figure 10.5 illustrates the progression of scar formation and transmural distribution in experimentally induced myocardial infarcts in rats [175, 176]. The so-called border zone is a region bordering the infarct scar which can be of variable thickness and is characterized by hypertrophied cardiomyocytes. In animal models, the enlargement of cardiomyocytes is associated with a decrease in capillary density.

Ventricular Remodeling

Studies in both animal models and humans have established that progressive changes take place in the architecture of the postinfarcted myocardium [177]. The changes within the affected chamber are not uniform; distinct differences exist with respect to both perfusion and wall stress, factors that dictate the remodeling processes. Experiments on rats have demonstrated that side-to-side slippage occurs during the first two days following coronary artery ligation, contributing to ventricular dilation when the infarction is large [177]. One month later, hypertrophy of the surviving cardiomyocytes can fully compensate for the loss of cardiomyocytes from the region if the infarct is small (about 38% of LV volume), but not when it is large (about 60%). In the latter case, myocardial mass undergoes a small reduction (10% in the case of an infarct affecting 60% of LV volume). These data are based on animal experiments. Humans do not survive infarcts as large as those noted above.

The process of postinfarction wound healing involves inflammation and macrophage activation; the latter is orchestrated by cytokines and chemokines [163]. As summarized by Lambert et al. [178], neutrophil infiltration occurs during the first day after infarction, followed by macrophages beginning on the third day after infarction. The latter migrate in response to monocyte chemotactic protein-1 released by ECs and secrete a variety of molecules necessary for angiogenesis, e.g., matrix metalloproteinases and cytokines.

Angiogenesis and Arteriogenesis

As previously stated, myocardial ischemia and its accompanying hypoxia are triggers for angiogenesis. When an infarction occurs, the surviving myocardium may experience limited or nonexistent ischemia, depending on its location (border or remote regions), and therefore may lack the molecular signals necessary to induce angiogenesis. To assess whether capillaries and arterioles grow after myocardial infarction, we quantified these vessels in the border and remote regions of rat LVs 4 weeks following coronary-artery ligation [179]. Despite a compensatory cardiomyocyte hypertrophy in the surviving free wall of hearts having undergone infarction, arteriolar length and volume densities were similar to those in controls, indicating that the level of arteriogenesis matched the magnitude of hypertrophy. DNA synthesis in coronary arterioles was increased about tenfold by 7 days after coronary artery ligation, and the increases occurred in both ECs and VSMCs. Consistent with these data, we found that the expression of both VEGFR-1 and VEGFR-2 was increased by the third day after coronary artery ligation, and this was followed by increases in the expression of angiopoietin-2 protein and its receptor, Tie-2. The finding that maximal coronary flow was reduced in both the LV free wall and the septum after infarction indicates that this limitation to perfusion is the consequence of a functional, rather than structural, impairment. Kalkman [180] also found that myocardial perfusion in this model was reduced 8 weeks after infarction.

Vascular Alterations in the Postinfarcted Myocardium

Changes in Vasoreactivity

As discussed earlier, ischemia, in the absence of MI, causes changes in the coronary vasculature. Changes also occur in the postinfarcted heart, as noted in both patients and experimental animals, and are likely influenced by a variety of factors, including myocardial remodeling and dysfunction. Data from swine indicate that coronary vasoconstriction induced by angiotensin II is reduced after myocardial infarction, despite an elevation in the levels of this vasoconstrictor [181]. The authors of that study suggested that the decreased response may be an adaptation that maintains adequate perfusion. Their subsequent work demonstrated that endothelin is also increased in the postinfarcted heart, and that blocking either the endothelin ET(A)/ET(B) or angiotensin II AT(1) receptor abolished the coronary vasodilation that characterizes the responses in noninfarcted hearts [182].

Structural Alterations

Studies carried out in experimental animals have revealed that intramyocardial coronary arteries and arterioles distal to epicardial artery occlusions are remodeled [34, 183]. In dogs, vascular remodeling was documented 6 weeks after myocardial infarction was induced in the resistance vessels of both the border and distal zones of the LV [183]. Vascular damage was shown to be related to myocardial cell injury more than 3 decades ago [184], with coronary occlusion for 20–180 min in dogs resulting in microvascular damage that was always associated with cardiomyocyte injury. However, the time course of the observed vascular and cardiomyocyte changes indicated that the former lagged behind the latter and, therefore, was not a primary cause of cardiomyocyte injury. Earlier, work by the same group had documented a relationship between the "no-reflow" phenomenon and capillary damage in dogs [185]. Specifically, occlusion of a coronary artery for a 40-min period followed by reflow resulted in uniform perfusion of the damaged myocardium, with no serious capillary damage being incurred. In contrast, occlusion for 90 min resulted in a failure of uniform perfusion (no-reflow) and in extensive capillary damage.

Compensatory Growth of Arterioles

Studies in experimental models have established that coronary resistance vessels in the myocardium can survive a large infarction [186, 187]. Kalkman [180] also found an increase in perivascular collagen, but no change in the tunica media, in hearts that had undergone myocardial infarction. Increases in both the volume percent of perivascular collagen and medial thickness in coronary arteries were documented in rats 6 weeks following myocardial infarction [188]. Taken together, these data indicate that structural and functional alterations contributed to the reduction in maximal myocardial perfusion in the postinfarcted heart. These changes can occur in remote regions of the ventricle.

Growth-Factor Changes

Growth-Factor Upregulation Is Transient After Myocardial Infarction

Acute myocardial infarction is characterized by a transient increase in growth-factor expression [81, 189–191]. In examining ventricular biopsy specimens from patients undergoing coronary bypass surgery, Lee and colleagues [81] found that specimens with evidence of acute ischemia (<48 h pre-surgery) or early infarction (<24 h pre-surgery) expressed the HIF-1α mRNA, whereas specimens from normal myocardium did not. VEGF mRNA was detected in the former but not the latter. Thus, HIF-1α is an early marker whose expression precedes that of VEGF. Growth-factor mRNA expression occurs early (24 h) after infarction and then declines, suggesting that it is limited to the subacute phase of MI [190]. Other observations made in that study indicate that levels of the VEGF-A mRNA and the VEGFR-1 protein increased threefold during this early phase and then declined to control levels. Similarly, levels of the angiopoietin-1 and -2 and the Tie-2 receptor mRNAs were elevated at 24 h post-MI, but not at the later time point. Levels of the VEGFR-2 mRNA were unchanged at this early time point and then dropped to values similar to or below those of controls; they never increased and were lower than those in controls after day 1. This is consistent with data from Dedkov et al. [187], in which arteriolar growth after myocardial infarction was associated with increases in VEGF receptors 1 and 2, angiopoietin 2, and Tie-2 expression during the first 2 weeks after coronary artery ligation (Fig. 10.6).

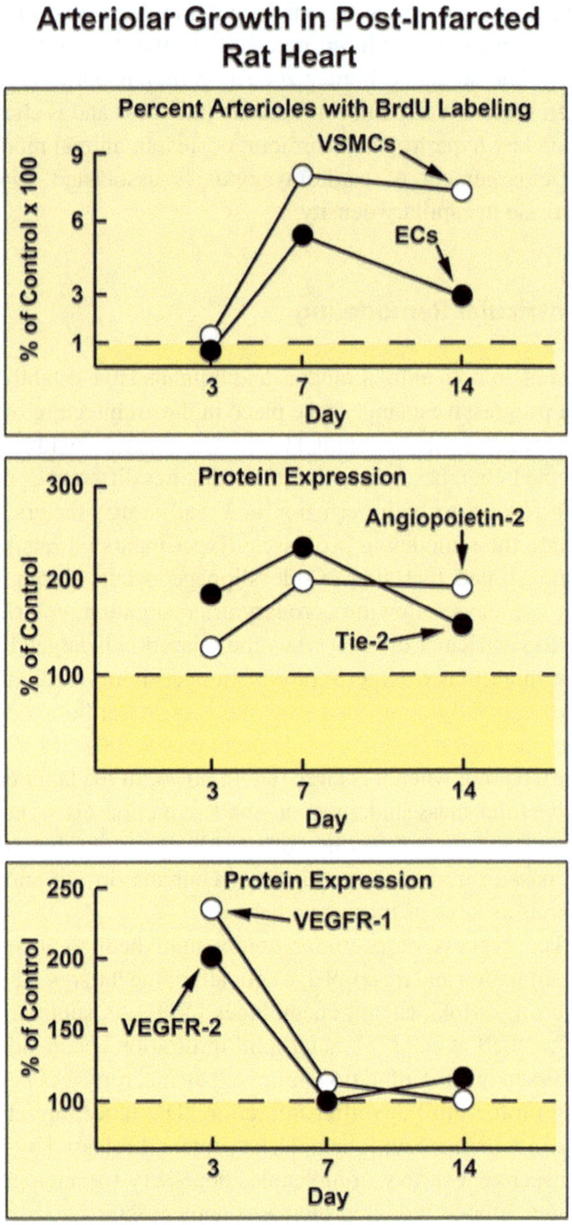

Fig. 10.6 Growth of coronary arterioles during the first 2 weeks following myocardial infarction, as indicated by large increases in the percentage of arterioles that contain proliferating endothelial cells (ECs) or vascular smooth muscle cells (VSMCs). Percentage growth was assessed based on labeling with a monoclonal antibody bromodeoxyuridine (BrdU), a synthetic (*top panel*). These increases at 7 days correspond to the peak expression of angiopoietin-2 and its receptor Tie-2 (*middle panel*). As seen in the *bottom panel*, peak expression of the VEGF receptors 1 and 2 proteins occurs 4 days earlier

Importance of VEGFR-1 Signaling

The VEGF mRNA is rapidly upregulated by transient ischemia 5–10 min in duration, as documented in rat hearts [192]. This increase was seen within 30 min of the ischemic episode and lasted for 3 h. Since similar results were obtained from hearts subjected to perfusion with a hypoxic perfusate, the authors suggested that the VEGF upregulation was a response to hypoxia. Support for this suggestion comes from the documentation, discussed in Chap. 9 (hypoxia), that VEGFR-1 plays a critical role in hypoxic induction of VEGF signaling. A key role for VEGFR-1 in both angiogenesis and arteriogenesis in the acutely infarcted heart has been detailed in a study on pigs [189], which revealed that adenovirus-mediated gene transfer of VEGF-A and VEGF-B_{186} (1) improved myocardial perfusion, (2) stimulated angiogenesis in the border zone of the infarct, and (3) enhanced collateral vessel formation. To determine the roles of VEGFR-1, VEGFR-2, and Neuropilin-1 (NrP-1), investigators injected competing, soluble forms of these receptors. These experiments indicated that angiogenesis during acute infarction is dependent on VEGFR-1 and NrP-1. The authors also demonstrated that VEGF-B_{186} has a strong antiapoptopic effect, and suggested that this signal may be transduced by a G-protein signaling pathway.

VEGF-B_{167} has also been found to enhance vascularization in the infarct region and the border zone, as demonstrated by experiments in which this splice variant was overexpressed in mice [193]. That study also noted that in VEGF-$B^{-/-}$ mice, vascular growth in the ischemic heart was impaired. They noted that while VEGF-B is important in revascularizing the ischemic heart, it does not play a role in the ischemic limb. VEGF-B and VEGFR-1 also contribute to the restoration of cardiac function after MI by preserving cardiac mass [191].

Reperfusion Injury: General Concepts

The idea that reperfusion can cause additional damage to the myocardium was first postulated by Jennings [194] a half century ago, when they noted four types of cardiac dysfunction (1) mechanical dysfunction (myocardial stunning) in the absence of irreversible damage; (2) impedance to blood flow, i.e., the inability to reperfuse a previously ischemic region; (3) the presence of reperfusion arrhythmias; and (4) lethal reperfusion injury. However, the very existence of lethal reperfusion injury was hotly investigated through the 1980s and 1990s. Although reperfusion caused rapid changes in morphology as the infarcted tissue swelled, it was argued that ischemia might have killed the tissue, and reperfusion simply added water that caused swelling. Reperfusion injury was established as playing a role in stunning when application of a free radical scavenger immediately prior to reperfusion was shown to attenuate the effects of stunning [195]. Proof of lethal reperfusion injury, however, required the application of an intervention just prior to reperfusion that would reduce infarct size. Although several candidate interventions were tested, they were all difficult to reproduce. The issue was finally settled when ischemic postconditioning was discovered [196] and could easily be reproduced (see postconditioning below). Reperfusion injury occurs because the ischemic area is hypoperfused even when blood flow in the major coronary arteries is restored, i.e., the microcirculation is involved. Thus, the term "no-reflow" was selected to denote compromised blood flow at the level of the microcirculation [185]. The presence of distinct regions of limited perfusion, as revealed in animal models of coronary artery occlusion and reperfusion, is associated with microvascular damage and a progressive decrease in the region's blood flow [185, 197, 198].

Inflammatory Injury and Reperfusion

Reperfusion may contribute to inflammatory injury in the postischemic myocardium [199–201]. Inflammation in this context is accompanied by the release of lytic enzymes from infiltrating neutrophils in response to chemoattractants, and by the release of oxygen-free radicals [202]. The activation of neutrophils that have migrated to the reperfused tissue (area at risk) produces superoxide, giving rise to hydrogen peroxide and hypochlorite, and these oxidants contribute to further infarction. Moreover, the release of proinflammatory mediators by neutrophils (e.g., leukotrienes, thromboxane, and platelet-activating factor) amplifies the inflammatory reaction. Neutrophils may also limit blood flow by blocking capillaries. Nearly 3 decades ago, the role of oxygen radicals in myocardial injury was demonstrated by Jolly and colleagues [203]; these investigators showed that coapplication of the scavenger enzymes superoxide dismutase and catalase before the onset of ischemia or 15 min before reperfusion reduced infarct size in dogs. Reperfusion injury can also be mediated by lipid peroxidation or calcium overload. The latter is associated with the initiation of ventricular tachycardia and fibrillation during reperfusion [204]. The notion that anti-inflammatory agents can reduce infarct size remains controversial, as it challenges the hypothesis that free radicals and/or neutrophils are the cause of reperfusion-associated pathogenesis [205]. Reperfusion injury is a topic of several reviews (see reviews by [161, 206–208]).

Impaired Myocardial Perfusion

Ischemia and reperfusion (IR) are limited by both structural and functional changes in the microvasculature, as illustrated in Fig. 10.7. Most of the abnormalities in reactivity of the coronary arteries and arterioles are due to endothelial dysfunction. For example, in the rat heart, IR attenuates acetylcholine-induced dilation, but not nitroglycerin-induced

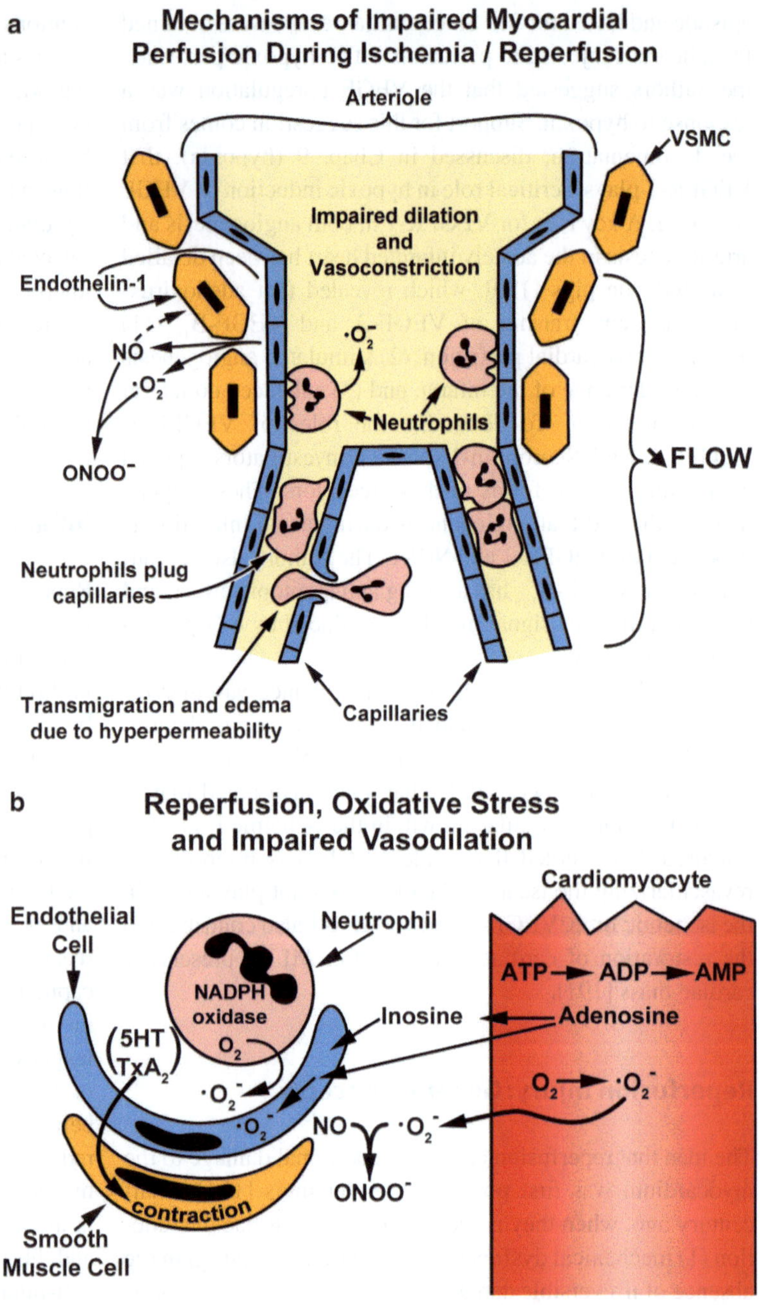

Fig. 10.7 (**a**) Impaired myocardial perfusion after ischemia/reperfusion is due to (1) reduced dilation and enhanced constriction of arterioles, (2) neutrophil adhesion to ECs, and the release of $\cdot O_2^-$ by these cells, (3) plugging of capillaries by neutrophils, and (4) the release of $\cdot O_2^-$ and endothelin-1 by ECs. The formation of ONOO– from O_2^- and NO limits the availability of the latter and thereby attenuates vasodilation. (**b**) The impairment of vasodilation is due to the interactions among several cell types. Both cardiomyocytes and neutrophils produce O_2^-. Cardiomyocytes also produce adenosine, which is deaminated to inosine. ECs take up both nucleotides. The impaired vasodilation and increased vasoconstriction (noted in the top figure and mediated by ECs/VSMCs) both contribute to the decrease in lumen diameter because they lead to a reduction in NO. Finally, VSMC contraction occurs in response to serotonin (SHT) and thromboxane (T_xA_2)

vasodilation [209]. The effects on coronary VSMCs are limited, which is consistent with the findings that nitroprusside elicits maximal vasodilation in porcine arterioles but that serotonin fails to do so [210]. This study provided evidence that IR alters the availability of NO by reducing levels of its cofactor, tetrahydrobiopterin. The preservation of VSMC function is also supported by the finding that vasodilation in response to the endothelium-independent vasodilator adenosine is not impaired after IR [211]. Data obtained from patients indicate that cardioplegia–reperfusion causes a release of COX-2 products, resulting in impaired release of NO, which in turn causes the cells to contract in response to serotonin [55]. This impairment of NO signaling has also been documented in a study on porcine coronary arterioles subjected to IR [212]. The data showed that arginase activity increases after IR, limiting the availability of L-arginine as a substrate for NOS, and thus also the production of NO in coronary arterioles. IR also enhanced the contractile response to endothelin-1, as a consequence of impaired release of NO and prostacyclin from the endothelin receptor; these impairments are associated with an increase in vasoconstrictor prostanoids [213].

Potential Mediators of Reperfusion Injury

Oxidative Stress

Hearse et al. [214] showed that anoxia in the absence of exogenous supplies of glucose causes enzyme release from the isolated, perfused rat heart. They found that reoxygenation after 7–8 hours triggered an immediate and massive increase in protein and enzyme release from the myocardium. They termed this the "oxygen paradox," and suggested that ROS might be responsible. The release of ROS in the ischemic myocardium occurs during reperfusion, resulting in oxidative stress [215, 216]; it constitutes a part of the oxygen paradox, with reoxygenation of the ischemic myocardium causing myocardial injury exceeding that incurred during the ischemic episode [206]. The release of free radicals occurs in the early phase of reperfusion, and reduces the availability of NO and its associated cardioprotective effects, e.g., inactivation of superoxide radicals, enhanced coronary flow, and inhibition of neutrophil accumulation [217]. Therefore, oxidative stress not only contributes directly to cardiomyocyte damage but also attenuates the increase in blood flow that is necessary to alleviate hypoperfusion and allows neutrophils to accumulate and thereby compromises perfusion.

A recent twist to the oxidative stress theory concerns the role of mitochondrial permeability transition pores (mPTPs) in reperfusion injury to the heart [218]. In injured cardiac muscle, oxygen radicals and high Ca^{2+} cause these pores to open, thus destroying the mitochondria and killing the cell. Blocking pore formation salvages a large amount of cardiac tissue after ischemia/reperfusion, indicating that this mechanism is a major mode of cell death, and a likely target for ROS. Ischemic pre- and postconditioning (see below) are both thought to protect the cell by preventing the opening of mPTPs during the first minutes of reperfusion. As mitochondria are destroyed by mPTP opening they release cytochrome C, causing slow apoptotic cell death; however, if enough mitochondria are destroyed, necrosis quickly ensues as a consequence of energy depletion.

The Calcium Paradox

Two types of injury that occur during reperfusion impair the mechanisms that regulate Ca^{2+} in the cardiomyocyte. In one, intracellular Ca^{2+} increases and, along with oxygen radicals, contributes to cardiomyocyte damage and death [219]. In the second, sarcolemmal damage occurs, and when myocardial reperfusion resumes, intracellular Ca^{2+} increases particularly abruptly [206]. This calcium paradox causes a Ca^{2+} overload in the cytoplasm and mitochondria, thereby inducing cell death. The importance of the calcium paradox in cardiomyocyte death was validated by experimental studies that demonstrated reductions in infarct size of as much as 50% when Ca^{2+} overload was pharmacologically attenuated by applying antagonists of the (1) Ca^{2+} ion channel, (2) mitochondrial Ca^{2+} uniporter, or (3) sodium-hydrogen exchanger (reviewed in [206]). Another phenomenon that contributes to ischemia–reperfusion injury is the pH paradox [220], i.e., the acidosis that occurs during ischemia protects cardiomyocytes from lethal injury by inhibiting degradative enzymes. However, the onset of reperfusion returns cellular pH to normal (isotonic) values, and may enhance mitochondrial permeability and activate myofibrillar ATPase, resulting in a decrease in the ATP supply. As noted above, any increase in intracellular Ca^{2+} will also contribute to mPTP opening.

Conclusions: Reperfusion Injury

Reperfusion following ischemia and infarction is necessary for limiting myocardial damage, yet it also triggers mediators of injury. Not only radicals generated by cardiomyocytes but also other agents of myocardial damage are generated, including inflammatory cells that block microvessels and release oxidants and ROS, thereby causing Ca^{2+} overload and altered vasoreactivity. Most important, however, is the effect of these substances on mPTPs; the opening of these pores triggers both apoptosis and necrosis in cardiomyocytes, and may account for a large portion of the irreversible injury that occurs in the reperfused heart.

Ischemic Preconditioning

Myocardial ischemic preconditioning (IPC), which consists of brief episodes of coronary occlusion and reperfusion, renders the heart more tolerant to ischemia and consequently limits the size of infarction. The fact that acute coronary occlusion is the leading cause of morbidity and mortality in the Western world [221] underscores the need for preventive measures with effects similar to these. Maroko and colleagues [222–224] were the first to explore the effectiveness of various interventions (i.e., the application of beta blockers, glucose–insulin–potassium, and hyaluronidase) in reducing infarct size, using dogs and surrogate markers of infarction. Although none of the interventions tested in this particular study were found to limit infarct size, a decade later Jennings and Reimer [3] provided the first evidence that early reperfusion could do so, and 3 years after that Murry et al. and Reimer et al. [225, 226] provided the first evidence, in dogs, that IPC enhances the myocardium's resistance to ischemia and thereby limits infarct size. This seminal finding has been affirmed in many human and animal studies, and the evidence has been extensively reviewed by Yellon and Downey [221] and Yang et al. [227]. IPC has been demonstrated in a variety of animal species: dog [226], mouse [228]

[229], rat [230], pig [231], rabbit [232], sheep [229], and chicken [230]. Notably, the second-fourth coronary occlusions were found to cause no further ATP depletion, providing the insight that energy metabolism in the ischemic myocardium is different after the first ischemic episode [225]. IPC consists of two phases that are regulated by distinct mechanisms (1) an early phase which develops within a few minutes of the exposure to the stimulus and lasts for 1–2 h and (2) a late phase that develops after 6 h or more and lasts several days [234, 235]. During the early phase, preexisting proteins are activated, whereas the late phase involves new synthesized cardioprotective proteins. The early phase of IPC limits infarct size but not postischemic contractile dysfunction. The late phase protects against both stunning and infarction, but is less potent than the early phase in limiting infarct size.

Experimental Evidence from Animal Studies

IPC Delays Infarct Development

Studies on experimental animals have provided consistent data establishing that IPC minimizes infarct size. The reductions measured were 40–60% in dogs [236], 42% in mice [228], 79% in swine [231], 49% in rats [230], 90% in rabbits [232], and 54% in sheep [229]. Several studies have demonstrated that IPC attenuates neutrophil accumulation in ischemic tissues in dogs [237, 238] and rats [239]. In addition to minimizing necrosis in the ischemic heart in this way, IPC also leads to a decrease in apoptosis [238–240], a form of cell death that has been found to occur primarily after reperfusion and along a time course that is slower than that of necrosis [241]. Experiments in a Langendorff-perfused heart revealed that EC apoptosis precedes cardiomyocyte apoptosis during reperfusion, indicating that the coronary vasculature may promote cardiomyocyte apoptosis by releasing proapoptotic proteins [242].

IPC Protects the Coronary Endothelium

Following reperfusion, vascular permeability increases, as does the number of inflammatory cells in the ischemic region. This suggests that endothelial dysfunction may be related to the vascular apoptosis and necrosis observed in the context of IR. The protective effect of IPC can in part be attributed to its effectiveness in reducing the generation of ROS by inflammatory cells, ECs, and cardiomyocytes [243–247]. The administration of superoxide dismutase in dogs with reperfused myocardial infarction reduced the extent of apoptosis by 50% [243]. Taken together, these data indicate that tissue responses to IR (1) involve both necrosis and apoptosis and (2) affect both the vascular endothelium and cardiomyocytes. Accordingly, the benefits of IPC appear to apply to both the coronary vasculature and the myocardium.

Ischemic vs. Hypoxic Preconditioning

In Chap. 9, the cardioprotective effects of hypoxic exposure were discussed. Hypoxic exposure is also a form of preconditioning. How similar the mechanisms underlying ischemic and hypoxic preconditioning are has been questioned [246]. To answer this question, Ostadalova and colleagues [247] found that mitochondrial K_{ATP} channels and NO in neonatal rats may be involved in the contractile adaptive mechanism associated with hypoxic but not IPC. Moreover, the greatest percent recovery was achieved when both hypoxic and IPC were applied. These results suggest that the two types of preconditioning include at least some separate, as well as complementary, mechanisms. As noted in Chap. 9, hypoxic preconditioning in adult rats not only increases the heart's tolerance to ischemia/reperfusion but also limits infarct size [248]. For example, rats exposed to chronic isobaric hypoxia for 3 weeks prior to myocardial IR had smaller infarcts [249]. Notably, this reduction, expressed as a percentage of the area at risk in rats exposed to intermittent hypoxia, was less after 35 days and absent by 90 days of normoxia [250]. That study also revealed that the ability of preexposure to hypoxia to limit infarct size was blunted if it was applied in the context of hypercapnia (CO_2=4.1%), a finding consistent with other data indicating that hypercapnia has an inhibitory effect on hypoxia-induced changes, e.g., pulmonary vascular remodeling [251].

Ischemic Preconditioning in Humans

Although clinical studies of IPC with infarction as an endpoint are limited for ethical and logistic reasons, a considerable volume of evidence indicates that IPC in humans has beneficial effects for acute ischemia. For example, patients who experience preinfarction angina have smaller infarcts and better outcome after thrombolytic therapy than patients who do not [202, 252–255]. Other support for preconditioning of the human myocardium comes from in vivo studies on the effects of (1) exercise, (2) angioplasty, and (3) surgery (reviewed in [221] and Tomai et al. [256]). Some patients experience the phenomenon of exercise warm-up, in which they develop angina when they first begin to exercise, but this initial pain is alleviated as they continue. The mechanisms responsible for this "first-effort angina" are not understood. Data from studies of angioplasty suggest that the procedure attenuates many or most indicators of myocardial ischemia. Specifically, when a first balloon inflation is carried out for 60–90 s, subsequent inflations do not evoke indicators of ischemia. Coronary bypass surgery has provided a unique opportunity to determine if preconditioning prior to ischemia is produced by cross-clamping. Preconditioning under this circumstance has been shown to minimize myocardial necrosis [257, 258]. In vitro studies on human muscle and cell preparations also indicate a role for preconditioning in reducing ischemia-induced injury. For example, studies by Ikonomidis and colleagues [259, 260] demonstrated that brief periods of simulated ischemia protected cardiomyocytes from injury, and that adenosine and PKC signaling play roles in this model of preconditioning. Human atrial muscle strips suspended in an organ bath also exhibited better mechanical function after a hypoxic insult if they had been subjected to simulated ischemia [261].

Conclusions

Considerable evidence from humans has revealed that preinfarction angina triggers mechanisms that may facilitate a reduction in infarct size, decrease the frequency of arrhythmias, and improve ventricular function. Moreover, patients with a history of preinfarction angina have better coronary flow following thrombolysis. Data from these studies also suggest that exercise may be an effective means of preconditioning. Despite substantial preclinical evidence supporting preconditioning, investigations on patients are yet to document, in clinical trials, a preconditioning mimetic agent that reduces infarct size.

Phases and Mechanisms Involved in Ischemic Preconditioning (See Reviews By [227, 262])

As noted more than 2 decades ago [263], many mechanisms could potentially explain the effectiveness of IPC. One among these is the slowing of energy metabolism, which would be consistent with the observation that ATP levels are higher in hearts subjected to IPC than hearts naïve to ischemia [264]. The observation that adenosine is elevated during ischemia led to a study on rabbit hearts, where IPC was found to greatly reduce infarct size, and two distinct, nonselective adenosine receptor antagonists each blocked the protective effect of IPC [265]. When either adenosine or an A_1-adenosine receptor selective adenosine agonist was added to a perfusate and introduced into the coronary circulation of an isolated rabbit heart prior to a 30-min coronary occlusion, the area affected by myocardial infarction was 25% of that in hearts from non-treated rabbits. Subsequent studies in rabbits [266], dogs [267], and swine [10] confirmed that adenosine plays a role in IPC. Although every Gi-coupled receptor tested in the heart triggered the preconditioned state [268], ligands of only four of these receptors were released during transient ischemia; therefore, only these receptors are capable of triggering preconditioning. The sections below review the data concerning the regulation of IPC with regard to its early and late phases.

Early Phase of IPC

The initiation of reperfusion is associated with H^+ washout from ischemic cells, an increase in pH, and the formation of mPTPs. When the mPTPs open, cytochrome C is released and mitochondrial electron transport becomes uncoupled from ATP synthesis. Thus, ATP production ceases and cardiomyocyte necrosis ensues. Given that IPC negates the formation of mPTPs, cardiocyte damage and necrosis are minimized. The specific differences between a cell that is preconditioned and one that is not clear, but one theory focuses on the ligand affinity of the adenosine A_{2B} receptors. According to it, IPC activates protein kinase C (PKC), which increases the affinity of A_{2B}, thus allowing adenosine to inhibit mPTP. The signaling pathway from the receptor to PKC involves the activation of eNOS and the consequent production of NO, which in turn activates protein kinase G (PKG) via guanylyl cyclase. PKG then phosphorylates a mitochondrial target, causing redox signaling and PKC activation [269]. Ultimately, the inhibition of mPTPs protects against reperfusion injury [270]. During the trigger phase of IPC, bradykinin and opioids are released, along with adenosine [271, 272], and each of these molecules target PKC via signaling pathways.

Delayed (Late) Phase of IPC

A second phase of IPC, noted 2 decades ago [234, 235], occurs when reperfusion occurs 24–48 h later than the initial preconditioning, and its effects can last for 3–4 days. The so-called "preinfarct angina," defined as angina chest pain 24–48 h prior to acute myocardial infarction, is a form of second window of preconditioning (SWOP), and is associated with better ejection fraction and survival [273], as well as fewer regional motion abnormalities [274]. This delayed IPC extends the window of cardioprotection by recruiting several signaling pathways (reviewed in [275]).

As reviewed by Bolli et al. [276], the mechanisms responsible for the delayed phase of IPC involve (1) the triggers eNOS-derived NO, ROS, and adenosine; (2) kinase activation by the triggering agents; (3) signal transduction to activate transcription factors (NF-κB, STAT 1/3); (4) upregulation of target genes; and finally (5) expression of the mediators of delayed IPC (iNOS, COX-2, HO-1, and antioxidant enzymes). The first four events occur on day 1 and the fifth on days 2–4. Twenty-four hours after exposure of the heart to an IPC protocol, iNOS is only modestly elevated, yet IPC fails to develop in its absence—which underscores its effectiveness in late IPC, i.e., its effect at low levels [163, 277]. Levels of the COX-2 protein are also elevated 24 h following the IPC protocol, and this is necessary for the cardioprotective effects of late IPC [278]. The signaling that triggers early IPC also appears to control iNOS levels, since blocking PKC or redox signaling for early IPC also blocked iNOS expression a day later [279].

Remote Preconditioning

One of the encouraging prospects for IPC is the phenomenon of remote ischemic conditioning, a concept first described by Przyklenk et al. [280]. This group's experiments in dogs revealed that ischemia in the territory of one coronary artery reduced subsequent potentially lethal ischemia in the territory of another coronary artery. Later studies (reviewed in [281]) have shown that remote IPC can be induced noninvasively by limb ischemia, to protect the myocardium. Such an approach can also be utilized for ischemic postconditioning (IPost), a topic reviewed by Wei [282]. The clinical effectiveness of remote conditioning is yet to be established, but it is attractive in that it could be routinely administered to patients suspected to have myocardial ischemia, using a simple blood-pressure cuff.

Conclusions: Ischemic Preconditioning
Many of the mechanisms involved in IPC-mediated attenuation of infarct size have been elucidated. First, triggers include adenosine, bradykinin, opioids, and sphingosine, and these must summate to induce the preconditioned state. Second, receptors that initiate certain signaling pathways (including the NOS, PKG, mitochondrial K_{ATP} channel, redox signaling, PKC, Akt, and ERK pathways) must be occupied. Finally, inhibition of lethal mPTPs must occur during the first few minutes of reperfusion.

Ischemic Postconditioning

IPC has limited application as a clinical entity because it must be initiated prior to the ischemic event that leads to myocardial infarction. In contrast, myocardial IPost can be administered at the onset of reperfusion, after a period of sustained ischemia. IPost consists of repeated brief occlusions of a coronary artery immediately following a prolonged coronary occlusion, and protects by the same mechanisms that contribute to IPC. Therefore, it becomes possible to confer myocardial protection pharmacologically (reviewed in [262, 283]), and in a clinical setting such as primary angioplasty. For a more complete review of IPost and its clinical possibilities, see Cohen and Downey [262], Ovize et al. [283] and Granfeldt et al. [284].

Experimental Animal Studies

Reduction of Infarct Size

Zhao et al. [196] compared IPost and IPC in dogs and found that the two interventions achieved comparable inhibition of myocardial injury, as judged by tissue edema, neutrophil accumulation, and size of the area at risk. Moreover, IPC and IPost have been documented to be equally effective in reducing infarct size, in a number of species including rabbits [285, 286], dogs [287], and rats [288]. The experiments in rabbits were confirmed numerous times in several laboratories (see review by [289]), and during the last decade a plethora of studies in rodents have documented a significant, even dramatic, reduction in infarct size after IPost. These data, as well as experimental protocols using both isolated and in vivo hearts, have been reviewed [284, 289]. Most studies found that IPost attenuated infarct size by about 20–40%. Notably, examples of data from in situ experiments [290–295] are in agreement with those from studies in which global ischemia was induced using a Langendorff preparation [296–299].

In their review, Skyschally and colleagues [289] point out that the algorithms of the IPost protocols utilized in the various animal studies affect the outcome of these studies. For example, if the ischemic period is prolonged, the infarct progresses to a point where tissue recovery due to conditioning is very limited, whereas if the ischemic period is shortened, the infarction that develops is limited and the potential for IPost-mediated protection is lost. Other critical variables include (1) the duration of the initial reperfusion period after the index of ischemia, (2) the number of occlusion cycles, and (3) the duration of each reperfusion period. In light of these considerations, it is notable that despite protocol differences in the studies surveyed, few failed to demonstrate a significant reduction in infarct size when IPost was applied.

Benefits of IPost for the Coronary Vasculature

The reduction in infarct size attributed to IPost is associated with improvements in both cardiac and coronary function. With respect to the former, an antiarrhythmic effect of IPost has been demonstrated in rats [300–303], cats [304], and dogs [287]. Also, IPost leads to ROS attenuation during IR [196] and after hypoxia and reoxygenation [305]. Animals subjected to IPost also were found to experience improvements in the coronary vasculature. Zhao et al. [196] found that endothelial function, as assessed by the maximal vasodilator response of the left anterior descending artery to acetylcholine, was greater in both IPC and IPost dogs. They also documented a decrease in neutrophil adherence and an accumulation of these cells in the left anterior descending coronary artery, a finding that is consistent with a decline in levels of P-selectin (a cell surface-localized carbohydrate-binding protein), which mediates cell–cell adhesion in the bloodstream.

Studies in Humans

To test the hypothesis that levels of creatine kinase (used clinically as an indicator of infarct size) are attenuated in patients, IPost records of 376 patients requiring multiple balloon inflations–deflations during primary angioplasty were compared to those of patients who required only minimal inflations or underwent direct stenting [286]. Peak creatine kinase release was 40% lower in the patients to whom four or more inflations were administered than in those administered only one to three. Subsequently, a review and meta-analysis of 6 studies on patients who underwent IPost conditioning during primary percutaneous coronary intervention concluded that these patients benefited from the treatment [306]. The six studies reviewed [307–312] included 244 patients. Of particular significance is the finding that patients who have undergone IPost have improved ST-segment resolution [308, 312], a greater reserve of coronary flow velocity [312] and improved endothelium-dependent vasodilation [309].

Mechanisms Underlying Ischemic Postconditioning

Cardioprotection by IPost involves several mechanisms that have been reviewed by Ovize et al. [283]. First, IPost leads to the formation and release of several autacoids and cytokines. Notably, classical autacoids trigger well-characterized mechanisms involving several receptor classes. For example, activation of the δ-opioid receptor during IPost reduces infarct size. This mechanism probably involves mPTP modulation [313], as mitochondrial K_{ATP} channels have been reported to trigger IPost in rat hearts [314]. Further evidence supporting the roles of opioids comes from several studies. In rats, IPost was shown to involve the preservation and activation of myocardial opioid content [315], and the beneficial effects of IPost (reductions in infarct size, caspase-3 activity, and apoptotic index) were abolished when the endogenous κ opioid receptor was inhibited by applying an antagonist [316]. Finally, the autacoid bradykinin also is cardioprotective in the IPost model, with its effects dependent on cyclooxygenase activation and prostacyclin release [317]. A second class of mechanism at play in IPost is the triggering of specific protein kinase cascades, some of which appear to offer protection both pre- and post-conditioning [318]. A third is the preservation of mitochondrial function. In mitochondria from IPost-treated myocardium, for example, tyrosine phosphorylation of STAT3 was enhanced and respiration via complex 1 and the capacity for calcium retention were better preserved [319]; these improvements in mitochondrial function were abrogated by STAT3 inhibition. mPTPs and K_{ATP} channels are considered "end effectors" in IPost [320]. Finally, IPost leads to the maintenance of acidosis, causing an accumulation of Na^+, and subsequently Ca^{2+} overload [283].

In 2007, Cohen et al. [321] proposed the pH hypothesis, which explains all of the above observations. Specifically, based on the observation that mPTPs open only at the onset of reperfusion because they are inhibited by acidosis during ischemia, these authors suggested that ischemia activates the signal cascade involved in IPC, with the latter proceeding up to the redox signaling step, which requires oxygen. In the untreated heart, oxygen becomes available for redox signaling and signal transduction is completed, but the mPTPs open before protection can be established. IPC protocols lead to "staccato" reperfusion, with only limited amounts of oxygen made available for redox signaling, while acidosis in the tissue remains high enough to keep mPTPs closed. The IPC signal cascade is activated only after several minutes of this limited flow, and inhibits mPTP once full reperfusion occurs. This explains why the algorithm of the protocol is critical: if the reperfusion periods are too short, oxygen levels are insufficient for redox signaling, whereas if the reperfusion periods are too long, mPTPs can open before the protective signal is transduced.

Conclusions: IPost-Mediated Protection

IPost is significant clinically because protection can be conferred to the heart at the onset of reperfusion following an ischemic insult. This is essential if IPost is to be used effectively to treat patients suffering from acute myocardial infarction. Understanding the pathways that transduce IPost will make it possible to apply this method in patients with coronary disease. It is notable that IPost may be transduced by the same signaling cascade as IPC (evidence for this is reviewed by [322]), and appears to involve (1) cell-surface receptors, i.e., those for adenosine, bradykinin/δ-opioid/NP; (2) a host of kinases; and (3) mitochondrial components (M_{ATP}/mPTP, PKC, and ROS).

References

1. Tomanek RJ, Grimes JC, Diana JN. Relationship between the magnitude of myocardial ischemia and ultrastructural alterations. Exp Mol Pathol. 1981;35:65–83.
2. Reimer KA, Jennings RB. The "wavefront phenomenon" of myocardial ischemic cell death. II. Transmural progression of necrosis within the framework of ischemic bed size (myocardium at risk) and collateral flow. Lab Invest. 1979;40:633–44.
3. Jennings RB, Reimer KA. Factors involved in salvaging ischemic myocardium: effect of reperfusion of arterial blood. Circulation. 1983;68:I25–36.
4. Kharbanda RK. Cardiac conditioning: a review of evolving strategies to reduce ischaemia-reperfusion injury. Heart. 2010;96:1179–86.
5. Stern MD, Silverman HS, Houser SR, Josephson RA, Capogrossi MC, Nichols CG, et al. Anoxic contractile failure in rat heart myocytes is caused by failure of intracellular calcium release due to alteration of the action potential. Proc Natl Acad Sci USA. 1988;85:6954–8.
6. Bing OH, Brooks WW, Messer JV. Heart muscle viability following hypoxia: protective effect of acidosis. Science. 1973; 180:1297–8.

7. Schmidt-Ott SC, Bletz C, Vahl C, Saggau W, Hagl S, Ruegg JC. Inorganic phosphate inhibits contractility and ATPase activity in skinned fibers from human myocardium. Basic Res Cardiol. 1990;85:358–66.
8. Canty Jr JM, Fallavollita JA. Hibernating myocardium. J Nucl Cardiol. 2005;12:104–19.
9. Heyndrickx GR, Millard RW, McRitchie RJ, Maroko PR, Vatner SF. Regional myocardial functional and electrophysiological alterations after brief coronary artery occlusion in conscious dogs. J Clin Invest. 1975;56:978–85.
10. Schulz R, Rose J, Post H, Heusch G. Involvement of endogenous adenosine in ischaemic preconditioning in swine. Pflugers Arch. 1995;430:273–82.
11. Fallavollita JA, Logue M, Canty Jr JM. Stability of hibernating myocardium in pigs with a chronic left anterior descending coronary artery stenosis: absence of progressive fibrosis in the setting of stable reductions in flow, function and coronary flow reserve. J Am Coll Cardiol. 2001;37:1989–95.
12. Depre C, Vatner SF. Cardioprotection in stunned and hibernating myocardium. Heart Fail Rev. 2007;12:307–17.
13. Sayen JJ, Sheldon WF, Peirce G, Kuo PT. Polarographic oxygen, the epicardial electrocardiogram and muscle contraction in experimental acute regional ischemia of the left ventricle. Circ Res. 1958;6:779–98.
14. Jennings RB, Kaltenbach JP, Sommers HM, Bahr GF, Wartman WB. Studies of the dying. The etiology of myocardial infarction. Boston: Little and Brown; 1963. p. 189–205.
15. Jennings RB, Reimer KA. The cell biology of acute myocardial ischemia. Annu Rev Med. 1991;42:225–46.
16. Jennings RB, Steenbergen Jr C, Reimer KA. Myocardial ischemia and reperfusion. Monogr Pathol. 1995;37:47–80.
17. Larsen BT, Gutterman DD. Hypoxia, coronary dilation, and the pentose phosphate pathway. Am J Physiol Heart Circ Physiol. 2006;290:H2169–71.
18. Close LA, Bowman PS, Paul RJ. Reoxygenation-induced relaxation of coronary arteries. A novel endothelium-dependent mechanism. Circ Res. 1994;74:870–81.
19. Lee YH, Kim JT, Kang BS. Mechanisms of relaxation of coronary artery by hypoxia. Yonsei Med J. 1998;39:252–60.
20. Gupte SA, Wolin MS. Hypoxia promotes relaxation of bovine coronary arteries through lowering cytosolic NADPH. Am J Physiol Heart Circ Physiol. 2006;290:H2228–38.
21. Frobert O, Haink G, Simonsen U, Gravholt CH, Levin M, Deussen A. Adenosine concentration in the porcine coronary artery wall and A2A receptor involvement in hypoxia-induced vasodilatation. J Physiol. 2006;570:375–84.
22. Wolin MS, Burke-Wolin TM, Mohazzab HK. Roles for NAD(P)H oxidases and reactive oxygen species in vascular oxygen sensing mechanisms. Respir Physiol. 1999;115:229–38.
23. Mohazzab KM, Kaminski PM, Wolin MS. NADH oxidoreductase is a major source of superoxide anion in bovine coronary artery endothelium. Am J Physiol. 1994;266:H2568–72.
24. Mohazzab HK, Kaminski PM, Fayngersh RP, Wolin MS. Oxygen-elicited responses in calf coronary arteries: role of H_2O_2 production via NADH-derived superoxide. Am J Physiol. 1996;270: H1044–53.
25. von Beckerath N, Cyrys S, Dischner A, Daut J. Hypoxic vasodilatation in isolated, perfused guinea-pig heart: an analysis of the underlying mechanisms. J Physiol. 1991;442:297–319.
26. Selwyn AP, Forse G, Fox K, Jonathan A, Steiner R. Patterns of disturbed myocardial perfusion in patients with coronary artery disease. Regional myocardial perfusion in angina pectoris. Circulation. 1981;64:83–90.
27. Sambuceti G, Marzilli M, Fedele S, Marini C, L'Abbate A. Paradoxical increase in microvascular resistance during tachycardia downstream from a severe stenosis in patients with coronary artery disease: reversal by angioplasty. Circulation. 2001;103: 2352–60.
28. Metais C, Bianchi C, Li J, Simons M, Sellke FW. Serotonin-induced human coronary microvascular contraction during acute myocardial ischemia is blocked by COX-2 inhibition. Basic Res Cardiol. 2001;96:59–67.
29. Kusmic C, Lazzerini G, Coceani F, Barsacchi R, L'Abbate A, Sambuceti G. Paradoxical coronary microcirculatory constriction during ischemia: a synergic function for nitric oxide and endothelin. Am J Physiol Heart Circ Physiol. 2006;291:H1814–21.
30. Duncker DJ, Bache RJ. Regulation of coronary vasomotor tone under normal conditions and during acute myocardial hypoperfusion. Pharmacol Ther. 2000;86:87–110.
31. Martinez-Lemus LA, Hill MA, Meininger GA. The plastic nature of the vascular wall: a continuum of remodeling events contributing to control of arteriolar diameter and structure. Physiology (Bethesda). 2009;24:45–57.
32. Mills I, Fallon JT, Wrenn D, Sasken H, Gray W, Bier J, et al. Adaptive responses of coronary circulation and myocardium to chronic reduction in perfusion pressure and flow. Am J Physiol. 1994;266:H447–57.
33. Pistea A, Bakker EN, Spaan JA, VanBavel E. Flow inhibits inward remodeling in cannulated porcine small coronary arteries. Am J Physiol Heart Circ Physiol. 2005;289:H2632–40.
34. Hong H, Aksenov S, Guan X, Fallon JT, Waters D, Chen C. Remodeling of small intramyocardial coronary arteries distal to a severe epicardial coronary artery stenosis. Arterioscler Thromb Vasc Biol. 2002;22:2059–65.
35. Sorop O, Merkus D, de Beer VJ, Houweling B, Pistea A, McFalls EO, et al. Functional and structural adaptations of coronary microvessels distal to a chronic coronary artery stenosis. Circ Res. 2008;102:795–803.
36. Chamuleau SA, Siebes M, Meuwissen M, Koch KT, Spaan JA, Piek JJ. Association between coronary lesion severity and distal microvascular resistance in patients with coronary artery disease. Am J Physiol Heart Circ Physiol. 2003;285:H2194–200.
37. Fearon WF, Aarnoudse W, Pijls NH, De Bruyne B, Balsam LB, Cooke DT, et al. Microvascular resistance is not influenced by epicardial coronary artery stenosis severity: experimental validation. Circulation. 2004;109:2269–72.
38. Ku DD. Coronary vascular reactivity after acute myocardial ischemia. Science. 1982;218:576–8.
39. Luo Y, Cha DG, Liu YL, Zhou SF. Coronary microcirculation changes during myocardial stunning in dogs. Cardiology. 2010;117:68–74.
40. Saito T, Fushimi E, Abe T, Kimura Y, Takahashi K, Kudo Y, et al. Augmented contractile response to endothelin and blunted endothelium-dependent relaxation in post-ischemic reperfused coronary arteries. Jpn Circ J. 1992;56:657–70.
41. Coughlan MG, Kenny D, Kampine JP, Bosnjak ZJ, Warltier DC. Differential sensitivity of proximal and distal coronary arteries to a nitric oxide donor following reperfusion injury or inhibition of nitric oxide synthesis. Cardiovasc Res. 1993;27:1444–8.
42. Symons JD, Schaefer S. Na(+)/H(+) exchange subtype 1 inhibition reduces endothelial dysfunction in vessels from stunned myocardium. Am J Physiol Heart Circ Physiol. 2001;281:H1575–82.
43. Wang QD, Uriuda Y, Pernow J, Hemsen A, Sjoquist PO, Ryden L. Myocardial release of endothelin (ET) and enhanced ET(A) receptor-mediated coronary vasoconstriction after coronary thrombosis and thrombolysis in pigs. J Cardiovasc Pharmacol. 1995;26:770–6.
44. Tsao PS, Aoki N, Lefer DJ, Johnson 3rd G, Lefer AM. Time course of endothelial dysfunction and myocardial injury during myocardial ischemia and reperfusion in the cat. Circulation. 1990;82:1402–12.
45. Fernandez N, Martinez MA, Climent B, Garcia-Villalon AL, Monge L, Sanz E, et al. Coronary reactivity to endothelin-1 during

partial ischemia and reperfusion in anesthetized goats. Role of nitric oxide and prostanoids. Eur J Pharmacol. 2002;457:161–8.
46. Heusch G, Deussen A, Thamer V. Cardiac sympathetic nerve activity and progressive vasoconstriction distal to coronary stenoses: feed-back aggravation of myocardial ischemia. J Auton Nerv Syst. 1985;13:311–26.
47. Aversano T, Klocke FJ, Mates RE, Canty JM Jr. Preload-induced alterations in capacitance-free diastolic pressure-flow relationship. Am J physiol. 1984;246(3Pt2):H410–17.
48. Lefer AM, Lefer DJ. The role of nitric oxide and cell adhesion molecules on the microcirculation in ischaemia-reperfusion. Cardiovasc Res. 1996;32:743–51.
49. Lefer AM, Campbell B, Scalia R, Lefer DJ. Synergism between platelets and neutrophils in provoking cardiac dysfunction after ischemia and reperfusion: role of selectins. Circulation. 1998;98:1322–8.
50. Pagliaro P, Chiribiri A, Mancardi D, Rastaldo R, Gattullo D, Losano G. Coronary endothelial dysfunction after ischemia and reperfusion and its prevention by ischemic preconditioning. Ital Heart J. 2003;4:383–94.
51. Kadletz M, Dignan RJ, Loesser KE, Hess ML, Wechsler AS. Ischemia and activated neutrophils alter coronary microvascular but not epicardial coronary artery reactivity. J Thorac Cardiovasc Surg. 1994;108:648–57.
52. Welbourn CR, Goldman G, Paterson IS, Valeri CR, Shepro D, Hechtman HB. Pathophysiology of ischaemia reperfusion injury: central role of the neutrophil. Br J Surg. 1991;78:651–5.
53. Yang BC, Nicolini FA, Nichols WW, Mehta JL. Decreased endothelium-dependent vascular relaxation following subtotal coronary artery occlusion in dogs. Free Radic Biol Med. 1993;14:295–302.
54. Sellke FW, Boyle Jr EM, Verrier ED. Endothelial cell injury in cardiovascular surgery: the pathophysiology of vasomotor dysfunction. Ann Thorac Surg. 1996;62:1222–8.
55. Metais C, Li J, Simons M, Sellke FW. Serotonin-induced coronary contraction increases after blood cardioplegia-reperfusion: role of COX-2 expression. Circulation. 1999;100:II328–34.
56. Kawata H, Sawatari K, Mayer Jr JE. Evidence for the role of neutrophils in reperfusion injury after cold cardioplegic ischemia in neonatal lambs. J Thorac Cardiovasc Surg. 1992;103:908–17. discussion 17–8.
57. Sellke FW, Quillen JE. Altered effects of vasopressin on the coronary circulation after ischemia. J Thorac Cardiovasc Surg. 1992;104:357–63.
58. Dagenais F, Cartier R, Hollmann C, Buluran J. Calcium-channel blockers preserve coronary endothelial reactivity after ischemia-reperfusion. Ann Thorac Surg. 1997;63:1050–6.
59. Kikkawa K, Murata S, Nagao T. Endothelium-dependent calcium-induced relaxation in the presence of Ca^{2+}-antagonists in canine depolarized coronary arteries. Br J Pharmacol. 1989;98:700–6.
60. Jayakody RL, Kappagoda CT, Senaratne MP, Sreeharan N. Absence of effect of calcium antagonists on endothelium-dependent relaxation in rabbit aorta. Br J Pharmacol. 1987;91:155–64.
61. Vanhoutte PM. Role of calcium and endothelium in hypertension, cardiovascular disease, and subsequent vascular events. J Cardiovasc Pharmacol. 1992;19 Suppl 3:S6–10.
62. Karasawa A, Kubo K. Protection by benidipine hydrochloride (KW-3049), a calcium antagonist, of ischemic kidney in rats via inhibitions of Ca-overload, ATP-decline and lipid peroxidation. Jpn J Pharmacol. 1990;52:553–62.
63. Clark RE, Magovern GJ, Christlieb IY, Boe S. Nifedipine cardioplegia experience: results of a 3-year cooperative clinical study. Ann Thorac Surg. 1983;36:654–63.
64. Christakis GT, Fremes SE, Weisel RD, Tittley JG, Mickle DA, Ivanov J, et al. Diltiazem cardioplegia. A balance of risk and benefit. J Thorac Cardiovasc Surg. 1986;91:647–61.
65. Kunsch C, Medford RM. Oxidative stress as a regulator of gene expression in the vasculature. Circ Res. 1999;85:753–66.
66. Miura H, Bosnjak JJ, Ning G, Saito T, Miura M, Gutterman DD. Role for hydrogen peroxide in flow-induced dilation of human coronary arterioles. Circ Res. 2003;92:e31–40.
67. Barlow RS, White RE. Hydrogen peroxide relaxes porcine coronary arteries by stimulating BKCa channel activity. Am J Physiol. 1998;275:H1283–9.
68. Liu Y, Bubolz AH, Mendoza S, Zhang DX, Gutterman DD. H_2O_2 is the transferrable factor mediating flow-induced dilation in human coronary arterioles. Circ Res. 2011;108:566–73.
69. Yada T, Shimokawa H, Hiramatsu O, Haruna Y, Morita Y, Kashihara N, et al. Cardioprotective role of endogenous hydrogen peroxide during ischemia-reperfusion injury in canine coronary microcirculation in vivo. Am J Physiol Heart Circ Physiol. 2006;291:H1138–46.
70. Feng J, Damrauer SM, Lee M, Sellke FW, Ferran C, Abid MR. Endothelium-dependent coronary vasodilatation requires NADPH oxidase-derived reactive oxygen species. Arterioscler Thromb Vasc Biol. 2010;30:1703–10.
71. Li J, De Leon H, Ueno T, Cui J, Coussement PK, King 3rd SB, et al. Vasomotor function of pig coronary arteries after chronic coronary occlusion. J Cardiovasc Pharmacol. 2003;41:600–8.
72. Li G, Xiao Y, Estrella JL, Ducsay CA, Gilbert RD, Zhang L. Effect of fetal hypoxia on heart susceptibility to ischemia and reperfusion injury in the adult rat. J Soc Gynecol Investig. 2003;10: 265–74.
73. Quillen JE, Sellke FW, Brooks LA, Harrison DG. Ischemia-reperfusion impairs endothelium-dependent relaxation of coronary microvessels but does not affect large arteries. Circulation. 1990;82:586–94.
74. Cannon 3rd RO, Camici PG, Epstein SE. Pathophysiological dilemma of syndrome X. Circulation. 1992;85:883–92.
75. Buffon A, Rigattieri S, Santini SA, Ramazzotti V, Crea F, Giardina B, et al. Myocardial ischemia-reperfusion damage after pacing-induced tachycardia in patients with cardiac syndrome X. Am J Physiol Heart Circ Physiol. 2000;279:H2627–33.
76. Chauhan A, Mullins PA, Taylor G, Petch MC, Schofield PM. Both endothelium-dependent and endothelium-independent function is impaired in patients with angina pectoris and normal coronary angiograms. Eur Heart J. 1997;18:60–8.
77. Maseri A, Crea F, Kaski JC, Crake T. Mechanisms of angina pectoris in syndrome X. J Am Coll Cardiol. 1991;17:499–506.
78. Konidala S, Gutterman DD. Coronary vasospasm and the regulation of coronary blood flow. Prog Cardiovasc Dis. 2004;46: 349–73.
79. Tun A, Khan IA. Myocardial infarction with normal coronary arteries: the pathologic and clinical perspectives. Angiology. 2001;52:299–304.
80. Masumoto A, Mohri M, Takeshita A. Three-year follow-up of the Japanese patients with microvascular angina attributable to coronary microvascular spasm. Int J Cardiol. 2001;81:151–6.
81. Saitoh S, Onogi F, Aikawa K, Mutor M, Saito T, Maehara K, Maruyama Y, Multiple endothelial injury in epicardial coronary artery induces downstresm microvascular spasm as well as remodeling partly via thromboxane A2. J Am Coll Cardiol. 2001;37:308–15.
82. VanBenthuysen KM, McMurtry IF, Horwitz LD. Reperfusion after acute coronary occlusion in dogs impairs endothelium-dependent relaxation to acetylcholine and augments contractile reactivity in vitro. J Clin Invest. 1987;79:265–74.

83. Lee SH, Wolf PL, Escudero R, Deutsch R, Jamieson SW, Thistlethwaite PA. Early expression of angiogenesis factors in acute myocardial ischemia and infarction. N Engl J Med. 2000;342:626–33.
84. Yamakawa M, Liu LX, Date T, Belanger AJ, Vincent KA, Akita GY, et al. Hypoxia-inducible factor-1 mediates activation of cultured vascular endothelial cells by inducing multiple angiogenic factors. Circ Res. 2003;93:664–73.
85. Kido M, Du L, Sullivan CC, Li X, Deutsch R, Jamieson SW, et al. Hypoxia-inducible factor 1-alpha reduces infarction and attenuates progression of cardiac dysfunction after myocardial infarction in the mouse. J Am Coll Cardiol. 2005;46:2116–24.
86. Shyu KG, Wang MT, Wang BW, Chang CC, Leu JG, Kuan P, et al. Intramyocardial injection of naked DNA encoding HIF-1alpha/VP16 hybrid to enhance angiogenesis in an acute myocardial infarction model in the rat. Cardiovasc Res. 2002;54:576–83.
87. Takeda K, Cowan A, Fong GH. Essential role for prolyl hydroxylase domain protein 2 in oxygen homeostasis of the adult vascular system. Circulation. 2007;116:774–81.
88. Jingjing L, Srinivasan B, Bian X, Downey HF, Roque RS. Vascular endothelial growth factor is increased following coronary artery occlusion in the dog heart. Mol Cell Biochem. 2000;214:23–30.
89. Li J, Brown LF, Hibberd MG, Grossman JD, Morgan JP, Simons M. VEGF, flk-1, and flt-1 expression in a rat myocardial infarction model of angiogenesis. Am J Physiol. 1996;270:H1803–11.
90. Heba G, Krzeminski T, Porc M, Grzyb J, Ratajska A, Dembinska-Kiec A. The time course of tumor necrosis factor-alpha, inducible nitric oxide synthase and vascular endothelial growth factor expression in an experimental model of chronic myocardial infarction in rats. J Vasc Res. 2001;38:288–300.
91. Schaper W. Collateral circulation: past and present. Basic Res Cardiol. 2009;104:5–21.
92. Berry C, Balachandran KP, L'Allier PL, Lesperance J, Bonan R, Oldroyd KG. Importance of collateral circulation in coronary heart disease. Eur Heart J. 2007;28:278–91.
93. Seiler C. The human coronary collateral circulation. Eur J Clin Invest. 2010;40:465–76.
94. Traupe T, Gloekler S, de Marchi SF, Werner GS, Seiler C. Assessment of the human coronary collateral circulation. Circulation. 2010;122:1210–20.
95. Fujita M, Tambara K. Recent insights into human coronary collateral development. Heart. 2004;90:246–50.
96. Meier P, Gloekler S, Zbinden R, Beckh S, de Marchi SF, Zbinden S, et al. Beneficial effect of recruitable collaterals: a 10-year follow-up study in patients with stable coronary artery disease undergoing quantitative collateral measurements. Circulation. 2007;116:975–83.
97. Cohen M, Rentrop KP. Limitation of myocardial ischemia by collateral circulation during sudden controlled coronary artery occlusion in human subjects: a prospective study. Circulation. 1986;74:469–76.
98. Cribier A, Korsatz L, Koning R, Rath P, Gamra H, Stix G, et al. Improved myocardial ischemic response and enhanced collateral circulation with long repetitive coronary occlusion during angioplasty: a prospective study. J Am Coll Cardiol. 1992;20:578–86.
99. Ohno A, Fujita M, Miwa K, Ejiri M, Asanoi H, Sasayama S. Importance of coronary collateral circulation for increased treadmill exercise capacity by nitrates in patients with stable effort angina pectoris. Cardiology. 1991;78:323–8.
100. Tanaka T, Fujita M, Nakae I, Tamaki S, Hasegawa K, Kihara Y, et al. Improvement of exercise capacity by sarpogrelate as a result of augmented collateral circulation in patients with effort angina. J Am Coll Cardiol. 1998;32:1982–6.
101. Fujita M, Yamanishi K, Inoko M, Miwa K. Preferential dilation of recipient coronary arteries of the collateral circulation by intracoronary administration of nitroglycerin. J Am Coll Cardiol. 1994;24:631–5.
102. Wustmann K, Zbinden S, Windecker S, Meier B, Seiler C. Is there functional collateral flow during vascular occlusion in angiographically normal coronary arteries? Circulation 2003;107:2213–20.
103. de Marchi SF, Gloekler S, Meier P, Traupe T, Steck H, Cook S, et al. Determinants of preformed collateral vessels in the human heart without coronary artery disease. Cardiology. 2011;118:198–206.
104. Schaper J, Mulch J, Winkler B, Schaper W. Ultrastructural, functional, and biochemical criteria for estimation of reversibility of ischemic injury: a study on the effects of global ischemia on the isolated dog heart. J Mol Cell Cardiol. 1979;11:521–41.
105. Fujita M, Ohno A, Wada O, Miwa K, Nozawa T, Yamanishi K, et al. Collateral circulation as a marker of the presence of viable myocardium in patients with recent myocardial infarction. Am Heart J. 1991;122:409–14.
106. Bexell D, Setser RM, Schoenhagen P, Lieber ML, Brener SJ, Ivanc TB, et al. Influence of coronary artery stenosis severity and coronary collateralization on extent of chronic myocardial scar: insights from quantitative coronary angiography and delayed-enhancement MRI. Open Cardiovasc Med J. 2008;2:79–86.
107. Habib GB, Heibig J, Forman SA, Brown BG, Roberts R, Terrin ML, et al. Influence of coronary collateral vessels on myocardial infarct size in humans. Results of phase I thrombolysis in myocardial infarction (TIMI) trial. The TIMI Investigators. Circulation. 1991;83:739–46.
108. Sheehan FH, Braunwald E, Canner P, Dodge HT, Gore J, Van Natta P, et al. The effect of intravenous thrombolytic therapy on left ventricular function: a report on tissue-type plasminogen activator and streptokinase from the Thrombolysis in Myocardial Infarction (TIMI Phase I) trial. Circulation. 1987;75:817–29.
109. Pohl T, Seiler C, Billinger M, Herren E, Wustmann K, Mehta H, et al. Frequency distribution of collateral flow and factors influencing collateral channel development. Functional collateral channel measurement in 450 patients with coronary artery disease. J Am Coll Cardiol. 2001;38:1872–8.
110. Ha JW, Cho SY, Jang YS, Chung N, Shim WH, Kim SS. Collateral circulation in total occlusion of the left anterior descending or right coronary artery. Yonsei Med J. 1994;35:132–41.
111. Werner GS, Surber R, Ferrari M, Fritzenwanger M, Figulla HR. The functional reserve of collaterals supplying long-term chronic total coronary occlusions in patients without prior myocardial infarction. Eur Heart J. 2006;27:2406–12.
112. Demirbag R, Gur M, Yilmaz R, Kunt AS, Erel O, Andac MH. Influence of oxidative stress on the development of collateral circulation in total coronary occlusions. Int J Cardiol. 2007;116:14–9.
113. Sahinarslan A, Kocaman SA, Topal S, Ercin U, Bukan N, Yalcin R, et al. Relation between serum monocyte chemoattractant protein-1 and coronary collateral development. Coron Artery Dis. 2010;21:455–9.
114. Lv S, Cheng G, Xu Y, Wang Y, Xu G. Relationship between serum thymosin beta4 levels and coronary collateral development. Coron Artery Dis. 2011;22:401–4.
115. Schaper W, Jageneau A, Xhonneux R. The development of collateral circulation in the pig and dog heart. Cardiologia. 1967;51:321–35.
116. Toyota E, Warltier DC, Brock T, Ritman E, Kolz C, O'Malley P, et al. Vascular endothelial growth factor is required for coronary collateral growth in the rat. Circulation. 2005;112:2108–13.
117. Carrao AC, Chilian WM, Yun J, Kolz C, Rocic P, Lehmann K, et al. Stimulation of coronary collateral growth by granulocyte stimulating factor: role of reactive oxygen species. Arterioscler Thromb Vasc Biol. 2009;29:1817–22.
118. Maxwell MP, Hearse DJ, Yellon DM. Species variation in the coronary collateral circulation during regional myocardial ischaemia: a critical determinant of the rate of evolution and extent of myocardial infarction. Cardiovasc Res. 1987;21:737–46.

119. Cohen MV, Downey JM, Sonnenblick EH, Kirk ES. The effects of nitroglycerin on coronary collaterals and myocardial contractility. J Clin Invest. 1973;52:2836–47.
120. Jugdutt BI, Becker LC, Hutchins GM, Bulkley BH, Reid PR, Kallman CH. Effect of intravenous nitroglycerin on collateral blood flow and infarct size in the conscious dog. Circulation. 1981;63:17–28.
121. Fujita M, McKown DP, McKown MD, Franklin D. Opening of coronary collaterals by repeated brief coronary occlusions in conscious dogs. Angiology. 1988;39:973–80.
122. Brazzamano S, Mays AE, Rembert JC, Greenfield Jr JC. Increase in collateral blood flow following repeated coronary artery occlusion and nitroglycerin administration. Circ Res. 1984;54:204–7.
123. Lohr NL, Warltier DC, Chilian WM, Weihrauch D. Haptoglobin expression and activity during coronary collateralization. Am J Physiol Heart Circ Physiol. 2005;288:H1389–95.
124. Yamamoto H, Tomoike H, Shimokawa H, Nabeyama S, Nakamura M. Development of collateral function with repetitive coronary occlusion in a canine model reduces myocardial reactive hyperemia in the absence of significant coronary stenosis. Circ Res. 1984;55:623–32.
125. Yamanishi K, Fujita M, Ohno A, Sasayama S. Importance of myocardial ischaemia for recruitment of coronary collateral circulation in dogs. Cardiovasc Res. 1990;24:271–7.
126. Schaper W, De Brabander M, Lewi P. DNA synthesis and mitoses in coronary collateral vessels of the dog. Circ Res. 1971;28:671–9.
127. Scheel KW, Galindez TA, Cook B, Rodriguez RJ, Ingram LA. Changes in coronary and collateral flows and adequacy of perfusion in the dog following one and three months of circumflex occlusion. Circ Res. 1976;39:654–8.
128. Scheel KW, Rodriguez RJ, Ingram LA. Directional coronary collateral growth with chronic circumflex occlusion in the dog. Circ Res. 1977;40:384–90.
129. Tomoike H, Inou T, Watanabe K, Mizukami M, Kikuchi Y, Nakamura M. Functional significance of collaterals during ameroid-induced coronary stenosis in conscious dogs. Interrelationships among regional shortening, regional flow and grade of coronary stenosis. Circulation. 1983;67:1001–8.
130. Gorge G, Schmidt T, Ito BR, Pantely GA, Schaper W. Microvascular and collateral adaptation in swine hearts following progressive coronary artery stenosis. Basic Res Cardiol. 1989;84:524–35.
131. Seko Y, Takahashi N, Shibuya M, Yazaki Y. Pulsatile stretch stimulates vascular endothelial growth factor (VEGF) secretion by cultured rat cardiac myocytes. Biochem Biophys Res Commun. 1999;254:462–5.
132. Zheng W, Seftor EA, Meininger CJ, Hendrix MJ, Tomanek RJ. Mechanisms of coronary angiogenesis in response to stretch: role of VEGF and TGF-beta. Am J Physiol Heart Circ Physiol. 2001;280:H909–17.
133. Zheng W, Christensen LP, Tomanek RJ. Stretch induces upregulation of key tyrosine kinase receptors in microvascular endothelial cells. Am J Physiol Heart Circ Physiol. 2004;287:H2739–45.
134. Lei L, Zhou R, Zheng W, Christensen LP, Weiss RM, Tomanek RJ. Bradycardia induces angiogenesis, increases coronary reserve, and preserves function of the postinfarcted heart. Circulation. 2004;110:796–802.
135. Lamping KG, Zheng W, Xing D, Christensen LP, Martins J, Tomanek RJ. Bradycardia stimulates vascular growth during gradual coronary occlusion. Arterioscler Thromb Vasc Biol. 2005;25:2122–7.
136. Ito WD, Arras M, Scholz D, Winkler B, Htun P, Schaper W. Angiogenesis but not collateral growth is associated with ischemia after femoral artery occlusion. Am J Physiol. 1997;273:H1255–65.
137. Pipp F, Boehm S, Cai WJ, Adili F, Ziegler B, Karanovic G, et al. Elevated fluid shear stress enhances postocclusive collateral artery growth and gene expression in the pig hind limb. Arterioscler Thromb Vasc Biol. 2004;24:1664–8.
138. Schaper W, Pipp F, Scholz D, Boehm S, Deindl E, Barancik M, et al. Physical forces and their translation into molecular mechanisms. Arteriogenesis. Boston: Kluwer Academic Publishing; 2004. p. 73–114.
139. Heil M, Schaper W. Influence of mechanical, cellular, and molecular factors on collateral artery growth (arteriogenesis). Circ Res. 2004;95:449–58.
140. Schaper W, Scholz D. Factors regulating arteriogenesis. Arterioscler Thromb Vasc Biol. 2003;23:1143–51.
141. Chilian WM, Mass HJ, Williams SE, Layne SM, Smith EE, Scheel KW. Microvascular occlusions promote coronary collateral growth. Am J Physiol. 1990;258:H1103–11.
142. Kersten JR, Pagel PS, Chilian WM, Warltier DC. Multifactorial basis for coronary collateralization: a complex adaptive response to ischemia. Cardiovasc Res. 1999;43:44–57.
143. van den Wijngaard JP, Schulten H, van Horssen P, Ter Wee RD, Siebes M, Post MJ, et al. Porcine coronary collateral formation in the absence of a pressure gradient remote of the ischemic border zone. Am J Physiol Heart Circ Physiol. 2011;300:H1930–7.
144. Lu H, Xu X, Zhang M, Cao R, Brakenhielm E, Li C, et al. Combinatorial protein therapy of angiogenic and arteriogenic factors remarkably improves collaterogenesis and cardiac function in pigs. Proc Natl Acad Sci USA. 2007;104:12140–5.
145. Carroll SM, White FC, Roth DM, Bloor CM. Heparin accelerates coronary collateral development in a porcine model of coronary artery occlusion. Circulation. 1993;88:198–207.
146. Herbert JM, Laplace MC, Maffrand JP. Effect of heparin on the angiogenic potency of basic and acidic fibroblast growth factors in the rabbit cornea assay. Int J Tissue React. 1988;10:133–9.
147. Bashkin P, Doctrow S, Klagsbrun M, Svahn CM, Folkman J, Vlodavsky I. Basic fibroblast growth factor binds to subendothelial extracellular matrix and is released by heparitinase and heparin-like molecules. Biochemistry. 1989;28:1737–43.
148. Gospodarowicz D, Cheng J. Heparin protects basic and acidic FGF from inactivation. J Cell Physiol. 1986;128:475–84.
149. Bombardini T, Picano E. The coronary angiogenetic effect of heparin: experimental basis and clinical evidence. Angiology. 1997;48:969–76.
150. Lazarous DF, Scheinowitz M, Shou M, Hodge E, Rajanayagam S, Hunsberger S, et al. Effects of chronic systemic administration of basic fibroblast growth factor on collateral development in the canine heart. Circulation. 1995;91:145–53.
151. Lazarous DF, Shou M, Scheinowitz M, Hodge E, Thirumurti V, Kitsiou AN, et al. Comparative effects of basic fibroblast growth factor and vascular endothelial growth factor on coronary collateral development and the arterial response to injury. Circulation. 1996;94:1074–82.
152. Rajanayagam MA, Shou M, Thirumurti V, Lazarous DF, Quyyumi AA, Goncalves L, et al. Intracoronary basic fibroblast growth factor enhances myocardial collateral perfusion in dogs. J Am Coll Cardiol. 2000;35:519–26.
153. Poling J, Szibor M, Schimanski S, Ingelmann ME, Rees W, Gajawada P, et al. Induction of smooth muscle cell migration during arteriogenesis is mediated by Rap2. Arterioscler Thromb Vasc Biol. 2011;31:2297–305.
154. Resnick N, Yahav H, Shay-Salit A, Shushy M, Schubert S, Zilberman LC, et al. Fluid shear stress and the vascular endothelium: for better and for worse. Prog Biophys Mol Biol. 2003;81:177–99.
155. Schierling W, Troidl K, Troidl C, Schmitz-Rixen T, Schaper W, Eitenmuller IK. The role of angiogenic growth factors in arteriogenesis. J Vasc Res. 2009;46:365–74.
156. Wu S, Wu X, Zhu W, Cai WJ, Schaper J, Schaper W. Immunohistochemical study of the growth factors, aFGF, bFGF,

PDGF-AB, VEGF-A and its receptor (Flk-1) during arteriogenesis. Mol Cell Biochem. 2010;343:223–9.
157. Patila T, Ikonen T, Rutanen J, Ahonen A, Lommi J, Lappalainen K, et al. Vascular endothelial growth factor C-induced collateral formation in a model of myocardial ischemia. J Heart Lung Transplant. 2006;25:206–13.
158. Carmeliet P, Moons L, Luttun A, Vincenti V, Compernolle V, De Mol M, et al. Synergism between vascular endothelial growth factor and placental growth factor contributes to angiogenesis and plasma extravasation in pathological conditions. Nat Med. 2001;7:575–83.
159. Pipp F, Heil M, Issbrucker K, Ziegelhoeffer T, Martin S, van den Heuvel J, et al. VEGFR-1-selective VEGF homologue PlGF is arteriogenic: evidence for a monocyte-mediated mechanism. Circ Res. 2003;92:378–85.
160. Jennings RB, Baum JH, Herdson PB. Fine structural changes in myocardial ischemic injury. Arch Pathol. 1965;79:135–43.
161. Buja LM, Weerasinghe P. Unresolved issues in myocardial reperfusion injury. Cardiovasc Pathol. 2010;19:29–35.
162. Buja LM, Vela D. Cardiomyocyte death and renewal in the normal and diseased heart. Cardiovasc Pathol. 2008;17:349–74.
163. Frangogiannis NG, Smith CW, Entman ML. The inflammatory response in myocardial infarction. Cardiovasc Res. 2002;53:31–47.
164. Bolli R, Dawn B, Tang XL, Qiu Y, Ping P, Xuan YT, et al. The nitric oxide hypothesis of late preconditioning. Basic Res Cardiol. 1998;93:325–38.
165. Bolli R, Marban E. Molecular and cellular mechanisms of myocardial stunning. Physiol Rev. 1999;79:609–34.
166. Kloner RA, Jennings RB. Consequences of brief ischemia: stunning, preconditioning, and their clinical implications: part 1. Circulation. 2001;104:2981–9.
167. Kloner RA, Jennings RB. Consequences of brief ischemia: stunning, preconditioning, and their clinical implications: part 2. Circulation. 2001;104:3158–67.
168. Cantin M, Leone A. Morphology of myocardial infarction. Methods Achiev Exp Pathol. 1981;10:244–84.
169. Jennings RB, Ganote CE. Structural changes in myocardium during acute ischemia. Circ Res. 1974;35 Suppl 3:156–72.
170. Herdson PB, Sommers HM, Jennings RB. A comparative study of the fine structure of normal and ischemic dog myocardium with special reference to early changes following temporary occlusion of a coronary artery. Am J Pathol. 1965;46:367–86.
171. Decker RS, Wildenthal K. Influence of methylprednisolone on ultrastructural and cytochemical changes during myocardial ischemia. Selective effects on various cell inclusions and organelles including lysosomes. Am J Pathol. 1978;92:1–22.
172. Rivas F, Cobb FR, Bache RJ, Greenfield Jr JC. Relationship between blood flow to ischemic regions and extent of myocardial infarction. Serial measurement of blood flow to ischemic regions in dogs. Circ Res. 1976;38:439–47.
173. Marcus ML, Tomanek RJ, Ehrhardt JC, Kerber RE, Brown DD, Abboud FM. Relationships between myocardial perfusion, myocardial necrosis, and technetium-99 m pyrophosphate uptake in dogs subjected to sudden coronary occlusion. Circulation. 1976;54:647–53.
174. Downey JM, Yoshida S, Harpen MD. A functional estimate of overlap between adjacent coronary circulations in the dog. Basic Res Cardiol. 1986;81:336–41.
175. Christensen LP, Zhang RL, Zheng W, Campanelli JJ, Dedkov EI, Weiss RM, et al. Postmyocardial infarction remodeling and coronary reserve: effects of ivabradine and beta blockade therapy. Am J Physiol Heart Circ Physiol. 2009;297:H322–30.
176. Zhang RL, Christensen LP, Tomanek RJ. Chronic heart rate reduction facilitates cardiomyocyte survival after myocardial infarction. Anat Rec (Hoboken). 2010;293:839–48.
177. Anversa P, Olivetti G, Capasso JM. Cellular basis of ventricular remodeling after myocardial infarction. Am J Cardiol. 1991;68:7D–16.
178. Lambert JM, Lopez EF, Lindsey ML. Macrophage roles following myocardial infarction. Int J Cardiol. 2008;130:147–58.
179. Dedkov EI, Zheng W, Christensen LP, Weiss RM, Mahlberg-Gaudin F, Tomanek RJ. Preservation of coronary reserve by ivabradine-induced reduction in heart rate in infarcted rats is associated with decrease in perivascular collagen. Am J Physiol Heart Circ Physiol. 2007;293:H590–8.
180. Kalkman EA, Bilgin YM, van Haren P, van Suylen RJ, Saxena PR, Schoemaker RG. Determinants of coronary reserve in rats subjected to coronary artery ligation or aortic banding. Cardiovasc Res. 1996;32:1088–95.
181. Merkus D, Haitsma DB, Sorop O, Boomsma F, de Beer VJ, Lamers JM, et al. Coronary vasoconstrictor influence of angiotensin II is reduced in remodeled myocardium after myocardial infarction. Am J Physiol Heart Circ Physiol. 2006;291:H2082–9.
182. de Beer VJ, Sorop O, Pijnappels DA, Dekkers DH, Boomsma F, Lamers JM, et al. Integrative control of coronary resistance vessel tone by endothelin and angiotensin II is altered in swine with a recent myocardial infarction. Am J Physiol Heart Circ Physiol. 2008;294:H2069–77.
183. Jugdutt BI, Menon V, Kumar D, Idikio H. Vascular remodeling during healing after myocardial infarction in the dog model: effects of reperfusion, amlodipine and enalapril. J Am Coll Cardiol. 2002;39:1538–45.
184. Kloner RA, Rude RE, Carlson N, Maroko PR, DeBoer LW, Braunwald E. Ultrastructural evidence of microvascular damage and myocardial cell injury after coronary artery occlusion: which comes first? Circulation. 1980;62:945–52.
185. Kloner RA, Ganote CE, Jennings RB. The "no-reflow" phenomenon after temporary coronary occlusion in the dog. J Clin Invest. 1974;54:1496–508.
186. Nelissen-Vrancken HJ, Debets JJ, Snoeckx LH, Daemen MJ, Smits JF. Time-related normalization of maximal coronary flow in isolated perfused hearts of rats with myocardial infarction. Circulation. 1996;93:349–55.
187. Dedkov EI, Zheng W, Tomanek RJ. Compensatory growth of coronary arterioles in postinfarcted heart: regional differences in DNA synthesis and growth factor/receptor expression patterns. Am J Physiol Heart Circ Physiol. 2006;291:H1686–93.
188. Sandmann S, Bohle RM, Dreyer T, Unger T. The T-type calcium channel blocker mibefradil reduced interstitial and perivascular fibrosis and improved hemodynamic parameters in myocardial infarction-induced cardiac failure in rats. Virchows Arch. 2000; 436:147–57.
189. Lahteenvuo JE, Lahteenvuo MT, Kivela A, Rosenlew C, Falkevall A, Klar J, et al. Vascular endothelial growth factor-B induces myocardium-specific angiogenesis and arteriogenesis via vascular endothelial growth factor receptor-1- and neuropilin receptor-1-dependent mechanisms. Circulation. 2009;119:845–56.
190. Siddiqui AJ, Fischer H, Widegren U, Grinnemo KH, Hao X, Mansson-Broberg A, et al. Depressed expression of angiogenic growth factors in the subacute phase of myocardial ischemia: a mechanism behind the remodeling plateau? Coronary artery disease. 2010;21:65–71.
191. Zentilin L, Puligadda U, Lionetti V, Zacchigna S, Collesi C, Pattarini L, et al. Cardiomyocyte VEGFR-1 activation by VEGF-B induces compensatory hypertrophy and preserves cardiac function after myocardial infarction. FASEB J. 2010;24:1467–78.
192. Hashimoto E, Ogita T, Nakaoka T, Matsuoka R, Takao A, Kira Y. Rapid induction of vascular endothelial growth factor expression by transient ischemia in rat heart. Am J Physiol. 1994;267: H1948–54.

193. Li X, Tjwa M, Van Hove I, Enholm B, Neven E, Paavonen K, et al. Reevaluation of the role of VEGF-B suggests a restricted role in the revascularization of the ischemic myocardium. Arterioscler Thromb Vasc Biol. 2008;28:1614–20.
194. Jennings RB, Sommers HM, Smyth GA, Flack HA, Linn H. Myocardial necrosis induced by temporary occlusion of a coronary artery in the dog. Arch Pathol. 1960;70:68–78.
195. Bolli R, Jeroudi MO, Patel BS, Aruoma OI, Halliwell B, Lai EK, et al. Marked reduction of free radical generation and contractile dysfunction by antioxidant therapy begun at the time of reperfusion. Evidence that myocardial "stunning" is a manifestation of reperfusion injury. Circ Res. 1989;65:607–22.
196. Zhao Y, Glesne D, Huberman E. A human peripheral blood monocyte-derived subset acts as pluripotent stem cells. Proc Natl Acad Sci USA. 2003;100:2426–31.
197. Ambrosio G, Weisman HF, Mannisi JA, Becker LC. Progressive impairment of regional myocardial perfusion after initial restoration of postischemic blood flow. Circulation. 1989;80:1846–61.
198. Schaper J, Schaper W. Reperfusion of ischemic myocardium: ultrastructural and histochemical aspects. J Am Coll Cardiol. 1983;1:1037–46.
199. Flaherty JT, Weisfeldt ML. Reperfusion injury. Free Radic Biol Med. 1988;5:409–19.
200. Lucchesi BR. Myocardial ischemia, reperfusion and free radical injury. Am J Cardiol. 1990;65:14I–23.
201. Ambrosio G, Tritto I. Reperfusion injury: experimental evidence and clinical implications. Am Heart J. 1999;138:S69–75.
202. Napoli C, Liguori A, Chiariello M, Di Ieso N, Condorelli M, Ambrosio G. New-onset angina preceding acute myocardial infarction is associated with improved contractile recovery after thrombolysis. Eur Heart J. 1998;19:411–9.
203. Jolly SR, Kane WJ, Bailie MB, Abrams GD, Lucchesi BR. Canine myocardial reperfusion injury. Its reduction by the combined administration of superoxide dismutase and catalase. Circ Res. 1984;54:277–85.
204. Brooks WW, Conrad CH, Morgan JP. Reperfusion induced arrhythmias following ischaemia in intact rat heart: role of intracellular calcium. Cardiovasc Res. 1995;29:536–42.
205. Reimer KA, Murry CE, Richard VJ. The role of neutrophils and free radicals in the ischemic-reperfused heart: why the confusion and controversy? J Mol Cell Cardiol. 1989;21:1225–39.
206. Yellon DM, Hausenloy DJ. Myocardial reperfusion injury. N Engl J Med. 2007;357:1121–35.
207. Vrints CJ. Pathophysiology of the no-reflow phenomenon. Acute Card Care. 2009;11:69–76.
208. Reffelmann T, Kloner RA. The no-reflow phenomenon: a basic mechanism of myocardial ischemia and reperfusion. Basic Res Cardiol. 2006;101:359–72.
209. Yasumura T, Aoki N, Yanagisawa A, Maki A, Shirato C, Ishikawa K. Effects of repeated brief episodes of ischemia and reperfusion in isolated perfused rat hearts. Heart Vessels. 1999;14:120–6.
210. Tiefenbacher CP, Chilian WM, Mitchell M, DeFily DV. Restoration of endothelium-dependent vasodilation after reperfusion injury by tetrahydrobiopterin. Circulation. 1996;94:1423–9.
211. Hashimoto K, Pearson PJ, Schaff HV, Cartier R. Endothelial cell dysfunction after ischemic arrest and reperfusion: a possible mechanism of myocardial injury during reflow. J Thorac Cardiovasc Surg. 1991;102:688–94.
212. Hein TW, Zhang C, Wang W, Chang CI, Thengchaisri N, Kuo L. Ischemia-reperfusion selectively impairs nitric oxide-mediated dilation in coronary arterioles: counteracting role of arginase. FASEB J. 2003;17:2328–30.
213. Climent B, Fernandez N, Sanz E, Sanchez A, Monge L, Garcia-Villalon AL, et al. Enhanced response of pig coronary arteries to endothelin-1 after ischemia-reperfusion. Role of endothelin receptors, nitric oxide and prostanoids. Eur J Pharmacol. 2005;524:102–10.
214. Hearse DJ, Humphrey SM, Chain EB. Abrupt reoxygenation of the anoxic potassium-arrested perfused rat heart: a study of myocardial enzyme release. J Mol Cell Cardiol. 1973;5:395–407.
215. Zweier JL, Flaherty JT, Weisfeldt ML. Direct measurement of free radical generation following reperfusion of ischemic myocardium. Proc Natl Acad Sci USA. 1987;84:1404–7.
216. Zweier JL. Measurement of superoxide-derived free radicals in the reperfused heart. Evidence for a free radical mechanism of reperfusion injury. J Biol Chem. 1988;263:1353–7.
217. Zweier JL, Talukder MA. The role of oxidants and free radicals in reperfusion injury. Cardiovasc Res. 2006;70:181–90.
218. Halestrap AP, Clarke SJ, Javadov SA. Mitochondrial permeability transition pore opening during myocardial reperfusion—a target for cardioprotection. Cardiovasc Res. 2004;61:372–85.
219. Altschuld R. Intracellular calcium regulatory systems during ischemia and reperfusion. Myocardial ischemia: mechanisms, reperfusion, protection. Basel: Birkhauser Verlag; 1996. p. 87–97.
220. Lemasters JJ, Bond J, Chacon E, Harper I, Kaplan S, Ohata H, et al. The pH paradox in ischemia-reperfusion injury to cardiomyocytes. Myocardial ischemia: mechanisms, reperfusion, protection. Basel: Birkhauser Verlag; 1996.
221. Yellon DM, Downey JM. Preconditioning the myocardium: from cellular physiology to clinical cardiology. Physiol Rev. 2003;83:1113–51.
222. Maroko PR, Kjekshus JK, Sobel BE, Watanabe T, Covell JW, Ross Jr J, et al. Factors influencing infarct size following experimental coronary artery occlusions. Circulation. 1971;43:67–82.
223. Maroko PR, Libby P, Bloor CM, Sobel BE, Braunwald E. Reduction by hyaluronidase of myocardial necrosis following coronary artery occlusion. Circulation. 1972;46:430–7.
224. Maroko PR, Libby P, Sobel BE, Bloor CM, Sybers HD, Shell WE, et al. Effect of glucose-insulin-potassium infusion on myocardial infarction following experimental coronary artery occlusion. Circulation. 1972;45:1160–75.
225. Reimer KA, Murry CE, Yamasawa I, Hill ML, Jennings RB. Four brief periods of myocardial ischemia cause no cumulative ATP loss or necrosis. Am J Physiol. 1986;251:H1306–15.
226. Murry CE, Jennings RB, Reimer KA. Preconditioning with ischemia: a delay of lethal cell injury in ischemic myocardium. Circulation. 1986;74:1124–36.
227. Yang X, Cohen MV, Downey JM. Mechanism of cardioprotection by early ischemic preconditioning. Cardiovasc Drugs Ther. 2010;24:225–34.
228. Sumeray MS, Yellon DM. Ischaemic preconditioning reduces infarct size following global ischaemia in the murine myocardium. Basic Res Cardiol. 1998;93:384–90.
229. Burns PG, Krunkenkamp IB, Calderone CA, Kirvaitis RJ, Gaudette GR, Levitsky S. Is the preconditioning response conserved in senescent myocardium? Ann Thorac Surg. 1996;61:925–9.
230. Li Y, Kloner RA. Cardioprotective effects of ischaemic preconditioning are not mediated by prostanoids. Cardiovasc Res. 1992;26:226–31.
231. Schott RJ, Rohmann S, Braun ER, Schaper W. Ischemic preconditioning reduces infarct size in swine myocardium. Circ Res. 1990;66:1133–42.
232. Cohen MV, Liu GS, Downey JM. Preconditioning causes improved wall motion as well as smaller infarcts after transient coronary occlusion in rabbits. Circulation. 1991;84:341–9.
233. Liang BT, Gross GJ. Direct preconditioning of cardiac myocytes via opioid receptors and KATP channels. Circ Res. 1999;84:1396–400.
234. Kuzuya T, Hoshida S, Yamashita N, Fuji H, Oe H, Hori M, et al. Delayed effects of sublethal ischemia on the acquisition of tolerance to ischemia. Circ Res. 1993;72:1293–9.
235. Marber MS, Latchman DS, Walker JM, Yellon DM. Cardiac stress protein elevation 24 hours after brief ischemia or heat stress is

associated with resistance to myocardial infarction. Circulation. 1993;88:1264–72.
236. Ovize M, Przyklenk K, Kloner RA. Partial coronary stenosis is sufficient and complete reperfusion is mandatory for preconditioning the canine heart. Circ Res. 1992;71:1165–73.
237. Bufkin BL, Shearer ST, Vinten-Johansen J, Duarte IG, Thourani VH, Nakamura M, et al. Preconditioning during simulated MIDCABG attenuates blood flow defects and neutrophil accumulation. Ann Thorac Surg. 1998;66:726–31. discussion 31–2.
238. Wang NP, Bufkin BL, Nakamura M, Zhao ZQ, Wilcox JN, Hewan-Lowe KO, et al. Ischemic preconditioning reduces neutrophil accumulation and myocardial apoptosis. Ann Thorac Surg. 1999;67:1689–95.
239. Nakamura M, Wang NP, Zhao ZQ, Wilcox JN, Thourani V, Guyton RA, et al. Preconditioning decreases Bax expression, PMN accumulation and apoptosis in reperfused rat heart. Cardiovasc Res. 2000;45:661–70.
240. Zhao ZQ, Vinten-Johansen J. Myocardial apoptosis and ischemic preconditioning. Cardiovasc Res. 2002;55:438–55.
241. Zhao ZQ, Velez DA, Wang NP, Hewan-Lowe KO, Nakamura M, Guyton RA, et al. Progressively developed myocardial apoptotic cell death during late phase of reperfusion. Apoptosis. 2001;6:279–90.
242. Scarabelli T, Stephanou A, Rayment N, Pasini E, Comini L, Curello S, et al. Apoptosis of endothelial cells precedes myocyte cell apoptosis in ischemia/reperfusion injury. Circulation. 2001;104:253–6.
243. Ambrosio G, Zweier JL, Becker LC. Apoptosis is prevented by administration of superoxide dismutase in dogs with reperfused myocardial infarction. Basic Res Cardiol. 1998;93:94–6.
244. Thourani VH, Nakamura M, Duarte IG, Bufkin BL, Zhao ZQ, Jordan JE, et al. Ischemic preconditioning attenuates postischemic coronary artery endothelial dysfunction in a model of minimally invasive direct coronary artery bypass grafting. J Thorac Cardiovasc Surg. 1999;117:383–9.
245. Hare JM. Oxidative stress and apoptosis in heart failure progression. Circ Res. 2001;89:198–200.
246. Tajima M, Katayose D, Bessho M, Isoyama S. Acute ischaemic preconditioning and chronic hypoxia independently increase myocardial tolerance to ischaemia. Cardiovasc Res. 1994;28:312–9.
247. Ostadalova I, Ostadal B, Jarkovska D, Kolar F. Ischemic preconditioning in chronically hypoxic neonatal rat heart. Pediatr Res. 2002;52:561–7.
248. Neckar J, Papousek F, Novakova O, Ost'adal B, Kolar F. Cardioprotective effects of chronic hypoxia and ischaemic preconditioning are not additive. Basic Res Cardiol. 2002;97:161–7.
249. Neckar J, Szarszoi O, Herget J, Ostadal B, Kolar F. Cardioprotective effect of chronic hypoxia is blunted by concomitant hypercapnia. Physiol Res. 2003;52:171–5.
250. Neckar J, Ostadal B, Kolar F. Myocardial infarct size-limiting effect of chronic hypoxia persists for five weeks of normoxic recovery. Physiol Res. 2004;53:621–8.
251. Ooi H, Cadogan E, Sweeney M, Howell K, O'Regan RG, McLoughlin P. Chronic hypercapnia inhibits hypoxic pulmonary vascular remodeling. Am J Physiol Heart Circ Physiol. 2000;278:H331–8.
252. Kloner RA, Shook T, Przyklenk K, Davis VG, Junio L, Matthews RV, et al. Previous angina alters in-hospital outcome in TIMI 4. A clinical correlate to preconditioning? Circulation. 1995;91:37–45.
253. Anzai T, Yoshikawa T, Asakura Y, Abe S, Meguro T, Akaishi M, et al. Effect on short-term prognosis and left ventricular function of angina pectoris prior to first Q-wave anterior wall acute myocardial infarction. Am J Cardiol. 1994;74:755–9.
254. Andreotti F, Pasceri V, Hackett DR, Davies GJ, Haider AW, Maseri A. Preinfarction angina as a predictor of more rapid coronary thrombolysis in patients with acute myocardial infarction. N Engl J Med. 1996;334:7–12.
255. Ishihara M, Sato H, Tateishi H, Kawagoe T, Shimatani Y, Kurisu S, et al. Implications of prodromal angina pectoris in anterior wall acute myocardial infarction: acute angiographic findings and long-term prognosis. J Am Coll Cardiol. 1997;30:970–5.
256. Tomai F, Crea F, Chiariello L, Gioffre PA. Ischemic preconditioning in humans: models, mediators, and clinical relevance. Circulation. 1999;100:559–63.
257. Jenkins DP, Pugsley WB, Alkhulaifi AM, Kemp M, Hooper J, Yellon DM. Ischaemic preconditioning reduces troponin T release in patients undergoing coronary artery bypass surgery. Heart. 1997;77:314–8.
258. Teoh LK, Grant R, Hulf JA, Pugsley WB, Yellon DM. The effect of preconditioning (ischemic and pharmacological) on myocardial necrosis following coronary artery bypass graft surgery. Cardiovasc Res. 2002;53:175–80.
259. Ikonomidis JS, Tumiati LC, Weisel RD, Mickle DA, Li RK. Preconditioning human ventricular cardiomyocytes with brief periods of simulated ischaemia. Cardiovasc Res. 1994;28:1285–91.
260. Ikonomidis JS, Shirai T, Weisel RD, Derylo B, Rao V, Whiteside CI, et al. Preconditioning cultured human pediatric myocytes requires adenosine and protein kinase C. Am J Physiol. 1997;272:H1220–30.
261. Walker DM, Marber MS, Walker JM, Yellon DM. Preconditioning in isolated superfused rabbit papillary muscles. Am J Physiol. 1994;266:H1534–40.
262. Cohen MV, Downey JM. Ischemic postconditioning: from receptor to end-effector. Antioxid Redox Signal. 2011;14:821–31.
263. Murry CE, Jennings RB, Reimer KA. New insights into potential mechanisms of ischemic preconditioning. Circulation. 1991;84:442–5.
264. Murry CE, Richard VJ, Reimer KA, Jennings RB. Ischemic preconditioning slows energy metabolism and delays ultrastructural damage during a sustained ischemic episode. Circ Res. 1990;66:913–31.
265. Liu GS, Thornton J, Van Winkle DM, Stanley AW, Olsson RA, Downey JM. Protection against infarction afforded by preconditioning is mediated by A1 adenosine receptors in rabbit heart. Circulation. 1991;84:350–6.
266. Tsuchida A, Miura T, Miki T, Shimamoto K, Iimura O. Role of adenosine receptor activation in myocardial infarct size limitation by ischaemic preconditioning. Cardiovasc Res. 1992;26:456–61.
267. Auchampach JA, Gross GJ. Adenosine A1 receptors, KATP channels, and ischemic preconditioning in dogs. Am J Physiol. 1993;264:H1327–36.
268. Cohen MV, Yang XM, Liu GS, Heusch G, Downey JM. Acetylcholine, bradykinin, opioids, and phenylephrine, but not adenosine, trigger preconditioning by generating free radicals and opening mitochondrial K(ATP) channels. Circ Res. 2001;89:273–8.
269. Costa AD, Garlid KD, West IC, Lincoln TM, Downey JM, Cohen MV, et al. Protein kinase G transmits the cardioprotective signal from cytosol to mitochondria. Circ Res. 2005;97:329–36.
270. Honda HM, Ping P. Mitochondrial permeability transition in cardiac cell injury and death. Cardiovasc Drugs Ther. 2006;20:425–32.
271. Downey JM, Krieg T, Cohen MV. Mapping preconditioning's signaling pathways: an engineering approach. Ann NY Acad Sci. 2008;1123:187–96.
272. Tissier R, Cohen MV, Downey JM. Protecting the acutely ischemic myocardium beyond reperfusion therapies: are we any closer to realizing the dream of infarct size elimination? Arch Mal Coeur Vaiss. 2007;100:794–802.
273. Ishihara M, Inoue I, Kawagoe T, Shimatani Y, Kurisu S, Nishioka K, et al. Diabetes mellitus prevents ischemic preconditioning in patients with a first acute anterior wall myocardial infarction. J Am Coll Cardiol. 2001;38:1007–11.

274. Noda T, Minatoguchi S, Fujii K, Hori M, Ito T, Kanmatsuse K, et al. Evidence for the delayed effect in human ischemic preconditioning: prospective multicenter study for preconditioning in acute myocardial infarction. J Am Coll Cardiol. 1999;34:1966–74.
275. Hausenloy DJ, Yellon DM. The second window of preconditioning (SWOP) where are we now? Cardiovasc Drugs Ther. 2010;24:235–54.
276. Bolli R, Li QH, Tang XL, Guo Y, Xuan YT, Rokosh G, et al. The late phase of preconditioning and its natural clinical application–gene therapy. Heart Fail Rev. 2007;12:189–99.
277. Guo Y, Jones WK, Xuan YT, Tang XL, Bao W, Wu WJ, et al. The late phase of ischemic preconditioning is abrogated by targeted disruption of the inducible NO synthase gene. Proc Natl Acad Sci USA. 1999;96:11507–12.
278. Shinmura K, Tang XL, Wang Y, Xuan YT, Liu SQ, Takano H, et al. Cyclooxygenase-2 mediates the cardioprotective effects of the late phase of ischemic preconditioning in conscious rabbits. Proc Natl Acad Sci USA. 2000;97:10197–202.
279. Xuan YT, Tang XL, Qiu Y, Banerjee S, Takano H, Han H, et al. Biphasic response of cardiac NO synthase isoforms to ischemic preconditioning in conscious rabbits. Am J Physiol Heart Circ Physiol. 2000;279:H2360–71.
280. Przyklenk K, Bauer B, Ovize M, Kloner RA, Whittaker P. Regional ischemic 'preconditioning' protects remote virgin myocardium from subsequent sustained coronary occlusion. Circulation. 1993;87:893–9.
281. Saxena P, Bala A, Campbell K, Meloni B, d'Udekem Y, Konstantinov IE. Does remote ischemic preconditioning prevent delayed hippocampal neuronal death following transient global cerebral ischemia in rats? Perfusion. 2009;24:207–11.
282. Wei M, Xin P, Li S, Tao J, Li Y, Li J, et al. Repeated remote ischemic postconditioning protects against adverse left ventricular remodeling and improves survival in a rat model of myocardial infarction. Circ Res. 2011;108:1220–5.
283. Ovize M, Baxter GF, Di Lisa F, Ferdinandy P, Garcia-Dorado D, Hausenloy DJ, et al. Postconditioning and protection from reperfusion injury: where do we stand? Position paper from the Working Group of Cellular Biology of the Heart of the European Society of Cardiology. Cardiovasc Res. 2010;87:406–23.
284. Granfeldt A, Lefer DJ, Vinten-Johansen J. Protective ischaemia in patients: preconditioning and postconditioning. Cardiovasc Res. 2009;83:234–46.
285. Yang XM, Proctor JB, Cui L, Krieg T, Downey JM, Cohen MV. Multiple, brief coronary occlusions during early reperfusion protect rabbit hearts by targeting cell signaling pathways. J Am Coll Cardiol. 2004;44:1103–10.
286. Darling CE, Solari PB, Smith CS, Furman MI, Przyklenk K. 'Postconditioning' the human heart: multiple balloon inflations during primary angioplasty may confer cardioprotection. Basic Res Cardiol. 2007;102:274–8.
287. Halkos ME, Kerendi F, Corvera JS, Wang NP, Kin H, Payne CS, et al. Myocardial protection with postconditioning is not enhanced by ischemic preconditioning. The Annals of thoracic surgery. 2004;78:961–9. discussion 9.
288. Tsang A, Hausenloy DJ, Mocanu MM, Yellon DM. Postconditioning: a form of "modified reperfusion" protects the myocardium by activating the phosphatidylinositol 3-kinase-Akt pathway. Circ Res. 2004;95:230–2.
289. Skyschally A, van Caster P, Iliodromitis EK, Schulz R, Kremastinos DT, Heusch G. Ischemic postconditioning: experimental models and protocol algorithms. Basic Res Cardiol. 2009;104:469–83.
290. Boengler K, Buechert A, Heinen Y, Roeskes C, Hilfiker-Kleiner D, Heusch G, et al. Cardioprotection by ischemic postconditioning is lost in aged and STAT3-deficient mice. Circ Res. 2008;102:131–5.
291. Heusch G, Buchert A, Feldhaus S, Schulz R. No loss of cardioprotection by postconditioning in connexin 43-deficient mice. Basic Res Cardiol. 2006;101:354–6.
292. Lim SY, Davidson SM, Hausenloy DJ, Yellon DM. Preconditioning and postconditioning: the essential role of the mitochondrial permeability transition pore. Cardiovasc Res. 2007;75:530–5.
293. Tsutsumi YM, Yokoyama T, Horikawa Y, Roth DM, Patel HH. Reactive oxygen species trigger ischemic and pharmacological postconditioning: in vivo and in vitro characterization. Life sciences. 2007;81:1223–7.
294. Gomez L, Paillard M, Thibault H, Derumeaux G, Ovize M. Inhibition of GSK3beta by postconditioning is required to prevent opening of the mitochondrial permeability transition pore during reperfusion. Circulation. 2008;117:2761–8.
295. Bouhidel O, Pons S, Souktani R, Zini R, Berdeaux A, Ghaleh B. Myocardial ischemic postconditioning against ischemia-reperfusion is impaired in ob/ob mice. Am J Physiol Heart Circ Physiol. 2008;295:H1580–6.
296. Kaljusto ML, Mori T, Mohammad Husain Rizvi S, Galagudza M, Frantzen ML, Valen G, et al. Postconditioning in rats and mice. Scand Cardiovasc J. 2006;40:334–41.
297. Nishino Y, Webb IG, Davidson SM, Ahmed AI, Clark JE, Jacquet S, et al. Glycogen synthase kinase-3 inactivation is not required for ischemic preconditioning or postconditioning in the mouse. Circ Res. 2008;103:307–14.
298. Przyklenk K, Maynard M, Darling CE, Whittaker P. Aging mouse hearts are refractory to infarct size reduction with post-conditioning. J Am Coll Cardiol. 2008;51:1393–8.
299. Xi L, Das A, Zhao ZQ, Merino VF, Bader M, Kukreja RC. Loss of myocardial ischemic postconditioning in adenosine A1 and bradykinin B2 receptors gene knockout mice. Circulation. 2008;118:S32–7.
300. Kloner RA, Rezkalla SH. Preconditioning, postconditioning and their application to clinical cardiology. Cardiovasc Res. 2006;70:297–307.
301. Kloner RA, Dow J, Bhandari A. Postconditioning markedly attenuates ventricular arrhythmias after ischemia-reperfusion. J Cardiovasc Pharmacol Ther. 2006;11:55–63.
302. Galagudza M, Kurapeev D, Minasian S, Valen G, Vaage J. Ischemic postconditioning: brief ischemia during reperfusion converts persistent ventricular fibrillation into regular rhythm. Eur J Cardiothorac Surg. 2004;25:1006–10.
303. Dow J, Bhandari A, Kloner RA. Ischemic postconditioning's benefit on reperfusion ventricular arrhythmias is maintained in the senescent heart. J Cardiovasc Pharmacol Ther. 2008;13:141–8.
304. Na HS, Kim YI, Yoon YW, Han HC, Nahm SH, Hong SK. Ventricular premature beat-driven intermittent restoration of coronary blood flow reduces the incidence of reperfusion-induced ventricular fibrillation in a cat model of regional ischemia. Am Heart J. 1996;132:78–83.
305. Sun HY, Wang NP, Kerendi F, Halkos M, Kin H, Guyton RA, et al. Hypoxic postconditioning reduces cardiomyocyte loss by inhibiting ROS generation and intracellular Ca^{2+} overload. Am J Physiol Heart Circ Physiol. 2005;288:H1900–8.
306. Hansen PR, Thibault H, Abdulla J. Postconditioning during primary percutaneous coronary intervention: a review and meta-analysis. Int J Cardiol. 2010;144:22–5.
307. Laskey WK. Brief repetitive balloon occlusions enhance reperfusion during percutaneous coronary intervention for acute myocardial infarction: a pilot study. Catheter Cardiovasc Interv. 2005;65:361–7.
308. Staat P, Rioufol G, Piot C, Cottin Y, Cung TT, L'Huillier I, et al. Postconditioning the human heart. Circulation. 2005; 112:2143–8.

309. Ma XJ, Zhang XH, Li CM, Luo M. Effect of postconditioning on coronary blood flow velocity and endothelial function in patients with acute myocardial infarction. Scand Cardiovasc J. 2006;40:327–33.
310. Yang XC, Liu Y, Wang LF, Cui L, Wang T, Ge YG, et al. Reduction in myocardial infarct size by postconditioning in patients after percutaneous coronary intervention. J Invasive Cardiol. 2007; 19:424–30.
311. Thibault H, Piot C, Staat P, Bontemps L, Sportouch C, Rioufol G, et al. Long-term benefit of postconditioning. Circulation. 2008;117:1037–44.
312. Laskey WK, Yoon S, Calzada N, Ricciardi MJ. Concordant improvements in coronary flow reserve and ST-segment resolution during percutaneous coronary intervention for acute myocardial infarction: a benefit of postconditioning. Catheter Cardiovasc Interv. 2008;72:212–20.
313. Jang Y, Xi J, Wang H, Mueller RA, Norfleet EA, Xu Z. Postconditioning prevents reperfusion injury by activating delta-opioid receptors. Anesthesiology. 2008;108:243–50.
314. Penna C, Mancardi D, Rastaldo R, Losano G, Pagliaro P. Intermittent activation of bradykinin B2 receptors and mitochondrial KATP channels trigger cardiac postconditioning through redox signaling. Cardiovasc Res. 2007;75:168–77.
315. Zatta AJ, Kin H, Yoshishige D, Jiang R, Wang N, Reeves JG, et al. Evidence that cardioprotection by postconditioning involves preservation of myocardial opioid content and selective opioid receptor activation. Am J Physiol Heart Circ Physiol. 2008;294: H1444–51.
316. Guo HT, Zhang RH, Zhang Y, Zhang LJ, Li J, Shi QX, Wang YM, Fan R, Bi H, Yin W, Pei JM. Endogenous k-opioid peptide mediates the cardioprotection induced by ischemic postconditioning. J Cardiovas Pharmacol. 2011;58:207–15.
317. Penna C, Mancardi D, Tullio F, Pagliaro P. Postconditioning and intermittent bradykinin induced cardioprotection require cyclooxygenase activation and prostacyclin release during reperfusion. Basic Res Cardiol. 2008;103:368–77.
318. Hausenloy DJ, Yellon DM. Survival kinases in ischemic preconditioning and postconditioning. Cardiovasc Res. 2006;70:240–53.
319. Heusch G, Skyoschally A, Schulz R. The insitu pig heart with regional ischemia/reperfusion-ready for translation. J Mol Cell Cardiol. 2011;50:951–63.
320. Kaur S, Jaggi AS, Singh N. Molecular aspects of ischaemic postconditioning. Fundam Clin Pharmacol. 2009;23:521–36.
321. Cohen MV, Yang XM, Downey JM. The pH hypothesis of postconditioning: staccato reperfusion reintroduces oxygen and perpetuates myocardial acidosis. Circulation. 2007;115: 1895–903.
322. Hausenloy DJ, Yellon DM. Preconditioning and postconditioning: underlying mechanisms and clinical application. Atherosclerosis. 2009;204:334–41.

11 Cardiac Hypertrophy

Abbreviations

DCM	Dilated cardiomyopathy
EC	Endothelial cell
HCM	Hypertrophic cardiomyopathy
LV	Left ventricle
LVH	Left ventricular hypertrophy
MCVR	Minimal coronary vascular resistance
RV	Right ventricle
SHR	Spontaneously hypertensive rat
VSMC	Vascular smooth muscle cell
WKY	Wistar Kyoto normotensive rat

Introduction

Adaptations of the coronary vasculature to cardiac hypertrophy are dependent, in part, on the stimulus that evokes the growth of the myocardium. It has become clear that myocardial perfusion and cardiac function are not necessarily compromised when the heart enlarges either during normal growth (Chap. 3) or under some conditions of increased work, e.g., exercise training (Chap. 8). Accordingly, the term "physiological hypertrophy" has sometimes been used to contrast cardiac enlargement that does not compromise cardiac function from one that does, i.e., "pathological hypertrophy." The response to aerobic exercise training evokes favorable adaptations that result in a phenotype called "athlete's heart" [1]. This physiological hypertrophy is induced by insulin-like growth factor-1 signaling pathways that also occur in pathological hypertrophy; however, physiological hypertrophy includes induction of cardiomyocyte growth via PI3K and Akt1 pathways, whereas the later may involve angiotensin II and endothelin-1 signaling. An important structural adaptation in physiological hypertrophy is vascular growth and/or remodeling that preserves coronary vasodilator reserve, as discussed in Chap. 8. The commonly observed absence of adequate vascular growth in pressure overload and cardiomyopathy contributes to decompensated cardiac hypertrophy. Moreover, enhanced systolic compression and/or altered vasoreactivity of arteries and arterioles in the hypertrophied heart can contribute to compromised ventricular function and consequently morbidity and mortality [2]. The major structural concern regarding coronary flow in the hypertrophied heart is whether arteries and arterioles increase their cross-sectional areas to compensate for increased cardiac mass. The cross-sectional areas of coronary ostia were found to increase with increasing heart mass up to 500 g in humans [3]. Subsequently, the increase in ostial size was found to occur only in the left, but not right coronary artery [4]. Analysis of epicardial arteries from patients with cardiac hypertrophy revealed a correlation of their diameters and heart mass [5]. Since these studies were limited to autopsy materials, the causes of hypertrophy were not distinguished. Moreover, only ostia or large epicardial arteries were included.

The vascular responses and alterations that occur with chronic hypoxia (Chap. 9) and myocardial infarction (Chap. 10) have already been discussed and are covered, and therefore are not included here. This chapter addresses the coronary vasculature in cardiac hypertrophy induced by (1) pressure overload, (2) volume overload, (3) thyroid hormones, and (4) that associated with cardiomyopathy. Although cardiac hypertrophy in response to various stimuli is a common adaptive response to increased work, the vascular responses are linked to mechanical and metabolic factors, as well as the type of ventricular remodeling (reviewed in [6–8]). Too often assumptions regarding characteristics of cardiac hypertrophy have been based on a single model of cardiac hypertrophy. For example, ischemic and reperfusion injury has been documented in rat hearts subjected to aortic banding [9–11] and too often the findings were considered as representative of all models of pressure overload [11]. In these instances, the findings were based on a model which produced a large degree of compensatory hypertrophy that is not necessarily seen in other forms of elevated pressure. Aortic banding and systemic hypertension also raise coronary

R.J. Tomanek, *Coronary Vasculature: Development, Structure-Function, and Adaptations*,
DOI 10.1007/978-1-4614-4887-7_11, © Springer Science+Business Media New York 2013

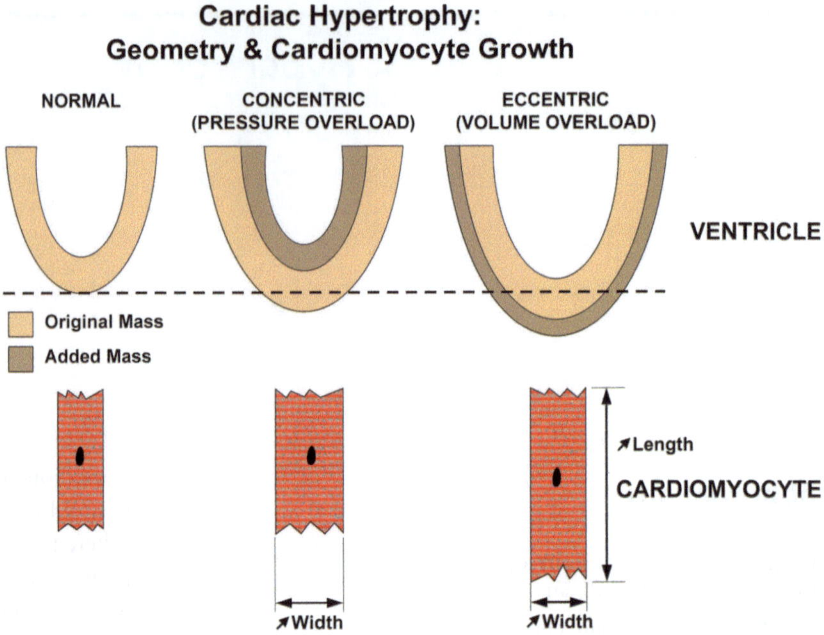

Fig. 11.1 Pressure overload causes a "concentric" type of hypertrophy characterized by increases in cardiomyocyte cross-sectional areas and minimal increases in cardiomyocyte length. In contrast, volume overload causes an "eccentric" type of hypertrophy by increasing both cardiomyocyte length and cross-sectional area. The increase in the latter is less than that which occurs in concentric hypertrophy

perfusion pressure, whereas valvular aortic stenosis does not. Thus, even within the category of pressure overload one must consider the specific model, i.e., aortic stenosis, renal hypertension, spontaneous hypertension. As discussed in this chapter, cardiac hypertrophy in response to volume overload, pressure overload, and thyroxine represents three fairly distinct models that involve different forms of ventricular remodeling. Accordingly, the differences in vascular responses and adaptations in these models should not be surprising. Moreover, the abruptness of the overload usually employed in experimental animals evokes a marked instantaneous increase in afterload that may cause inflammatory changes in the myocardium that are not associated with pressure overload in patients.

As illustrated in Fig. 11.1, one major difference between myocardial remodeling in response to enhanced afterload (pressure) vs. enhanced preload (volume) is that remodeling involves concentric hypertrophy in the former and eccentric hypertrophy in the latter (reviewed in [12, 13]). Concentric hypertrophy is due to lateral expansion of cardiomyocytes with little or no increase in their lengths. In contrast, eccentric hypertrophy is a consequence of similar increases in both cross-sectional areas (or diameters) and length of cardiomyocytes [14, 15]. This model of hypertrophy is also contrasted with that which occurs during enhanced afterload in that fibrosis and inflammation are not characteristic and there is less apoptosis. Moreover, pressure- and volume-induced cardiac hypertrophies are characterized by distinct molecular phenotypes and patterns of peptide growth factor induction [16]. For example, FGF-1 mRNA is increased only in the volume overload model of hypertrophy, whereas fetal gene mRNAs are elevated only in the pressure overload model. A comprehensive review [8] of the effects of hypertrophy on the coronary circulation includes a comparison of the various models of hypertrophy, whereas a more recent review is focused on microvascular dysfunction in patients with left ventricular hypertrophy [17].

Pressure Overload in Humans

Systemic hypertension subjects the left ventricle (LV) to an increased afterload, which lead to concentric hypertrophy that, if proportional to the degree of increased pressure, maintains the normal relationship between wall thickness and the radius of the ventricle's lumen and a normal stroke volume. These adaptations in slowly developing hypertension facilitate normal contractile indices (reviewed in [18]). In contrast, impairment of diastolic filling occurs relatively early in hypertensive states and is correlated with the degree of hypertension. Prolongation of elevated arterial pressure results in ventricular dilatation and fibrosis that increases ventricular stiffness. In the heart facing persistent hypertension, increased wall stress and impaired systolic function develop and microvascular alterations develop. The rat heart subjected to chronic pressure overload induced by renal hypertension has been shown to experience after potentials which predispose the hypertrophied cardiomyocytes to arrhythmias [19]. The coronary vasculature is also directly affected by the increase in blood pressure, as evidenced by an increase in stiffness of large arteries, small artery remodeling, and changes in the architecture of the microvasculature [20].

The coronary circulation is affected not only by cardiomyocyte hypertrophy and interstitial fibrosis but also by changes in coronary vessel reactivity and perivascular fibrosis. As noted by Vatner and Hittinger [21], hypertrophy induced by increased afterload is associated with LV diastolic and systolic dysfunction, ischemia, and impaired endomyocardial coronary reserve. If sufficient, these effects can lead to heart failure. In dogs with hypertension-induced heart failure, connective tissue was shown to increase about 15-fold in the endomyocardial region of the LV along with an exhaustion of coronary vasodilator reserve in this region [22].

Coronary Reserve Impairment in Humans with Pressure Overload

In humans, long-term hypertension has repeatedly been shown to cause a decrease in coronary flow reserve. Coronary vasodilator flow reserve (difference between maximal and resting flow) is a parameter that indicates the capacity of the coronary circulation to meet the O_2 demands of increased workloads of the heart; it depends both on resting and maximal flows. This means that if flow is increased under basal conditions then maximal flow will need to reach a higher level than if resting flow was at more normal levels (see review by [23]). Thus, there are two ways that coronary vasodilator reserve can be compromised (1) if coronary maximal flow is limited, e.g., by a failure of the resistance vessels to expand during hypertrophy and (2) if maximal flow is preserved but resting flow is increased to meet metabolic demands, e.g., when basal heart rate is increased. Impairment of the microcirculation in humans occurs early in the process of hypertensive heart disease and is characterized by vascular remodeling resulting in thickening of the arteriolar wall, even in the absence of ventricular hypertrophy [24]. An elevated resting coronary flow was found in men with hypertension and LVH, which contributed to impaired coronary vasodilator reserve [25]. Moreover, the left main coronary artery cross-sectional area in the hypertensive group was less than that in normotensive subjects.

The decrease in maximal coronary flow, indicated by elevated coronary vascular resistance, has been shown to be most marked in patients with the greatest degree of aortic stenosis [26]. This study also revealed that coronary vascular reserve was more severely impaired in the subendocardial layers than in the subepicardial layers in aortic stenosis. In addition to the degree of aortic stenosis, the severity of coronary vascular reserve impairment was also related to hemodynamic load on the LV and the reduced diastolic perfusion time. A study of 25 patients with systemic hypertension and ventricular hypertrophy concluded that myocardial ischemia is linked to impaired endothelium-independent vasodilation of coronary resistance arteries and to the increased minimal coronary vascular resistance [27]. Patients with ischemia had significantly lower coronary vascular reserve values than patients without ischemia, and coronary vascular reserve was inversely related to the percent of coronary artery stenosis (CAS). This study underscored the contribution of vascular

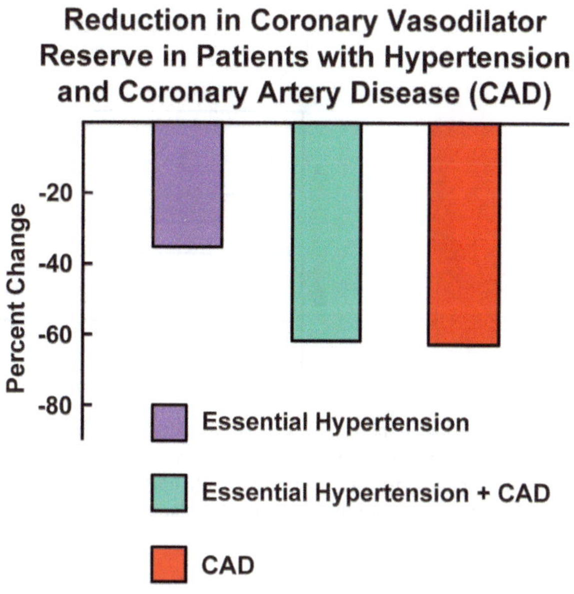

Fig. 11.2 Vasodilator reserve in patients is reduced more by coronary artery disease (CAD) than by hypertension. Moreover, the reduction in coronary vasodilator reserve is similar in patients with CAD and those with both hypertension and CAD. Figure is based on data from Strauer [32]

remodeling and plaque formation to myocardial ischemia in hypertensive patients.

LVH and Hypertension as Contributors to Impaired Coronary Reserve

During the last 2 decades, it has become evident that perfusion abnormalities in patients with hypertension are due to both the effects of myocardial hypertrophy and remodeling of arteries/arterioles, as well as interstitial and perivascular fibrosis [28, 29] (Fig. 11.3). Thus, multiple factors need to be addressed in evaluating the status of the coronary circulation in pressure overload hypertrophy. These include locally generated substances, e.g., locally produced angiotensin II, endothelin, vasoconstrictor prostaglandins, and importantly cytokines from resident inflammatory cells and endothelial cells (ECs), which in turn affect cardiomyocytes and various vascular cells (reviewed in [30]). These substances not only promote vasoconstriction but also cause vascular smooth muscle cell (VSMC) hypertrophy and perivascular collagen deposition.

Strauer [31] showed that both hypertension and coronary artery disease contribute to the decline in coronary vasodilator reserve of hypertensive patients. He found that coronary vasodilator reserve was 30% lower in hypertensive patients with hypertrophy, but without coronary artery disease, whereas in patients with both hypertensive hypertrophy and coronary stenosis, the decline in coronary vasodilator reserve was reduced by 60% (Fig. 11.2). Even in the absence of large coronary artery disease, patients can experience pacing-induced

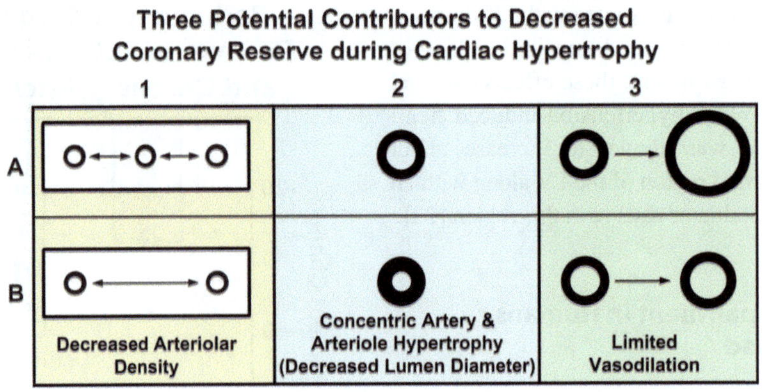

Fig. 11.3 Cardiac hypertrophy can be associated with anatomical (1 & 2) and functional (3) changes in coronary arteries and arterioles, as shown in panel (**b**) and contrasted with normal hearts in panel (**a**). (1) The absence of or limitations in arteriolar growth decrease their numerical densities. (2) A reduction in lumen diameter of coronary arteries and arterioles may occur with chronic hypertension and thereby limit maximal flow. (3) Similarly, maximal coronary flow can be limited if vasodilator responses of these vessels are impaired

angina and a subnormal increase in coronary flow [33, 34]. Coronary vascular reserve in patients with hypertension is impaired in proportion to the extent of the myocardial hypertrophy [35].

Hypertensive patients with LVH have markedly decreased coronary vascular reserve, whereas those with normal heart mass present with moderate decreases in this parameter [36]. When hypertensive patients were treated for at least 1 year, coronary vascular reserve was normalized only in the patients in whom LVH was reversed. Nevertheless, hypertension is a determinant of coronary vasodilator reserve as demonstrated by studies in patients with borderline hypertension and no evidence of LVH [37, 38]. Moreover, in patients with arterial hypertension, minimal coronary vascular resistance correlated positively with mean arteriolar wall area and the mean area of arteriolar fibrosis [29]. When hypertensive patients were treated for 12 months with the ACE inhibitor, perindopril maximal coronary blood flow and coronary reserve increased by 54 and 67%, respectively [39]. Although LV mass decreased by 11%, periarteriolar collagen area regressed by 54% and is the most likely structural basis for the improvement in coronary flow and reserve.

Contributors to Coronary Vasodilation Abnormalities Associated with LVH and Hypertension

Impairment of coronary vasoreactivity in patients with hypertension and LVH has also been documented and may be a contributor to a decreased vasodilator reserve. Patients with hypertension demonstrated impaired vasodilation in response to increases in coronary flow during a cold pressor test [40]. When flow velocity was increased, both proximal and distal segments of coronary arteries constricted, rather than dilated. Patients with essential hypertension and LVH demonstrated marked attenuation of endothelium-dependent vasodilation to acetylcholine, but not to adenosine, an endothelium-independent vasodilator [41]. Consistent with these data, a study on 100 patients showed that the presence of LVH in hypertensive patients was associated with attenuated endothelium-dependent and -independent coronary flow reserve, since hypertension in the absence of LVH did not cause a significant impairment [42]. Attenuation of the vasodilator response to both acetylcholine and adenosine in patients with concentric hypertrophy due to pressure overload has also been documented [43]. Advanced age and hypercholesterolemia have been found to selectively impair relaxation of coronary epicardial arteries [44]. However, the response to acetylcholine in hypertensive patients without evidence of LVH was normal, thus documenting the role of LVH in abnormalities of vasodilation. Finally, a reduction in the lumens of small intramyocardial arteries has been documented in hypertensive patients [45], a finding that indicates a structural basis for the decrement in coronary vasodilator reserve.

Coronary Collaterals in Pressure Overloaded Hearts

Postmortem examinations, more than a half century ago, suggested that the frequency of intercoronary anastomoses is greater in hypertrophied hearts [46, 47], an observation that implied that collaterals might compensate for the increased cardiac mass. However, decades later, pressure–flow relationships in adenosine-vasodilated, blood-perfused normal and collateral zones in dogs with renal hypertension and LVH were found to be similar to those of control dogs [48]. Thus, these data suggested that collateral resistance is not altered by hypertension and LVH. Another study regarding collateral flow in dog hearts hypertrophied by pressure overload concluded that the increased pressure and wall stress did not cause significant collateral growth [49]. Thus, the data in these two studies indicate that the functional capacity of collateral vessels was not enhanced by pressure overload and the presence of LVH.

Pressure Overload in Experimental Animals

Perfusion Abnormalities: Canine, Porcine, and Canine Studies

Reduction in Maximal Myocardial Perfusion

Myocardial perfusion abnormalities due to LVH and hypertension (induced by aortic constriction, renal hypertension, or perinephritic hypertension) have been documented in numerous studies [22, 50–63]. Melvin Marcus and his colleagues defined some key abnormalities that occur in the coronary circulation of dogs with LVH induced by renal hypertension [53, 54, 57, 58, 64]. Using the 1-kidney, 1 clip renal vascular hypertension model, they documented a 70% increase in minimal coronary vascular resistance/100 g ventricle (MCVR) in the hypertensive dogs with LVH (HT-LVH) with no change in total LV resistance [53]. O'Keefe et al. [59] found a similar increase in minimal coronary vascular resistance (84%) in dogs 6 weeks after banding the aorta. Findings from these studies indicated that the cross-sectional area of the coronary vasculature does not increase in response to a 50% increase in ventricular mass.

In dogs with 1-kidney, 1-wrap (Page) hypertension, myocardial oxygen consumption (MVO_2) was increased by administration of dobutamine, a β-receptor agonist [65]. Coronary blood flow and MVO_2 were similar in the normotensive and hypertensive dogs, and adenosine release was the same at similar MVO_2 and coronary blood flows for both groups. Therefore, the authors concluded that the higher coronary vascular resistance in the hypertensive dogs is not the consequence of a reduced release of adenosine.

Changes in Flow Distribution

Abnormalities of coronary blood flow in the heart hypertrophied by pressure overload are usually noted during stress and are most severe in the endomyocardium [22, 51, 60, 61, 66–70]. Dogs with LVH due to aortic stenosis experience a reduction in endomyocardial/epimyocardial blood flow during strenuous exercise [50] and a failure of endomyocardial flow to increase during the higher demand for O_2 [55]. Similar data have been derived from experiments on pigs [67] and cats [70]. Moreover, dogs with pressure overload-induced LVH subjected to atrial pacing failed to increase flow to the endomyocardium [69, 71]. Flow distribution during tachycardia favors the epimyocardium, causing hypoperfusion of the endomyocardium [50], which also is characterized by a deterioration of contractile function [69]. Data from pigs with RV pressure overload created by banding the pulmonary artery indicated that during tachycardia (pacing up to 225 beats/min), the increases in blood flow to the endomyocardium and midmyocardium were lower than in the control pigs, and that endomyocardial/epimyocardial flow ratio decreased to near unity [72]. This contrasted with transmural perfusion gradients favoring the endomyocardium in the control group.

Factors Contributing to Hypoperfusion in the Hypertrophied Heart

As previously indicated, a lower length density and impaired vasodilation of resistance vessels are factors that limit maximal myocardial perfusion in hearts hypertrophied in response to pressure overload. Experiments by Bache's group [63] on dogs with aortic constriction and LVH explored other factors that contribute to hypoperfusion. First, they found that when these dogs were subjected to a bout of exercise on a treadmill, their heart rates were increased more and their myocardial O_2 consumption was 52% greater than control dogs exercising at the same intensity. This greater O_2 demand was associated with a large decrease in endomyocardial/epimyocardial flow ratio in the dogs with LVH. Second, they noted that back pressure (coronary pressure at zero flow) during total coronary artery occlusion in these dogs was significantly increased, compared to the controls [73]. This regional perfusion and work mismatch was accompanied by increased end-diastolic pressure both at rest and during graded exercise stress to maximal heart rate and striking perturbations of the calculated extravascular impedance to flow. Thus, this study provided evidence that exaggerated enhancement of filling pressure during exercise in dogs with LVH contributes to impaired myocardial perfusion due, in part, to changes in extravascular compression that oppose flow. Finally, in a subsequent study, these authors addressed the contribution of extravascular compressive forces to endomyocardial hypoperfusion during exercise [74]. Dogs with LVH and their controls had similar increases in myocardial perfusion and similar endomyocardial/epimyocardial blood flow ratios during adenosine infusion. However, when adenosine was infused during exercise, heart rate doubled causing a redistribution of myocardial perfusion and a more marked decline in endomyocardial/epimyocardial flow ratio than that recorded in control dogs. This exaggerated decline in endomyocardial perfusion during exercise was attributed to increased extravascular compressive forces resulting from a greater decrease in diastolic duration and a greater increase in LV end-diastolic pressure.

Elevated Arterial Pressure and Myocardial Hypertrophy Each Influence Perfusion

Valvular aortic stenosis has either no effect on coronary pressure or may slightly decrease perfusion pressure, if severe. In contrast, experimental models in which the occlusion is placed above the coronary ostia cause an increase in coronary artery pressure in addition to evoking LV pressure overload. To determine the effects of pressure overload on the LV in the absence of increased coronary pressure, Alyono [75] placed a noncoronary cusp to affect aortic valve stenosis in dogs aged 6–8 weeks. When the dogs reached adulthood, myocardial blood flow was elevated at rest and attenuated during maximal vasodilation compared to the non-hypertrophic hearts of control dogs. During tachycardia, increases in myocardial perfusion were subnormal in the dogs with LVH; the smallest increases occurred in the endomyocardium. Therefore, pressure overload, in the absence of hypertension, compromised myocardial perfusion in this model.

Role of Myocardial Hypertrophy in Ischemia and Infarction

To test the hypothesis that the presence of LVH and hypertension (HT) causes a larger infarct during myocardial ischemia, dogs with HT and LVH were subjected to sudden coronary occlusion [53]. Indeed, the area of myocardial ischemia was greater in these dogs than in the normotensive controls. However, over a 48-h period, collateral blood flow increased to a similar level in the HT-LVH and control dogs, and the reduction in flow in response to coronary occlusion was similar in the two groups. Therefore, the greater ischemia that occurred in the HT-LVH group could not be attributed to a lower level of flow from collateral channels. Later it was found that in hearts hypertrophied in response to renal hypertension the infarct size in the mid- and endomyocardium relative to the risk area was greater than in normotensive dogs [58]. Most important was the finding that postcoronary artery occlusion mortality was threefold higher in the HT-LVH dogs [57]. Subsequently, it was discovered that the wave front of infarction was accelerated in dogs with HT-LVH and that this wave front could be attenuated by reducing arterial pressure during the first hour of coronary occlusion [76]. Vulnerability to myocardial hypoperfusion of the hypertrophied heart in dogs with aortic constriction was documented by Bache et al. [63]. In the presence of various degrees of CAS, both control and LVH dogs experienced a gradient of hypoperfusion from epicardium to endocardium during exercise. However, at each level of CAS, flow to the endomyocardium was less in the dogs with LVH. Surprisingly, dogs with LVH of 12-month duration by aortic constriction are able to recover from myocardial ischemia as effectively as their non-hypertrophic controls [77].

Regression of Myocardial Hypertrophy and Myocardial Perfusion

The effects of LVH regression on myocardial perfusion abnormalities was investigated by removing the pressure overload and causing a 50% reduction of the increase in LV mass [71]. This degree of LVH regression caused normalization of both endo- and epimyocardial blood flows during maximal coronary vasodilation. However, flow during pacing failed to increase in either of these myocardial regions. Since flow during maximal vasodilation was normal when LVH partially regressed, the authors concluded that coronary vascular capacity was normalized and that functional vascular compressive forces were responsible for the flow limitations that occurred during rapid pacing.

Structural Changes in Hearts with Perfusion Abnormalities Due to Pressure Overload

My colleagues and I used morphometry to determine the coronary arterial hierarchy in relation to the enhanced MCVR in dogs with renal hypertension-induced LVH [78]. A 27% increase in LV mass occurred after short-term (6 weeks) renal hypertension and LVH (HT-LVH), and was associated with a 67% increase in MCVR. The wall/lumen ratios were similar in all size classes of arterioles and arteries. The increase in the percent of collagen in the tunica media of epicardial arteries did not cause inward remodeling as lumen diameter in these vessels was increased in the HT-LVH dogs. Thus, the data suggested that the marked increase in MCVR was due to a lack of growth of the resistance vessels. Next, as summarized in Fig. 11.4, we studied dogs with long-term (7 months) hypertension, which resulted in a 46% increase in LV mass (compared to only a 27% increase that occurred after 6 weeks) and found that a substantial growth of the resistance vessels had occurred during long-term hypertension, since (1) total MCVR was significantly lower and (2) MCVR/100 g was no longer significantly elevated [80]. Indeed, arteriolar density in the epimyocardium and endomyocardium was virtually identical in the hypertensive and normotensive dogs and tended to be higher in the midmyocardium of the hypertensive group. The diameter size profile of arterioles of the two groups was similar, with a tendency of more small arterioles in the hypertensive group, a finding indicative of arteriogenesis. In contrast, capillary growth did not fully compensate for the increase in LV mass, as indicated by a tendency for lower values for capillary length density, which were significant in the midmyocardium and endomyocardium [81]. However, total capillary length was 40% higher in the HT-LVH dogs, a finding that documents a substantial capillary growth during the 7-month period of hypertension, which we estimated to be 1/5 of the total absolute capillary length. This study demonstrated that the coronary microcirculation has a remarkable capacity to remodel in the setting of long-term hypertension and hypertrophy.

Arteriolar growth and remodeling in the pressure overloaded RV of pigs has also been reported [82]. A complete computerized reconstruction of RV branches was established and flows were computed throughout the reconstructed trees based on conversion of mass and momentum. The data revealed that flow rate was increased in large arteries in the

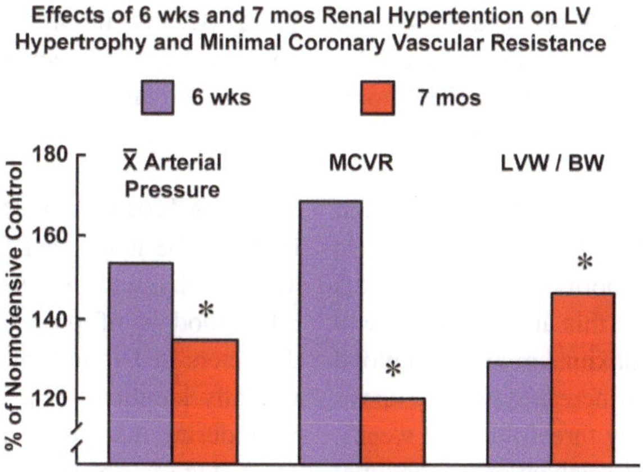

Fig. 11.4 A comparison of minimal coronary vascular resistance (MCVR) in dogs with hypertension for 6 weeks or 7 months. The data indicate that mean arterial pressure and MCVR (pressure/maximal flow) are high at 6 weeks, but fall significantly by 7 months, despite a further increase in LVW/BW (left ventricular weight adjusted for body weight). These data suggest that compensatory growth of coronary resistance vessels occurred over time, enabling the improvement in myocardial perfusion. Data derived from Tomanek et al. [78] and Tomanek et al. [79]

hypertrophied RV and normalized in intramyocardial arteries; the latter was due to an increase in the number of arterioles. This analysis of the coronary hierarchy demonstrated that perfusion in the arteriolar and capillary beds are compensated in this model of RV hypertrophy. Data from the RV of pigs with pulmonary hypertension indicates that all segments of the coronary arterial tree grew during the development of RV hypertrophy and that as a consequence coronary resistance was decreased [83]. Subsequently, remodeling of the right main coronary artery in this model was documented [84]. Both lumen diameter and flow increased during a 4-week pressure overload by banding of the pulmonary artery and the increases were associated with increased levels of ROS. Thus, ROS appears to have a beneficial effect in promoting growth of the coronary vasculature during pressure overload. However, the downside of ROS generation is that endothelial function becomes compromised due, in part, to perturbations of eNOS function.

Hypertension Modulates Coronary Microvascular Function

Urbieta Caceres et al. [85] tested the hypothesis that hypertension modulates microvascular function in hearts with a chronic CAS. Pigs with chronic renovascular hypertension (HT) or with CAS or both (HT+CAS) were studied. Microvascular (arterioles/small arteries) density was reduced in swine with CAS, but not in swine with HT or HT+CAS. Arteriolar/small artery density, compared to the controls, was lower in pigs with CAS, but not in those with HT or CAS+HT. In the area of risk, HT enhanced interstitial fibrosis and inflammation. Although the former is clearly a factor that limits cardiac function, the later may facilitate microvascular proliferation [86]. The investigators concluded that the coexistence of early renovascular hypertension exacerbated myocardial fibrosis and coronary vascular remodeling and that these changes were not secondary to a decline in vascular density, but rather the extracellular changes, i.e., inflammation and fibrosis.

Pressure Overload in Spontaneously Hypertensive Rats

Vascular Growth and Myocardial Perfusion

The development of LVH in the spontaneously hypertensive rats (SHR) model of hypertension is gradual, as evidenced by 14%, 28%, and 29% increases in LV mass at 3, 7, and 15 months, respectively [87]. Friberg [88] found that MCVR in isolated hearts was about twofold greater in SHR than in the normotensive WKY at the age of 4 months. We found that MCVR/g at 7 months was elevated, but declined by 15 months to values similar to the normotensive, WKY rats. However, MCVR/g continued to be elevated in 14-month-old stroke-prone SHR that had developed a much more severe cardiac hypertrophy. These data indicate that growth of resistance vessels (1) compensates for the LVH once it is stabilized, but (2) is inadequate when hypertension and hypertrophy are severe. Using a miniature, pulsed Doppler flowmeter, we found that a decrement in peak/rest blood flow velocity and repayment/debt area ratios were lower in SHR during the period of developing LVH, but increased in 12-month-old SHR with stabilized LVH to values similar to normotensive WKY [89]. Capillary growth between 7 and 15 months was also normalized as indicated by values for numerical and surface densities of these vessels, as well as intercapillary distances that were similar to the normotensive WKY group [90], a finding verified by a subsequent study [91]. However, capillary density in stroke-prone SHR continues to be depressed as late as 40 weeks of age [92]. Work by Vitullo et al. [93] also demonstrated a decline in maximal myocardial perfusion in SHR between ages 4 and 11 months that was associated with a decline in arteriolar density as well as higher wall/lumen/ratios in SHR compared to WKY. The latter was due to an increase in wall thickness.

McAinsh et al. [94] analyzed VEGF mRNA expression and found that in 4-month-old SHR, the expression levels are not elevated above those of the normotensive WKY rats and that this failure of activation of this angiogenic growth factor is associated with impaired maximal myocardial blood flow. By 28 weeks, VEGF mRNA is increased twofold above that of WKY and is increased nearly threefold at 32 weeks. These time points correspond to normalization of maximal coronary blood flow in SHR noted above.

Hypertension and Coronary Vessel Reactivity

In addition to structural changes in the coronary vasculature of SHR, changes in vascular reactivity also contribute to impairments in coronary flow. Kushibiki et al. [95] reported that aldosterone-induced arteriolar vasoconstriction was 1.6 times greater in SHR than in age-matched WKY and was associated with higher angiotensin II type-1 receptor (AT1R) mRNA. AT1R blockade abolished aldosterone-activated vasoconstriction. Regression of structural changes in the coronary vasculature by antihypertensive treatment (SHR) is suggested as the basis for improving maximal myocardial perfusion [96]. To distinguish the effect of hypertension from LVH, we treated SHR with hydralazine from the time of weaning (1 month) until they were 7 or 8 months of age, corresponding to the age when LVH peaks [97]. This antihypertensive drug maintained arterial blood pressures in the normotensive range, but had little effect on LV mass. Nevertheless, MCVR/g and total MCVR were significantly lower in the treated SHR and did not differ from the values recorded in WKY. Moreover, MCVR/g was also reduced in the non-hypertrophied RV of SHR by lowering arterial blood pressure. These data document an elevated blood pressure as a contributor to the increased MCVR/g that occurs in SHR during the development of LVH.

In SHR, coronary flow in response to serotonin was reduced in a dose-dependent manner, whereas in normotensive WKY rats, the response was increased flow [98]. When the cyclooxygenase inhibitor indomethacin was injected, the decrease in coronary flow was prevented. The investigators concluded that the decrease in coronary flow in response to serotonin could be due to (1) direct vasoconstriction, (2) endothelial dysfunction, or (3) effects on cardiac performance. SHR have also been found to be more sensitive to excess salt than the normotensive WKY [99]. Although excess salt in the diet of these two strains elevated arterial pressure only slightly, it increased both interstitial and perivascular collagen deposition, and decreased maximal coronary flow in response to dipyridamole in SHR, but not in WKY. Because the maximal coronary flow was impaired in both the hypertrophied LV and the non-hypertrophied RV, the investigators concluded that hypertension-induced fibrosis contributed to attenuated coronary blood flow.

SHR as a Model of Hypertension and LVH

It should be noted that SHR is a genetic model of cardiac hypertrophy, and therefore it differs in some respects from other models of pressure overload. First, cardiomyocyte diameters in 1-month-old SHR and their WKY controls are virtually identical [90], although heart weight is greater in SHR during the prehypertensive stage [100]. Therefore, the early stage is not associated with cardiac hypertrophy, but rather a greater number of cardiomyocytes in SHR, a consequence of hyperplasia. Second, eccentric, rather than concentric, cardiac hypertrophy characterizes SHR, as indicated by LV pressure–volume curves [101]. On the other hand, this model is more similar to idiopathic hypertension in humans, because blood pressure increases and cardiac hypertrophy develops gradually.

Pressure Overload in Rodents and Rabbits

Renal Hypertension

Rats with one-kidney, one clip hypertension had significant decrements in capillary density despite evidence of capillary growth, i.e., increased total capillary length and capillary/cardiomyocyte ratio [102]. Even a modest increase in heart weight in this model caused a 21% decrease in capillary density in the endomyocardium [103]. Renal hypertension in rats induced by the two-kidney, one-clip method was associated with closely related increases in blood pressure and LV mass, and resulted in an increase in MCVR/g and a decrease in maximal coronary flow [104, 105]. Similar results were obtained in another study that used this model of hypertension [106]. In rabbits with 1-kidney, 1-clip hypertension, arteriolar densities were reduced, causing an increase in the percent of perfused arterioles [107]. The latter normalized resting flow, but maximal myocardial perfusion would be likely attenuated. Both impaired LV function and coronary flow during anoxia were demonstrated in working isolated hearts from rats with renal hypertension [108]. These impairments occurred after only 6 days of hypertension and persisted during at least the 10 week duration of the studies. Thus, impaired coronary vasodilator reserve is an early response to hypertension and is associated with impaired ventricular function [109]. Similarly, in rats with deoxycorticosterone acetate-salt hypertension of 18 weeks duration, minimal RV and LV coronary vascular resistance per tissue mass was elevated, although endomyocardial/epimyocardial flow ratios were similar to the normotensive rats [110]. The relationship between perivascular fibrosis and impaired maximal coronary flow and vasodilator reserve, noted in humans (described earlier in this chapter), is also suggested by data from experimental animals [111]. In rats with renovascular hypertension, a reduction in coronary perivascular collagen with captopril (an ACE inhibitor) treatment could, like in humans, be responsible for the improved coronary flow and reserve.

Aortic Constriction

In guinea pigs, aortic banding caused inward remodeling of coronary arterioles and reduced reactive hyperemia, i.e., both peak flow and debt repayment were attenuated [112]. Similarly aortic constriction in rats has been shown to decrease coronary vasodilator reserve [113–115] and the reactive hyperemic response [113]. Coronary arterioles were remodeled, as evidenced by increased wall/lumen ratios and an increase in perivascular collagen [114, 115]. The reversibility of this remodeling was documented by removing the aortic band and finding that coronary reserve and the arteriolar structural changes were normalized after 4–10 weeks [113–115]. The normalization of impaired autoregulation in rats after debanding was found to depend on the duration of the pressure overload [116]. When the aorta was constricted for 4 weeks, the coronary autoregulation gain was normalized by the fourth week after debanding, whereas it remained unchanged in the rats that had been banded for 10 weeks. A marked reduction in coronary vasodilator reserve in mice with pressure overload has also been demonstrated [117]. Moreover, vasodilation in response to endothelium-dependent (acetylcholine) and endothelium-independent (sodium nitroprusside and adenosine) mediators was decreased. Aortic constriction in mice has been shown to impair coronary arteriolar dilations to acetylcholine and adenosine and to enhance constriction in response to endothelin-1 (Guangrong Lu, personal communication). Three to five weeks after banding, the medial layer of arterioles was thickened and perivascular fibrosis was present. Accordingly, these data support the conclusion that both structural and functional impairments occur in the coronary vasculature in hearts hypertrophied by pressure overload due to aortic constriction.

Maximal Coronary Perfusion and Vascular Growth

Hypertension and Cardiac Hypertrophy Limit Vasodilator Reserve

Dissociation Of Pressure Overload and Cardiac Hypertrophy

Long-term pressure overload in humans is usually characterized by a decreased coronary vasodilator reserve, a finding that indicates that the cross-sectional area of the coronary vasculature has not increased in proportion to the increase in cardiac mass. As noted earlier, the reduction in coronary vasodilator reserve can occur if the resistance vessels (1) do not grow in proportion to the magnitude of myocardial hypertrophy, (2) undergo a concentric medial hypertrophy (inward remodeling), or (3) experience attenuation of their dilator responses (by either a structural or functional change). It has been documented that both hypertension and cardiac hypertrophy may limit coronary vasodilator reserve [118]. Moreover, we found that cardiac hypertrophy and hypertension can be dissociated [97, 119]. For example, when SHR were treated with a dose of α-methyldopa that failed to significantly reduce arterial pressure, LVH was attenuated [119]. Similarly, a reduction in arterial pressure in SHR with hydralazine and normalization of coronary vasodilator reserve had only a minimal effect on LV weight [97]. Arterial pressure was normalized in SHR by either hydralazine or captopril (an ACE inhibitor), but only the later reduced LV mass [120]. Maximal coronary perfusion was normalized by captopril and slightly improved by hydralazine, whereas capillary density was increased only by captopril. These data indicate that the improvement in myocardial perfusion is a consequence of both lowering arterial pressure and LV mass. In contrast, capillary density is dependent on LV mass. To disassociate the effects of elevated blood pressure and cardiac hypertrophy on coronary vasodilator reserve, Wicker and Tarazi [121] decreased arterial pressure with captopril and then discontinued treatment, allowing pressure to rise. RV minimal coronary vascular resistance rose as pressure increased, but RV mass remained normal, indicating that the increase in resistance was related to elevated arterial pressure.

The effects of arterial pressure and LV mass and their interactions in determining maximal coronary flow was addressed by Kobayashi et al. [122]. They compared rats with (1) LVH and normal arterial pressure, (2) small hearts and normal arterial pressure, (3) both LVH and hypertension (SHR-stroke prone), and (4) normotensive rats with no LVH. Their data revealed that maximal coronary perfusion is a function of arterial pressure/LV weight, a finding that indicates that elevated arterial pressure helps maintain maximal myocardial perfusion.

Pressure Overload Induces Structural Changes in Coronary Arteries

Rats with pressure overload due to aortic banding were found to have medial hypertrophy and perivascular fibrosis of coronary arteries [115]. When β-aminopropionitrile was administered to inhibit collagen deposition, perivascular collagen decreased to the levels of sham rats, but arterial wall/lumen ratios were not altered and peak flow reactive/resting ratios did not improve. However, when the pressure overload was reversed by debanding and the anti-collagen treatment administered, wall/lumen ratios were normalized and peak reactive/resting flow ratio values were similar to the sham group. These data indicate that wall/lumen ratio rather than perivascular collagen is a key determinant of peak coronary flow. Similar conclusions were reached in a study of SHR treated with the ACE inhibitor, lisinopril; the data showed that normalization of coronary vasodilator reserve occurred only in rats in which coronary artery wall thickness was reduced [123].

Coronary Reserve and Cardiomyocyte Vulnerability

Because LVH limits maximal coronary flow, we tested the hypothesis that a decreased coronary vascular reserve enhances the vulnerability of cardiomyocytes to acute hypoxia in SHR [124]. Electron micrographs revealed that a 20-min period of hypoxia (7% O_2 resulting in a 70% decrease in PO_2) caused intracellular and T-tubule swelling, and mitochondrial damage. In normotensive rats with normal LV mass, cardiomyocyte damage was limited or nonexistent with a similar reduction in PO_2. When LV mass in SHR was reduced by a 3-month captopril treatment, coronary reserve was improved and cardiomyocyte damage in response to acute hypoxia was negligible.

Limitations in Capillary Growth

The long-held opinion that myocardial capillaries do not proliferate or that the proliferation is insignificant when the heart is overloaded by pressure was based on Wearn's work more than a half century ago [125, 126]. Subsequently, Mandache [127] and Ljungqvist [128] reported that, based on electron microscopy and [^{3}H] thymidine labeling, they could not find any evidence for capillary proliferation in hearts hypertrophied by either aortic constriction or renal hypertension. However, only one time point was investigated, which was a limitation of these studies. The finding that capillary/fiber ratio in the hypertrophied RV in dogs with pulmonary artery constriction was not increased after 1–5 months of pressure overload also implied that capillary proliferation does not occur in this model [129]. A decline in capillary density in pressure overloaded hearts in rats, pigs, cats, dogs, and rabbits has been reported by many investigators [78, 81, 102, 130–138]. Under this circumstance, diffusion distance for O_2 and capillary domains (the tissue served by a capillary) are increased [139]. For example, Henquell [140] reported a 2.44 μm increase in diffusion distance in rat hearts with a 43% renal hypertension-induced cardiac hypertrophy. However, the earlier assumption that no capillary growth occurs during this type of cardiac enlargement has not stood the test of time, since many studies have provided evidence that capillary growth can occur in this model. A number of factors (discussed below) serve as determinants of capillary growth and include the duration of the pressure overload, the magnitude of the cardiac hypertrophy, and the specific model of hypertension studied.

Compensatory Capillary Growth

Capillary Proliferation

Even 4 and 5 decades ago, growth of myocardial capillaries in models of pressure overload was recognized [130, 141, 142]. My colleagues and I followed the course of cardiac hypertrophy in SHR from 1 to 15 months and discovered that capillary density is lowest and cardiomyocyte diameter greatest at 7 months [90]. Stabilization of the hypertrophy between 7 and 15 months corresponded to a normalization of capillary density and intercapillary distance. Proliferation of capillary endothelial cells, based on [^{3}H] thymidine labeling, was increased twofold at 12 months. These data indicate that compensatory growth occurs in this model and that it corresponds to a period of stabilized cardiac hypertrophy. Subsequent work by Rakusan et al. [91] demonstrated that compared to normotensive WKY, SHR, aged 7 months have (1) lower capillary densities in both the epimyocardium and endomyocardium and (2) larger arteriolar and venular capillary domains. As defined in Chap. 3, arteriolar and venular capillary domains are the areas surrounding a capillary that is closest to an arteriolar and venule, respectively. The myocardial angiogenesis in the SHR model of hypertrophy was also documented by Anversa et al. [143], who employed electron microscopy to document accelerated capillary growth between 21 and 45 days of postnatal life. Taken together, these data indicate that capillary growth occurs during the early stage of developing cardiac hypertrophy and after its stabilization. Myocardial angiogenesis in this model has been shown to correlate with marked increases in VEGF mRNA [144].

Sympathetic Inhibition of Capillary Proliferation

The role of sympathetic nerve activity in hypertension-induced cardiac hypertrophy was addressed in studies in my laboratory [79, 145]. In SHR, chemical sympathectomy from birth increased capillary density, without limiting the increase in cardiac mass or the magnitude of arterial pressure [79]. Capillary diameters and intercapillary distances were also similar to those of the WKY control group. These data support the conclusion that sympathetic nerves inhibit capillary proliferation in this model of hypertension. Regional sympathectomy in renal hypertensive rats also had a marked effect on capillary growth, as evidenced by a 30% increase in capillary density and a 21% decrease in intercapillary distance [145]. This improvement in capillary growth in hypertensive rats after sympathectomy may be due to the effect of sympathectomy in limiting the decrease in VEGF gene and protein expression that has been documented in chronic renal failure in rats [146]. These investigators suggested that myocardial VEGF is decreased because of overactivity of the sympathetic nervous system, and that this deficit limits capillary growth. Another finding in our studies is that sympathectomy increases mitochondrial growth in cardiomyocytes during hypertension-induced cardiac hypertrophy [79, 147]. These findings support the conclusion that sympathetic activity negatively affects O_2 utilization of cardiomyocytes since it increases O_2 diffusion distance and limits mitochondrial growth necessary for the greater O_2 demands of increased cardiomyocyte mass.

Increased Capillary Volume Via Remodeling

Capillary length density is important because it is a determinant of diffusion distance. Another important determinant of regional flow is capillary diameter. Under some conditions, capillaries remodel to increase their diameters and consequently capillary volume density, as indicated by the following examples. Although young rats with renal hypertension did not experience an increase in total myocardial capillary length, capillary volume density was increased to the level of that of normotensive controls [133]. Morphometric analysis revealed that capillary remodeling occurred in both the endo- and epi-myocardium and resulted in an increased capillary lumen volume and surface area densities. Thus, adaptation in this model of renal hypertension that resulted in a 30% increase in LV mass involved an increase in capillary lumen cross-sectional area rather than an increase in capillary length density. Since the number of endothelial cells was not increased, the adaptation occurred as a result of an increase in capillary endothelial cell length. This type of remodeling has also been observed by us in a model of gradual coronary artery occlusion during estrogen therapy; estrogen therapy did not increase capillary length density, but caused an increase in volume density as a consequence of an increase in mean capillary diameter [148].

Pressure Overload in the Young

Data from Experimental Animals

This topic is also addressed in Chap. 3. Several studies examined the effect of pressure overload-induced LVH in young humans and animals. Vascular growth is more robust in the young. For example, the angiogenic response in the myocardium of young animals [130, 149] and humans [150, 151] is generally equal or nearly proportional to the magnitude of the hypertrophy. Even when a twofold increase in LV mass occurred in neonatal rats after banding the aorta to increase afterload, capillary density was normal [152]. Although puppies with constriction of the aorta at 8–10 weeks of age demonstrated a modest, 10–15%, decrease in capillary density, capillary diameter increased, resulting in normal capillary volume density [134]. Moreover, growth of the arteriolar bed compensated for the magnitude of LVH as documented by arteriolar densities that were similar to the controls. Aortic constriction in 10-week old lambs resulted in a smaller decline in maximal flow conductance than that observed in adult sheep with aortic constriction [149]. Young dogs (aged 1–12 months) with RV pressure overload, induced by banding of the pulmonary artery, had peak hyperemic responses that were similar to those of nonbanded control dogs [153]. Moreover, minimal coronary vascular resistance in the pressure-overloaded right ventricles was lower than that of the controls. These data lead to the conclusion that coronary vascular growth in the young can compensate for cardiac hypertrophy and thereby enable a hyperemic response proportional to the magnitude of the hypertrophy. However, several studies have shown that the endomyocardial/epimyocardial flow ratio is decreased in puppies with pressure overload due to aortic banding [66, 154, 155].

Data from Humans

Rakusan and colleagues [151] used morphometric analyses to determine the degree of capillary growth in infants (<1 year), children (9–14 years), and adults (15–30 years) with congenital aortic stenosis (Fig. 11.5). Age-matched control tissue samples were obtained from individuals who died with no known left ventricular disease. The data revealed that capillary density and domain area were similar in hearts with congenital aortic stenosis and the age-matched controls. Thus, capillary growth in hearts in which pressure overload was imposed during development was fully compensatory despite twofold to threefold increases in heart mass. However, in hearts of adults with acquired, rather than congenital, aortic valve disease, capillary density was 25% lower and capillary domain area 36% greater than that of age-matched controls. A comparison of these parameters in adults with (1) congenital coarctation and coronary hypertension and (2) aortic valve stenosis and normal coronary artery pressure indicated that the groups were similar, a finding that rules out elevated coronary pressure as a modifier of capillary growth during congenital pressure overload. An earlier study [150] also indicated normal capillary growth in infants and children with various congenital cardiac malformations.

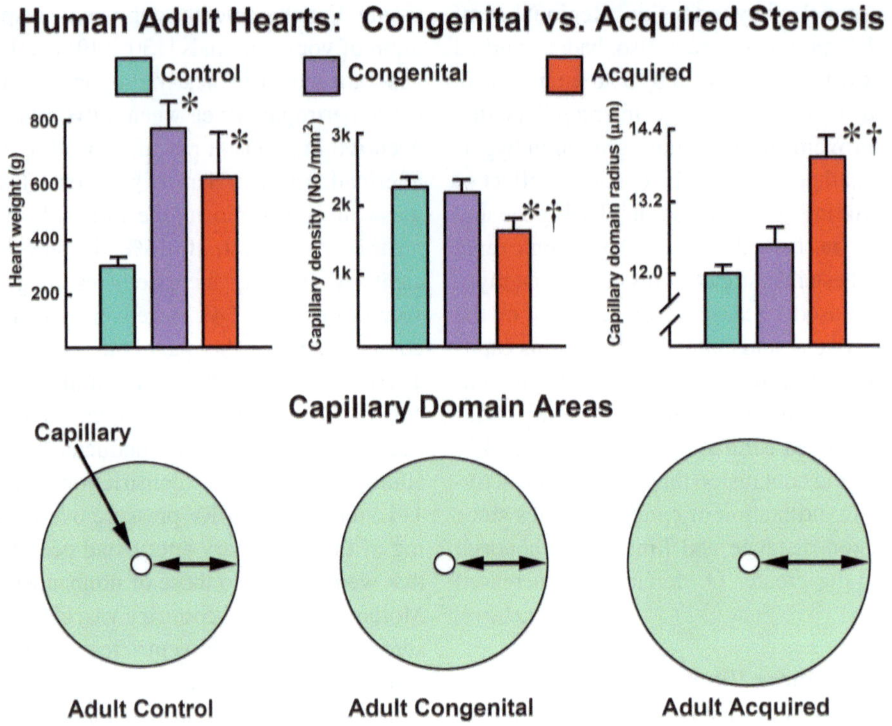

Fig. 11.5 In human adults, myocardial capillary density and capillary domain radius (a measure of diffusion distance) were preserved when the aortic valve stenosis was congenital, but not when it was acquired. The green circles represent the tissue area served by one capillary; the *arrows* indicate the radius of the capillary domain. These data were derived from Rakusan et al. [151]

> **Conclusions: Pressure Overload Hypertrophy**
> Coronary angiogenesis and arteriogenesis are usually limited when cardiac hypertrophy develops in response to increased afterload. Perfusion abnormalities are a consequence of both increased ventricular mass and hemodynamics associated with increased coronary pressure (Fig. 11.5). Several factors known to limit coronary reserve and maximal flow include (1) inadequate vascular growth, (2) perivascular fibrosis, (3) inward remodeling of resistance vessels, and (4) limited vasodilator responses.

Volume Overload

As shown in mice, the cardiac phenotype of an increased preload (volume overload) differs from that of increased afterload (pressure overload via aortic stenosis) by its lack of fibrosis and inflammation, little apoptosis, and better function [15]. Volume overload, unlike pressure overload, did not result in disturbed intracellular calcium cycling. Moreover, gene array analysis showed a different expression pattern between the two models of hypertrophy. Ventricular function may be normal even in long-term volume overload as occurs in aortocaval fistulas [156]. Chronic mitral valve regurgitation in dogs was characterized by increased end diastolic pressure, stroke volume as a consequence of increased diastolic filling due to ventricular remodeling [157]. LV stiffness was decreased, as indicated by the modulus of chamber stiffness of 2.9 vs. 7.1 in the control dogs. As noted earlier, the ventricular remodeling that occurs during chronic volume overload differs from that which characterizes chronic pressure overload, e.g., the former results in eccentric hypertrophy due to a substantial longitudinal cardiomyocyte growth only, whereas the latter causes a concentric hypertrophy. Another difference between the two models is that collagen is the major contributor to fibrosis in pressure overload, whereas volume overload is characterized by an abnormal extracellular matrix production, with a relative abundance of non-collagen proteins [158]. These structural differences may affect the vascular responses in the two models, and are therefore mentioned here.

One of the complicating factors regarding volume overload-induced cardiac hypertrophy is that it is "not a single entity, but rather a variety of hemodynamic conditions" [13]. The extremes of volume overload include the low pressure type, e.g., mitral valve regurgitation and the high pressure types, e.g., aortic valve regurgitation. Different ventricular geometries and different degrees of ventricular hypertrophy develop in these types of overload.

Microvascular Growth

Most studies have found that capillary growth in the heart hypertrophied by volume overload is proportional to the increase in cardiac mass. One study in rats reported that myocardial capillary endothelial cells proliferate as early as 1 week following creation of an aortocaval shunt [159]. Another study found that a large (70%) increase in LV mass in response to an aortocaval shunt was accompanied by sufficient angiogenesis to preserve O_2 distances [139]. Consistent with this finding, my colleagues and I [160] found that capillary volume densities in all regions of the volume-overloaded and hypertrophied LV (55% increase in mass) were similar to the controls. Our data also documented a fully compensatory growth of arterioles as evidenced by the finding that their length density and diameter frequency distributions were similar to those of the sham controls. Similarly, dog hearts with aortocaval fistulas were also found to have capillary density values that did not differ from those of their control counterparts [161]. An earlier study on dogs with arterial-venous shunts reported a small (11%) reduction in capillary density in the endomyocardium, but not in the mid- or epimyocardium [162]. Taken together, these studies indicate that growth of microvessels compensates for the increase in myocardial mass that occurs during volume overload of the ventricle. Other studies have found that although capillary growth occurred in rats with volume overload induced by aortocaval fistula in rats [163] or aortic valve lesion in dogs [164], it did not compensate for the magnitude of cardiac hypertrophy. In the study with volume overload in rats, heart weight increased by 60% during the first month after surgery and capillary density grew in proportion to the magnitude of the hypertrophy. However, by the end of the second month, capillary density decreased, despite no further increase in heart weight. A study on volume overload induced by an aortic valve lesion in rabbits reported that capillary growth did not fully compensate for the 36% increase in heart weight [164]. However, when chronic bradycardia was induced (by pacing at about 55% of the normal heart rate in the rabbits with valve lesions), capillary density increased to values above that of the non-paced, non-lesion controls.

Similarly, hypochromic microcytic anemia (another model of volume overload) due to a diet deficient in iron and copper, which caused a 65% increase in RV weight, was accompanied by a substantial (60%) increase in total capillary length and a significant increase in capillary diameter [165]. The combined increases in capillary diameter and length density resulted in 65% increase in capillary volume density in the RV. These data indicate that the compensatory response of capillaries to the increases in heart mass included both angiogenesis and remodeling, each of which contributed to an increase in capillary volume.

Coronary Vasodilator Reserve and Maximal Flow

Preservation of Maximal Coronary Flow

Chronic volume overload was produced in 1–2-year-old Beagles by a surgical shunt between the left subclavian artery and the left atrial appendage, which caused significant increases in left ventricular end diastolic volume and stroke volume [166]. The procedure affected a 36% increase in LV mass 10 weeks after the surgery, without signs of heart failure. The increase in myocardial perfusion in response to exercise stress was greater in the volume overload group than the controls. In dogs with LV hypertrophy due to the presence of aortocaval fistulas, minimal coronary vascular resistance, measured during exercise and adenosine administration, was not different from those of controls [167]. However, the endomyocardial/epimyocardial ratio was lower in the dogs with aortocaval fistulas during exercise alone or exercise and adenosine infusion. The investigators concluded that this abnormality is secondary to hemodynamic considerations, e.g., the combined effects of high O_2 demand and low diastolic pressures, rather than to the presence of hypertrophy. Gascho and colleagues [168] subjected dogs to volume overload by creating a complete heart block that resulted in a 49% increase in LV mass. Minimal coronary vascular resistance, determined during maximal vasodilation induced by adenosine infusion, was similar in these dogs and their non-overloaded controls, indicating that maximal flow was not compromised in this type of cardiac hypertrophy. In another model of volume overload, i.e., mitral valve regurgitation, Carabello et al. [169] demonstrated that baseline and maximal blood flows were normal, despite the fact that all indices of ventricular function were reduced [170].

The magnitude of the hypertrophy, coupled with its duration, may affect the ability of the coronary vasculature to adapt to volume overload. Twelve months after the imposition of an arterio-venous shunt, a group of dogs with a mean 67% increase in heart mass had attenuated values of coronary vasodilator reserve, whereas a group with a mean 32% increase in LV mass demonstrated normal values for this parameter [171]. Part of the limited coronary vasodilator reserve was attributed to the higher coronary flows during baseline conditions. However, Wahlander et al. [106] found MCVR to be normal, despite a 72% increase in LV mass 4 weeks following the creation of an A–V fistula. Volume overload, produced by an arteriovenous fistula between the iliac vessels in dogs, was found to increase coronary blood flow and myocardial O_2 consumption at rest and to decrease coronary vascular resistance [171]. Thus, coronary flow and O_2 consumption per gram of myocardium were similar in dogs with and without hypertension and LVH. Coronary reserve, determined by the percent increase in flow during reactive hyperemia, was decreased in a group of dogs with marked LVH (67%), but not in those with a more moderate (43%) LVH. Taken together, these studies indicate that coronary vascular growth in volume overload induced LVH is compensatory in moderate, but not marked LVH.

Defects in Maximal Flow in Hearts with Valve and Septal Defects

Another form of volume overload occurs in patients with atrial septal defects. Although myocardial perfusion and arterial pressures in these patients were normal at rest, their coronary hyperemic response to 20 s occlusions was 44% lower than in patients with no RV abnormalities [172]. This finding indicates an attenuated coronary reserve in these patients. However, not all experimental models of volume overload induced by valvular regurgitation cause the abnormalities seen in hearts with pressure overload. Tricuspid regurgitation, induced in dogs, increased the weights of the right atrium and RV by 77% and 30%, respectively [173]. However, MCVR was normal in the right atrium despite the large increase in mass and was only slightly increased in the RV.

In conclusion, volume overload-induced ventricular hypertrophy is characterized by some degree of compensatory coronary vascular growth that may facilitate normal maximal coronary blood flow. As noted earlier, the effects on the heart are not identical in the several different types of volume overload. Thus, the various hemodynamic variables must be taken into account. However, in general the coronary circulation adapts better to volume than to pressure overload.

Hyperthyroidism

Thyroid hormones T_3 (triiodothyromine) and T_4 (L-thyroxine) induce physiological hypertrophy by mechanisms that maintain the physiological cardiac phenotype (reviewed in [174]) and cause cardiomyocyte enlargement that resembles that which occurs during physiological growth [156]. The signaling pathways activated during thyroid hormone-induced cardiac hypertrophy preserve cell survival, maintain the normal cardiomyocyte protein expression and prevent the development of fibrosis. Work in my lab demonstrated that age does not preclude a hypertrophic response to T_4 [175], which is in contrast to some forms of cardiac hypertrophy evoked by pressure [176–178] or volume overload [179, 180]. Thyroxine hormone administration in experimental animals and in patients has been shown to maintain normal cardiovascular function, a finding that has occasionally been used to support its clinical potential (reviewed by [181]). A unique aspect of thyroid hormone-induced cardiac hypertrophy is that it is accompanied by a substantial neovascularization that is initiated on a cell surface receptor on integrin αVβ3. The neovascular response in this model of cardiac hypertrophy is consistent with an increase in O_2 required by the increased cardiac metabolism. The result is the activation of several angiogenic genes including VEGF and FGF-2 [182].

Thyroid Hormone-induced Coronary Angiogenesis and Arteriogenesis

Compensated Coronary Microvascular Growth

Administration of thyroxine to both young and adult rats has been shown to evoke compensatory growth of myocardial capillaries [137, 183–189]. A 35–40% increase in LV weight in (1 month) or adult (5 month) rats, respectively, occurred when they were treated with thyroxine for 2 months and was associated with an increase in capillary density of 35% in young and 16% in adult rats [183]. These anatomic adaptations were associated with a normal peak flow/resting flow ratio of about 2.2 in both age groups, which was similar to the control rats, a finding that indicates coronary reserve was not compromised in this model of cardiac hypertrophy. Friberg [88] measured coronary flow in isolated rat hyperthyroid hearts. He found that flows at low arterial pressures were similar to those of non-hypertrophied hearts, whereas hearts from SHR had impaired flows. Similarly, thyroxine-induced cardiac hypertrophy in pigs was characterized by a decrease in minimal coronary vascular resistance and a significant growth of arterioles and capillaries that matched the magnitude of the hypertrophy [190]. Mall and colleagues [137] reported that thyroxine-treated rats displayed a robust capillary growth as indicated by a 38% increase in capillary/cardiomyocyte ratio and a 35% increase in LV mass. Another study found that capillary growth, based on capillary volume density, compensated for the thyroxine-induced LV hypertrophy [191]. In contrast, a study on T_4-induced hypertrophy in rabbits found that myocardial perfusion demands were met by increases in the percent of arterioles and capillaries that were perfused, rather than by increases in the density these vessels [192].

As noted in Chap. 7, my colleagues and I tested the hypothesis that coronary angiogenesis in this model of hypertrophy is not significantly altered in old rats [186]. Thyroxine induced a similar increase in heart weight in 8 month (47%) and 24 month (44%) rats. Maximal myocardial perfusion in diastolic arrested hearts was similar in the thyroxine-treated rats and their age-matched controls. This finding and the data demonstrating similar capillary volume and surface densities and intercapillary distances indicate a proportional growth of the coronary vasculature in the treated and age-matched controls. Consistent with these data, Heron and Rakusan [193] found that capillary density and capillary domain area in hearts of rats treated with T_3 were normal despite a 53% increase in absolute LV weight and an 83% increase in heart weight/body weight ratio.

Direct Effects of Thyroxine on Coronary Vascularization

We tested the hypothesis that angiogenesis in the heart is initiated with the onset of T_4 treatment rather than after cardiac hypertrophy has begun developing. Using bromodeoxyuridine labeling of capillary endothelial cells, we found that their proliferation occurs during the first 24 h of T_4 treatment and is accompanied by a slight increase in FGF-2 mRNA and then a doubling of this growth factor at 48 h [187, 188]. By distinguishing arteriolar and venular capillary profiles after 4 days of treatment with thyroxine with histochemical methods, we were able to show that the proliferation of capillaries occurred predominantly at the venular sites. That capillary density increased after 5 days of treatment, prior to notable cardiac hypertrophy, supports the hypothesis that angiogenesis in this model is a response to thyroxine rather than to the hypertrophy [187]. During the next 5 days of treatment and development of cardiac hypertrophy, capillary growth continued and facilitated a density similar to the non-hypertrophic controls. Growth of the capillary bed in response to thyroxine has been shown to occur via thyroid hormone receptor TRβ, as documented in experiments on mice with knockouts of this receptor [194]. In these mice, capillary densities were lower than in the wild-type mice and their isolated ECs were unable to form capillary networks. The study also established that VEGFR-2 is a receptor controlled by thyroxine 3 in coronary ECs.

A Thyroid Hormone Analog is Angiogenic and Arteriogenic

A synthetic thyroid hormone analog, 3,5-diiodothyropropionic acid (DITPA) became available in the 1990s and was found to improve cardiac output and the rate of LV relaxation in the postinfarcted rat heart [195], and to decrease LV end-diastolic pressure [196]. Since that time, DITPA has been documented as a postinfarction treatment modality that increases eNOS protein expression in cultured ECs, and enhances both aortic vasodilation in response to either acetylcholine or isoproterenol in rats with a myocardial infarction [197]. Its role in reducing infarct size and promoting angiogenesis and arteriogenesis is discussed in Chap. 12 [189, 198–202].

Capillary Growth in the Hypothyroid State

Since hypothyroidism is characterized by a relative bradycardia and therefore a prolongation of diastole, we tested the hypothesis that this hemodynamic effect would facilitate capillary growth, despite the virtual absence of thyroid hormones in experimental hypothyroidism [175]. New Zealand white rabbits received a diet containing propylthiouracil, which reduced T_4 levels below the sensitivity of the assay and decreased heart rate by 17%. Minimal coronary vascular resistance was similar in the hypothyroid and euthyroid rabbits, whereas capillary length density in the midmyocardium and endomyocardium was higher in hearts from hypothyroid rabbits. We then subjected the hypothyroid rabbits to experimental, Page, renal hypertension (one-kidney, one-wrap) and found that, compared to their euthyroid hypertensive counterparts, they had lower mean arterial pressures, lower minimal coronary vascular resistance per heart mass, and greater values for capillary length densities. Myocardial capillary growth in hypothyroid and hyperthyroid rats has also been documented, despite the fact that hypothyroid rat hearts were smaller and hyperthyroid rat hearts larger than their euthyroid counterparts [193]. Additional studies then demonstrated that hypothyroidism in neonatal rats attenuates arteriolar growth, but not capillary growth, whereas hyperthyroidism stimulates growth of both types of vessels [203]. Vascularization in embryonic hearts was also found to occur independently of thyroxine [204]. Taken together, these studies support the conclusion that while thyroxine affects coronary vascular growth, it is not essential for the growth of capillaries. In contrast, hypothyroidism in adult rats results in a decline in the number of smallest coronary arterioles, but their number is restored when the vasodilator dipyridamole is administered concomitantly with the propylthiouracil that causes the reduction in thyroid hormones [205]. These findings suggest that enhanced myocardial perfusion, a consequence of dipyridamole administration, may be responsible for preventing the arteriolar loss that occurs with a decline or loss of thyroid hormones.

Conclusions: Hyperthyroid-Induced Cardiac Hypertrophy

Thyroid hormones induce angiogenesis and arteriogenesis, as well as cardiac hypertrophy. The extent of this vascular growth exceeds that which occurs in any other model of cardiac enlargement, and indicates that the vascular growth is fully compensatory. A thyroid hormone analog has been shown to be effective in inducing capillary growth in the infarcted heart, a finding associated with upregulation of angiogenic growth factors.

Cardiomyopathy

Hypertrophic cardiomyopathies (HCM) and dilated cardiomyopathies (DCM) are characterized by circulatory abnormalities which are not necessarily a consequence of the magnitude of the hypertrophy. HCM is an autosomal dominant disease that is characterized by mutations in sarcomeric proteins that cause hypercontractility [206]. DCM is a phenotype that results from diverse mutations (e.g., components of the membrane-scaffolding apparatus, reduced myofilament activation, transcription proteins, and nuclear envelope proteins). DCM can be either genetic or acquired. Left ventricular hypertrophy in HCM may be a response to an increase in cytosolic free Ca^{2+} or diastolic dysfunction, whereas the phenotype of DCM may be a consequence of decreased force transmission leading to LV chamber dilation [207].

Hypertrophic Cardiomyopathy

Myocardial ischemia is recognized as an aspect of the pathophysiology of HCM, but has been underappreciated [208]. The authors note that cardiovascular magnetic resonance data indicate an association between ischemia, myocardial fibrosis, and LV remodeling. These patients have impaired hyperemic myocardial blood flow [209, 210] and a lower endomyocardial/epimyocardial flow ratio, causing an under perfusion of the endomyocardium [210]. The flow impairment has been shown to be related to contractile dysfunction [209], and microcirculatory abnormalities have been proposed as contributors to the HCM phenotype [211–213]. Thus, blunted blood flow in response to adenosine provides evidence of possible coronary microvascular dysfunction in some patients with HCM [208].

Maximal myocardial blood flow and coronary vascular reserve data from 51 HCM patients has documented these variables as good predictors of favorable or unfavorable outcomes as defined by the New York Heart Association classification [214]. The follow-up, during an 8-year period, indicated that mortality was highest in the patients with the lowest myocardial blood flows. Two structural defects that may contribute to myocardial ischemia in patients with HCM are (1) hypertrophy of the walls of arterioles affecting a narrowing of their lumens [215] and (2) the lower capillary density in the hypertrophied regions of the ventricle [216, 217], which limits O_2 availability to the cardiomyocytes by increasing diffusion distances. The reduction in coronary arteriole diameters due to remodeling has been noted in regions of myocardial ischemia by several investigators, but the genesis of the remodeling is yet to be delineated (reviewed in [218]). Still another structural liability in HCM is myocardial fibrosis, which has been shown to limit myocardial perfusion at rest [219].

Dilated Cardiomyopathy

Myocardial Ischemia

Similar to HCM, myocardial ischemia is common in patients with DCM and may play an important role in the development of DCM. Accordingly, it has been suggested that anti-ischemic therapy may improve LV function and clinical outcomes in these patients (reviewed in [220]). Johnson and Palacios [221] noted that the most common cause of a form of DCM is ischemic cardiomyopathy, which develops from "multiple infarctions caused by coronary artery disease." Impaired coronary vascular reserve is frequently observed in patients with DCM [222–226], and predicts poor outcomes in these patients [223, 226]. Impaired coronary reserve is thought to prevent recovery of ventricular function in patients with hypertensive DCM [226]. Additionally, there is evidence that coronary vascular reserve is an independent predictor of long-term prognosis of atherosclerosis [227] and that coronary flow reserve correlates with dP/dt [224]. Although myocardial ischemia and a limited coronary vascular reserve are usual components of DCM, cause and effect has not been established. One frequent view, expressed decades ago, was that perfusion abnormalities are secondary to the structural and functional changes in the myocardium, e.g., increased wall stress and poor neovascularization of the hypertrophied myocardium. However, subsequent work revealed that vascular changes, including vascular remodeling or impaired vasomotion, may be primary, rather than secondary to the myocardial alterations [228].

Alterations in Vascular Function

A role for coronary microvascular dysfunction in DCM, as noted by Neglia and L'Abbate [229], has been implied by a number of studies. A relationship between myocardial perfusion and microvascular dysfunction was discovered in a study on DCM patients [230]. Infusion of acetylcholine, an endothelium-dependent vasodilator, affected a >2-fold increase in flow in non-DCM patients, but failed to significantly increase flow in DCM patients. The response to adenosine, an endothelium-independent vasodilator, was only about one-half that of the controls. Endothelial dysfunction associated with decreased NO has also been demonstrated in a mouse model of DCM [231]. In patients with DCM, inflammation has been implicated in abnormal coronary blood flow, as indicated by the discovery that the maximal flows and osteopontin, a marker of inflammation, are inversely related and that osteopontin correlates with plasma renin activity [225]. A role for adenosine $A2_A$ receptor gene polymorphism in impaired coronary flow reserve was demonstrated in a study on 80 DCM patients [232]. The findings showed that while the genetic polymorphism of $A2_A$ does not play a role in the susceptibility of DCM, it limits coronary flow reserve by blunting the coronary vasodilator response during dipyridamole infusion. A role for microvascular spasm in myocardial ischemia in cardiomyopathies was suggested 3 decades ago by Factor and Sonnenblick [233], based on their finding that of β-blockers prevented microvascular spasms in Syrian hamsters with cardiomyopathy.

Structural Alterations

A decrement in the length density of the smallest arterioles (6–20 μm) has been suggested to be the anatomical basis for the limited coronary vasodilator reserve in patients with DCM [234]. Moreover, arterioles <50 μm in diameter were characterized by an incomplete layer of smooth muscle cells. Changes in the capillary bed of patients with DCM have also been suggested to be closely related to vasodilator reserve [235, 236]. An increase in the irregularity of capillary spacing, a decrease in capillary density, and an increase in intercapillary distances were documented in histological sections from DCM patients [235]. Although coronary reserve and myocardial capillary density have been found to be significantly correlated in patients with DCM [236], the contribution of a decreased capillary density to coronary vasodilator reserve is not likely. Nevertheless, diffusion distances from capillaries are important for O_2 diffusion and irregular spacing of capillaries may contribute to pockets of tissue hypoxia within the myocardium.

Animal Models of Cardiomyopathy

Animal Models of DCM

Depending on the strain, Syrian hamsters develop either HCM or DCM, both of which are characterized by the development of cardiac hypertrophy; however, in the DCM hamsters, the hypertrophy regresses by 6 months [237]. Fibrosis is extensive in DCM hearts, as indicated by the percent of the myocardium consisting of connective tissue, which is about 25-fold greater than that of control hamsters [238]. Capillary density in the DCM Syrian hamster heart is reduced [238] and flow distribution is altered due to increased transit times in specific regions of the myocardium [239]. The authors suggested that incidences of hypoperfusion, which last from 1 to 10 s, may be due to spasms of precapillary vessels. The coronary vasculature in this type of cardiomyopathy is hyperactive; there is a 50% lower bradykinin-induced relaxation and a 1.7-fold greater thromboxane-induced resistance in 2-month-old Syrian hamsters with DCM [213]. Another study has shown that in both 4-and 6-month-old hamsters with DCM, resting and maximal blood flow is impaired, the number of cardiomyocytes is reduced, and the extent of fibrosis is increased [240].

Increased Vasoreactivity and Spasms

Microvascular spasm—a likely cause of focal ischemia and necrosis—develops as early as 1 month of age in Syrian hamsters and has been proposed as a cause of myocardial necrosis in cardiomyopathic hamsters [241]. Evidence for this hypothesis comes from data indicating focal narrowing of microvessels that is prevented by early treatment with verapamil. Such spasms are associated with focal fibrosis and cell loss [242]. Subsequently, Conway et al. [243] found that MCVR during vasopressin infusion was nearly fourfold greater in young Syrian cardiomyopathic hamsters that were undergoing myocardial necrosis compared to their older counterparts that were in a quiescent phase of the disease. A probable cause of increased vasoreactivity in this model is enhanced vascular renin–angiotensin activity and endothelial cell dysfunction related to oxidative stress [213].

Ischemic Cardiomyopathy in Mice

Ischemic cardiomyopathy in mice is characterized by an increase in ventricular dilation, a decrease in fractional shortening, and eventual heart failure [244]. Inactivation of PHD (prolyl hydroxylase domain-containing protein), which is the site of HIF-1α hydroxylation (discussed in Chap. 9), caused changes similar to those of ischemic cardiomyopathy that develop over time [245]. The finding that capillary density is increased as a consequence of HIF activation [245] suggests that ischemia might be due to changes in precapillary vessels.

> **Conclusions: Cardiomyopathies**
> A limited hyperemic response and episodes of myocardial ischemia may contribute to cardiomyopathies. Both structural (failure of compensatory arterial growth) and functional (impaired vasodilation) vascular abnormalities occur in cardiomyopathies, especially DCM. The perturbations of vascular abnormalities observed in humans are recapitulated in many animal models of cardiomyopathy.

Mechanisms of Angiogenesis and Arteriogenesis During Cardiac Hypertrophy

As discussed in Chap. 1, and also noted in other chapters of this book, vascular growth is stimulated by metabolic (primarily hypoxia) and mechanical (primarily shear stress and stretch) factors. The roles of these influences in angiogenesis and arteriogenesis of the hypertrophied heart may be modified by other factors associated with specific types of hypertrophies. Nevertheless, as already noted, coronary vessels can, under the right conditions, grow and remodel when the heart enlarges. Although both shear stress and stretch stimulate vascular growth by triggering growth factors and other signaling molecules (reviewed in [6, 246]), there are differences between the two mechanical forces. With the development of cardiac hypertrophy, blood flow must increase to provide sufficient O_2 to cardiomyocytes. The flow-associated shear stress is a force that causes cellular and extracellular changes through multiple sensing mechanisms, including integrins, ion channels, G protein receptors and G proteins, PECAM, and tyrosine kinase receptors [247]. ECs respond differently to specific types of shear stresses, i.e., laminar, disturbed, or oscillatory. Flow/shear stress and cyclic stretch in vessels containing smooth muscle affect both the endothelium and the adjacent VSMCs, and therefore there are similarities in the effects involving mechanotransduction in both. However, as discussed below, the effects also differ with regard to cell type and specific mechanical force.

Flow and Shear Stress in Coronary Angiogenesis and Arteriogenesis

Responses of ECs

ECs undergo DNA synthesis in response to enhanced flow or turbulence and flattening (Fig. 11.6). Cardiac hypertrophy in response to exercise, hypoxia, and hypothyroidism is characterized by vascular growth (reviewed in [6, 248]). When rabbits with renal hypertension and a moderate (27%) LVH were administered dipyridamole for 2 months, capillary length density (total capillary length in a volume of tissue) in the endomyocardium was increased by 33% [249]. Each injection of dipyridamole elevated blood flow by 60% after 1 h, which then returned gradually to baseline levels over the next 5 h. These findings are consistent with previous studies that have reported increased capillary growth in response to dipyridamole in normotensive rats [250, 251] and in response to adenosine in normotensive rabbits [252].

ECs sense shear stress via integrins, PECAM-1, thyrosine kinase receptors, the glycocalyx, G-proteins, and ion channels; signals are then transmitted to the nucleus via eNOS, Ca^{2+}, and kinases (Fig. 11.6). Shear stress-induced EC proliferation has been shown to produce an enhanced and sustained ERK ½ phosphorylation [253]. These experiments, which employed variable flow profiles and hence variable shear stress, demonstrate that even a short burst of impulse flow is a potent mitogenic stimulus in ECs. ROS facilitates the induction of the c-fos oncogene [254] and increases ICAM-1 mRNA [255], an adhesion molecule that facilitates attachment of ECs during their assembly into vascular tubes. Suggested reviews of this topic: Skalak [256]; Ishida [257].

Responses of VSMCs

Flow has long been recognized as a modulator of vessel diameter. A prime example of the role of flow and shear stress is coronary collateral growth involving remodeling [258]. Shear stress increases with increase in flow in the collateral vessels when one of its parent vessels is occluded, a topic that was discussed in Chap. 10. Shear stress triggers mechanoreceptors including cell membrane receptors, ion channels, cell surface glycocalyx, and integrins, which then activate signaling messengers, e.g., NO, Ca^{2+}, and kinases [259]. Shear stress in small coronary arteries is regulated by NO release from ECs, whereas NO has only minimal effects in arterioles [260].

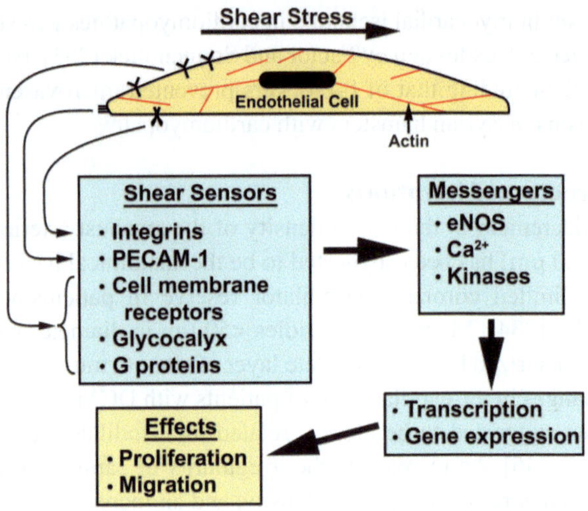

Fig. 11.6 Shear stress applied to the luminal cell surface of endothelial cells is sensed by cell membrane components, such as tyrosine kinase receptors and ion channels. Cytoskeletal filaments, including actin, are interconnected to membrane proteins throughout the cell and are also responsive to shear stress; they align in the direction of the shear. PECAM-1 is located at junctions between endothelial cells; its expression is required for shear-induced ERK phosphorylation. Mechanotransduction involves messengers, which lead to the induction of transcription factors and the gene expression of angiogenic factors

Cyclic Stretch (Cyclic Strain) in Coronary Angiogenesis and Arteriogenesis

Response of Endothelial Cells

The ventricular walls of the volume-overloaded heart are subjected to stretch resulting from the eccentric hypertrophy and the increased diastolic volume that characterize this model. The evidence that stretch plays a role in angiogenesis is supported by our in vitro studies. When the conditioned media from isolated cardiomyocytes subjected to cyclic stretch were added to cultures of microvascular endothelial cells, their proliferation, migration, and tube formation were significantly increased [261]. VEGF mRNA and protein expression were increased twofold in the conditioned media; when VEGF neutralizing antibodies were added to the media, the proliferative response of the microvascular ECs was greatly reduced. We then subjected the isolated microvascular ECs to cyclic stretch and found that VEGFR-2, Tie-1, Tie-2, angiopoietin-1, and -2 proteins were elevated and that proliferation migration and tube formation of these cells were significantly increased [262]. These data demonstrate that cyclic stretch provides angiogenic signaling by enhancing both paracrine and autocrine signaling and facilitates the angiogenic potential of coronary microvascular ECs.

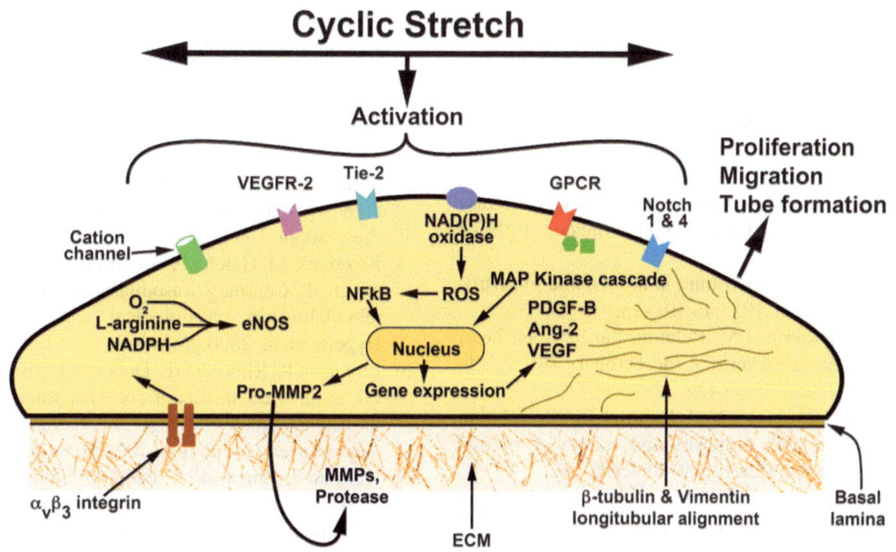

Fig. 11.7 Cyclic stretch is an important activator of events that enable endothelial cell proliferation, migration, and vascular tube formation. The cell membrane detects hemodynamic forces via mechanosensory signaling systems: tyrosine kinase receptors, ion channels, G protein receptors (GPCR), and integrins. This detection activates second messengers, including mitogen-activated protein (MA)) kinase, and leads to an increase in transcription factors and consequently gene expression of key angiogenic factors, e.g., PDGF-B, angiopoietin-2 (Ang-2), and VEGF. The release of matrix metalloproteinases (MMPs) enables degradation of the extracellular matrix, thus facilitating endothelial cell migration

As illustrated in Fig. 11.7, cyclic stretch activates kinase receptors, G protein-coupled receptors, and integrins that cause an ensuing intracellular cascade involving MAP kinases. EC proliferation and migration are facilitated by intracellular rearrangement of the cytoskeleton and MMP-mediated changes in the extracellular matrix. Endothelial nitric oxide synthase (eNOS) mRNA and protein are upregulated by cyclic stretch [263]. Cyclic stretch-activated upregulation of eNOS is mediated by an increase in intracellular Ca^{2+} through stretch-activated channels during an early phase, followed by a later phase of PI3K/Akt activation [264]. An endothelial-derived hyperpolarizing factor synthase/cytochrome P 450 has been shown to be a mechanosensitive gene product that is responsive to cyclic stretch [265]. This factor is significant because it regulates multiple signaling pathways that promote EC proliferation [266] and angiogenesis [267]. Suggested reviews for this topic are Skalak and Price [256] and Cummins et al. [268]

Vascular Smooth Muscle Cells

Stretch activates molecules not only in ECs but also in VSMCs. The latter are influenced by both the molecules secreted by ECs (paracrine effect) and by direct mechanical influences of the stretch (reviewed in [256, 269]). RhoA expression in VSMCs is a key response to stretch that mediates downstream effectors including MAPKs (reviewed in [270]). Most of the data are based on static stretch of isolated cells and therefore do not reflect the in vivo situation and the influence of cyclic stretch. Although stretch of isolated VSMCs induces their proliferation and migration, this effect does not usually occur in vivo because of the influence of ECs and because the degree of cyclic stretch is much less than that utilized by in vitro studies using static stretch. Cyclic stretch has been shown to induce EC locomotion, in part, by the dynamic regulation of syndecan-4 [271] and by activation of protein kinase C delta [272]. The latter implies a link between the cyclic stretch and actin fibers that facilitate migration.

Conclusions Regarding a Role of Mechanical Factors in Angiogenesis and Arteriogenesis

Both flow-mediated shear stress and cyclic stretch are hemodynamic forces that can trigger changes in ECs and VSMCs causing vascular growth and remodeling. Increases in coronary blood flow, which occur in some models of cardiac hypertrophy (namely thyroxine and exercise), are the most likely activators of both angiogenesis and arteriogenesis in these models. The shear stress that occurs in developing collateral vessels when an artery undergoes narrowing is another example of flow-mediated vascular growth. In contrast, enhanced cyclic stretch that occurs in the volume-overloaded ventricle provides the impetus for angiogenesis and most likely arteriogenesis.

References

1. Weeks KL, McMullen JR. The athlete's heart vs. the failing heart: can signaling explain the two distinct outcomes? Physiology. 2011;26:97–105.
2. Sheridan DJ, McAinsh A, O'Gorman DJ. The coronary circulation in cardiac hypertrophy. J Cardiovasc Pharmacol. 1993;22 Suppl 6:S18–28.
3. Vogelberg K. Caliber of coronary ostium in normal and hypertrophic hearts. Z Kreislaufforsch. 1957;46:101–15.
4. Paulsen S, Vetner M, Hagerup LM. Relationship between heart weight and the cross sectional area of the coronary ostia. Acta Pathol Microbiol Scand A. 1975;83:429–32.
5. Hutchins GM, Bulkley BH, Miner MM, Boitnott JK. Correlation of age and heart weight with tortuosity and caliber of normal human coronary arteries. Am Heart J. 1977;94:196–202.
6. Tomanek RJ, Torry RJ. Growth of the coronary vasculature in hypertrophy: mechanisms and model dependence. Cell Mol Biol Res. 1994;40:129–36.
7. Tomanek R, Dedkov E. Angiogenesis and arteriogenesis in cardiac hypertrophy in angiogenesis. Modern concepts in angiogenesis. London: Imperial College Press; 2007. p. 253–80.
8. Bache RJ. Effects of hypertrophy on the coronary circulation. Prog Cardiovasc Dis. 1988;30:403–40.
9. Anderson PG, Allard MF, Thomas GD, Bishop SP, Digerness SB. Increased ischemic injury but decreased hypoxic injury in hypertrophied rat hearts. Circ Res. 1990;67:948–59.
10. Menasche P, Grousset C, Apstein CS, Marotte F, Mouas C, Piwnica A. Increased injury of hypertrophied myocardium with ischemic arrest: preservation with hypothermia and cardioplegia. Am Heart J. 1985;110:1204–9.
11. Allard MF, Lopaschuk GD. Ischemia and reperfusion injury in the hypertrophied heart. Myocardial ischemia: mechanisms, reperfusion, protection. Basel/Switzerland: Burkhauser Verlag; 1996. p. 423–41.
12. Carabello BA. Concentric versus eccentric remodeling. J Card Fail. 2002;8:S258–63.
13. Carabello BA. Models of volume overload hypertrophy. J Card Fail. 1996;2:55–64.
14. Hatt PY, Rakusan K, Gastineau P, Laplace M. Morphometry and ultrastructure of heart hypertrophy induced by chronic volume overload (aorto-caval fistula in the rat). J Mol Cell Cardiol. 1979;11:989–98.
15. Toischer K, Rokita AG, Unsold B, Zhu W, Kararigas G, Sossalla S, et al. Differential cardiac remodeling in preload versus afterload. Circulation. 2010;122:993–1003.
16. Calderone A, Takahashi N, Izzo Jr NJ, Thaik CM, Colucci WS. Pressure- and volume-induced left ventricular hypertrophies are associated with distinct myocyte phenotypes and differential induction of peptide growth factor mRNAs. Circulation. 1995; 92:2385–90.
17. Camici PG, Olivotto I, Rimoldi OE. The coronary circulation and blood flow in left ventricular hypertrophy. J Mol Cell Cardiol. 2012;52:857–64.
18. Vogt M, Motz WH, Schwartzkopf B, Strauer BE. Pathophysiology and clinical aspects of hypertensive hypertrophy. Eur Heart J. 1993;14(Suppl D):2–7.
19. Aronson RS. Afterpotentials and triggered activity in hypertrophied myocardium from rats with renal hypertension. Circ Res. 1981;48:720–7.
20. Struijker Boudier HA, Cohuet GM, Baumann M, Safar ME. The heart, macrocirculation and microcirculation in hypertension: a unifying hypothesis. J Hypertens Suppl. 2003;21:S19–23.
21. Vatner SF, Hittinger L. Coronary vascular mechanisms involved in decompensation from hypertrophy to heart failure. J Am Coll Cardiol. 1993;22:34A–40.
22. Hittinger L, Mirsky I, Shen YT, Patrick TA, Bishop SP, Vatner SF. Hemodynamic mechanisms responsible for reduced subendocardial coronary reserve in dogs with severe left ventricular hypertrophy. Circulation. 1995;92:978–86.
23. Hoffman JI. Maximal coronary flow and the concept of coronary vascular reserve. Circulation. 1984;70:153–9.
24. Strauer BE, Schwartzkopff B. Left ventricular hypertrophy and coronary microcirculation in hypertensive heart disease. Blood Press Suppl. 1997;2:6–12.
25. Kozakova M, Galetta F, Gregorini L, Bigalli G, Franzoni F, Giusti C, et al. Coronary vasodilator capacity and epicardial vessel remodeling in physiological and hypertensive hypertrophy. Hypertension. 2000;36:343–9.
26. Rajappan K, Rimoldi OE, Dutka DP, Ariff B, Pennell DJ, Sheridan DJ, et al. Mechanisms of coronary microcirculatory dysfunction in patients with aortic stenosis and angiographically normal coronary arteries. Circulation. 2002;105:470–6.
27. Kataoka T, Hamasaki S, Ishida S, Saihara K, Okui H, Fukudome T, et al. Contribution of increased minimal coronary resistance and attenuated vascular adaptive remodeling to myocardial ischemia in patients with systemic hypertension and ventricular hypertrophy. Am J Cardiol. 2004;94:484–7.
28. Schwartzkopff B, Mundhenke M, Strauer BE. Remodelling of intramyocardial arterioles and extracellular matrix in patients with arterial hypertension and impaired coronary reserve. Eur Heart J. 1995;16(Suppl I):82–6.
29. Schwartzkopff B, Motz W, Frenzel H, Vogt M, Knauer S, Strauer BE. Structural and functional alterations of the intramyocardial coronary arterioles in patients with arterial hypertension. Circulation. 1993;88:993–1003.
30. Weber KT, Anversa P, Armstrong PW, Brilla CG, Burnett Jr JC, Cruickshank JM, et al. Remodeling and reparation of the cardiovascular system. J Am Coll Cardiol. 1992;20:3–16.
31. Strauer BE. Left ventricular hypertrophy, myocardial blood flow and coronary flow reserve. Cardiology. 1992;81:274–82.
32. Strauer BE. The concept of coronary flow reserve. J Cardiovasc Pharmacol. 1992;19 Suppl 5:S67–80.
33. Brush Jr JE, Cannon 3rd RO, Schenke WH, Bonow RO, Leon MB, Maron BJ, et al. Angina due to coronary microvascular disease in hypertensive patients without left ventricular hypertrophy. N Engl J Med. 1988;319:1302–7.
34. Houghton JL, Frank MJ, Carr AA, von Dohlen TW, Prisant LM. Relations among impaired coronary flow reserve, left ventricular hypertrophy and thallium perfusion defects in hypertensive patients without obstructive coronary artery disease. J Am Coll Cardiol. 1990;15:43–51.
35. Olsen MH, Wachtell K, Meyer C, Hove JD, Palmieri V, Dige-Petersen H, et al. Association between vascular dysfunction and reduced myocardial flow reserve in patients with hypertension: a LIFE substudy. J Hum Hypertens. 2004;18:445–52.
36. Antony I, Nitenberg A, Foult JM, Aptecar E. Coronary vasodilator reserve in untreated and treated hypertensive patients with and without left ventricular hypertrophy. J Am Coll Cardiol. 1993;22:514–20.
37. Kozakova M, Palombo C, Pratali L, Pittella G, Galetta F, L'Abbate A. Mechanisms of coronary flow reserve impairment in human hypertension. An integrated approach by transthoracic and transesophageal echocardiography. Hypertension. 1997;29:551–9.
38. Palombo C, Kozakova M, Magagna A, Bigalli G, Morizzo C, Ghiadoni L, et al. Early impairment of coronary flow reserve and increase in minimum coronary resistance in borderline hypertensive patients. J Hypertens. 2000;18:453–9.
39. Schwartzkopff B, Brehm M, Mundhenke M, Strauer BE. Repair of coronary arterioles after treatment with perindopril in hypertensive heart disease. Hypertension. 2000;36:220–5.
40. Nitenberg A, Antony I, Aptecar E, Arnoult F, Lerebours G. Impairment of flow-dependent coronary dilation in hypertensive

patients. Demonstration by cold pressor test induced flow velocity increase. Am J Hypertens. 1995;8:13S–8.
41. Treasure CB, Klein JL, Vita JA, Manoukian SV, Renwick GH, Selwyn AP, et al. Hypertension and left ventricular hypertrophy are associated with impaired endothelium-mediated relaxation in human coronary resistance vessels. Circulation. 1993; 87:86–93.
42. Hamasaki S, Al Suwaidi J, Higano ST, Miyauchi K, Holmes Jr DR, Lerman A. Attenuated coronary flow reserve and vascular remodeling in patients with hypertension and left ventricular hypertrophy. J Am Coll Cardiol. 2000;35:1654–60.
43. Sekiya M, Funada J, Suzuki J, Watanabe K, Miyagawa M, Akutsu H. The influence of left ventricular geometry on coronary vasomotion in patients with essential hypertension. Am J Hypertens. 2000; 13:789–95.
44. Zeiher AM, Drexler H, Saurbier B, Just H. Endothelium-mediated coronary blood flow modulation in humans. Effects of age, atherosclerosis, hypercholesterolemia, and hypertension. J Clin Invest. 1993;92:652–62.
45. Tanaka M, Fujiwara H, Onodera T, Wu DJ, Matsuda M, Hamashima Y, et al. Quantitative analysis of narrowings of intramyocardial small arteries in normal hearts, hypertensive hearts, and hearts with hypertrophic cardiomyopathy. Circulation. 1987;75:1130–9.
46. Blumgart HL. Studies on the relation of the clinical manifestations of angina pectoris, coronary thrombosis and myocardial infarction to the pathological findings. Am Heart J. 1940;19:1–91.
47. Zoll PM, Wessler S, Schlesinger MJ. Interarterial coronary anastomoses in the human heart, with particular reference to anemia and relative cardiac anoxia. Circulation. 1951;4:797–815.
48. Harrison DG, Barnes DH, Hiratzka LF, Eastham CL, Kerber RE, Marcus ML. The effect of cardiac hypertrophy on the coronary collateral circulation. Circulation. 1985;71:1135–45.
49. Scheel KW, Eisenstein BL, Ingram LA. Coronary, collateral, and perfusion territory responses to aortic banding. Am J Physiol. 1984;246:H768–75.
50. Bache RJ, Vrobel TR, Ring WS, Emery RW, Andersen RW. Regional myocardial blood flow during exercise in dogs with chronic left ventricular hypertrophy. Circ Res. 1981;48:76–87.
51. Bache RJ, Vrobel TR, Arentzen CE, Ring WS. Effect of maximal coronary vasodilation on transmural myocardial perfusion during tachycardia in dogs with left ventricular hypertrophy. Circ Res. 1981;49:742–50.
52. Bache RJ, Alyono D, Sublett E, Dai XZ. Myocardial blood flow in left ventricular hypertrophy developing in young and adult dogs. Am J Physiol. 1986;251:H949–56.
53. Mueller TM, Marcus ML, Kerber RE, Young JA, Barnes RW, Abboud FM. Effect of renal hypertension and left ventricular hypertrophy on the coronary circulation in dogs. Circ Res. 1978;42:543–9.
54. Mueller TM, Tomanek RJ, Kerber RE, Marcus ML. Myocardial infarction in dogs with chronic hypertension and left ventricular hypertrophy. Am J Physiol. 1980;239:H731–5.
55. Bache RJ, Arentzen CE, Simon AB, Vrobel TR. Abnormalities in myocardial perfusion during tachycardia in dogs with left ventricular hypertrophy: metabolic evidence for myocardial ischemia. Circulation. 1984;69:409–17.
56. Bache RJ, Dai XZ, Alyono D, Vrobel TR, Homans DC. Myocardial blood flow during exercise in dogs with left ventricular hypertrophy produced by aortic banding and perinephritic hypertension. Circulation. 1987;76:835–42.
57. Koyanagi S, Eastham CL, Harrison DG, Marcus ML. Increased size of myocardial infarction in dogs with chronic hypertension and left ventricular hypertrophy. Circ Res. 1982;50:55–62.
58. Koyanagi S, Eastham C, Marcus ML. Effects of chronic hypertension and left ventricular hypertrophy on the incidence of sudden cardiac death after coronary artery occlusion in conscious dogs. Circulation. 1982;65:1192–7.
59. O'Keefe DD, Hoffman JI, Cheitlin R, O'Neill MJ, Allard JR, Shapkin E. Coronary blood flow in experimental canine left ventricular hypertrophy. Circ Res. 1978;43:43–51.
60. Hittinger L, Shannon RP, Bishop SP, Gelpi RJ, Vatner SF. Subendomyocardial exhaustion of blood flow reserve and increased fibrosis in conscious dogs with heart failure. Circ Res. 1989;65:971–80.
61. Hittinger L, Shannon RP, Kohin S, Manders WT, Kelly P, Vatner SF. Exercise-induced subendocardial dysfunction in dogs with left ventricular hypertrophy. Circ Res. 1990;66:329–43.
62. Hittinger L, Shen YT, Patrick TA, Hasebe N, Komamura K, Ihara T, et al. Mechanisms of subendocardial dysfunction in response to exercise in dogs with severe left ventricular hypertrophy. Circ Res. 1992;71:423–34.
63. Bache RJ, Wright L, Laxson DD, Dai XZ. Effect of coronary stenosis on myocardial blood flow during exercise in the chronically pressure-overloaded hypertrophied left ventricle. Circulation. 1990;81:1967–73.
64. Marcus ML. The coronary circulation in health and disease. New York: McGraw-Hill; 1983.
65. Ely SW, Sun CW, Knabb RM, Gidday JM, Rubio R, Berne RM. Adenosine and metabolic regulation of coronary blood flow in dogs with renal hypertension. Hypertension. 1983;5:943–50.
66. Rembert JC, Kleinman LH, Fedor JM, Wechsler AS, Greenfield Jr JC. Myocardial blood flow distribution in concentric left ventricular hypertrophy. J Clin Invest. 1978;62:379–86.
67. White FC, Sanders M, Peterson T, Bloor CM. Ischemic myocardial injury after exercise stress in the pressure-overloaded heart. Am J Pathol. 1979;97:473–88.
68. Vatner SF, Shannon R, Hittinger L. Reduced subendocardial coronary reserve. A potential mechanism for impaired diastolic function in the hypertrophied and failing heart. Circulation. 1990;81:III8–14.
69. Nakano K, Corin WJ, Spann Jr JF, Biederman RW, Denslow S, Carabello BA. Abnormal subendocardial blood flow in pressure overload hypertrophy is associated with pacing-induced subendocardial dysfunction. Circ Res. 1989;65:1555–64.
70. Breisch EA, Houser SR, Carey RA, Spann JF, Bove AA. Myocardial blood flow and capillary density in chronic pressure overload of the feline left ventricle. Cardiovasc Res. 1980;14:469–75.
71. Ishihara K, Zile MR, Nagatsu M, Nakano K, Tomita M, Kanazawa S, et al. Coronary blood flow after the regression of pressure-overload left ventricular hypertrophy. Circ Res. 1992;71:1472–81.
72. Manohar M, Parks CM, Busch MA, Bisgard GE. Transmural coronary vasodilator reserve and flow distribution in unanesthetized calves sojourning at 3500 m. J Surg Res. 1985;39:499–509.
73. Duncker DJ, Zhang J, Pavek TJ, Crampton MJ, Bache RJ. Effect of exercise on coronary pressure-flow relationship in hypertrophied left ventricle. Am J Physiol. 1995;269:H271–81.
74. Duncker DJ, Stubenitsky R, Verdouw PD. Role of adenosine in the regulation of coronary blood flow in swine at rest and during treadmill exercise. Am J Physiol. 1998;275:H1663–72.
75. Alyono D, Anderson RW, Parrish DG, Dai XZ, Bache RJ. Alterations of myocardial blood flow associated with experimental canine left ventricular hypertrophy secondary to valvular aortic stenosis. Circ Res. 1986;58:47–57.
76. Dellsperger KC, Clothier JL, Koyanagi S, Inou T, Marcus ML. Effects of coronary artery occlusion in animals with hypertension and left ventricular hypertrophy. J Cardiovasc Pharmacol. 1991;17 Suppl 2:S40–5.
77. Gaasch WH, Zile MR, Hoshino PK, Weinberg EO, Rhodes DR, Apstein CS. Tolerance of the hypertrophic heart to ischemia. Studies in compensated and failing dog hearts with pressure overload hypertrophy. Circulation. 1990;81:1644–53.
78. Tomanek RJ, Palmer PJ, Peiffer GL, Schreiber KL, Eastham CL, Marcus ML. Morphometry of canine coronary arteries, arterioles, and capillaries during hypertension and left ventricular hypertrophy. Circ Res. 1986;58:38–46.

79. Tomanek RJ. Sympathetic nerves modify mitochondrial and capillary growth in normotensive and hypertensive rats. J Mol Cell Cardiol. 1989;21:755–64.
80. Tomanek RJ, Schalk KA, Marcus ML, Harrison DG. Coronary angiogenesis during long-term hypertension and left ventricular hypertrophy in dogs. Circ Res. 1989;65:352–9.
81. Tomanek RJ, Wessel TJ, Harrison DG. Capillary growth and geometry during long-term hypertension and myocardial hypertrophy in dogs. Am J Physiol. 1991;261:H1011–8.
82. Huo Y, Linares CO, Kassab GS. Capillary perfusion and wall shear stress are restored in the coronary circulation of hypertrophic right ventricle. Circ Res. 2007;100:273–83.
83. Kassab GS, Imoto K, White FC, Rider CA, Fung YC, Bloor CM. Coronary arterial tree remodeling in right ventricular hypertrophy. Am J Physiol. 1993;265:H366–75.
84. Lu X, Dang CQ, Guo X, Molloi S, Wassall CD, Kemple MD, et al. Elevated oxidative stress and endothelial dysfunction in right coronary artery of right ventricular hypertrophy. J Appl Physiol. 2011;110:1674–81.
85. Urbieta Caceres VH, Lin J, Zhu XY, Favreau FD, Gibson ME, Crane JA, et al. Early experimental hypertension preserves the myocardial microvasculature but aggravates cardiac injury distal to chronic coronary artery obstruction. Am J Physiol Heart Circ Physiol. 2011;300:H693–701.
86. Liu J, Agarwal S. Mechanical signals activate vascular endothelial growth factor receptor-2 to upregulate endothelial cell proliferation during inflammation. J Immunol. 2010;185:1215–21.
87. Wangler RD, Peters KG, Marcus ML, Tomanek RJ. Effects of duration and severity of arterial hypertension and cardiac hypertrophy on coronary vasodilator reserve. Circ Res. 1982;51:10–8.
88. Friberg P. Diastolic characteristics and cardiac energetics of isolated hearts exposed to volume and pressure overload. Cardiovasc Res. 1988;22:329–39.
89. Peters KG, Wangler RD, Tomanek RJ, Marcus ML. Effects of long-term cardiac hypertrophy on coronary vasodilator reserve in SHR rats. Am J Cardiol. 1984;54:1342–8.
90. Tomanek RJ, Searls JC, Lachenbruch PA. Quantitative changes in the capillary bed during developing, peak, and stabilized cardiac hypertrophy in the spontaneously hypertensive rat. Circ Res. 1982;51:295–304.
91. Rakusan K, Cicutti N, Kazda S, Turek Z. Effect of nifedipine on coronary capillary geometry in normotensive and hypertensive rats. Hypertension. 1994;24:205–11.
92. Koyama T, Gao M, Batra S, Togashi H, Saito H. Myocyte hypertrophy and capillarization in spontaneously hypertensive stroke-prone rats. Adv Exp Med Biol. 1997;411:365–8.
93. Vitullo JC, Penn MS, Rakusan K, Wicker P. Effects of hypertension and aging on coronary arteriolar density. Hypertension. 1993;21:406–14.
94. McAinsh AM, Geyer M, Fandrey J, Ruegg JC, Wiesner RJ. Expression of vascular endothelial growth factor during the development of cardiac hypertrophy in spontaneously hypertensive rats. Mol Cell Biochem. 1998;187:141–6.
95. Kushibiki M, Yamada M, Oikawa K, Tomita H, Osanai T, Okumura K. Aldosterone causes vasoconstriction in coronary arterioles of rats via angiotensin II type-1 receptor: influence of hypertension. Eur J Pharmacol. 2007;572:182–8.
96. Friberg P, Nordlander M. Influence of long-term antihypertensive therapy on cardiac function, coronary flow and myocardial oxygen consumption in spontaneously hypertensive rats. J Hypertens. 1986;4:165–73.
97. Tomanek RJ, Wangler RD, Bauer CA. Prevention of coronary vasodilator reserve decrement in spontaneously hypertensive rats. Hypertension. 1985;7:533–40.
98. Luscher TF, Rubanyi GM, Aarhus LL, Edoute Y, Vanhoutte PM. Serotonin reduces coronary flow in the isolated heart of the spontaneously hypertensive rat. J Hypertens Suppl. 1986;4:S148–50.
99. Varagic J, Frohlich ED, Diez J, Susic D, Ahn J, Gonzalez A, et al. Myocardial fibrosis, impaired coronary hemodynamics, and biventricular dysfunction in salt-loaded SHR. Am J Physiol Heart Circ Physiol. 2006;290:H1503–9.
100. Yamori Y, Mori C, Nishio T, Ooshima A, Horie R, Ohtaka M, et al. Cardiac hypertrophy in early hypertension. Am J Cardiol. 1979;44:964–9.
101. Nordlander M, Wahlander H, Friberg P. Myocardial and vascular structural adaptation to chronic pressure overload. J Cardiovasc Pharmacol. 1987;10 Suppl 6:S51–61.
102. Kayar SR, Weiss HR. Diffusion distances, total capillary length and mitochondrial volume in pressure-overload myocardial hypertrophy. J Mol Cell Cardiol. 1992;24:1155–66.
103. Michel JB, Salzmann JL, Ossondo Nlom M, Bruneval P, Barres D, Camilleri JP. Morphometric analysis of collagen network and plasma perfused capillary bed in the myocardium of rats during evolution of cardiac hypertrophy. Basic Res Cardiol. 1986;81:142–54.
104. Wicker P, Tarazi RC, Kobayashi K. Coronary blood flow during the development and regression of left ventricular hypertrophy in renovascular hypertensive rats. Am J Cardiol. 1983;51:1744–9.
105. Kobayashi N, Kobayashi K, Kouno K, Yagi S, Matsuoka H. Effect of benidipine on microvascular remodeling and coronary flow reserve in two-kidney, one clip Goldblatt hypertension. J Hypertens. 1997;15:1285–94.
106. Wahlander H, Haraldsson B, Friberg P. Myocardial capillary diffusion capacity in rat hearts with cardiac hypertrophy due to pressure and volume overload. Am J Physiol. 1993;265:H61–8.
107. Cimini CM, Weiss HR. Microvascular morphometry and perfusion in renal hypertension-induced cardiac hypertrophy. Am J Physiol. 1988;255:H1384–90.
108. Alfaro A, Schaible TF, Malhotra A, Yipintsoi T, Scheuer J. Impaired coronary flow and ventricular function in hearts of hypertensive rats. Cardiovasc Res. 1983;17:553–61.
109. Wicker P, Abdul-Samad M, Rakusan K, Tarazi RC, Healy B. Effects of chronic exercise on the coronary circulation in conscious rats with renovascular hypertension. Hypertension. 1987;10:74–81.
110. Yamamoto J, Tsuchiya M, Saito M, Ikeda M. Cardiac contractile and coronary flow reserves in deoxycorticosterone acetate-salt hypertensive rats. Hypertension. 1985;7:569–77.
111. Jalil JE, Janicki JS, Pick R, Weber KT. Coronary vascular remodeling and myocardial fibrosis in the rat with renovascular hypertension. Response to captopril. Am J Hypertens. 1991; 4:51–5.
112. Kingsbury MP, Turner MA, Flores NA, Bovill E, Sheridan DJ. Endogenous and exogenous coronary vasodilatation are attenuated in cardiac hypertrophy: a morphological defect? J Mol Cell Cardiol. 2000;32:527–38.
113. Sato F, Isoyama S, Takishima T. Normalization of impaired coronary circulation in hypertrophied rat hearts. Hypertension. 1990;16:26–34.
114. Ito N, Isoyama S, Takahashi T, Takishima T. Coronary dilator reserve and morphological changes after relief of pressure-overload in rats. J Mol Cell Cardiol. 1993;25:3–14.
115. Isoyama S, Ito N, Satoh K, Takishima T. Collagen deposition and the reversal of coronary reserve in cardiac hypertrophy. Hypertension. 1992;20:491–500.
116. Sato F, Isoyama S, Takishima T. Effects of duration of pressure overload on the reversibility of impaired coronary autoregulation in rats. Int J Cardiol. 1992;37:131–43.
117. Hartley CL. 31st Annual International Conference of the IEEE EMBS. Minneapolis, MN, USA 2009. p. 1094.
118. Harrison DG, Marcus ML, Dellsperger KC, Lamping KG, Tomanek RJ. Pathophysiology of myocardial perfusion in hypertension. Circulation. 1991;83:III14–8.

119. Tomanek RJ, Davis JW, Anderson SC. The effects of alpha-methyldopa on cardiac hypertrophy in spontaneously hypertensive rats: ultrastructural, stereological, and morphometric analysis. Cardiovasc Res. 1979;13:173–82.
120. Canby CA, Tomanek RJ. Role of lowering arterial pressure on maximal coronary flow with and without regression of cardiac hypertrophy. Am J Physiol. 1989;257:H1110–8.
121. Wicker P, Tarazi RC. Right ventricular coronary flow in arterial hypertension. Am Heart J. 1985;110:845–50.
122. Kobayashi K, Tarazi RC, Lovenberg W, Rakusan K. Coronary blood flow in genetic cardiac hypertrophy. Am J Cardiol. 1984;53:1360–4.
123. Brilla CG, Janicki JS, Weber KT. Impaired diastolic function and coronary reserve in genetic hypertension. Role of interstitial fibrosis and medial thickening of intramyocardial coronary arteries. Circ Res. 1991;69:107–15.
124. Canby CA, Tomanek RJ. Regression of ventricular hypertrophy abolishes cardiocyte vulnerability to acute hypoxia. Anat Rec. 1990;226:198–206.
125. Wearn JT. Alterations in the heart accompanying growth and hypertrophy. Bull Johns Hopkins Hosp. 1941;68:363.
126. Roberts J, Wearn J. Quantitative changes in the capillary-muscle relationship in human hearts during normal growth and hypertrophy. Am Heart J. 1941;21:617–33.
127. Mandache E, Unge G, Ljungqvist A. Myocardial blood capillary reaction in various forms of cardiac hypertrophy. An electron microscopical investigation in the rat. Virchows Arch B Cell Pathol. 1972;11:97–110.
128. Ljungqvist A, Unge G. The proliferative activity of the myocardial tissue in various forms of experimental cardiac hypertrophy. Acta Pathol Microbiol Scand [A]. 1973;81:233–40.
129. Murray PA, Baig H, Fishbein MC, Vatner SF. Effects of exerimental right ventricular hypertrophy on myocardial blood flow in conscious dogs. J Clin Invest. 1979;64:421–7.
130. Rakusan K, du Mesnil de Rochemont W, Braasch W, Tschopp H, Bing RJ. Capacity of the terminal vascular bed during normal growth, in cardiomegaly, and in cardiac atrophy. Circ Res. 1967;21:209–15.
131. Lund DD, Tomanek RJ. Myocardial morphology in spontaneously hypertensive and aortic-constricted rats. Am J Anat. 1978;152: 141–51.
132. Tillmanns H, Neumann FJ, Parekh N, Zimmermann R, Tiefenbacher C, Dorigo O, et al. Microcirculation in the hypertrophic and ischemic heart. Eur J Clin Pharmacol. 1990;39 Suppl 1:S9–12.
133. Wiener J, Giacomelli F, Loud AV, Anversa P. Morphometry of cardiac hypertrophy induced by experimental renal hypertension. Am J Cardiol. 1979;44:919–29.
134. Bishop SP, Powell PC, Hasebe N, Shen YT, Patrick TA, Hittinger L, et al. Coronary vascular morphology in pressure-overload left ventricular hypertrophy. J Mol Cell Cardiol. 1996;28:141–54.
135. Breisch EA, White FC, Nimmo LE, Bloor CM. Cardiac vasculature and flow during pressure-overload hypertrophy. Am J Physiol. 1986;251:H1031–7.
136. Breisch EA, White FC, Bloor CM. Myocardial characteristics of pressure overload hypertrophy. A structural and functional study. Lab Invest. 1984;51:333–42.
137. Mall G, Zimmer G, Baden S, Mattfeldt T. Capillary neoformation in the rat heart—stereological studies on papillary muscles in hypertrophy and physiologic growth. Basic Res Cardiol. 1990;85:531–40.
138. White FC, Nakatani Y, Nimmo L, Bloor CM. Compensatory angiogenesis during progressive right ventricular hypertrophy. Am J Cardiovasc Pathol. 1992;4:51–68.
139. Batra S, Rakusan K. Geometry of capillary networks in volume overloaded rat heart. Microvasc Res. 1991;42:39–50.
140. Henquell L, Honig CR. Intercapillary distances and capillary reserve in right and left ventricles: significance for control of tissue po2. Microvasc Res. 1976;12:35–41.
141. Arai S, Machida A, Nakamura T. Myocardial structure and vascularization of hypertrophied hearts. Tohoku J Exp Med. 1968;95:35–54.
142. Henquell L, Odoroff CL, Honig CR. Intercapillary distance and capillary reserve in hypertrophied rat hearts beating in situ. Circ Res. 1977;41:400–8.
143. Anversa P, Melissari M, Beghi C, Olivetti G. Structural compensatory mechanisms in rat heart in early spontaneous hypertension. Am J Physiol. 1984;246:H739–46.
144. Gu JW, Fortepiani LA, Reckelhoff JF, Adair TH, Wang J, Hall JE. Increased expression of vascular endothelial growth factor and capillary density in hearts of spontaneously hypertensive rats. Microcirculation. 2004;11:689–97.
145. Torry RJ, Connell PM, O'Brien DM, Chilian WM, Tomanek RJ. Sympathectomy stimulates capillary but not precapillary growth in hypertrophic hearts. Am J Physiol. 1991;260:H1515–21.
146. Amann K, Odoni G, Benz K, Campean V, Jacobi J, Hilgers KF, et al. Sympathetic blockade prevents the decrease in cardiac VEGF expression and capillary supply in experimental renal failure. Am J Physiol Renal Physiol. 2011;300:F105–12.
147. Tomanek RJ, Carlson DW, Palmer PJ, Bhatnagar RK. Role of sympathetic nerves during developing cardiac hypertrophy in Grollman hypertensive rats. Am J Physiol. 1987;253:H818–25.
148. Lamping KG, Christensen LP, Tomanek RJ. Estrogen therapy induces collateral and microvascular remodeling. Am J Physiol Heart Circ Physiol. 2003;285:H2039–44.
149. Flanagan MF, Aoyagi T, Currier JJ, Colan SD, Fujii AM. Effect of young age on coronary adaptations to left ventricular pressure overload hypertrophy in sheep. J Am Coll Cardiol. 1994;24: 1786–96.
150. Hort W, Severidt HJ. Capillarization and microscopic changes in the myocardium in congenital heart defects. Virchows Arch Pathol Anat Physiol Klin Med. 1966;341:192–203.
151. Rakusan K, Flanagan MF, Geva T, Southern J, Van Praagh R. Morphometry of human coronary capillaries during normal growth and the effect of age in left ventricular pressure-overload hypertrophy. Circulation. 1992;86:38–46.
152. Batra S, Rakusan K, Campbell SE. Geometry of capillary networks in hypertrophied rat heart. Microvasc Res. 1991;41:29–40.
153. Botham MJ, Lemmer JH, Gerren RA, Long RW, Behrendt DM, Gallagher KP. Coronary vasodilator reserve in young dogs with moderate right ventricular hypertrophy. Ann Thorac Surg. 1984;38:101–7.
154. Holtz J, Restorff WV, Bard P, Bassenge E. Transmural distribution of myocardial blood flow and of coronary reserve in canine left ventricular hypertrophy. Basic Res Cardiol. 1977;72:286–92.
155. Einzig S, Leonard JJ, Tripp MR, Lucas RV, Swayze CR, Fox IJ. Changes in regional myocardial blood flow and variable development of hypertrophy after aortic banding in puppies. Cardiovasc Res. 1981;15:711–23.
156. Liu Z, Hilbelink DR, Gerdes AM. Regional changes in hemodynamics and cardiac myocyte size in rats with aortocaval fistulas. 2. Long-term effects. Circ Res. 1991;69:59–65.
157. Zile MR, Tomita M, Nakano K, Mirsky I, Usher B, Lindroth J, et al. Effects of left ventricular volume overload produced by mitral regurgitation on diastolic function. Am J Physiol. 1991;261:H1471–80.
158. Borer JS, Truter S, Herrold EM, Falcone DJ, Pena M, Carter JN, et al. Myocardial fibrosis in chronic aortic regurgitation: molecular and cellular responses to volume overload. Circulation. 2002;105:1837–42.
159. Kawamura K, Tohda K, Kobayashi M, Masuda H, Shozawa T. Fine structure of capillary proliferation in myocardium of volume overloaded rats. Adv Exp Med Biol. 1990;277:387–94.

160. Chen Y, Torry RJ, Baumbach GL, Tomanek RJ. Proportional arteriolar growth accompanies cardiac hypertrophy induced by volume overload. Am J Physiol. 1994;267:H2132–7.
161. Legault F, Rouleau JL, Juneau C, Rose C, Rakusan K. Functional and morphological characteristics of compensated and decompensated cardiac hypertrophy in dogs with chronic infrarenal aortocaval fistulas. Circ Res. 1990;66:846–59.
162. Thomas DP, Phillips SJ, Bove AA. Myocardial morphology and blood flow distribution in chronic volume-overload hypertrophy in dogs. Basic Res Cardiol. 1984;79:379–88.
163. Ratajska A, Fiejka E, Maksymowicz M, Gawlik Z. Tunnel capillaries in hypertrophied myocardium of rats with aorto-caval fistula. Basic Res Cardiol. 1993;88:120–9.
164. Wright AJ, Hudlicka O, Brown MD. Beneficial effect of chronic bradycardial pacing on capillary growth and heart performance in volume overload heart hypertrophy. Circ Res. 1989;64:1205–12.
165. Olivetti G, Lagrasta C, Quaini F, Ricci R, Moccia G, Capasso JM, et al. Capillary growth in anemia-induced ventricular wall remodeling in the rat heart. Circ Res. 1989;65:1182–92.
166. Hultgren PB, Bove AA. Myocardial blood flow and mechanics in volume overload-induced left ventricular hypertrophy in dogs. Cardiovasc Res. 1981;15:522–8.
167. Badke FR, White FC, Le Winter M, Covell J, Andres J, Bloor C. Effects of experimental volume-overload hypertrophy on myocardial blood flow and cardiac function. Am J Physiol. 1981;241:H564–70.
168. Gascho JA, Mueller TM, Eastham C, Marcus ML. Effect of volume-overload hypertrophy on the coronary circulation awake dogs. Cardiovasc Res. 1982;16:288–92.
169. Carabello BA, Nakano K, Ishihara K, Kanazawa S, Biederman RW, Spann Jr JF. Coronary blood flow in dogs with contractile dysfunction due to experimental volume overload. Circulation. 1991;83:1063–75.
170. Carabello BA, Nakano K, Corin W, Biederman R, Spann Jr JF. Left ventricular function in experimental volume overload hypertrophy. Am J Physiol. 1989;256:H974–81.
171. Marchetti GV, Merlo L, Noseda V, Visioli O. Myocardial blood flow in experimental cardiac hypertrophy in dogs. Cardiovasc Res. 1973;7:519–27.
172. Doty DB, Wright CB, Hiratzka LF, Eastham CL, Marcus ML. Coronary reserve in volume-induced right ventricular hypertrophy from atrial septal defect. Am J Cardiol. 1984;54:1059–63.
173. Bauman RP, Rembert JC, Greenfield Jr JC. Myocardial blood flow in awake dogs with chronic tricuspid regurgitation. Basic Res Cardiol. 1998;93:63–9.
174. Ojamaa K. Signaling mechanisms in thyroid hormone-induced cardiac hypertrophy. Vasc Pharmacol. 2010;52:113–9.
175. Tomanek RJ, Barlow PA, Connell PM, Chen Y, Torry RJ. Effects of hypothyroidism and hypertension on myocardial perfusion and vascularity in rabbits. Am J Physiol. 1993;265:H1638–44.
176. Capasso JM, Malhotra A, Scheuer J, Sonnenblick EH. Myocardial biochemical, contractile, and electrical performance after imposition of hypertension in young and old rats. Circ Res. 1986;58:445–60.
177. Tomanek RJ, Aydelotte MR. Late onset renal hypertension in old rats alters left ventricular structure and function. Am J Physiol. 1992;262:H531–8.
178. Tomanek RJ, Aydelotte MR, Butters CA. Late-onset renal hypertension in old rats alters myocardial microvessels. Am J Physiol. 1990;259:H1681–7.
179. Isoyama S, Grossman W, Wei JY. Effect of age on myocardial adaptation to volume overload in the rat. J Clin Invest. 1988;81:1850–7.
180. Walford GD, Spurgeon HA, Lakatta EG. Diminished cardiac hypertrophy and muscle performance in older compared with younger adult rats with chronic atrioventricular block. Circ Res. 1988;63:502–11.
181. Galli E, Pingitore A, Iervasi G. The role of thyroid hormone in the pathophysiology of heart failure: clinical evidence. Heart Fail Rev. 2010;15:155–69.
182. Luidens MK, Mousa SA, Davis FB, Lin HY, Davis PJ. Thyroid hormone and angiogenesis. Vasc Pharmacol. 2010;52:142–5.
183. Chilian WM, Wangler RD, Peters KG, Tomanek RJ, Marcus ML. Thyroxine-induced left ventricular hypertrophy in the rat. Anatomical and physiological evidence for angiogenesis. Circ Res. 1985;57:591–8.
184. Wachtlova M, Ostadal B, Mares V. Thyroxine-induced cardiomegaly in rats of different age. Physiol Bohemoslov. 1985;34:385–94.
185. Heron MI, Kolar F, Papousek F, Rakusan K. Early and late effect of neonatal hypo- and hyperthyroidism on coronary capillary geometry and long-term heart function in rat. Cardiovasc Res. 1997;33:230–40.
186. Tomanek RJ, Connell PM, Butters CA, Torry RJ. Compensated coronary microvascular growth in senescent rats with thyroxine-induced cardiac hypertrophy. Am J Physiol. 1995;268:H419–25.
187. Tomanek RJ, Busch TL. Coordinated capillary and myocardial growth in response to thyroxine treatment. Anat Rec. 1998;251:44–9.
188. Tomanek RJ, Doty MK, Sandra A. Early coronary angiogenesis in response to thyroxine: growth characteristics and upregulation of basic fibroblast growth factor. Circ Res. 1998;82:587–93.
189. Tomanek RJ, Zimmerman MB, Suvarna PR, Morkin E, Pennock GD, Goldman S. A thyroid hormone analog stimulates angiogenesis in the post-infarcted rat heart. J Mol Cell Cardiol. 1998;30:923–32.
190. Breisch EA, White FC, Hammond HK, Flynn S, Bloor CM. Myocardial characteristics of thyroxine stimulated hypertrophy. A structural and functional study. Basic Res Cardiol. 1989;84:345–58.
191. Craft-Cormney C, Hansen JT. Early ultrastructural changes in the myocardium following thyroxine-induced hypertrophy. Virchows Arch B Cell Pathol Incl Mol Pathol. 1980;33:267–73.
192. Weiss HR, Grover GJ. T4-induced cardiac hypertrophy and the perfused and total microvasculature of the heart. Can J Physiol Pharmacol. 1987;65:1848–55.
193. Heron MI, Rakusan K. Geometry of coronary capillaries in hyperthyroid and hypothyroid rat heart. Am J Physiol. 1994;267:H1024–31.
194. Makino A, Suarez J, Wang H, Belke DD, Scott BT, Dillmann WH. Thyroid hormone receptor-beta is associated with coronary angiogenesis during pathological cardiac hypertrophy. Endocrinology. 2009;150:2008–15.
195. Pennock GD, Raya TE, Bahl JJ, Goldman S, Morkin E. Combination treatment with captopril and the thyroid hormone analogue 3,5-diiodothyropropionic acid. A new approach to improving left ventricular performance in heart failure. Circulation. 1993;88:1289–98.
196. Mahaffey KW, Raya TE, Pennock GD, Morkin E, Goldman S. Left ventricular performance and remodeling in rabbits after myocardial infarction. Effects of a thyroid hormone analogue. Circulation. 1995;91:794–801.
197. Spooner PH, Thai HM, Goldman S, Gaballa MA. Thyroid hormone analog, DITPA, improves endothelial nitric oxide and beta-adrenergic mediated vasorelaxation after myocardial infarction. J Cardiovasc Pharmacol. 2004;44:453–9.
198. Zheng W, Weiss RM, Wang X, Zhou R, Arlen AM, Lei L. et al. DITPA stimulates arteriolar growth and modifies myocardial postinfarction remodeling. Am J Physiol. 286:H1994–2000, 2004.
199. Liu Y, Wang D, Redetzke RA, Sherer BA, Gerdes AM. Thyroid hormone analog 3,5-diiodothyropropionic acid promotes healthy vasculature in the adult myocardium independent of thyroid

effects on cardiac function. Am J Physiol Heart Circ Physiol. 2009;296:H1551–7.
200. Arsanjani R, McCarren M, Bahl JJ, Goldman S. Translational potential of thyroid hormone and its analogs. J Mol Cell Cardiol. 2011;51(4):506–11.
201. Wang X, Zheng W, Christensen LP, Tomanek RJ. DITPA stimulates bFGF, VEGF, angiopoietin, and Tie-2 and facilitates coronary arteriolar growth. Am J Physiol Heart Circ Physiol. 2003;284:H613–8.
202. Zheng W, Weiss RM, Wang X, Zhou R, Arlen AM, Lei L, et al. DITPA stimulates arteriolar growth and modifies myocardial postinfarction remodeling. Am J Physiol Heart Circ Physiol. 2004;286:H1994–2000.
203. Heron MI, Rakusan K. Short- and long-term effects of neonatal hypo- and hyperthyroidism on coronary arterioles in rat. Am J Physiol. 1996;271:H1746–54.
204. Rongish BJ, Torry RJ, Tomanek RJ. Coronary neovascularization of embryonic rat hearts cultured in oculo is independent of thyroid hormones. Am J Physiol. 1995;268:H811–6.
205. Liu Y, Sherer BA, Redetzke RA, Gerdes AM. Regulation of arteriolar density in adult myocardium during low thyroid conditions. Vasc Pharmacol. 2010;52:146–50.
206. Watkins H, Ashrafian H, Redwood C. Inherited cardiomyopathies. N Engl J Med. 2011;364:1643–56.
207. Fatkin D, Graham RM. Molecular mechanisms of inherited cardiomyopathies. Physiol Rev. 2002;82:945–80.
208. Maron MS, Olivotto I, Maron BJ, Prasad SK, Cecchi F, Udelson JE, et al. The case for myocardial ischemia in hypertrophic cardiomyopathy. J Am Coll Cardiol. 2009;54:866–75.
209. Timmer SA, Germans T, Gotte MJ, Russel IK, Lubberink M, Ten Berg JM, et al. Relation of coronary microvascular dysfunction in hypertrophic cardiomyopathy to contractile dysfunction independent from myocardial injury. Am J Cardiol. 2011;107:1522–8.
210. Knaapen P, Germans T, Camici PG, Rimoldi OE, ten Cate FJ, ten Berg JM, et al. Determinants of coronary microvascular dysfunction in symptomatic hypertrophic cardiomyopathy. Am J Physiol Heart Circ Physiol. 2008;294:H986–93.
211. Rossi MA. Microvascular changes as a cause of chronic cardiomyopathy in Chagas' disease. Am Heart J. 1990;120:233–6.
212. Parodi O, Sambuceti G. The role of coronary microvascular dysfunction in the genesis of cardiovascular diseases. Q J Nucl Med. 1996;40:9–16.
213. Escobales N, Crespo MJ. Early pathophysiological alterations in experimental cardiomyopathy: the Syrian cardiomyopathic hamster. P R Health Sci J. 2008;27:307–14.
214. Cecchi F, Olivotto I, Gistri R, Lorenzoni R, Chiriatti G, Camici PG. Coronary microvascular dysfunction and prognosis in hypertrophic cardiomyopathy. N Engl J Med. 2003;349:1027–35.
215. Maron BJ. Hypertrophic cardiomyopathy. Lancet. 1997;350:127–33.
216. Johansson B, Morner S, Waldenstrom A, Stal P. Myocardial capillary supply is limited in hypertrophic cardiomyopathy: a morphological analysis. Int J Cardiol. 2008;126:252–7.
217. Moon J, Cho IJ, Shim CY, Ha JW, Jang Y, Chung N, et al. Abnormal myocardial capillary density in apical hypertrophic cardiomyopathy can be assessed by myocardial contrast echocardiography. Circ J. 2010;74:2166–72.
218. Cecchi F, Sgalambro A, Baldi M, Sotgia B, Antoniucci D, Camici PG, et al. Microvascular dysfunction, myocardial ischemia, and progression to heart failure in patients with hypertrophic cardiomyopathy. J Cardiovasc Transl Res. 2009;2:452–61.
219. Aquaro GD, Todiere G, Barison A, Strata E, Marzilli M, Pingitore A, et al. Myocardial blood flow and fibrosis in hypertrophic cardiomyopathy. J Card Fail. 2011;17:384–91.
220. Fang W, Zhang J, He ZX. Myocardial ischemia in patients with dilated cardiomyopathy. Nucl Med Commun. 2010;31:981–4.
221. Johnson RA, Palacios I. Dilated cardiomyopathies of the adult (first of two parts). N Engl J Med. 1982;307:1051–8.
222. Inoue T, Sakai Y, Morooka S, Hayashi T, Takayanagi K, Yamanaka T, et al. Coronary flow reserve in patients with dilated cardiomyopathy. Am Heart J. 1993;125:93–8.
223. Rigo F, Gherardi S, Galderisi M, Sicari R, Picano E. The independent prognostic value of contractile and coronary flow reserve determined by dipyridamole stress echocardiography in patients with idiopathic dilated cardiomyopathy. Am J Cardiol. 2007;99:1154–8.
224. Morales MA, Neglia D, L'Abbate A. Reduction of myocardial blood flow reserve in idiopathic dilated cardiomyopathy without overt heart failure and its relation with functional indices: an echo-Doppler and positron emission tomography study. J Cardiovasc Med (Hagerstown). 2008;9:778–82.
225. Del Ry S, Giannessi D, Maltinti M, Cabiati M, Prontera C, Iervasi A, et al. Increased plasma levels of osteopontin are associated with activation of the renin-aldosterone system and with myocardial and coronary microvascular damage in dilated cardiomyopathy. Cytokine. 2010;49:325–30.
226. Pereira VF, de Carvalho Frimm C, Rodrigues AC, Curi M. Coronary reserve impairment prevents the improvement of left ventricular dysfunction and adversely affects the long-term outcome of patients with hypertensive dilated cardiomyopathy. J Am Soc Hypertens. 2010;4:14–21.
227. Britten MB, Zeiher AM, Schachinger V. Microvascular dysfunction in angiographically normal or mildly diseased coronary arteries predicts adverse cardiovascular long-term outcome. Coron Artery Dis. 2004;15:259–64.
228. L'Abbate A, Sambuceti G, Neglia D. Myocardial perfusion and coronary microcirculation: from pathophysiology to clinical application. J Nucl Cardiol. 2002;9:328–37.
229. Neglia D, L'Abbate A. Coronary microvascular dysfunction and idiopathic dilated cardiomyopathy. Pharmacol Rep. 2005; 57(Suppl):151–5.
230. Treasure CB, Vita JA, Cox DA, Fish RD, Gordon JB, Mudge GH, et al. Endothelium-dependent dilation of the coronary microvasculature is impaired in dilated cardiomyopathy. Circulation. 1990;81:772–9.
231. Drelicharz L, Kozlovski V, Skorka T, Heinze-Paluchowska S, Jasinski A, Gebska A, et al. NO and PGI(2) in coronary endothelial dysfunction in transgenic mice with dilated cardiomyopathy. Basic Res Cardiol. 2008;103:417–30.
232. Andreassi MG, Laghi Pasini F, Picano E, Capecchi PL, Pompella G, Foffa I, et al. Adenosine A2(A) receptor gene polymorphism (1976C>T) affects coronary flow reserve response during vasodilator stress testing in patients with non ischemic-dilated cardiomyopathy. Pharmacogenet Genomics. 2011;21:469–75.
233. Factor SM, Sonnenblick EH. Hypothesis: is congestive cardiomyopathy caused by a hyperreactive myocardial microcirculation (microvascular spasm)? Am J Cardiol. 1982;50:1149–52.
234. Laguens R, Alvarez P, Vigliano C, Cabeza Meckert P, Favaloro L, Diez M, et al. Coronary microcirculation remodeling in patients with idiopathic dilated cardiomyopathy. Cardiology. 2011;119:191–6.
235. Karch R, Neumann F, Ullrich R, Neumuller J, Podesser BK, Neumann M, et al. The spatial pattern of coronary capillaries in patients with dilated, ischemic, or inflammatory cardiomyopathy. Cardiovasc Pathol. 2005;14:135–44.
236. Tsagalou EP, Anastasiou-Nana M, Agapitos E, Gika A, Drakos SG, Terrovitis JV, et al. Depressed coronary flow reserve is associated with decreased myocardial capillary density in patients with heart failure due to idiopathic dilated cardiomyopathy. J Am Coll Cardiol. 2008;52:1391–8.
237. Whitmer JT. Energy metabolism and mechanical function in perfused hearts of Syrian hamsters with dilated or hypertrophic cardiomyopathy. J Mol Cell Cardiol. 1986;18:307–17.

238. Hirata Y, Soeki T, Akaike M, Sakai Y, Igarashi T, Sata M. Synthetic prostacycline agonist, ONO-1301, ameliorates left ventricular dysfunction and cardiac fibrosis in cardiomyopathic hamsters. Biomed Pharmacother. 2009;63:781–6.
239. Figulla HR, Vetterlein F, Glaubitz M, Kreuzer H. Inhomogenous capillary flow and its prevention by verapamil and hydralazine in the cardiomyopathic Syrian hamster. Circulation. 1987;76:208–16.
240. Khalife WI, Tang YD, Kuzman JA, Thomas TA, Anderson BE, Said S, et al. Treatment of subclinical hypothyroidism reverses ischemia and prevents myocyte loss and progressive LV dysfunction in hamsters with dilated cardiomyopathy. Am J Physiol Heart Circ Physiol. 2005;289:H2409–15.
241. Factor SM, Minase T, Cho S, Dominitz R, Sonnenblick EH. Microvascular spasm in the cardiomyopathic Syrian hamster: a preventable cause of focal myocardial necrosis. Circulation. 1982;66:342–54.
242. Sonnenblick EH, Fein F, Capasso JM, Factor SM. Microvascular spasm as a cause of cardiomyopathies and the calcium-blocking agent verapamil as potential primary therapy. Am J Cardiol. 1985;55:179B–84.
243. Conway RS, Natelson BH, Chen WH, Ting W. Enhanced coronary vasoconstriction in the Syrian myopathic hamster supports the microvascular spasm hypothesis. Cardiovasc Res. 1994; 28:320–4.
244. Minamishima YA, Moslehi J, Bardeesy N, Cullen D, Bronson RT, Kaelin Jr WG. Somatic inactivation of the PHD2 prolyl hydroxylase causes polycythemia and congestive heart failure. Blood. 2008;111:3236–44.
245. Moslehi J, Minamishima YA, Shi J, Neuberg D, Charytan DM, Padera RF, et al. Loss of hypoxia-inducible factor prolyl hydroxylase activity in cardiomyocytes phenocopies ischemic cardiomyopathy. Circulation. 2010;122:1004–16.
246. Lehoux S, Tedgui A. Signal transduction of mechanical stresses in the vascular wall. Hypertension. 1998;32:338–45.
247. Li YS, Haga JH, Chien S. Molecular basis of the effects of shear stress on vascular endothelial cells. J Biomech. 2005;38:1949–71.
248. Hudlicka O, Brown M, Egginton S. Angiogenesis in skeletal and cardiac muscle. Physiol Rev. 1992;72:369–417.
249. Torry RJ, O'Brien DM, Connell PM, Tomanek RJ. Dipyridamole-induced capillary growth in normal and hypertrophic hearts. Am J Physiol. 1992;262:H980–6.
250. Tornling G. Capillary neoformation in the heart of dipyridamole-treated rats. Acta Pathol Microbiol Immunol Scand A. 1982;90: 269–71.
251. Mall G, Schikora I, Mattfeldt T, Bodle R. Dipyridamole-induced neoformation of capillaries in the rat heart. Quantitative stereological study on papillary muscles. Lab Invest. 1987;57: 86–93.
252. Ziada AM, Hudlicka O, Tyler KR, Wright AJ. The effect of long-term vasodilatation on capillary growth and performance in rabbit heart and skeletal muscle. Cardiovasc Res. 1984;18:724–32.
253. Bao X, Lu C, Frangos JA. Mechanism of temporal gradients in shear-induced ERK1/2 activation and proliferation in endothelial cells. Am J Physiol Heart Circ Physiol. 2001;281:H22–9.
254. Hsieh HJ, Cheng CC, Wu ST, Chiu JJ, Wung BS, Wang DL. Increase of reactive oxygen species (ROS) in endothelial cells by shear flow and involvement of ROS in shear-induced c-fos expression. J Cell Physiol. 1998;175:156–62.
255. Chiu JJ, Wung BS, Shyy JY, Hsieh HJ, Wang DL. Reactive oxygen species are involved in shear stress-induced intercellular adhesion molecule-1 expression in endothelial cells. Arterioscler Thromb Vasc Biol. 1997;17:3570–7.
256. Skalak TC, Price RJ. The role of mechanical stresses in microvascular remodeling. Microcirculation. 1996;3:143–65.
257. Ishida T, Takahashi M, Corson MA, Berk BC. Fluid shear stress-mediated signal transduction: how do endothelial cells transduce mechanical force into biological responses? Ann N Y Acad Sci. 1997;811:12–23. discussion –4.
258. Troidl K, Ruding I, Cai WJ, Mucke Y, Grossekettler L, Piotrowska I, et al. Actin-binding rho activating protein (Abra) is essential for fluid shear stress-induced arteriogenesis. Arterioscler Thromb Vasc Biol. 2009;29:2093–101.
259. Shi ZD, Tarbell JM. Fluid flow mechanotransduction in vascular smooth muscle cells and fibroblasts. Ann Biomed Eng. 2011; 39:1608–19.
260. Stepp DW, Nishikawa Y, Chilian WM. Regulation of shear stress in the canine coronary microcirculation. Circulation. 1999;100: 1555–61.
261. Zheng W, Seftor EA, Meininger CJ, Hendrix MJ, Tomanek RJ. Mechanisms of coronary angiogenesis in response to stretch: role of VEGF and TGF-beta. Am J Physiol Heart Circ Physiol. 2001;280:H909–17.
262. Zheng W, Christensen LP, Tomanek RJ. Stretch induces upregulation of key tyrosine kinase receptors in microvascular endothelial cells. Am J Physiol Heart Circ Physiol. 2004;287:H2739–45.
263. Awolesi MA, Sessa WC, Sumpio BE. Cyclic strain upregulates nitric oxide synthase in cultured bovine aortic endothelial cells. J Clin Invest. 1995;96:1449–54.
264. Takeda H, Komori K, Nishikimi N, Nimura Y, Sokabe M, Naruse K. Bi-phasic activation of eNOS in response to uni-axial cyclic stretch is mediated by differential mechanisms in BAECs. Life Sci. 2006;79:233–9.
265. Fisslthaler B, Popp R, Michaelis UR, Kiss L, Fleming I, Busse R. Cyclic stretch enhances the expression and activity of coronary endothelium-derived hyperpolarizing factor synthase. Hypertension. 2001;38:1427–32.
266. Fleming I, Fisslthaler B, Michaelis UR, Kiss L, Popp R, Busse R. The coronary endothelium-derived hyperpolarizing factor (EDHF) stimulates multiple signalling pathways and proliferation in vascular cells. Pflugers Arch. 2001;442:511–8.
267. Munzenmaier DH, Harder DR. Cerebral microvascular endothelial cell tube formation: role of astrocytic epoxyeicosatrienoic acid release. Am J Physiol Heart Circ Physiol. 2000;278:H1163–7.
268. Cummins PM, von Offenberg Sweeney N, Killeen MT, Birney YA, Redmond EM, Cahill PA. Cyclic strain-mediated matrix metalloproteinase regulation within the vascular endothelium: a force to be reckoned with. Am J Physiol Heart Circ Physiol. 2007;292:H28–42.
269. Haga JH, Li YS, Chien S. Molecular basis of the effects of mechanical stretch on vascular smooth muscle cells. J Biomech. 2007;40:947–60.
270. Halka AT, Turner NJ, Carter A, Ghosh J, Murphy MO, Kirton JP, et al. The effects of stretch on vascular smooth muscle cell phenotype in vitro. Cardiovasc Pathol. 2008;17:98–102.
271. Li L, Chaikof EL. Mechanical stress regulates syndecan-4 expression and redistribution in vascular smooth muscle cells. Arterioscler Thromb Vasc Biol. 2002;22:61–8.
272. Li C, Wernig F, Leitges M, Hu Y, Xu Q. Mechanical stress-activated PKCdelta regulates smooth muscle cell migration. FASEB J. 2003;17:2106–8.

Therapy for the Coronary Circulation

12

Abbreviations

EC	Endothelial cell
EPC	Endothelial progenitor cell
FGF	Fibroblast growth factor
G-CSF	Granulocyte-colony stimulating factor
HIF	Hypoxia inducible factor
MCP-1	Monocyte chemoattractant-1
MSC	Mesenchymal stem cell
SDF-1	Stromal-derived factor
VEGF	Vascular endothelial growth factor
VSMC	Vascular smooth muscle cell

Introduction

Enhancement of Myocardial Perfusion

The need to maintain or enhance myocardial perfusion is apparent from the many conditions in which coronary vascular reserve is limited or flow is impeded to the extent that ischemia and death can occur. Examples, as described in the preceding chapters of this book, include coronary anomalies, changes associated with aging, coronary artery disease, cardiac hypertrophy, and coronary vascular dysfunction. The classical treatments are pharmacological or mechanical revascularization therapies. Pharmacological approaches are aimed at reducing O_2 demand, increasing its utilization, or enhancing myocardial perfusion by improving vascular reactivity. Surgical or percutaneous mechanical interventions are used to correct coronary anomalies, open occluded channels, or provide vascular bypass for severely occluded arteries. More recently gene and cell therapy have been proposed as ways of increasing vascular capacity to prevent ischemic events. These approaches have great potential. The goal of this chapter is to summarize the effects of pharmacological, gene, protein, and stem cell therapies on myocardial perfusion.

There are two ways that therapies may enhance myocardial perfusion. First, they may improve the dilatory responses of coronary arteries and arterioles by delivering specific pharmacological agents, genes, or proteins, either directly or via stem or putative progenitor cells. Second, they may evoke vascular growth and/or remodeling and thereby increase the volume of the coronary vascular bed. The latter may occur by (1) stimulating vascular sprouting or intussusceptive vessel branching (angiogenesis), (2) forming arterioles from capillaries or remodeling existing arterioles to increase their diameters (arteriogenesis), or (3) adding cells to the vasculature to form new vessels (vasculogenesis).

Gene and Protein Therapy: Clinical Trials

VEGF Gene and Protein Therapy

Many clinical trials have been conducted by administering vascular endothelial growth factor (VEGF) via intramyocardial injections or percutaneously; the findings of these studies have been reviewed [1–4] and are summarized in Table 12.1. Intramyocardial injections of plasmid-encoded $VEGF_{165}$ were utilized in numerous studies in an attempt to improve myocardial perfusion and/or decrease the frequency of angina [5–11]. Most of the unblinded, nonrandomized studies documented improvement in these parameters. In two of the seven studies, however, myocardial perfusion was not improved [8, 12] and in one study [5] adenovirus $VEGF_{165}$ was found to be more effective than plasmid $VEGF_{165}$. A double-blind study on 178 patients reported that recombinant $VEGF_{165}$ attenuated ischemia, but did not improve exercise tolerance [13]. Although some studies indicate that gene therapy with $VEGF_{165}$ may be useful in patients with coronary artery disease, interest in this topic has diminished. Treatment with adenovirus $VEGF_{121}$ was shown to improve exercise-induced ischemia [14] in one study of 67 patients, but not in another study of 17 patients [15]. Plasmid VEGF-B (earlier called VEGF-2) was found to be effective in reducing

R.J. Tomanek, *Coronary Vasculature: Development, Structure-Function, and Adaptations*,
DOI 10.1007/978-1-4614-4887-7_12,

Table 12.1 VEGF therapy for myocardial ischemia in patients with coronary artery disease

Growth factor	Route (*n*)	Results	References
rhVEGF-A_{165}	IC, i.v. (178)	VEGF attenuated ischemia, no improvement in exercise tolerance	Henry et al. [13]
Plasmid $VEGF_{165}$	IM (6)	Myocardial perfusion improved in 4 of 6 patients	Sylven et al. [11]
Plasmid $VEGF_{165}$	IM (20)	Increased collateral filling, decreased ischemic abnormalities	Symes et al. [10]
Plasmid $VEGF_{165}$	IM (93)	No change in perfusion at 3 or 6 months	Stewart et al. [8]
Adenovirus $VEGF_{165}$ plasmid $VEGF_{165}$	IC (103)	Better myocardial perfusion with Ad-VEGF	Hedman et al. [5]
Plasmid $VEGF_{165}$	IM (80)	No improvement in stress-induced perfusion, but improved wall motion	Kastrup et al. [6]
Plasmid $VEGF_{165}$	IM (40)	Ameliorated stress-induced abnormalities	Gyongyosi et al. [7]
Plasmid $VEGF_{165}$	IM (35)	Decreased myocardial ischemia	Tio et al. [9]
Plasmid $VEGF_{165}$	IM (32)	No improvement in perfusion	Ripa et al. [12]
Adenovirus $VEGF_{121}$	IM (67)	Ameliorated exercise ischemia	Stewart et al. [14]
Adenovirus $VEGF_{121}$	IM (17)	No improvement in exercise capacity or myocardial perfusion	Kastrup et al. [15]
Plasmid VEGF-2(B)	IM (20)	Reduced angina class (1 & 2 year follow-up)	Losordo et al. [16]; Fortuin et al. [17]; Reilly et al. [18]

IC intracoronary; *IM* intramyocardial; *IV* intravenous

Table 12.2 FGF therapy for myocardial ischemia in patients with coronary artery disease

Growth factor	Admin. route (*n*)	Results	References
rFGF-2[a]	IM (24)	Improved myocardial perfusion with high dose, and ameliorated symptoms of ischemia	Laham et al. [21]; Ruel et al. [221]
rFGF-2	IC (337)	No improvement in exercise test or perfusion	Simons et al. [23]
Ad5FGF-4	IC (52)	Trend toward improved myocardial perfusion	Grines et al. [25]
Plasmid $VEGF_{165}$/FGF-2	IC (33)	No improvement in myocardial perfusion, but improved exercise tolerance	Kukula et al. [222]

IC intracoronary; *IM* intramyocardial
[a]Phase I and a follow-up study

angina in an unblinded study that included 20 patients and follow-up after 1 and 2 years [16–18]. A double-blind randomized trial was terminated due to lack of efficacy. In conclusion, the potentially favorable effects of VEGF treatments have not been sufficiently addressed and the previous studies have not been uniform in terms of selection of patients, methods of testing, time points after treatment, and criteria for effectiveness.

FGF Gene and Protein Therapy

Many studies have utilized fibroblast growth factor (FGF) with the goal of promoting myocardial angiogenesis in patients with myocardial ischemia (Table 12.2). However, not all provided direct evidence of enhanced perfusion or vascularization, since their measurements were limited to ventricular function or exercise capacity. Improved perfusion with FGF-2 therapy was reported in three studies [19–21], a fourth found evidence for a reduction in ischemic area [22], and a fifth found a reduction in angina symptoms [23]. FGF-4 gene therapy has been reported to affect some favorable outcomes, i.e., improvements in stress-induced myocardial perfusion and angina class [24], and a reduction in myocardial ischemia [25]. However, blinded studies have not provided encouraging data, a finding that diminishes enthusiasm for FGF gene or protein therapy.

Gene and Protein Therapy: Experimental Animals

FGF Therapy

During the 1990s, several laboratories were able to demonstrate the usefulness of FGF therapy for the ischemic myocardium. Several studies were conducted in Unger's laboratory. The first of these showed that in dogs with regional myocardial ischemia due to an ameroid constrictor on a coronary artery, a sponge containing recombinant FGF-2 positioned over the ischemic region of the left ventricle (LV) caused vascular smooth muscle cell (VSMC) hyperplasia [26]. In contrast, FGF-2-saturated sponges on the nonischemic myocardium had no effect, thus suggesting that the effects of FGF-2 were dependent on an ischemic environment. In another study, using the same model, they delivered FGF-2 by daily bolus injections to the collateral-dependent region of the LV [27]. Important findings from this study included increases in vascular density and EC DNA synthesis, and a greater maximal collateral coronary blood flow. The latter may have been due, in part, to an acute vasodilatory effect of FGF-2. Collateral development in response to daily FGF-2 bolus injections in dogs with ischemia was also reported in another study by these investigators [28]. In contrast, FGF-1 delivered continuously into the coronary artery had no effect on collateral flow in this model [29]. In a porcine model of ischemia, FGF-2 was delivered to the ischemic region via heparin-alginate beads that were placed on the gradually occluded circumflex artery and the non-occluded LAD [30]. This periadventitial administration of FGF-2 caused a fourfold reduction in infarct size and improvements in cardiac function and blood flow to the ischemic region. The use of plasmid DNA encoding FGF-2 was found to be more effective than FGF-2 protein in improving regional myocardial perfusion. Consistent with these data are those from dogs with acute myocardial infarction [31]. Gene transfer of FGF-5 in the ischemic heart also was effective in the amelioration of both myocardial perfusion and cardiac function abnormalities [32]. Two weeks after injecting a recombinant adenovirus expressing human FGF-5, regional abnormalities in blood flow during stress were attenuated and were associated with angiogenesis.

VEGF Therapy

Studies in both canine and porcine models have documented increased collateral blood flow in the ischemic region of the heart following VEGF therapy. In dogs with gradual occlusion of a coronary artery, VEGF administered into the occluded vessel during a 28-day period enhanced coronary blood flow by 40% and increased the number of precapillary vessels with diameters >20 μm by 89% [33]. Pearlman and colleagues [34] demonstrated that VEGF was able to increase collateral blood flow and reduce the size of the ischemic zone in a porcine model of chronic myocardial ischemia. These effects were associated with a better ejection fraction and regional wall thickening. However, pericardial delivery of adenoviral-mediated gene transfer of VEGF did not increase collateral perfusion in the ischemic dog model [35]. As noted in Chap. 7, angiogenesis is impaired during aging and the impairment in the heart of senescent rats has been reported to be associated with a downregulation of VEGF/VEGFR-2 signaling [36]. However, intramyocardial injections of $VEGF_{165}$ in senescent rats increased both capillary and arteriolar density to levels comparable to those in young (3 month) rats. Intramyocardial injections of naked DNA encoding hypoxia-inducible factor-1α/VP16 (a hybrid transcription factor) were reported to increase capillary density and regional myocardial blood flow in rats with acute myocardial infarction (MI) [37]. The potency of this hybrid and VEGF were shown to be similar.

Experimental studies that have explored growth factor and cytokine therapy for MI have usually focused on cardiomyocyte survival and/or cardiac function (see review by [38]). In addition to the growth factor studies cited above, platelet-derived growth factor (PDGF-AB) has been found to decrease infarct size and stimulate angiogenesis when injected into the rat heart immediately after coronary occlusion [39]. Similarly, such early treatment with stromal-derived growth factor-1 (SDF-1) increased capillary density in the infarcted rat heart [40]. In that study, SDF-1 was delivered by intramyocardial injection of mesenchymal cells. Both neovascularization and enhancement of $CD45^+$ and $CD34^+$ cells were found 6 and 30 days following subcutaneous injections of parathyroid hormone after coronary artery occlusion in mice [41].

Endothelial Stem and Progenitor Cell Therapies

Putative Endothelial Progenitor Cells: Description

Endothelial Progenitor Cell Markers

The idea that putative progenitor cells (EPCs), e.g., angioblasts, in the adult can form new vessels is primarily a product of the 1990s. Vasculogenesis, the differentiation of putative EPCs and their coalescence to form blood vessels, is now a generally recognized process (reviewed in [42]). Although there is no consensus as to the origin of these cells, they have most commonly been reported to arise from bone marrow and the vascular wall. These precursors may be the progeny of more than one cell type [43]. The first cell surface markers associated with circulating putative EPCs were found to express the surface markers, $CD34^+/VEGF\text{-}2^+$ [44]. They were shown to be derived from bone and to colonize endothelial flow surfaces on vascular prostheses [45]. The CD34 marker is found on isolated hematopoietic cells (reviewed in [46]). Some studies show CD133 as an additional (or alternate) marker [47], but one that represents fewer circulating cells than those with $CD34^+/VEGF\text{-}2^+$ [48]. Despite some questions concerning the more immature marker, CD133, there is now good documentation that $CD34^+$ or $CD133^+$ cells are enriched for endothelial cell (EC) lineage potential and can form endothelium both in vitro and in vivo [49–52]. In addition, coexpression of CD34 and CD133 and/or VEGFR-2 with c-kit (CD117) CD31 (PECAM) or CD146 (VE-cadherin), among other cell surface proteins, has been reported to be indicative of an EPC phenotype [53].

Not all $CD34^+$ cells function as putative EPCs, but rather subsets like $CD34^+/VEGFR\text{-}2^+$ appear to be the more enriched fraction [54]. In addition, Friedrich et al. [55] identified a population of $CD34^-/133^+$ progenitors that differentiates into $CD34^+/133^+$ cells. These home rapidly into sites of limb ischemia and are more potent in vascular repair. Others have found that $CD14^+$ cells (monocytes) purified from peripheral blood mononuclear cells and cultured in EC growth media express CD45, but also vWF and VEGFR-2 [56]. However, many believe that these are not true endothelial cells (ECs).

Circulating ECs were reported as early as the 1970s [57] and their presence can cause confusion when attempting to identify circulating putative EPCs. A recent polychromatic flow cytometry study purports to distinguish between them [58] and indicates that both circulating ECs and Endothelial colony-forming cells (ECFCs) (or putative EPCs) are rare in the peripheral blood of healthy adults. The latter cell type has been found to be postnatally vasculogenic when transplanted into a matrix scaffold [59]. Unfortunately, despite hundreds of studies, there is no consensus as to the phenotype of circulating cells that are EC progenitors. The contradictory conclusions from many reports have led to arguments both for and against expression of CD34, CD133, and VEGFR-2 as markers of EC progenitor cells. These contradictions suggest that EPC phenotype is plastic and depends on its environment and the physiological status of the organism.

Endothelial Progenitor Cells: Multiple Types

Cells termed "EPCs" in the literature include true endothelial progenitor cells (EPCs), proangiogenic hematopoietic stem and/or progenitor cells, monocytes, macrophages, and other blood cells, as well as the rare circulating endothelial cell. ECFCs have been identified in human peripheral blood and umbilical cord blood [60]. These cells appear to meet many of the characteristics of EPCs proposed by various investigators; most importantly they are able to produce endothelial cell progeny that form vascular tubes in vitro and contribute to the endothelial lining of vascular structures in vivo [61].

Resident and Circulating EC Progenitors

Origin of Progenitors

Putative EPCs have multiple origins and have been shown to have the capacity of self-renewal, clonogenecity, and differentiation [62]. Romagnani and colleagues [63] discovered a novel population of peripheral blood mononuclear cells that expressed CD14 and VEGFR-2 (flk-1), as well as low levels of CD34 by using a sensitive technique, i.e., a combination of immunofluorescence and immunomagnetism. These cells, derived from bone marrow and peripheral blood, proliferated and differentiated into ECs, osteoblasts, adipocytes, and neural cells. More than a decade ago, it was found that 5% of the circulating ECs in subjects that received a bone marrow transplantation from a gender-mismatched donor 5–20 months earlier were derived from the donor (transplanted) cells [64]. Endothelial outgrowth from the blood samples cultured for a month was 50-fold greater in the donor-genotype ECs than in the recipient-genotype ECs. The authors concluded that most circulating ECs originate from vessel walls and have a relatively limited growth capacity. In contrast, the cells derived from transplantable marrow-derived cells have a greater proliferative rate and appear to be derived from circulating angioblasts.

Myocardial Niches

Vascular progenitor cells have been shown to exist in various organs (reviewed in [65, 66]). The presence of resident progenitor cells in the adult heart has been documented in several studies, e.g., Messina et al. [67], Barile et al. [68] and Bearzi et al. [69]. The adult human internal thoracic artery has been found to contain mural $CD34^+$ cells in both the endothelial layer and a transitional area between the tunica media and adventitia [70]. In ring assays of the artery, these cells formed capillary sprouts and were positive for markers of activated ECs, i.e., VE-cadherin, CEACAM-1 (cell adhesion molecules). A review by Torsney and Xu [66] points to evidence that blood vessels contain resident progenitor cells, including "EPCs," mesenchymal, stromal, $Sca^{-/+}$, and $CD34^+$ cells.

In patients with myocardial infarction, administration of autologous bone marrow cells or $CD133^+$-enriched bone marrow-derived cells was found to improve ejection fraction 4–6 months later [71, 72] and to decrease perfusion defects [72]. Bone marrow-derived cell therapy was also shown to decrease infarct size in a study of randomly assigned patients [73, 74], as well as in a double-blind, placebo study [75]. In contrast, another study that administered mononuclear bone marrow cells to a group of randomly assigned patients failed to find a decrease in infarction size [76]. Three studies that randomized patients into treatment and control groups reported improvements in perfusion defects after treatment with bone marrow- or peripheral blood-derived mononuclear cells [73, 77, 78]. Three months after administration of the cells, perfusion in the infarct region was enhanced compared to patients who received standard therapy [73]. Consistent with this finding, coronary flow reserve 4 months following treatment with these cell types was significantly improved [77].

Mesenchymal Stem Cells

Mesenchymal stem cells (MSCs) are important because they home to various tissues, particularly when injury occurs [79]. Although human MSCs are usually isolated from bone marrow, they are also present in other sites, e.g., adipose tissue and perivascular cells [80]. MSCs have been utilized for tissue repair in many studies; those concerning systematically administered MSCs and their therapeutic benefits have been reviewed by Chamberlain et al. [79]. MSCs injected into mouse hearts were found to differentiate into ECs, pericytes, VSMCs, and cardiomyocytes [81], and a perivascular origin of MSCs has been indicated, since cells of perivascular origin expressed MSC markers and migrated in culture [80]. Thus, blood vessels harbor a reserve of progenitor cells. Adhesion of MSCs appears to be an endothelial-dependent process and is sensitive to activators of both MSCs and ECs [82]. These activators include tumor necrosis factor-α (TNF-α) and interleukin-1β (IL-1β), which are released

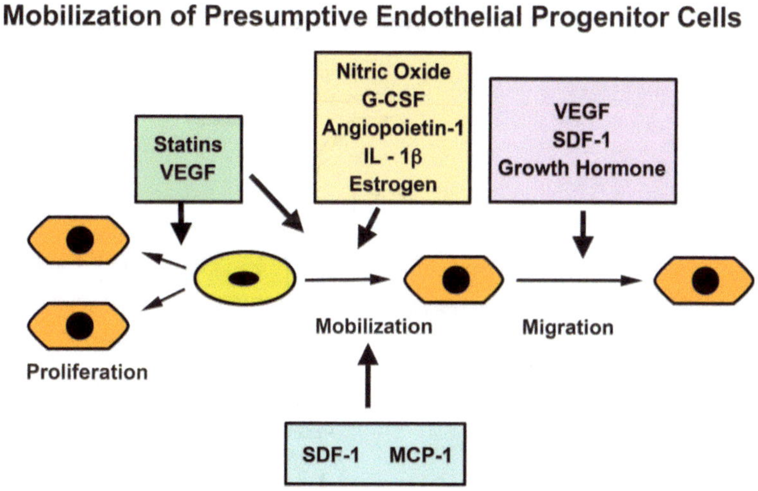

Fig. 12.1 Molecules known to mobilize presumptive endothelial progenitor cells. Additionally, the proliferation and migration of these cells require signaling via growth factors and serum-derived factor-1 (SDF-1) and monocyte chemoattractant-1 factor (MCP-1). Statins have also been shown to stimulate proliferation of presumptive endothelial progenitor cells

during myocardial infarction [83]. Most importantly, when implanted into the myocardium, MSCs secrete large amounts of both angiogenic and antiapoptotic factors [84]. For example, they secrete 5 times as much FGF as mononuclear cells commonly used in regenerative therapy. Injection of MSCs into the myocardium of rats with dilated cardiomyopathy resulted in a marked increase in capillary density, decreased left ventricular (LV) end-diastolic pressure, and increased maximum dP/dt [84].

Monocytes

Monocytes ($CD14^+/CD45^+$) include a subpopulation of multipotent cells that are capable of in vitro differentiation [85] and can restore LV function after myocardial infarction (MI) in experimental animals [86]. Moreover, human bone marrow $CD14^+/C34^-$ cells have been found to enhance reendothelialization following balloon injury to the carotid artery [87]. In acute MI, the number of circulating $CD14^+$/VEGFR-2^+ cells was shown to increase and to stimulate formation of capillary-like structures from human microvascular endothelial cells [88]. When human-activated macrophages were injected into rat hearts following MI, vascularization, cardiac remodeling, and function were improved [89]. Moreover, monocytes are key players in collateral arteriogenesis since they attach to the vessel wall and secrete growth factors, thereby degrading enzymes and survival factors [90]. These data underscore the potential of monocyte therapy for coronary vessels, but as paracrine agents rather than putative EPCs. There is limited evidence that they contribute substantially to neovascularization.

Mobilization of Bone- or Blood-Derived Putative EPCs

As illustrated in Fig. 12.1, a variety of molecules mobilize putative EPCs. These include VEGF [44, 91, 92], nitric oxide [93, 94], estrogen [95], granulocyte-colony-stimulating factor (G-CSF) [96] interleukin-1β [97], stromal-derived factor-1 (SDF-1) [92, 98], and monocyte chemoattractant protein-1 (MCP-1) [87]. VEGF also evokes proliferation of putative EPCs [92]. Interestingly, statins stimulate both mobilization and proliferation of these cells [99–102]. Many of the molecules that promote mobilization are activated by ischemia or hypoxia. One study that documented this adaptation involved patients with symptomatic coronary artery disease. These patients were subjected to a single bout of exercise of sufficient magnitude to induce myocardial ischemia [103]. Two to six hours after the exercise bout, the serum concentration of VEGF was increased, whereas granulocyte macrophage colony-stimulating factor, FGF-2 and tumor necrosis factor-α remained unchanged. The number of circulating mononuclear cells was increased and was maximal between 24 and 48 h post-exercise. The effectiveness of G-CSF in neovascularization was addressed in a randomized double-blind study in which G-CSF or placebo was administered to patients ($n=18$) with chronic angina [104]. However, the treatment did not improve myocardial perfusion or angina. Failure to improve these parameters may have been due to an unfavorable cytokine milieu, as indicated by a lack of change in VEGF and PDGF levels and a decrease in angiopoietin-1, interleukin-8, and tumor necrosis factor-α levels. Unfortunately, the many studies that have addressed putative EPC mobilization have shed little light on the biology of circulating progenitor cells. Since there is a lack of consensus as to the identity of "EPCs," a conclusion regarding this issue is not warranted at this time.

Paracrine Effects of Cell Therapy

There is now considerable evidence that paracrine and autocrine mechanisms may be key factors in revascularization, as well as in repair of the heart [105]. A key finding in this

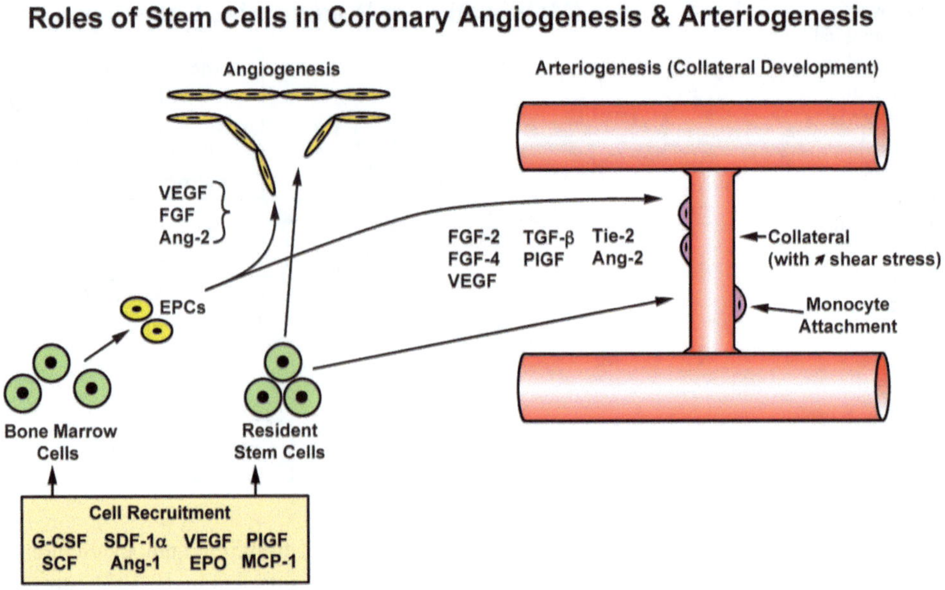

Fig. 12.2 Brief summary of the contributions of bone marrow cells and resident stem cells in myocardial angiogenesis and collateral development, as may occur in the context of ischemia and infarction. Recruitment of these cells occurs in response to the growth factors VEGF, placental growth factor (PlGF), and angiopoietin-1 (Ang-1), as well as to granulocyte colony-stimulating factor (G-CSF), stromal-derived factor-1α (SDF-1α), synergistic colony-stimulating factor (SCF), erythropoietin (EPO), and monocyte chemoattractant protein-1 (MCP-1). The angiogenic and arteriogenic events are facilitated by several growth factors, and collateral vessel development is linked to monocyte attachment and the presence of increased shear stress

regard is that recruited bone marrow-derived circulating cells summoned by VEGF serve to enhance in situ proliferation of endothelial cells by secreting angiogenic factors [106]. The study showed that the recruited circulating cells were retained in close proximity to angiogenic vessels and that their retention was mediated by SDF-1. Indeed, the release of cytokines and growth factors from stem and progenitor cells is beneficial even in the absence of cell incorporation into the tissue. This is a critical point, since putative EPCs only rarely incorporate into the growing vasculature of adults, for example, in hindlimb ischemic muscles and tumors [107] and in the heart [108]. Enhancement of angiogenesis due to the release of cytokines and growth factors, particularly VEGF and SDF-1 from putative EPCs (expressing VEGFR-2, VE-cadherin, eNOS, and von Willebrand factor), has been documented [92]. The expression profile of cytokines in these cells derived from human peripheral blood revealed that VEGF-B, SDF-1, and IGF-1 mRNA levels were higher than in human umbilical vein endothelial cells (HUVECs) or human microvascular ECs. Paralleling the higher mRNA levels in these cells derived from human peripheral blood was a greater release of VEGF-B, SDF-1, and insulin-like growth factor-1 protein into the culture medium. The release of these proteins was shown to enhance the migration of mature ECs and tissue resident cardiac progenitor cells. Further documentation of the importance of paracrine signaling in mediating bone marrow cell therapy for ischemic tissues comes from data indicating that bone marrow stromal cells express genes encoding a broad spectrum of arteriogenic cytokines, many of which, namely VEGF-A, FGFs 2 and 7, interleukin-1 and -6, PlGF, tumor necrosis factor-α, and TGF-β, are induced in the context of hypoxia [109]. In addition, secretion of MCP-1 appears to be an essential component of bone marrow cell-induced vascularization [110].

To release these and other angiogenic and arteriogenic factors on site, putative EPCs must migrate to ischemic foci (Fig. 12.2). In this regard, CD18 (integrin β-2), a cell surface protein that interacts with intercellular adhesion molecule-1 (ICAM-1), has been shown to mediate both the recruitment of putative EPCs and their subsequent stimulation of capillary growth at the border zone of a myocardial infarct in mice [111]. Homing of putative EPCs derived from human blood is dependent on an ischemic stimulus, as shown in experiments in which these cells were radioactively labeled and injected into athymic nude rats 24 h after infarction [112]. Their incorporation in the rats with infarction was double that of sham-operated rats. Non-adipocyte stromal cells have also been shown to be a source of angiogenic factors, i.e., VEGF, hepatocyte growth factor, and TGF-β [113]. When non-adipocyte stromal cells were cultured in a hypoxic environment, VEGF secretion increased fivefold. Moreover, when the conditioned medium from these hypoxic cell cultures was added to EC cultures, their growth increased and apoptosis decreased.

A novel avenue for cell therapy in acute myocardial infarction was recently documented [114] through a phase

I clinical trial that included patients with ST-segment elevation (an indication of myocardial ischemia) after infarction. An allogenic bone marrow-derived stem cell product that is non-immunogenic, can suppress activated T-cell proliferation, and has both anti-inflammatory and angiogenic properties, was administered to the coronary artery adventitia. Administration of 50 million cells was optimal for increasing ejection fraction and stroke volume, especially in patients with the lowest ejection fractions. Although this study did not address the effects of this treatment on myocardial perfusion, it underscores the importance of paracrine effects of bone marrow-derived cells in the restoration of cardiac function after myocardial infarction.

The lack of convincing evidence for substantial donor-recipient chimerism in various tissues in most studies calls attention to mechanisms other than the trans-differentiation of cells injected into the blood stream that could ultimately be harnessed for use in stem cell therapies [115]. It is evident that stem cells secrete an abundance of chemokines, growth factors, cytokines, bioactive lipids, and microvesicles [116–118]. Moreover, there is good evidence that infusion of conditioned media from stem cells or delivery via microvesicles has the same regenerative potential as infusion of intact cells capable of secreting paracrine factors [114, 117, 119]. A recent editorial by Leistner and Zeiher [120] points out that both age and risk factors for coronary artery disease impair both the functional capacity and paracrine activity of isolated bone-marrow-derived cells. Thus, data from patients should be analyzed with regard to specificity of disease, age, and any other data that characterizes a given patient. Comorbidity in patient populations is likely a major factor affecting the inconsistent results in clinical trials.

Cell-Based Therapy for Ischemia and Myocardial Infarction

Introduction

Although cell-based therapy for myocardial infarction has been largely focused on the cardiomyocyte and ventricular remodeling, with an endpoint of improved ventricular function, neovascularization and vascular remodeling are two promising areas that have been addressed in clinical and animal studies. One goal, stressed in many studies, has been the induction of stem and progenitor cells into cardiomyocytes, vascular smooth muscle cells (VSMCs), and endothelial cells (ECs). As reviewed by Laflamme et al. [121], a wide range of cell types have been employed in an attempt to attenuate myocardial injury after ischemia. These have included bone marrow-derived hematopoietic cells, putative EPCs, mesenchymal cells, resident cardiac progenitor cells, and embryonic stem cells.

Cell Therapy for Myocardial Ischemia

Studies on Patients

Treatment of chronic myocardial ischemia has been addressed by several studies. Injection of bone marrow-derived non-nuclear cells via a percutaneous catheter has been found to improve exercise time and/or myocardial perfusion [122–124]. Direct intramural injection of bone marrow-derived mononuclear cells during coronary artery bypass surgery has also demonstrated improvements in myocardial perfusion [125–127]. Long-term follow-up indicates that the procedure is both feasible and safe [128]. More recent data provide evidence that a population of c-Kit$^+$ cells that also express VEGFR-2 are stored in a niche in vascular walls [129]. Their administration near a critical stenosis in a canine artery was found to contribute to the formation of large conductive vessels forming a "biological coronary bypass." In a randomized, double-blind, placebo-controlled study, bone marrow-derived cells were injected in 50 patients with chronic myocardial ischemia; the study concluded that the angina score was improved, and more importantly that significant improvements in myocardial perfusion and exercise time occurred in the treated patients [130]. Similarly, a double-blind randomized phase II study injected autologous CD34$^+$ cells into the hearts of 167 patients with refractory angina [131]. The patients that received this cell therapy had a lower frequency of angina and an increased exercise tolerance at 6 and 12 months after treatment. Moreover, another study reported improvement in myocardial perfusion in patients undergoing incomplete coronary bypass grafting who received an injection of autologous bone marrow cells [132].

Autologous bone marrow cells were injected into the endomyocardium of patients with severe chronic coronary artery disease [133]. In patients randomized to receive the cells the peri-infarct region was reduced by 24% 6 months after treatment. A phase I clinical trial using autologous c-Kit$^+$ lineage negative cells in patients with ischemic cardiomyopathy was launched in 2011 [134]. Intracoronary infusion of these cardiac stem cells in seven randomly assigned patients with old myocardial infarcts in whom MRI data was available infarct size was reduced by 24% and 30% at 4 months and 1 year, respectively, after treatment. LV ejection fraction in the 16 treated patients improved by 27% 4 months after cell infusion.

Studies on Experimental Animals

Neovascularization of the myocardium of experimental animals occurred when CD31$^+$ (PECAM) mononuclear cells were transplanted into ischemic porcine hearts [135]. In this study, the cells were introduced when an ameroid occluder was placed on the left circumflex coronary artery causing chronic (4 weeks) ischemia. Capillary density in the ischemic myocardium was about double that of ischemic untreated pigs. A parallel study in rats also indicated a greater capillary density in the treated group, as well as an attenuation of fibrosis. Intracoronary injections of cardiac progenitor cells revealed limited differentiation, but was shown to have a paracrine effect in rats with old infarctions [136]. Implantation of autologous bone marrow cells into the ischemic rat heart also caused angiogenesis and was associated with enhanced IL-1β and cytokine-induced neutrophil chemoattractant levels [137]. Transplantation of bone marrow-derived cells into the chronically ischemic myocardium of pigs resulted in a greater arteriolar density in both the area at risk and the nonischemic region [138].

Cell Therapy for Acute Myocardial Infarction

Studies on Patients

Putative EPCs derived from bone marrow or the peripheral circulation have been grafted into patients with acute MI to improve myocardial perfusion and ventricular function. These clinical trials taken together indicate that treatment with bone marrow-derived cells during the acute phase of MI may be effective in reducing infarct size and improving myocardial perfusion. A meta-analysis of 18 studies, which collectively included 999 patients with ischemic heart disease who received bone marrow cells (including mononuclear cells, mesenchymal cells, and bone marrow-derived circulating progenitor cells) concluded that this type of therapy leads to a modest decrease in infarct size [139]. Myocardial ischemia provides a milieu conducive to activation of progenitor cells, as observed in patients with acute MI [140]. Blood samples obtained 1–5 days after acute MI revealed a 3.4-fold increase in the number of Oct-4$^+$ very small embryonic-like stem cells, compared to the levels in control subjects. These cells were characterized by cardiac lineage (GATA-4, Nkx 2.5/Csx & MEF2C) and EC (VE-cadherin) markers. The mobilization of very small embryonic stem cells expressing pluripotent markers (Oct-$^{4+}$ SSEA-4$^+$), early cardiac and endothelial markers, and the chemokine receptor (CXCR4) have been discovered in patients with acute MI [140]. The finding that these cells were few in number in patents >50 years of age suggests that their mobilization is limited by the aging process. Again, as noted earlier in this chapter, a lack of agreement in studies on patients is not surprising considering the diverse populations included. A review of the studies during the 2000s led to the conclusion that the variable results are due to differences in cell types used for treatment, the timing, and approach to cell transplantation [141]. Infarct size is a prime example of a parameter that is difficult to measure accurately, and is influenced by the time intervening between the ischemic event and the measurement.

Studies on Experimental Animals

A study more than a decade ago reported that introducing lineage-negative bone marrow cells into the border region of a myocardial infarct in mice resulted in a newly formed myocardium with blood vessels [142]. That same year, Kocher et al. [50] published a paper documenting a role for the GATA-2/CD117^{Dim} cell fraction of the bone-derived CD34$^+$ population in angiogenesis during MI in rats. They showed that capillary density in the infarct zone was threefold to fivefold greater than in the hearts of rats that received CD34+/CD117^{Dim} cells. This cell population migrated to the ischemic myocardium, and its presence was associated with reduced cardiomyocyte apoptosis in the zone with hypertrophied cardiomyocytes bordering the infarct. Similarly, transplantation of autologous bone marrow-derived cells into the ischemic myocardium of swine or nude rats was shown to increase capillary density [135]. Goodell and colleagues [143] provided evidence that bone marrow stem cells in mice contribute to both repair and neovascularization of the myocardium after ischemic injury. These investigators also demonstrated that highly enriched hematopoietic stem cells transplanted into the ischemic myocardium 60 min after occlusion and reperfusion migrated into the ischemic myocardium and to blood vessels [144]. EC engraftment was noted primarily in small vessels. The adult bone marrow-derived very small embryonic-like cells (noted above) that are mobilized during MI in humans have also been found in mouse bone marrow and peripheral blood [145]. Intramyocardial injection of these cells in mice with MI resulted in improved LV ejection fraction and improved myocardial contractility.

G-CSF-based stem cell mobilization has shown promise for myocardial revascularization [142, 146]. More recently, Theiss et al. [147] provided evidence that homing of bone-marrow-derived cells after myocardial infarction requires the SDF-1/CXCR4 axis. CXCR4 is the α-chemokine receptor that is specific for SDF-1 (stromal-derived factor), and as noted earlier SDF-1 facilitates retention of bone marrow-derived circulating cells at angiogenic sites [106]. Their experiments in mice revealed that the increase in capillary density in the infarct border zone and improved myocardial perfusion in response to G-CSF treatment did not occur when CXCR4 was antagonized. Moreover, infarct size was increased by this antagonism. Blockage of CXCR4 at low doses augments mobilization of bone-marrow cells, whereas its continuous infusion causes an increase in infarct size [148].

These data document important roles for both G-CSF and SDF-1/CXCR4 in neovascularization after MI.

The formation of a coronary artery by progenitor cells was reported in a study in which these cells were injected in the proximity of the occlusion site of a coronary artery [108]. c-Kit$^+$ cardiac progenitor cells were activated with insulin-like growth factor-1 and hepatocyte growth factor prior to their injection. These cells divided and differentiated into ECs and VSMCs, and the lineages appeared to be mediated by SDF-1, which was induced by (HIF-1α). The formation of these vessels, along with that of arterioles, was associated with a large increase in coronary blood flow. Moreover, infarct size was reduced by the cell transplantation. Incorporation of human umbilical cord blood-derived EC progenitor cells into the microvessels of hearts with acute infarctions has also been demonstrated [149]. The treated rats experienced enhanced microvessel formation, less fibrosis, and a significant improvement in global heart function. These findings are consistent with earlier work that demonstrated incorporation of umbilical-derived cells into the infarcted regions of mouse hearts where they were associated with angiogenesis and improved remodeling [150]. In mice subjected to coronary artery ligation, treatment with either VEGFR-2$^-$ or VEGFR-2$^+$ cells had favorable effects on myocardial remodeling and cardiac function [151]. However, the effects of VEGFR-2$^+$ grafts were greater and most importantly increased myocardial vascularity.

Prospects for Cell Therapy

The great hope of cell therapy for heart disease remains to be realized. The most encouraging signs come from studies that have documented paracrine effects of bone-derived cells. Malliaras et al. [152] noted that the "spotty trajectory of cell therapy to date" is due to an inadequacy of more systematic approaches. With regard to the debate between those who advocate large-scale outcome trials and others who favor a "back to the bench approach," one must admit that the knowledge of stem and progenitor cells still remains inadequate, which supports the admonition that more preclinical studies should be conducted. Based on encouraging results from studies that have shown these cells to have positive paracrine effects on neovascularization, this role appears more important than incorporation of these cells into vessels or assembly into new vascular channels (vasculogenesis). One of the most encouraging signs for cell therapy is the progress in manipulating stem and progenitor cells to become more effective in coronary angiogenesis and arteriogenesis. In reviewing the role of adult bone marrow stem cells in the repair of the ischemic myocardium, Charwat et al. [153] concluded: "further clinical research should aim to optimize the cell types utilized and their delivery mode, and pinpoint optimal time of cell transplantation." This admonition is well founded considering the many variables that have not been controlled in clinical and even in experimental animal studies.

Pharmacotherapy

This section reviews studies that have utilized approaches other than direct gene or growth factor administration, in which coronary vascular growth and/or improved perfusion was facilitated in ischemic and infarcted hearts. Unfortunately, these approaches have not received sufficient attention in the literature, in spite of the fact that many have been found to increase endogenous growth-promoting factors, including angiogenic and arteriogenetic growth factors.

Thyroid Hormones

Thyroid hormones have been shown to induce vasodilation and enhance myocardial function [154]. The stimulation of myocardial angiogenesis in the nonischemic heart was documented in my laboratory [155–157]. Based on the data from these studies, discussed in Chap. 11, we explored the therapeutic merits of thyroxine therapy for the infarcted heart. We administered the thyroid hormone analog, diodothyroproprionic acid (DITPA), to rats for a period of 10 days following myocardial infarction [158]. Capillary length density in the surviving myocardium of the LV was higher in the DITPA-treated group and correlated with infarct size, i.e., hearts with the largest infarcts had the greatest capillary growth. Subsequently, we demonstrated coronary arteriolar growth in nonischemic, noninfarcted rat hearts that were treated daily for 3 weeks with DITPA [159]. Most importantly, data from that study documented upregulation of FGF-2, $VEGF_{164}$, $VEGF_{188}$, angiopoietin, and Tie-2. Therefore, DITPA treatment was not limited to the enhancement of a single growth factor, but rather increased the levels of the three families of growth factors that play roles in angiogenesis. A similar treatment in rats with myocardial infarction also revealed arteriolar growth in the surviving myocardium [160]. During the first week following infarction the expressions of FGF-2, VEGF, and Tie-2 increased in the non-treated rats. Although DITPA did not increase VEGF and Tie-2 above the expression evoked by infarction, it did enhance FGF-2 expression and it blunted the increase in the size of the region of kinesis (region of infarct expansion). These findings indicate that this thyroid hormone analog plays an important role in arteriolar growth and LV remodeling.

Heart Rate Reduction

A high heart rate enhances the probability of mortality due to cardiovascular events [161], and increases in heart rate have been found to precede episodes of angina and myocardial ischemia [162, 163]. Heart rate reduction has long been considered an important therapeutic tool because it reduces oxygen consumption. Moreover, it increases the diastolic interval and therefore the window during which nearly all myocardial perfusion occurs. Having shown that chronic reduction of heart rate with the K_{ATP} channel antagonist, alinidine, enhances capillary growth in normal rat hearts by a VEGF mechanism [160], we induced myocardial infarctions in rats, aged 4 months, and treated them with alinidine for a period of 4 weeks. The treated rats experienced significant capillary and arteriolar growth and preservation of coronary reserve [164]. These improvements in vascularity and blood flow were associated with elevations in VEGF, VEGFR-2, and FGF-2 protein expression during the first week of treatment and a continued elevation in VEGF after 3 weeks of therapy. Subsequently, we conducted heart rate reduction experiments in middle-aged rats with myocardial infarctions using ivabradine, a selective inhibitor of the I_f current in sinoatrial cells [165]. The 4-week treatment resulted in a decrease in perivascular fibrosis in arterioles and preservation of coronary reserve compared to the non-treated rats with MI. Later we showed that heart rate reduction with either ivabradine or the beta blocker, atenolol, preserved coronary vascular dilator reserve and attenuated coronary arteriolar fibrosis [166]. Furthermore, cardiomyocyte survival in the infarct region was increased and infarct expansion attenuated by ivabradine and atenolol [167].

We [168, 169] and others [170] have documented growth factor and receptor upregulation in cardiomyocytes and coronary ECs subjected to cyclic stretch. These in vitro findings indicate that stretch of coronary microvascular cells enhances the expression of VEGF and VEGFR-2 [169]. To test the hypothesis that bradycardia can evoke arteriolar and collateral growth in model of gradually developed ischemia, we placed an ameroid occluder on coronary arteries of dogs with normal heart rates and on their counterparts with bradycardia evoked by atrioventricular nodal ablation. A comparison of the collateral-dependent and -independent regions of the LV-revealed capillary density was reduced in the group with ameroid constriction and normal heart rates, whereas it was normal in the dogs with bradycardia. The increase in myocardial perfusion in response to adenosine was normal in the bradycardia group, but reduced in the dogs with normal heart rates. Substantial arteriolar growth occurred in the collateral-dependent myocardium of the bradycardia group as evidenced by arteriolar length densities that were 80% greater than in the control dogs with coronary constriction. These benefits of bradycardia were associated with increased VEGF expression in the collateral-dependent regions.

In conclusion, these findings provide strong evidence that heart rate reduction plays an important role in postinfarction therapy of the coronary circulation. Taken together, the data suggest that stretch of cardiomyocytes and ECs activates key angiogenic growth factors and receptors. Although favorable changes can be induced in both young and middle-aged rats, the effects of aging limit the arteriolar growth that characterizes young treated animals. Thus, the effects of aging need to be considered in studies on myocardial ischemia and infarction, which primarily affect middle-aged and older individuals. Given the well-recognized roles of mechanical factors in vascular growth, noted in Chaps. 1 and 11 (reviewed in [171, 172]), their roles as primary angiogenic and arteriogenic stimuli should be tested in research addressing improvements in the coronary circulation.

Erythropoietin

Erythropoietin (EPO) and VEGF have been shown to have equal angiogenic potential [173]. Binding of EPO to its receptors, which are found on the surface of several cell types including ECs, activates several signaling pathways that together upregulate eNOS transcription and cyclooxygenase [174]. The resulting increase in NO facilitates the mobilization of putative EPCs [175] by increasing SDF-1 in the setting of ischemia–reperfusion [174]. As recently reviewed [174], many animal experiments have demonstrated that exogenous EPO can (1) mobilize cells that limit infarct size, (2) stimulate neovascularization, and (3) reduce adverse remodeling. For example, administering human recombinant EPO to rats with acute MI reduced apoptosis, the area at risk, and infarct size [176]. In this model, EPO also enhanced capillary density [177]. Similarly, in dogs with an acute myocardial infarction EPO not only limited infarct size but also increased the number of $CD24^+$ cells in the myocardium, capillary density, and myocardial perfusion [178]. A study in rats with post-MI heart failure concluded that the neovascularization resulting from EPO treatment was a consequence of increased bone marrow cell recruitment and increased VEGF expression in the myocardium [179]. Enhanced EPO associated with angiogenesis after MI has been demonstrated in other rodent studies [180, 181]; however, the effects depend on an ischemic environment [181].

A protective effect of EPO in patients is suggested by the relationship between the levels of EPO and a smaller infarct size [182]. Moreover, in patients with acute MI, EPO levels were found to correlate with the percentage of $CD34^+CD133^+VEGFR\text{-}2^+$ cells [183]. Data from studies on humans with myocardial ischemia and acute infarction have shown that EPO administration is safe but the findings with respect to therapeutic efficacy have been variable (reviewed in [174]). This variability may be due, at least in part, to the endpoints assessed, dosages employed, and patient selection.

Estrogen

Clinical trials testing the efficacy of estrogen hormone therapy in protecting the hearts of postmenopausal women against heart disease have not provided significant evidence that such treatment is clearly beneficial [184]. However, more encouraging data have come from studies addressing estrogen's protection against ischemia and reperfusion injury. All estrogen receptor (ER) subtypes confer cardioprotective effects against ischemia/reperfusion injury (reviewed in [185]). The biological effects of estrogen in the heart are primarily mediated by ERs located on cardiomyocytes [186]. Although it would appear that the protective effects are mediated directly within the cardiomyocyte, a role for eNOS is also indicated [185]. Blocking NOS in ovariectomized mice prevented the protective effect of estrogen receptor treatments; the treatment benefits were associated with an increase in protein S-nitrosylation [187]. The high prevalence of syndrome X (characterized by normal angiograms, but angina pectoris and a positive response to stress tests) in postmenopausal women suggests that estrogen deficiency may play role in this syndrome [188, 189].

Only a few studies have addressed the effects of estrogen therapy on the coronary circulation of patients. Short-term oral estrogen replacement therapy in postmenopausal women failed to improve myocardial perfusion at rest or in response to adenosine [190]. However, these women were healthy with no indication of family coronary artery disease. In contrast, in a study of randomized, double-blind, placebo-controlled patients, improvement in endothelial-dependent dilation and a reduction in perfusion abnormalities in patients with increased estradiol levels were documented after hormone therapy [191]. Knuuti et al. [192] tested the hypothesis that estrogen can improve coronary vascular reserve in patients with myocardial ischemia. They administered 17β-estradiol in combination with drospirenone (a new progestin) to postmenopausal women with angina pectoris for a 6-week treatment period and found that the treatment group had a myocardial perfusion reserve that was 24% higher than the placebo group. Animal studies have also provided evidence that estrogen favorably affects the coronary vasculature. Estrogen treatment of male rats was shown to protect against reperfusion arrhythmias following severe myocardial ischemia [193]. Another study of ovariectomized rats found that an increase in coronary artery myogenic tone was normalized with estradiol [194]. Moreover, estrogen replacement therapy caused enhancement of coronary artery vasorelaxation in response to bradykinin. Finally, my colleagues and I [195] provided evidence that estrogen replacement therapy in ovariectomized rabbits with ameroid occlusion of a coronary artery induced collateral and microvascular remodeling. Coronary (conductance flow/pressure) to the collateral-dependent myocardium was higher both at rest and during maximal vasodilation in treated vs. nontreated ovariectomized rabbits with ameroid-induced ischemia. The treatment also increased capillary diameters and volume density in both the collateral-dependent and -independent regions. Taken together, these findings suggest that estrogen therapy may be useful in preventing or reversing myocardial perfusion abnormalities.

Other Cardiovascular Medications

Miura and Saku [196] suggested that conventional medication with drugs, such as statins and/or ACE inhibitors, should be included in clinical trials because of their angiogenic effects. Statins rapidly activate the downstream signaling components of Akt/PKB (which plays a key role in cell proliferation, survival, and angiogenesis) in ECs and accelerate the formation of vascular structures both in vitro and in vivo [197]. Their inhibitory effect on HMG-CoA reductase (a rate controlling enzyme for cholesterol metabolism) has a biphasic dose-dependent effect on angiogenesis, i.e., it is angiogenic at low doses and antiangiogenic at high doses [198]. As noted by Sodha et al. [199], statins may improve EC function as documented in a porcine model of chronic ischemia, yet not affect collateral-dependent perfusion [200]. For example, a high dose of atorvastatin in pigs improved hypercholesterolemic coronary endothelial dysfunction, but not collateral-dependent myocardial perfusion [200]. Moreover, this treatment reduced VEGF expression and increased endostatin expression.

The key role of NO in vessel formation and reactivity also deserves consideration in the search for pharmacological agents for ischemic heart therapy. There is evidence that sodium nitrite augments myocardial perfusion in the ischemic heart [180]; however, further work is needed to determine the applicability of sodium nitrite in therapy [199]. A single i.v. injection of recombinant human interleukin-2 used to treat mice following MI affected a 34% increase in capillary density and enhanced EC proliferation in the border region of the infarct scar [201].

Stimulation of Coronary Collateral Growth

The importance of the collateral circulation in preventing myocardial ischemia, as occurs during brief coronary occlusion or during exercise [202], is well recognized (see Chaps. 4, 5, 8, and 10 in this book). Therefore, efforts to increase the size and numbers of collateral vessels are important clinical goals. Stimulation of coronary collateral growth is especially relevant for patients with intractable angina pectoris who are not candidates for coronary artery bypass grafts or percutaneous coronary intervention [202]. Collateral growth is usually a remodeling phenomenon, but also occurs de novo. In either situation, the growth involves both ECs and VSMCs and therefore differs from angiogenesis which does not include the latter. This section reviews the human and animal studies that have attempted to enhance the development of coronary collateral growth.

Studies in Patients

Attempts to promote collateral growth in patients with coronary artery disease are summarized in Table 12.3. Four of the studies used granulocyte monocyte colony-stimulating factor (GM-CSF) or G-CSF. These cytokines promote the growth, differentiation, and release of hematopoietic progenitor cells [203]. GM-CSF is upregulated in ECs in response to shear stress [204], prolongs the life cycle of monocytes and macrophages, and enhances collateral growth in a rabbit hindlimb ischemia model [205]. The four studies cited here [206–208], were conducted by the same group of investigators who demonstrated that (1) during coronary occlusion collateral flow index (collateral flow as a percentage of normal flow) and ST segment elevation were improved and (2) collateral flow index correlated with the number of circulating monocytes. Table 12.3 also includes three studies [209–211] that used exercise training as a treatment modality. Among these, one reported improvement in collateral flow index after a 3-month training program [209]. Another evaluated patients who exercised regularly for 1 year and adhered to a low fat diet [210]. Angiographic data failed to detect evidence of improved collateralization in this group compared to a non-treated control group. However, exercise in combination with a low fat diet retarded the development of coronary artery lesions. Exercise training was also found to enhance the effects of dipyridamole treatment on collateral flow [211]. Finally, collateral flow index was shown to be improved in patients who underwent enhanced counterpulsation therapy over a 4-week period [212].

Studies in Experimental Animals

Stem and Progenitor Cells

One of the earliest studies to address the role of autologous bone marrow cells in collateral perfusion in the ischemic heart revealed that these cells secrete the angiogenic and arteriogenic factors, VEGF and MCP-1, respectively [213]. In pigs, injection of the autologous bone marrow cells into the myocardial ischemic zone 4 weeks after ameroid constriction of the left circumflex coronary artery increased collateral flow—both at rest and during adenosine infusion—and also improved function of the ischemic myocardium. Subsequent studies have tested the efficacy of treatment with specific subpopulations of bone marrow cells. MSCs are an important source of paracrine factors that play a role in myocardial protection, vascular regeneration, and angiogenesis [214–216], and are able to differentiate into an EC phenotype and ultimately improve vascular density in chronic

Table 12.3 Studies on coronary collateral development in patients with coronary artery disease

Treatment	Number of patients	Findings	References
GM-CSF (SC-2 weeks) SC	21	Improved collateral flow index during coronary occlusion	Seiler et al. [206]
GM-CSF (SC-2 weeks)	14	Improved collateral flow index during coronary occlusion	Zbinden et al. [207]
G-CSF (SC-2 weeks)	52	Improved collateral flow index and ST segment	Meier et al. [223]
GM-CSF (SC-2 weeks)	21	Collateral flow index correlates with number of blood monocytes	Zbinden et al. [208]
External counterpulsation[a] 3 h (randomly allocated over 4 weeks)	20	Improved collateral flow index	Gloekler et al. [212]
Exercise training (3 months)	40	Improved collateral flow index	Zbinden et al. [209]
Exercise + dipyridamole (8 weeks)	30	Dipyridamole increased collateral flow; exercise potentiated the effect	Belardinelli et al. [211]
Exercise (>3 h/week)	56	No change in collateral formation	Niebauer et al. [210]

GM-CSF granulocyte macrophage colony-stimulating factor; *G-CSF* granulocyte-stimulating factor; *SC* subcutaneous
[a]A technique applied during diastole to increase myocardial blood flow and oxygen demand

myocardial ischemia [217]. Transplantation of CD31$^+$ mononuclear cells in the context of myocardial ischemia in pigs, due to gradual coronary occlusion, also induced collateral growth [135].

The role of multipotent MSCs in coronary collateral development was pursued by studies in Chilian's lab [218]. First they showed that treatment of rat MSCs with epidermal growth factor (EGF) caused an increase in their adhesion to ECs as a consequence of increased expression of intracellular adhesion and vascular cell molecules. They then evaluated the effectiveness of MSCs in stimulating collateral growth by injecting these cells into the LV lumen of rats that were subjected to repetitive episodes of myocardial ischemia. Coronary collateral growth was based on the flow ratio of collateral-dependent and collateral-independent zone flows. Compared to the non-treated controls, animals injected with untreated and treated MSCs exhibited 1.4-fold and 2.1-fold increases, respectively, in collateral flow. More recently, the Chilian laboratory [219] generated a vascular progenitor-type cell they termed "induced vascular progenitor cell" by reprogramming rat vascular ECs with Oct4, Klf4, Sox2, and c-Myc. These cells stimulated coronary collateral growth and had the capacity to differentiate into either ECs or VSMCs. When implanted into the ischemic myocardium, they engrafted into blood vessels, increased coronary collateral flow, and improved cardiac function more than native ECs and mesenchymal cells.

Cytokine-Induced Collateral Growth in a Hind-Limb Ischemic Model

Because the hindlimb model of ischemia is easier to manipulate, most studies have employed it to study collateral growth. A summary of cytokines that have been shown to stimulate arteriogenesis in this model was published in a review by Schirmer et al. [220]. Many of the molecules that are arteriogenic in this model may act by mobilizing bone marrow cells, either directly or indirectly, by interacting with MCP-1. Compared to the more controversial studies on human coronary collateral growth, the data from the hindlimb ischemia model reveal that many growth factors (FGFs, VEGF, PlGF, TNFα, angiopoietin-1, PDGF, and TGFβ) are arteriogenic.

Concluding Remarks

As discussed in this chapter, many approaches to improving myocardial perfusion and cardiac function have been tested. With regard to myocardial perfusion, which is the focus of this chapter, therapeutic angiogenesis is the most frequently mentioned approach. This phenomenon involves ECs and the formation of branches in the microvasculature. However, arteriogenesis, especially coronary collateral development, requires other mechanisms, and therefore specific therapeutic approaches. Arteriogenesis needs to be a prime goal of coronary therapy because arterioles are the main structures for the local delivery of blood within the myocardium. A second goal of therapy should be improving vascular function. Correcting endothelial dysfunction has considerable merit because vasoactive responses are important for the regulation of myocardial perfusion. Therefore, even though single therapeutic approaches may be valuable, they are unlikely to improve all aspects of the coronary circulation. Cell therapy has merit as indicated by both clinical trials and experimental data from studies on animals. Although incorporation of stem or progenitor cells into the vasculature can occur, it is usually limited. However, the treatment with these cells has merit because they deliver factors that promote vascularization and improve vascular function. The paracrine benefit of these cells is also documented by studies that have utilized their conditioned media to treat the heart. An approach to coronary therapy that has not received sufficient attention is that of pharmacologically or physiologically activating endogenous factors, e.g., growth factors that are capable of improving the coronary circulation via functional or structural changes. Stretch of the myocardium caused by bradycardia and enhancement of flow and shear stress are examples of mechanical factors that have been proven to be angiogenic and arteriogenic.

The future of therapy for myocardial ischemia and infarction depends on several considerations. First, preclinical studies are needed to more fully address mechanisms that underlie improved coronary vessel responses and the enhancement of myocardial perfusion. In this regard, the animal models must be appropriate, e.g., testing of middle-aged and older animals that reflect the human condition when ischemia and infarction are most prevalent. Second, studies need to focus on the coronary circulation as an endpoint rather than limiting the data to improvements in cardiac function. Third, attention should be given to long-term benefits of the various therapies, since early improvements may be transient. Finally, combined therapeutic approaches may prove beneficial. For example, gene or protein therapy may be enhanced if combined with exercise training.

References

1. Gupta R, Tongers J, Losordo DW. Human studies of angiogenic gene therapy. Circ Res. 2009;105:724–36.
2. Kastrup J. Gene therapy and angiogenesis in patients with coronary artery disease. Exp Rev Cardiovasc Ther. 2010;8:1127–38.
3. Lavu M, Gundewar S, Lefer DJ. Gene therapy for ischemic heart disease. J Mol Cell Cardiol. 2011;50:742–50.
4. Eibel B, Rodrigues CG, Giusti II, Nesralla IA, Prates PR, Sant'Anna RT, et al. Gene therapy for ischemic heart disease: review of clinical trials. Rev Bras Cir Cardiovasc. 2011;26:635–46.
5. Hedman M, Hartikainen J, Syvanne M, Stjernvall J, Hedman A, Kivela A, et al. Safety and feasibility of catheter-based local intracoronary vascular endothelial growth factor gene transfer in the prevention of postangioplasty and in-stent restenosis and in the treatment of chronic myocardial ischemia: phase II results of the Kuopio Angiogenesis Trial (KAT). Circulation. 2003;107:2677–83.
6. Kastrup J, Jorgensen E, Ruck A, Tagil K, Glogar D, Ruzyllo W, et al. Direct intramyocardial plasmid vascular endothelial growth factor-A165 gene therapy in patients with stable severe angina pectoris A randomized double-blind placebo-controlled study: the Euroinject One trial. J Am Coll Cardiol. 2005;45:982–8.
7. Gyongyosi M, Khorsand A, Zamini S, Sperker W, Strehblow C, Kastrup J, et al. NOGA-guided analysis of regional myocardial perfusion abnormalities treated with intramyocardial injections of plasmid encoding vascular endothelial growth factor A-165 in patients with chronic myocardial ischemia: subanalysis of the EUROINJECT-ONE multicenter double-blind randomized study. Circulation. 2005;112:I157–65.
8. Stewart DJ, Kutryk MJ, Fitchett D, Freeman M, Camack N, Su Y, et al. VEGF gene therapy fails to improve perfusion of ischemic myocardium in patients with advanced coronary disease: results of the NORTHERN trial. Mol Ther. 2009;17:1109–15.
9. Tio RA, Tan ES, Jessurun GA, Veeger N, Jager PL, Slart RH, et al. PET for evaluation of differential myocardial perfusion dynamics after VEGF gene therapy and laser therapy in end-stage coronary artery disease. J Nucl Med. 2004;45:1437–43.
10. Symes JF, Losordo DW, Vale PR, Lathi KG, Esakof DD, Mayskiy M, et al. Gene therapy with vascular endothelial growth factor for inoperable coronary artery disease. Ann Thorac Surg. 1999;68:830–6. discussion 6–7.
11. Sylven C, Sarkar N, Ruck A, Drvota V, Hassan SY, Lind B, et al. Myocardial Doppler tissue velocity improves following myocardial gene therapy with VEGF-A165 plasmid in patients with inoperable angina pectoris. Coron Artery Dis. 2001;12:239–43.
12. Ripa RS, Wang Y, Jorgensen E, Johnsen HE, Hesse B, Kastrup J. Intramyocardial injection of vascular endothelial growth factor-A165 plasmid followed by granulocyte-colony stimulating factor to induce angiogenesis in patients with severe chronic ischaemic heart disease. Eur Heart J. 2006;27:1785–92.
13. Henry TD, Annex BH, McKendall GR, Azrin MA, Lopez JJ, Giordano FJ, et al. The VIVA trial: Vascular endothelial growth factor in Ischemia for Vascular Angiogenesis. Circulation. 2003;107:1359–65.
14. Stewart DJ, Hilton JD, Arnold JM, Gregoire J, Rivard A, Archer SL, et al. Angiogenic gene therapy in patients with nonrevascularizable ischemic heart disease: a phase 2 randomized, controlled trial of AdVEGF(121) (AdVEGF121) versus maximum medical treatment. Gene Ther. 2006;13:1503–11.
15. Kastrup J, Jorgensen E, Fuchs S, Nikol S, Botker HE, Gyongyosi M, et al. A randomised, double-blind, placebo-controlled, multicentre study of the safety and efficacy of BIOBYPASS (AdGVVEGF121.10NH) gene therapy in patients with refractory advanced coronary artery disease: the NOVA trial. EuroIntervention. 2011;6:813–8.
16. Losordo DW, Vale PR, Hendel RC, Milliken CE, Fortuin FD, Cummings N, et al. Phase 1/2 placebo-controlled, double-blind, dose-escalating trial of myocardial vascular endothelial growth factor 2 gene transfer by catheter delivery in patients with chronic myocardial ischemia. Circulation. 2002;105:2012–8.
17. Fortuin FD, Vale P, Losordo DW, Symes J, DeLaria GA, Tyner JJ, et al. One-year follow-up of direct myocardial gene transfer of vascular endothelial growth factor-2 using naked plasmid deoxyribonucleic acid by way of thoracotomy in no-option patients. Am J Cardiol. 2003;92:436–9.
18. Reilly JP, Grise MA, Fortuin FD, Vale PR, Schaer GL, Lopez J, et al. Long-term (2-year) clinical events following transthoracic intramyocardial gene transfer of VEGF-2 in no-option patients. J Interv Cardiol. 2005;18:27–31.
19. Schumacher B, Stegmann T, Pecher P. The stimulation of neoangiogenesis in the ischemic human heart by the growth factor FGF: first clinical results. J Cardiovasc Surg (Torino). 1998;39:783–9.
20. Sellke FW, Laham RJ, Edelman ER, Pearlman JD, Simons M. Therapeutic angiogenesis with basic fibroblast growth factor: technique and early results. Ann Thorac Surg. 1998;65:1540–4.
21. Laham RJ, Sellke FW, Edelman ER, Pearlman JD, Ware JA, Brown DL, et al. Local perivascular delivery of basic fibroblast growth factor in patients undergoing coronary bypass surgery: results of a phase I randomized, double-blind, placebo-controlled trial. Circulation. 1999;100:1865–71.
22. Laham RJ, Chronos NA, Pike M, Leimbach ME, Udelson JE, Pearlman JD, et al. Intracoronary basic fibroblast growth factor (FGF-2) in patients with severe ischemic heart disease: results of a phase I open-label dose escalation study. J Am Coll Cardiol. 2000;36:2132–9.
23. Simons M, Annex BH, Laham RJ, Kleiman N, Henry T, Dauerman H, et al. Pharmacological treatment of coronary artery disease with recombinant fibroblast growth factor-2: double-blind, randomized, controlled clinical trial. Circulation. 2002;105:788–93.
24. Henry TD, Grines CL, Watkins MW, Dib N, Barbeau G, Moreadith R, et al. Effects of Ad5FGF-4 in patients with angina: an analysis of pooled data from the AGENT-3 and AGENT-4 trials. J Am Coll Cardiol. 2007;50:1038–46.
25. Grines CL, Watkins MW, Mahmarian JJ, Iskandrian AE, Rade JJ, Marrott P, et al. A randomized, double-blind, placebo-controlled trial of Ad5FGF-4 gene therapy and its effect on myocardial perfusion in patients with stable angina. J Am Coll Cardiol. 2003; 42:1339–47.
26. Banai S, Jaklitsch MT, Casscells W, Shou M, Shrivastav S, Correa R, et al. Effects of acidic fibroblast growth factor on normal and ischemic myocardium. Circ Res. 1991;69:76–85.
27. Unger EF, Banai S, Shou M, Lazarous DF, Jaklitsch MT, Scheinowitz M, et al. Basic fibroblast growth factor enhances myocardial collateral flow in a canine model. Am J Physiol. 1994;266:H1588–95.
28. Lazarous DF, Shou M, Scheinowitz M, Hodge E, Thirumurti V, Kitsiou AN, et al. Comparative effects of basic fibroblast growth factor and vascular endothelial growth factor on coronary collateral development and the arterial response to injury. Circulation. 1996;94:1074–82.
29. Unger EF, Banai S, Shou M, Jaklitsch M, Hodge E, Correa R, et al. A model to assess interventions to improve collateral blood flow: continuous administration of agents into the left coronary artery in dogs. Cardiovasc Res. 1993;27:785–91.
30. Harada K, Grossman W, Friedman M, Edelman ER, Prasad PV, Keighley CS, et al. Basic fibroblast growth factor improves myocardial function in chronically ischemic porcine hearts. J Clin Invest. 1994;94:623–30.

31. Liu Y, Sun L, Huan Y, Zhao H, Deng J. Effects of basic fibroblast growth factor microspheres on angiogenesis in ischemic myocardium and cardiac function: analysis with dobutamine cardiovascular magnetic resonance tagging. Eur J Cardiothorac Surg. 2006;30:103–7.
32. Giordano FJ, Ping P, McKirnan MD, Nozaki S, DeMaria AN, Dillmann WH, et al. Intracoronary gene transfer of fibroblast growth factor-5 increases blood flow and contractile function in an ischemic region of the heart. Nat Med. 1996;2:534–9.
33. Banai S, Jaklitsch MT, Shou M, Lazarous DF, Scheinowitz M, Biro S, et al. Angiogenic-induced enhancement of collateral blood flow to ischemic myocardium by vascular endothelial growth factor in dogs. Circulation. 1994;89:2183–9.
34. Pearlman JD, Hibberd MG, Chuang ML, Harada K, Lopez JJ, Gladstone SR, et al. Magnetic resonance mapping demonstrates benefits of VEGF-induced myocardial angiogenesis. Nat Med. 1995;1:1085–9.
35. Lazarous DF, Shou M, Stiber JA, Hodge E, Thirumurti V, Goncalves L, et al. Adenoviral-mediated gene transfer induces sustained pericardial VEGF expression in dogs: effect on myocardial angiogenesis. Cardiovasc Res. 1999;44:294–302.
36. Besse S, Boucher F, Linguet G, Riou L, De Leiris J, Riou B, et al. Intramyocardial protein therapy with vascular endothelial growth factor (VEGF-165) induces functional angiogenesis in rat senescent myocardium. J Physiol Pharmacol. 2010;61:651–61.
37. Shyu KG, Wang MT, Wang BW, Chang CC, Leu JG, Kuan P, et al. Intramyocardial injection of naked DNA encoding HIF-1alpha/VP16 hybrid to enhance angiogenesis in an acute myocardial infarction model in the rat. Cardiovasc Res. 2002;54:576–83.
38. Hwang H, Kloner RA. Improving regenerating potential of the heart after myocardial infarction: factor-based approach. Life Sci. 2010;86:461–72.
39. Edelberg JM, Lee SH, Kaur M, Tang L, Feirt NM, McCabe S, et al. Platelet-derived growth factor-AB limits the extent of myocardial infarction in a rat model: feasibility of restoring impaired angiogenic capacity in the aging heart. Circulation. 2002;105:608–13.
40. Zhao T, Zhang D, Millard RW, Ashraf M, Wang Y. Stem cell homing and angiomyogenesis in transplanted hearts are enhanced by combined intramyocardial SDF-1alpha delivery and endogenous cytokine signaling. Am J Physiol Heart Circ Physiol. 2009;296:H976–86.
41. Zaruba MM, Huber BC, Brunner S, Deindl E, David R, Fischer R, et al. Parathyroid hormone treatment after myocardial infarction promotes cardiac repair by enhanced neovascularization and cell survival. Cardiovasc Res. 2008;77:722–31.
42. Schatteman GC, Awad O. Hemangioblasts, angioblasts, and adult endothelial cell progenitors. Anat Rec A Discov Mol Cell Evol Biol. 2004;276:13–21.
43. Ribatti D. The discovery of endothelial progenitor cells. An historical review. Leuk Res. 2007;31:439–44.
44. Asahara T, Takahashi T, Masuda H, Kalka C, Chen D, Iwaguro H, et al. VEGF contributes to postnatal neovascularization by mobilizing bone marrow-derived endothelial progenitor cells. EMBO J. 1999;18:3964–72.
45. Shi Q, Rafii S, Wu MH, Wijelath ES, Yu C, Ishida A, et al. Evidence for circulating bone marrow-derived endothelial cells. Blood. 1998;92:362–7.
46. Fadini GP, Losordo D, Dimmeler S. Critical reevaluation of endothelial progenitor cell phenotypes for therapeutic and diagnostic use. Circ Res. 2012;110:624–37.
47. Gehling UM, Ergun S, Schumacher U, Wagener C, Pantel K, Otte M, et al. In vitro differentiation of endothelial cells from AC133-positive progenitor cells. Blood. 2000;95:3106–12.
48. Yamahara K, Itoh H. Potential use of endothelial progenitor cells for regeneration of the vasculature. Ther Adv Cardiovasc Dis. 2009;3:17–27.
49. Masuda H, Alev C, Akimaru H, Ito R, Shizuno T, Kobori M, et al. Methodological development of a clonogenic assay to determine endothelial progenitor cell potential. Circ Res. 2011;109:20–37.
50. Kocher AA, Schuster MD, Szabolcs MJ, Takuma S, Burkhoff D, Wang J, et al. Neovascularization of ischemic myocardium by human bone-marrow-derived angioblasts prevents cardiomyocyte apoptosis, reduces remodeling and improves cardiac function. Nat Med. 2001;7:430–6.
51. Kawamoto A, Iwasaki H, Kusano K, Murayama T, Oyamada A, Silver M, et al. CD34-positive cells exhibit increased potency and safety for therapeutic neovascularization after myocardial infarction compared with total mononuclear cells. Circulation. 2006;114:2163–9.
52. Ramos AL, Darabi R, Akbarloo N, Borges L, Catanese J, Dineen SP, et al. Clonal analysis reveals a common progenitor for endothelial, myeloid, and lymphoid precursors in umbilical cord blood. Circ Res. 2010;107:1460–9.
53. Padfield GJ, Newby DE, Mills NL. Understanding the role of endothelial progenitor cells in percutaneous coronary intervention. J Am Coll Cardiol. 2010;55:1553–65.
54. Madeddu P, Emanueli C, Pelosi E, Salis MB, Cerio AM, Bonanno G, et al. Transplantation of low dose CD34+KDR+ cells promotes vascular and muscular regeneration in ischemic limbs. FASEB J. 2004;18:1737–9.
55. Friedrich EB, Walenta K, Scharlau J, Nickenig G, Werner N. CD34-/CD133+/VEGFR-2+ endothelial progenitor cell subpopulation with potent vasoregenerative capacities. Circ Res. 2006;98:e20–5.
56. Urbich C, Heeschen C, Aicher A, Dernbach E, Zeiher AM, Dimmeler S. Relevance of monocytic features for neovascularization capacity of circulating endothelial progenitor cells. Circulation. 2003;108:2511–6.
57. Weber G, Losi M, Toti P, Vatti R. Circulating endothelial-like cells in arterial peripheral blood of hypercholesterolemic rabbits. Artery. 1979;5:29–36.
58. Mund JA, Estes ML, Yoder MC, Ingram Jr DA, Case J. Flow cytometric identification and functional characterization of immature and mature circulating endothelial cells. Arterioscler Thromb Vasc Biol. 2012;32:1045–53.
59. Richardson MR, Yoder MC. Endothelial progenitor cells: quo vadis? J Mol Cell Cardiol. 2011;50:266–72.
60. Yoder MC. Is endothelium the origin of endothelial progenitor cells? Arterioscler Thromb Vasc Biol. 2010;30:1094–103.
61. Hirschi KK, Ingram DA, Yoder MC. Assessing identity, phenotype, and fate of endothelial progenitor cells. Arterioscler Thromb Vasc Biol. 2008;28:1584–95.
62. Urbich C, Dimmeler S. Endothelial progenitor cells: characterization and role in vascular biology. Circ Res. 2004;95:343–53.
63. Romagnani P, Annunziato F, Liotta F, Lazzeri E, Mazzinghi B, Frosali F, et al. CD14+CD34low cells with stem cell phenotypic and functional features are the major source of circulating endothelial progenitors. Circ Res. 2005;97:314–22.
64. Lin Y, Weisdorf DJ, Solovey A, Hebbel RP. Origins of circulating endothelial cells and endothelial outgrowth from blood. J Clin Invest. 2000;105:71–7.
65. Bautch VL. Stem cells and the vasculature. Nat Med. 2011;17:1437–43.
66. Torsney E, Xu Q. Resident vascular progenitor cells. J Mol Cell Cardiol. 2011;50:304–11.
67. Messina E, De Angelis L, Frati G, Morrone S, Chimenti S, Fiordaliso F, et al. Isolation and expansion of adult cardiac stem cells from human and murine heart. Circulation Res. 2004;95:911–21.
68. Barile L, Messina E, Giacomello A, Marban E. Endogenous cardiac stem cells. Prog Cardiovasc Dis. 2007;50:31–48.
69. Bearzi C, Rota M, Hosoda T, Tillmanns J, Nascimbene A, De Angelis A, et al. Human cardiac stem cells. Proc Natl Acad Sci USA. 2007;104:14068–73.

70. Zengin E, Chalajour F, Gehling UM, Ito WD, Treede H, Lauke H, et al. Vascular wall resident progenitor cells: a source for postnatal vasculogenesis. Development. 2006;133:1543–51.
71. Wollert KC, Meyer GP, Lotz J, Ringes-Lichtenberg S, Lippolt P, Breidenbach C, et al. Intracoronary autologous bone-marrow cell transfer after myocardial infarction: the BOOST randomised controlled clinical trial. Lancet. 2004;364:141–8.
72. Bartunek J, Vanderheyden M, Vandekerckhove B, Mansour S, De Bruyne B, De Bondt P, et al. Intracoronary injection of CD133-positive enriched bone marrow progenitor cells promotes cardiac recovery after recent myocardial infarction: feasibility and safety. Circulation. 2005;112:I178–83.
73. Strauer BE, Brehm M, Zeus T, Kostering M, Hernandez A, Sorg RV, et al. Repair of infarcted myocardium by autologous intracoronary mononuclear bone marrow cell transplantation in humans. Circulation. 2002;106:1913–8.
74. Schachinger V, Assmus B, Britten MB, Honold J, Lehmann R, Teupe C, et al. Transplantation of progenitor cells and regeneration enhancement in acute myocardial infarction: final one-year results of the TOPCARE-AMI Trial. J Am Coll Cardiol. 2004;44:1690–9.
75. Janssens S, Dubois C, Bogaert J, Theunissen K, Deroose C, Desmet W, et al. Autologous bone marrow-derived stem-cell transfer in patients with ST-segment elevation myocardial infarction: double-blind, randomised controlled trial. Lancet. 2006;367: 113–21.
76. Lunde K, Solheim S, Aakhus S, Arnesen H, Abdelnoor M, Egeland T, et al. Intracoronary injection of mononuclear bone marrow cells in acute myocardial infarction. N Engl J Med. 2006;355:1199–209.
77. Assmus B, Schachinger V, Teupe C, Britten M, Lehmann R, Dobert N, et al. Transplantation of Progenitor Cells and Regeneration Enhancement in Acute Myocardial Infarction (TOPCARE-AMI). Circulation. 2002;106:3009–17.
78. Chen SL, Fang WW, Ye F, Liu YH, Qian J, Shan SJ, et al. Effect on left ventricular function of intracoronary transplantation of autologous bone marrow mesenchymal stem cell in patients with acute myocardial infarction. Am J Cardiol. 2004;94:92–5.
79. Chamberlain G, Fox J, Ashton B, Middleton J. Concise review: mesenchymal stem cells: their phenotype, differentiation capacity, immunological features, and potential for homing. Stem Cells. 2007;25:2739–49.
80. Crisan M, Yap S, Casteilla L, Chen CW, Corselli M, Park TS, et al. A perivascular origin for mesenchymal stem cells in multiple human organs. Cell stem cell. 2008;3:301–13.
81. Gojo S, Gojo N, Takeda Y, Mori T, Abe H, Kyo S, et al. In vivo cardiovasculogenesis by direct injection of isolated adult mesenchymal stem cells. Exp Cell Res. 2003;288:51–9.
82. Segers VF, Van Riet I, Andries LJ, Lemmens K, Demolder MJ, De Becker AJ, et al. Mesenchymal stem cell adhesion to cardiac microvascular endothelium: activators and mechanisms. Am J Physiol Heart Circ Physiol. 2006;290:H1370–7.
83. Frangogiannis NG, Smith CW, Entman ML. The inflammatory response in myocardial infarction. Cardiovasc Res. 2002;53:31–47.
84. Nagaya N, Kangawa K, Itoh T, Iwase T, Murakami S, Miyahara Y, et al. Transplantation of mesenchymal stem cells improves cardiac function in a rat model of dilated cardiomyopathy. Circulation. 2005;112:1128–35.
85. Zhao Y, Glesne D, Huberman E. A human peripheral blood monocyte-derived subset acts as pluripotent stem cells. Proc Natl Acad Sci USA. 2003;100:2426–31.
86. Dresske B, El Mokhtari NE, Ungefroren H, Ruhnke M, Plate V, Janssen D, et al. Multipotent cells of monocytic origin improve damaged heart function. Am J Transplant. 2006;6:947–58.
87. Fujiyama S, Amano K, Uehira K, Yoshida M, Nishiwaki Y, Nozawa Y, et al. Bone marrow monocyte lineage cells adhere on injured endothelium in a monocyte chemoattractant protein-1-dependent manner and accelerate reendothelialization as endothelial progenitor cells. Circ Res. 2003;93:980–9.
88. Bruno S, Bussolati B, Scacciatella P, Marra S, Sanavio F, Tarella C, et al. Combined administration of G-CSF and GM-CSF stimulates monocyte-derived pro-angiogenic cells in patients with acute myocardial infarction. Cytokine. 2006;34:56–65.
89. Leor J, Rozen L, Zuloff-Shani A, Feinberg MS, Amsalem Y, Barbash IM, et al. Ex vivo activated human macrophages improve healing, remodeling, and function of the infarcted heart. Circulation. 2006;114:I94–100.
90. van Royen N, Piek JJ, Schaper W, Fulton WF. A critical review of clinical arteriogenesis research. J Am Coll Cardiol. 2009;55:17–25.
91. Kalka C, Masuda H, Takahashi T, Gordon R, Tepper O, Gravereaux E, et al. Vascular endothelial growth factor(165) gene transfer augments circulating endothelial progenitor cells in human subjects. Circ Res. 2000;86:1198–202.
92. Urbich C, Aicher A, Heeschen C, Dernbach E, Hofmann WK, Zeiher AM, et al. Soluble factors released by endothelial progenitor cells promote migration of endothelial cells and cardiac resident progenitor cells. J Mol Cell Cardiol. 2005;39:733–42.
93. Ziche M, Morbidelli L. Nitric oxide and angiogenesis. J Neurooncol. 2000;50:139–48.
94. Aicher A, Heeschen C, Mildner-Rihm C, Urbich C, Ihling C, Technau-Ihling K, et al. Essential role of endothelial nitric oxide synthase for mobilization of stem and progenitor cells. Nat Med. 2003;9:1370–6.
95. Strehlow K, Werner N, Berweiler J, Link A, Dirnagl U, Priller J, et al. Estrogen increases bone marrow-derived endothelial progenitor cell production and diminishes neointima formation. Circulation. 2003;107:3059–65.
96. Takahashi T, Kalka C, Masuda H, Chen D, Silver M, Kearney M, et al. Ischemia- and cytokine-induced mobilization of bone marrow-derived endothelial progenitor cells for neovascularization. Nat Med. 1999;5:434–8.
97. Amano K, Okigaki M, Adachi Y, Fujiyama S, Mori Y, Kosaki A, et al. Mechanism for IL-1 beta-mediated neovascularization unmasked by IL-1 beta knock-out mice. J Mol Cell Cardiol. 2004;36:469–80.
98. Yamaguchi J, Kusano KF, Masuo O, Kawamoto A, Silver M, Murasawa S, et al. Stromal cell-derived factor-1 effects on ex vivo expanded endothelial progenitor cell recruitment for ischemic neovascularization. Circulation. 2003;107:1322–8.
99. Vasa M, Fichtlscherer S, Adler K, Aicher A, Martin H, Zeiher AM, et al. Increase in circulating endothelial progenitor cells by statin therapy in patients with stable coronary artery disease. Circulation. 2001;103:2885–90.
100. Llevadot J, Murasawa S, Kureishi Y, Uchida S, Masuda H, Kawamoto A, et al. HMG-CoA reductase inhibitor mobilizes bone marrow–derived endothelial progenitor cells. J Clin Invest. 2001;108:399–405.
101. Walter DH, Rittig K, Bahlmann FH, Kirchmair R, Silver M, Murayama T, et al. Statin therapy accelerates reendothelialization: a novel effect involving mobilization and incorporation of bone marrow-derived endothelial progenitor cells. Circulation. 2002;105:3017–24.
102. Dimmeler S, Aicher A, Vasa M, Mildner-Rihm C, Adler K, Tiemann M, et al. HMG-CoA reductase inhibitors (statins) increase endothelial progenitor cells via the PI 3-kinase/Akt pathway. J Clin Invest. 2001;108:391–7.
103. Adams V, Lenk K, Linke A, Lenz D, Erbs S, Sandri M, et al. Increase of circulating endothelial progenitor cells in patients with coronary artery disease after exercise-induced ischemia. Arterioscler Thromb Vasc Biol. 2004;24:684–90.
104. Chih S, Macdonald PS, McCrohon JA, Ma D, Moore J, Feneley MP, et al. Granulocyte colony stimulating factor in chronic angina

to stimulate neovascularisation: a placebo controlled crossover trial. Heart. 2012;98:282–90.

105. Gnecchi M, Zhang Z, Ni A, Dzau VJ. Paracrine mechanisms in adult stem cell signaling and therapy. Circ Res. 2008;103:1204–19.
106. Grunewald M, Avraham I, Dor Y, Bachar-Lustig E, Itin A, Jung S, et al. VEGF-induced adult neovascularization: recruitment, retention, and role of accessory cells. Cell. 2006;124:175–89.
107. Ziegelhoeffer T, Fernandez B, Kostin S, Heil M, Voswinckel R, Helisch A, et al. Bone marrow-derived cells do not incorporate into the adult growing vasculature. Circ Res. 2004;94:230–8.
108. Tillmanns J, Rota M, Hosoda T, Misao Y, Esposito G, Gonzalez A, et al. Formation of large coronary arteries by cardiac progenitor cells. Proc Natl Acad Sci USA. 2008;105:1668–73.
109. Kinnaird T, Stabile E, Burnett MS, Lee CW, Barr S, Fuchs S, et al. Marrow-derived stromal cells express genes encoding a broad spectrum of arteriogenic cytokines and promote in vitro and in vivo arteriogenesis through paracrine mechanisms. Circ Res. 2004;94:678–85.
110. Schatteman GC, Awad O, Nau E, Wang C, Jiao C, Tomanek RJ, et al. Lin- cells mediate tissue repair by regulating MCP-1/CCL-2. Am J Pathol. 2010;177:2002–10.
111. Wu Y, Ip JE, Huang J, Zhang L, Matsushita K, Liew CC, et al. Essential role of ICAM-1/CD18 in mediating EPC recruitment, angiogenesis, and repair to the infarcted myocardium. Circ Res. 2006;99:315–22.
112. Aicher A, Brenner W, Zuhayra M, Badorff C, Massoudi S, Assmus B, et al. Assessment of the tissue distribution of transplanted human endothelial progenitor cells by radioactive labeling. Circulation. 2003;107:2134–9.
113. Rehman J, Li J, Parvathaneni L, Karlsson G, Panchal VR, Temm CJ, et al. Exercise acutely increases circulating endothelial progenitor cells and monocyte-/macrophage-derived angiogenic cells. J Am Coll Cardiol. 2004;43:2314–8.
114. Penn MS, Ellis S, Gandhi S, Greenbaum A, Hodes Z, Mendelsohn FO, et al. Adventitial delivery of an allogeneic bone marrow-derived adherent stem cell in acute myocardial infarction: phase I clinical study. Circ Res. 2012;110:304–11.
115. Ratajczak MZ, Shin DM, Liu R, Mierzejewska K, Ratajczak J, Kucia M, et al. Very small embryonic/epiblast-like stem cells (VSELs) and their potential role in aging and organ rejuvenation—an update and comparison to other primitive small stem cells isolated from adult tissues. Aging. 2012;4(4):235–46.
116. Ratajczak J, Miekus K, Kucia M, Zhang J, Reca R, Dvorak P, et al. Embryonic stem cell-derived microvesicles reprogram hematopoietic progenitors: evidence for horizontal transfer of mRNA and protein delivery. Leukemia. 2006;20:847–56.
117. Gatti S, Bruno S, Deregibus MC, Sordi A, Cantaluppi V, Tetta C, et al. Microvesicles derived from human adult mesenchymal stem cells protect against ischaemia-reperfusion-induced acute and chronic kidney injury. Nephrol Dial Transplant. 2011;26:1474–83.
118. Beaudoin AR, Grondin G. Shedding of vesicular material from the cell surface of eukaryotic cells: different cellular phenomena. Biochim Biophys Acta. 1991;1071:203–19.
119. Herrera MB, Fonsato V, Gatti S, Deregibus MC, Sordi A, Cantarella D, et al. Human liver stem cell-derived microvesicles accelerate hepatic regeneration in hepatectomized rats. J Cell Mol Med. 2010;14:1605–18.
120. Leistner DM, Zeiher AM. Novel avenues for cell therapy in acute myocardial infarction. Circ Res. 2012;110:195–7.
121. Laflamme MA, Zbinden S, Epstein SE, Murry CE. Cell-based therapy for myocardial ischemia and infarction: pathophysiological mechanisms. Annu Rev Pathol. 2007;2:307–39.
122. Perin EC, Dohmann HF, Borojevic R, Silva SA, Sousa AL, Mesquita CT, et al. Transendocardial, autologous bone marrow cell transplantation for severe, chronic ischemic heart failure. Circulation. 2003;107:2294–302.
123. Tse HF, Kwong YL, Chan JK, Lo G, Ho CL, Lau CP. Angiogenesis in ischaemic myocardium by intramyocardial autologous bone marrow mononuclear cell implantation. Lancet. 2003;361:47–9.
124. Beeres SL, Bax JJ, Kaandorp TA, Zeppenfeld K, Lamb HJ, Dibbets-Schneider P, et al. Usefulness of intramyocardial injection of autologous bone marrow-derived mononuclear cells in patients with severe angina pectoris and stress-induced myocardial ischemia. Am J Cardiol. 2006;97:1326–31.
125. Hamano K, Nishida M, Hirata K, Mikamo A, Li TS, Harada M, et al. Local implantation of autologous bone marrow cells for therapeutic angiogenesis in patients with ischemic heart disease: clinical trial and preliminary results. Jpn Circ J. 2001;65:845–7.
126. Briguori C, Reimers B, Sarais C, Napodano M, Pascotto P, Azzarello G, et al. Direct intramyocardial percutaneous delivery of autologous bone marrow in patients with refractory myocardial angina. Am Heart J. 2006;151:674–80.
127. Fuchs S, Kornowski R, Weisz G, Satler LF, Smits PC, Okubagzi P, et al. Safety and feasibility of transendocardial autologous bone marrow cell transplantation in patients with advanced heart disease. Am J Cardiol. 2006;97:823–9.
128. Tse HF, Lau CP. Therapeutic angiogenesis with bone marrow–derived stem cells. J Cardiovasc Pharmacol Ther. 2007;12:89–97.
129. Hosoda T. C-kit-positive cardiac stem cells and myocardial regeneration. Am J Cardiovasc Dis. 2012;2:58–67.
130. van Ramshorst J, Bax JJ, Beeres SL, Dibbets-Schneider P, Roes SD, Stokkel MP, et al. Intramyocardial bone marrow cell injection for chronic myocardial ischemia: a randomized controlled trial. JAMA. 2009;301:1997–2004.
131. Losordo DW, Henry TD, Davidson C, Sup Lee J, Costa MA, Bass T, et al. Intramyocardial, autologous CD34+ cell therapy for refractory angina. Circ Res. 2011;109:428–36.
132. Gowdak LH, Schettert IT, Rochitte CE, Lisboa LA, Dallan LA, Cesar LA, et al. Early increase in myocardial perfusion after stem cell therapy in patients undergoing incomplete coronary artery bypass surgery. J Cardiovasc Transl Res. 2011;4:106–13.
133. Chan CW, Kwong YL, Kwong RY, Lau CP, Tse HF. Improvement of myocardial perfusion reserve detected by cardiovascular magnetic resonance after direct endomyocardial implantation of autologous bone marrow cells in patients with severe coronary artery disease. J Cardiovasc Magn Reson. 2010;12:6.
134. Bolli R, Chugh AR, D'Amario D, Loughran JH, Stoddard MF, Ikram S, et al. Cardiac stem cells in patients with ischaemic cardiomyopathy (SCIPIO): initial results of a randomised phase 1 trial. Lancet. 2011;378:1847–57.
135. Kawamoto A, Tkebuchava T, Yamaguchi J, Nishimura H, Yoon YS, Milliken C, et al. Intramyocardial transplantation of autologous endothelial progenitor cells for therapeutic neovascularization of myocardial ischemia. Circulation. 2003;107:461–8.
136. Tang XL, Rokosh G, Sanganalmath SK, Yuan F, Sato H, Mu J, et al. Intracoronary administration of cardiac progenitor cells alleviates left ventricular dysfunction in rats with a 30-day-old infarction. Circulation. 2010;121:293–305.
137. Kobayashi T, Hamano K, Li TS, Katoh T, Kobayashi S, Matsuzaki M, et al. Enhancement of angiogenesis by the implantation of self bone marrow cells in a rat ischemic heart model. J Surg Res. 2000;89:189–95.
138. Schneider C, Jaquet K, Geidel S, Rau T, Malisius R, Boczor S, et al. Transplantation of bone marrow-derived stem cells improves myocardial diastolic function: strain rate imaging in a model of hibernating myocardium. J Am Soc Echocardiogr. 2009;22:1180–9.
139. Abdel-Latif A, Bolli R, Tleyjeh IM, Montori VM, Perin EC, Hornung CA, et al. Adult bone marrow-derived cells for cardiac repair: a systematic review and meta-analysis. Arch Intern Med. 2007;167:989–97.
140. Wojakowski W, Tendera M, Kucia M, Zuba-Surma E, Paczkowska E, Ciosek J, et al. Mobilization of bone marrow-derived Oct-4+

SSEA-4+ very small embryonic-like stem cells in patients with acute myocardial infarction. J Am Coll Cardiol. 2009;53:1–9.
141. Dai W, Kloner RA. Bone marrow-derived cell transplantation therapy for myocardial infarction: lessons learned and future questions. Am J Transplant. 2011;11:2297–301.
142. Orlic D, Kajstura J, Chimenti S, Jakoniuk I, Anderson SM, Li B, et al. Bone marrow cells regenerate infarcted myocardium. Nature. 2001;410:701–5.
143. Goodell MA, Jackson KA, Majka SM, Mi T, Wang H, Pocius J, et al. Stem cell plasticity in muscle and bone marrow. Ann N Y Acad Sci. 2001;938:208–18. discussion 18–20.
144. Jackson KA, Majka SM, Wang H, Pocius J, Hartley CJ, Majesky MW, et al. Regeneration of ischemic cardiac muscle and vascular endothelium by adult stem cells. J Clin Invest. 2001;107: 1395–402.
145. Wojakowski W, Kucia M, Zuba-Surma E, Jadczyk T, Ksiazek B, Ratajczak MZ, et al. Very small embryonic-like stem cells in cardiovascular repair. Pharmacol Ther. 2011;129:21–8.
146. Deindl E, Zaruba MM, Brunner S, Huber B, Mehl U, Assmann G, et al. G-CSF administration after myocardial infarction in mice attenuates late ischemic cardiomyopathy by enhanced arteriogenesis. FASEB J. 2006;20:956–8.
147. Theiss HD, Vallaster M, Rischpler C, Krieg L, Zaruba MM, Brunner S, et al. Dual stem cell therapy after myocardial infarction acts specifically by enhanced homing via the SDF-1/CXCR4 axis. Stem Cell Res. 2011;7:244–55.
148. Jujo K, Hamada H, Iwakura A, Thorne T, Sekiguchi H, Clarke T, et al. CXCR4 blockade augments bone marrow progenitor cell recruitment to the neovasculature and reduces mortality after myocardial infarction. Proc Natl Acad Sci USA. 2010;107: 11008–13.
149. Hu CH, Li ZM, Du ZM, Zhang AX, Rana JS, Liu DH, et al. Expanded human cord blood-derived endothelial progenitor cells salvage infarcted myocardium in rats with acute myocardial infarction. Clin Exp Pharmacol Physiol. 2010;37:551–6.
150. Ma N, Stamm C, Kaminski A, Li W, Kleine HD, Muller-Hilke B, et al. Human cord blood cells induce angiogenesis following myocardial infarction in NOD/scid-mice. Cardiovasc Res. 2005;66:45–54.
151. Mauritz C, Martens A, Rojas SV, Schnick T, Rathert C, Schecker N, et al. Induced pluripotent stem cell (iPSC)-derived Flk-1 progenitor cells engraft, differentiate, and improve heart function in a mouse model of acute myocardial infarction. Eur Heart J. 2011;32:2634–41.
152. Malliaras K, Kreke M, Marban E. The stuttering progress of cell therapy for heart disease. Clin Pharmacol Ther. 2011;90:532–41.
153. Charwat S, Gyongyosi M, Lang I, Graf S, Beran G, Hemetsberger R, et al. Role of adult bone marrow stem cells in the repair of ischemic myocardium: current state of the art. Exp Hematol. 2008;36:672–80.
154. Liu Z, Gerdes AM. Influence of hypothyroidism and the reversal of hypothyroidism on hemodynamics and cell size in the adult rat heart. J Mol Cell Cardiol. 1990;22:1339–48.
155. Chilian WM, Wangler RD, Peters KG, Tomanek RJ, Marcus ML. Thyroxine-induced left ventricular hypertrophy in the rat. Anatomical and physiological evidence for angiogenesis. Circ Res. 1985;57:591–8.
156. Tomanek RJ, Connell PM, Butters CA, Torry RJ. Compensated coronary microvascular growth in senescent rats with thyroxine-induced cardiac hypertrophy. Am J Physiol. 1995;268:H419–25.
157. Tomanek RJ, Doty MK, Sandra A. Early coronary angiogenesis in response to thyroxine: growth characteristics and upregulation of basic fibroblast growth factor. Circ Res. 1998;82:587–93.
158. Tomanek RJ, Busch TL. Coordinated capillary and myocardial growth in response to thyroxine treatment. Anat Rec. 1998;251: 44–9.
159. Wang X, Zheng W, Christensen LP, Tomanek RJ. DITPA stimulates bFGF, VEGF, angiopoietin, and Tie-2 and facilitates coronary arteriolar growth. Am J Physiol Heart Circ Physiol. 2003;284:H613–8.
160. Zheng W, Weiss RM, Wang X, Zhou R, Arlen AM, Lei L, et al. DITPA stimulates arteriolar growth and modifies myocardial postinfarction remodeling. Am J Physiol Heart Circ Physiol. 2004;286:H1994–2000.
161. Laperche T, Logeart D, Cohen-Solal A, Gourgon R. Potential interests of heart rate lowering drugs. Heart. 1999;81:336–41.
162. Quyyumi AA, Wright CA, Mockus LJ, Fox KM. Mechanisms of nocturnal angina pectoris: importance of increased myocardial oxygen demand in patients with severe coronary artery disease. Lancet. 1984;1:1207–9.
163. Panza JA, Diodati JG, Callahan TS, Epstein SE, Quyyumi AA. Role of increases in heart rate in determining the occurrence and frequency of myocardial ischemia during daily life in patients with stable coronary artery disease. J Am Coll Cardiol. 1992;20:1092–8.
164. Lei L, Zhou R, Zheng W, Christensen LP, Weiss RM, Tomanek RJ. Bradycardia induces angiogenesis, increases coronary reserve, and preserves function of the postinfarcted heart. Circulation. 2004;110:796–802.
165. Dedkov EI, Zheng W, Christensen LP, Weiss RM, Mahlberg-Gaudin F, Tomanek RJ. Preservation of coronary reserve by ivabradine-induced reduction in heart rate in infarcted rats is associated with decrease in perivascular collagen. Am J Physiol Heart Circ Physiol. 2007;293:H590–8.
166. Christensen LP, Zhang RL, Zheng W, Campanelli JJ, Dedkov EI, Weiss RM, et al. Postmyocardial infarction remodeling and coronary reserve: effects of ivabradine and beta blockade therapy. Am J Physiol Heart Circ Physiol. 2009;297:H322–30.
167. Zhang RL, Christensen LP, Tomanek RJ. Chronic heart rate reduction facilitates cardiomyocyte survival after myocardial infarction. Anat Rec (Hoboken). 2010;293:839–48.
168. Zheng W, Seftor EA, Meininger CJ, Hendrix MJ, Tomanek RJ. Mechanisms of coronary angiogenesis in response to stretch: role of VEGF and TGF-beta. Am J Physiol Heart Circ Physiol. 2001;280:H909–17.
169. Zheng W, Christensen LP, Tomanek RJ. Differential effects of cyclic and static stretch on coronary microvascular endothelial cell receptors and vasculogenic/angiogenic responses. Am J Physiol Heart Circ Physiol. 2008;295:H794–800.
170. Seko Y, Takahashi N, Shibuya M, Yazaki Y. Pulsatile stretch stimulates vascular endothelial growth factor (VEGF) secretion by cultured rat cardiac myocytes. Biochem Biophys Res Commun. 1999;254:462–5.
171. Hudlicka O, Brown M, Egginton S. Angiogenesis in skeletal and cardiac muscle. Physiol Rev. 1992;72:369–417.
172. Tomanek RJ, Torry RJ. Growth of the coronary vasculature in hypertrophy: mechanisms and model dependence. Cell Mol Biol Res. 1994;40:129–36.
173. Jaquet K, Krause K, Tawakol-Khodai M, Geidel S, Kuck KH. Erythropoietin and VEGF exhibit equal angiogenic potential. Microvasc Res. 2002;64:326–33.
174. Tilling L, Clapp B. Erythropoietin: a future therapy for failing hearts? Heart Fail Rev. 2011;16(6):503–8.
175. Santhanam AV, d'Uscio LV, Peterson TE, Katusic ZS. Activation of endothelial nitric oxide synthase is critical for erythropoietin-induced mobilization of progenitor cells. Peptides. 2008;29:1451–5.
176. Moon C, Krawczyk M, Ahn D, Ahmet I, Paik D, Lakatta EG, et al. Erythropoietin reduces myocardial infarction and left ventricular functional decline after coronary artery ligation in rats. Proc Natl Acad Sci USA. 2003;100:11612–7.
177. van der Meer P, Lipsic E, Henning RH, Boddeus K, van der Velden J, Voors AA, et al. Erythropoietin induces neovascularization and

improves cardiac function in rats with heart failure after myocardial infarction. J Am Coll Cardiol. 2005;46:125–33.
178. Hirata A, Minamino T, Asanuma H, Fujita M, Wakeno M, Myoishi M, et al. Erythropoietin enhances neovascularization of ischemic myocardium and improves left ventricular dysfunction after myocardial infarction in dogs. J Am Coll Cardiol. 2006;48:176–84.
179. Westenbrink BD, Lipsic E, van der Meer P, van der Harst P, Oeseburg H, Du Marchie Sarvaas GJ, et al. Erythropoietin improves cardiac function through endothelial progenitor cell and vascular endothelial growth factor mediated neovascularization. Eur Heart J. 2007;28:2018–27.
180. Nishiya D, Omura T, Shimada K, Matsumoto R, Kusuyama T, Enomoto S, et al. Effects of erythropoietin on cardiac remodeling after myocardial infarction. J Pharmacol Sci. 2006;101:31–9.
181. Westenbrink BD, Oeseburg H, Kleijn L, van der Harst P, Belonje AM, Voors AA, et al. Erythropoietin stimulates normal endothelial progenitor cell-mediated endothelial turnover, but attributes to neovascularization only in the presence of local ischemia. Cardiovasc Drugs Ther. 2008;22:265–74.
182. Namiuchi S, Kagaya Y, Ohta J, Shiba N, Sugi M, Oikawa M, et al. High serum erythropoietin level is associated with smaller infarct size in patients with acute myocardial infarction who undergo successful primary percutaneous coronary intervention. J Am Coll Cardiol. 2005;45:1406–12.
183. Ferrario M, Massa M, Rosti V, Campanelli R, Ferlini M, Marinoni B, et al. Early haemoglobin-independent increase of plasma erythropoietin levels in patients with acute myocardial infarction. Eur Heart J. 2007;28:1805–13.
184. Booth EA, Lucchesi BR. Estrogen-mediated protection in myocardial ischemia-reperfusion injury. Cardiovasc Toxicol. 2008;8:101–13.
185. Deschamps AM, Murphy E, Sun J. Estrogen receptor activation and cardioprotection in ischemia reperfusion injury. Trends Cardiovasc Med. 2010;20:73–8.
186. Lizotte E, Grandy SA, Tremblay A, Allen BG, Fiset C. Expression, distribution and regulation of sex steroid hormone receptors in mouse heart. Cell Physiol Biochem. 2009;23:75–86.
187. Lin J, Steenbergen C, Murphy E, Sun J. Estrogen receptor-beta activation results in S-nitrosylation of proteins involved in cardioprotection. Circulation. 2009;120:245–54.
188. Kaski JC. Overview of gender aspects of cardiac syndrome X. Cardiovasc Res. 2002;53:620–6.
189. Kaski JC. Cardiac syndrome X in women: the role of oestrogen deficiency. Heart. 2006;92 Suppl 3:iii5–9.
190. Peterson LR, Eyster D, Davila-Roman VG, Stephens AL, Schechtman KB, Herrero P, et al. Short-term oral estrogen replacement therapy does not augment endothelium-independent myocardial perfusion in postmenopausal women. Am Heart J. 2001;142:641–7.
191. Emre A, Sahin S, Erzik C, Nurkalem Z, Oz D, Cirakoglu B, et al. Effect of hormone replacement therapy on plasma lipoproteins and apolipoproteins, endothelial function and myocardial perfusion in postmenopausal women with estrogen receptor-alpha IVS1-397 C/C genotype and established coronary artery disease. Cardiology. 2006;106:44–50.
192. Knuuti J, Kalliokoski R, Janatuinen T, Hannukainen J, Kalliokoski KK, Koskenvuo J, et al. Effect of estradiol-drospirenone hormone treatment on myocardial perfusion reserve in postmenopausal women with angina pectoris. Am J Cardiol. 2007;99:1648–52.
193. Wang Y, Wang Q, Zhao Y, Gong D, Wang D, Li C, et al. Protective effects of estrogen against reperfusion arrhythmias following severe myocardial ischemia in rats. Circ J. 2010;74:634–43.
194. Mericli M, Nadasy GL, Szekeres M, Varbiro S, Vajo Z, Matrai M, et al. Estrogen replacement therapy reverses changes in intramural coronary resistance arteries caused by female sex hormone depletion. Cardiovasc Res. 2004;61:317–24.
195. Lamping KG, Christensen LP, Tomanek RJ. Estrogen therapy induces collateral and microvascular remodeling. Am J Physiol Heart Circ Physiol. 2003;285:H2039–44.
196. Miura S, Saku K. Regulation of angiogenesis and angiogenic factors by cardiovascular medications. Curr Pharm Des. 2007;13:2113–7.
197. Kureishi Y, Luo Z, Shiojima I, Bialik A, Fulton D, Lefer DJ, et al. The HMG-CoA reductase inhibitor simvastatin activates the protein kinase Akt and promotes angiogenesis in normocholesterolemic animals. Nat Med. 2000;6:1004–10.
198. Weis M, Heeschen C, Glassford AJ, Cooke JP. Statins have biphasic effects on angiogenesis. Circulation. 2002;105:739–45.
199. Sodha NR, Chu LM, Boodhwani M, Sellke FW. Pharmacotherapy for end-stage coronary artery disease. Expert Opin Pharmacother. 2010;11:207–13.
200. Boodhwani M, Nakai Y, Voisine P, Feng J, Li J, Mieno S, et al. High-dose atorvastatin improves hypercholesterolemic coronary endothelial dysfunction without improving the angiogenic response. Circulation. 2006;114:I402–8.
201. Bouchentouf M, Williams P, Forner KA, Cuerquis J, Michaud V, Paradis P, et al. Interleukin-2 enhances angiogenesis and preserves cardiac function following myocardial infarction. Cytokine. 2011;56:732–8.
202. Fujita M, Sasayama S. Coronary collateral growth and its therapeutic application to coronary artery disease. Circ J. 2010;74:1283–9.
203. Hubel K, Dale DC, Liles WC. Therapeutic use of cytokines to modulate phagocyte function for the treatment of infectious diseases: current status of granulocyte colony-stimulating factor, granulocyte-macrophage colony-stimulating factor, macrophage colony-stimulating factor, and interferon-gamma. J Infect Dis. 2002;185:1490–501.
204. Kosaki K, Ando J, Korenaga R, Kurokawa T, Kamiya A. Fluid shear stress increases the production of granulocyte-macrophage colony-stimulating factor by endothelial cells via mRNA stabilization. Circ Res. 1998;82:794–802.
205. Buschmann IR, Hoefer IE, van Royen N, Katzer E, Braun-Dulleaus R, Heil M, et al. GM-CSF: a strong arteriogenic factor acting by amplification of monocyte function. Atherosclerosis. 2001;159:343–56.
206. Seiler C, Pohl T, Wustmann K, Hutter D, Nicolet PA, Windecker S, et al. Promotion of collateral growth by granulocyte-macrophage colony-stimulating factor in patients with coronary artery disease: a randomized, double-blind, placebo-controlled study. Circulation. 2001;104:2012–7.
207. Zbinden S, Zbinden R, Meier P, Windecker S, Seiler C. Safety and efficacy of subcutaneous-only granulocyte-macrophage colony-stimulating factor for collateral growth promotion in patients with coronary artery disease. J Am Coll Cardiol. 2005;46:1636–42.
208. Zbinden R, Vogel R, Meier B, Seiler C. Coronary collateral flow and peripheral blood monocyte concentration in patients treated with granulocyte-macrophage colony stimulating factor. Heart. 2004;90:945–6.
209. Zbinden R, Zbinden S, Meier P, Hutter D, Billinger M, Wahl A, et al. Coronary collateral flow in response to endurance exercise training. Eur J Cardiovasc Prev Rehabil. 2007;14:250–7.
210. Niebauer J, Hambrecht R, Marburger C, Hauer K, Velich T, von Hodenberg E, et al. Impact of intensive physical exercise and low-fat diet on collateral vessel formation in stable angina pectoris and angiographically confirmed coronary artery disease. Am J Cardiol. 1995;76:771–5.
211. Belardinelli R, Paolini I, Cianci G, Piva R, Georgiou D, Purcaro A. Exercise training intervention after coronary angioplasty: the ETICA trial. J Am Coll Cardiol. 2001;37:1891–900.
212. Gloekler S, Meier P, de Marchi SF, Rutz T, Traupe T, Rimoldi SF, et al. Coronary collateral growth by external counterpulsation: a randomised controlled trial. Heart. 2010;96:202–7.

213. Fuchs S, Baffour R, Zhou YF, Shou M, Pierre A, Tio FO, et al. Transendocardial delivery of autologous bone marrow enhances collateral perfusion and regional function in pigs with chronic experimental myocardial ischemia. J Am Coll Cardiol. 2001;37:1726–32.
214. Tang YL, Zhao Q, Qin X, Shen L, Cheng L, Ge J, et al. Paracrine action enhances the effects of autologous mesenchymal stem cell transplantation on vascular regeneration in rat model of myocardial infarction. Ann Thorac Surg. 2005;80:229–36. discussion 36–7.
215. Tang J, Xie Q, Pan G, Wang J, Wang M. Mesenchymal stem cells participate in angiogenesis and improve heart function in rat model of myocardial ischemia with reperfusion. Eur J Cardiothorac Surg. 2006;30:353–61.
216. Gnecchi M, He H, Liang OD, Melo LG, Morello F, Mu H, et al. Paracrine action accounts for marked protection of ischemic heart by Akt-modified mesenchymal stem cells. Nat Med. 2005;11:367–8.
217. Silva GV, Litovsky S, Assad JA, Sousa AL, Martin BJ, Vela D, et al. Mesenchymal stem cells differentiate into an endothelial phenotype, enhance vascular density, and improve heart function in a canine chronic ischemia model. Circulation. 2005;111:150–6.
218. Belmadani S, Matrougui K, Kolz C, Pung YF, Palen D, Prockop DJ, et al. Amplification of coronary arteriogenic capacity of multipotent stromal cells by epidermal growth factor. Arterioscler Thromb Vasc Biol. 2009;29:802–8.
219. Yin L, Ohanyan V, Pung YF, Delucia A, Bailey E, Enrick M, et al. Induction of vascular progenitor cells from endothelial cells stimulates coronary collateral growth. Circ Res. 2012;110:241–52.
220. Schirmer SH, van Nooijen FC, Piek JJ, van Royen N. Stimulation of collateral artery growth: travelling further down the road to clinical application. Heart. 2009;95:191–7.
221. Ruel M, Laham RJ, Parker JA, Post MJ, Ware JA, Simons M, et al. Long-term effects of surgical angiogenic therapy with fibroblast growth factor 2 protein. J Thorac Cardiovasc Surg. 2002;124:28–34.
222. Kukula K, Chojnowska L, Dabrowski M, Witkowski A, Chmielak Z, Skwarek M, et al. Intramyocardial plasmid-encoding human vascular endothelial growth factor A165/basic fibroblast growth factor therapy using percutaneous transcatheter approach in patients with refractory coronary artery disease (VIF-CAD). Am Heart J. 2011;161:581–9.
223. Meier P, Gloekler S, de Marchi SF, Indermuehle A, Rutz T, Traupe T, et al. Myocardial salvage through coronary collateral growth by granulocyte colony-stimulating factor in chronic coronary artery disease: a controlled randomized trial. Circulation. 2009;120:1355–63.

Index

R.J. Tomanek, *Coronary Vasculature: Development, Structure-Function, and Adaptations*, DOI 10.1007/978-1-4614-4887-7, © Springer Science+Business Media New York 2013

MIX
Papier aus verantwortungsvollen Quellen
Paper from responsible sources
FSC® C105338

If you have any concerns about our products,
you can contact us on
ProductSafety@springernature.com

In case Publisher is established outside the EU,
the EU authorized representative is:
Springer Nature Customer Service Center GmbH
Europaplatz 3, 69115 Heidelberg, Germany

Printed by Libri Plureos GmbH
in Hamburg, Germany